Jopling's

Handbook of
Leprosy

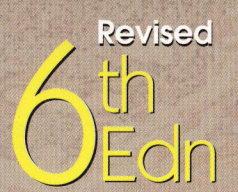
Revised 6th Edn

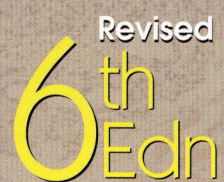

Jopling's Handbook of Leprosy

Editors

Kabir Sardana MD, DNB, MNAMS
Professor of Skin and VD
Central Health Services
Ministry of Health and Family Welfare
Department of Dermatology, Venereology and Leprosy
Dr Ram Manohar Lohia Hospital and
Postgraduate Institute of Medical Education and
Research, New Delhi
Professor of Dermatology, Indraprastha University
Associate Professor of Dermatology, Delhi University

Ananta Khurana MD, DNB, MNAMS
Associate Professor
Department of Dermatology, Venereology and Leprosy
Dr Ram Manohar Lohia Hospital and
Postgraduate Institute of Medical Education and Research
New Delhi

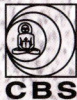

CBS Publishers & Distributors Pvt Ltd

New Delhi • Bengaluru • Chennai • Kochi • Kolkata • Mumbai
Hyderabad • Jharkhand • Nagpur • Patna • Pune • Uttarakhand

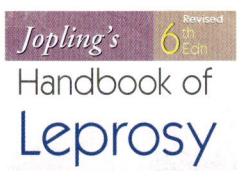

Jopling's Handbook of Leprosy
Revised 6th Edn

Disclaimer
Science and technology are constantly changing fields. New research and experience broaden the scope of information and knowledge. The editors have tried their best in giving information available to them while preparing the material for this book. Although all efforts have been made to ensure optimum accuracy of the material, yet it is quite possible some errors might have been left uncorrected. The publisher, the printer and the editors will not be held responsible for any inadvertent errors or inaccuracies.

ISBN: 978-93-89688-11-5

Copyright © Editors and Publisher

Revised Sixth Edition: 2021
First Edition: 1971
Second Edition: 1978
Third Edition: 1984
Fourth Edition: 1988
Fifth Edition: 1996
Sixth Edition: 2020
The Fifth Edition of the book was brought out by CBS Publishers & Distributors under the arrangement with WH Jopling and AC McDougall (1995).

All rights reserved. No part of this book may be reproduced or transmitted in any form or by any means, electronic or mechanical, including photocopying, recording, or any information storage and retrieval system without permission, in writing, from the authors and the publisher.

Published by **Satish Kumar Jain** and produced by **Varun Jain** for

CBS Publishers & Distributors Pvt Ltd
4819/XI Prahlad Street, 24 Ansari Road, Daryaganj, New Delhi 110 002, India
Ph: 011-23289259, 23266861, 23266867   Fax: 011-23243014   Website: www.cbspd.com
e-mail: delhi@cbspd.com; cbspubs@airtelmail.in.

Corporate Office: 204 FIE, Industrial Area, Patparganj, Delhi 110 092
Ph: 011-4934 4934   Fax: 011-4934 4935   e-mail: publishing@cbspd.com; publicity@cbspd.com

Branches

- **Bengaluru:** Seema House 2975, 17th Cross, K.R. Road,
  Banasankari 2nd Stage, Bengaluru 560 070, Karnataka, India
  Ph: +91-80-26771678/79   Fax: +91-80-26771680   e-mail: bangalore@cbspd.com
- **Chennai:** 7, Subbaraya Street, Shenoy Nagar, Chennai 600 030, Tamil Nadu, India
  Ph: +91-44-26680620, 26681266   Fax: +91-44-42032115   e-mail: chennai@cbspd.com
- **Kochi:** 42/1325, 1326, Power House Road, Opp KSEB, Power House, Ernakulam 682 018, Kerala, India
  Ph: +91-484-4059061-65/67   Fax: +91-484-4059065   e-mail: kochi@cbspd.com
- **Kolkata:** 6/B, Ground Floor, Rameswar Shaw Road, Kolkata-700 014, West Bengal, India
  Ph: +91-33-22891126, 22891127, 22891128   e-mail: kolkata@cbspd.com
- **Mumbai:** PWD Shed. Gala no. 25/26, Ramchandra Bhatt Marg, Next to JJ Hospital Gate no. 2,
  Opp. Union Bank of India, Noorbaug Mumbai-400009, Maharashtra, India
  Ph: 022-66661880/89   Mob: 0-8424005858   e-mail: mumbai@cbspd.com

Representatives

• **Hyderabad**	0-9885175004	• **Jharkhand**	0-9811541605	• **Nagpur**	0-9421945513	
• **Patna**	0-9334159340	• **Pune**	0-9623451994	• **Uttarakhand**	0-9716462459	

Printed at Manipal Technologies Limited, Manipal, Karnataka, India

to
Mohandas Karamchand Gandhi

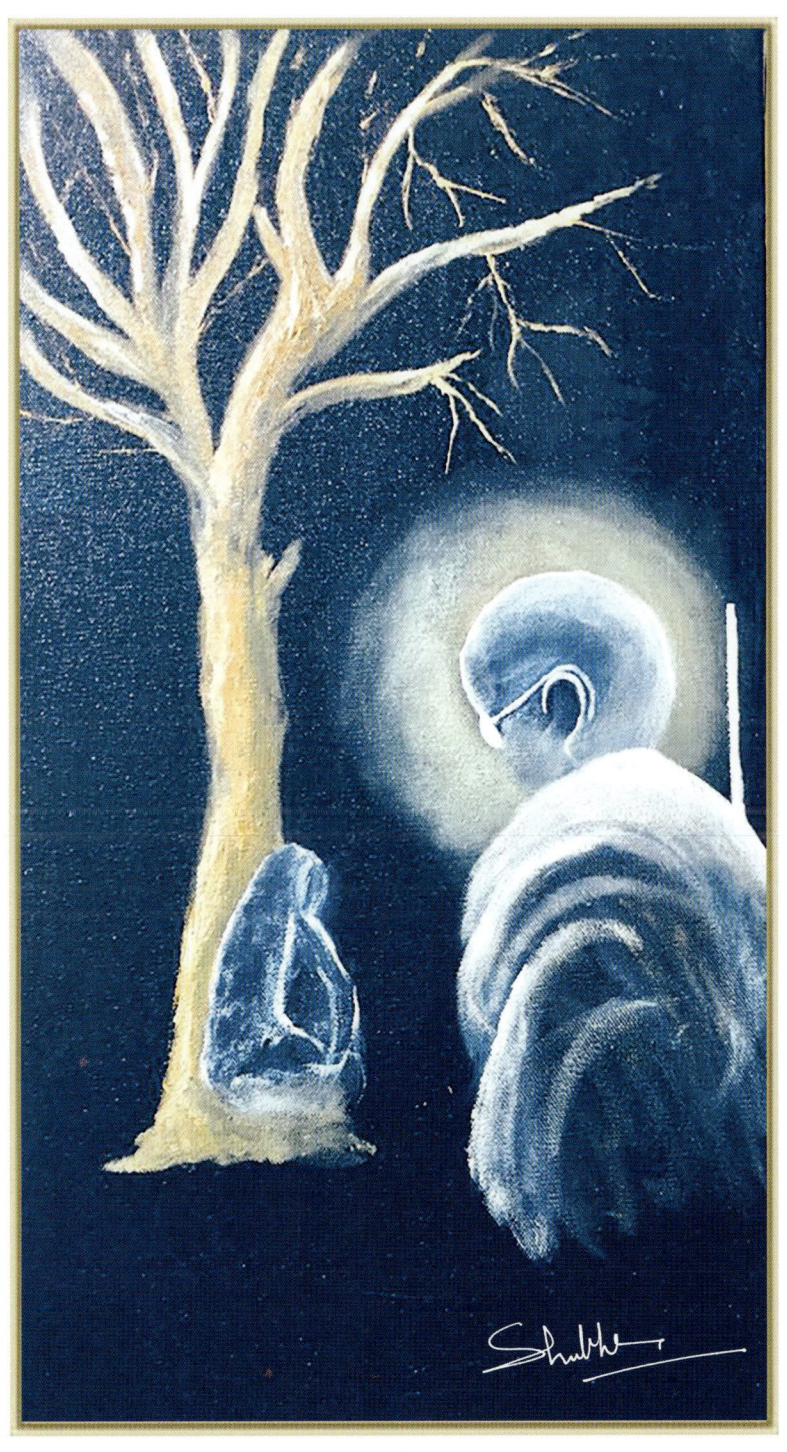

who devoted his life to the care and rehabilitation of leprosy patients.

List of Contributors

Ananta Khurana MD, DNB, MNAMS
Associate Professor
Department of Dermatology,
Venereology and Leprosy
Dr Ram Manohar Lohia Hospital and
Postgraduate Institute of Medical Education and
Research, New Delhi

Anil Dhal MS
Former: Professor of Excellence
Department of Orthopedics
Maulana Azad Medical College and Associated
LN & GB Pant Hospitals, New Delhi

Aparna Govindan MD
Associate Professor
Department of Pathology
Government Medical College
Kozhikode

Atul Shah MS
Ex-Professor of Plastic Surgery
Grant Medical College and Sir J J Group of
Hospitals and Consultant Plastic Surgeon
Nanavati Super Specialty Hospital
Mumbai

Babu Govindan MPT (Ortho)
Physiotherapist
Training Coordinator
The Leprosy Mission Hospital, Naini
Prayagraj, Uttar Pradesh

Chetan Rajput MD
Associate Professor
SBH Govt Medical College
Dhule, Maharashtra

C Ruth Butlin MRCGP, MA, MBBCh
Retired staff of the Leprosy Mission International
Honorary Medical Advisor to DBLM Hospital
Bangladesh
Mailing Address: 42 Old Drive, Polegate
East Sussex, BN 26 5ES, UK

David Scollard MD, PhD
Former Director
National Hansen's Disease Programs (USA)
Co-Editor, International Textbook of Leprosy

Debajyoti Chatterjee MD, DM (Histopathology)
Assistant Professor
Department of Histopathology
Post-Graduate Institute of Medical Education
and Research (PGIMER)
Chandigarh, India

Divya Kamat MD
Senior Resident
Department of Dermatology, Venerelogy and
Leprology, Post-Graduate Institute of Medical
Education and Research (PGIMER)
Chandigarh, India

Gaurish R Laad MD
Consultant Dermatologist
Sushruta Nursing Home
Ponda, Goa

Jaison A Barreto MD, PhD
Chief of Epidemiology
Lauro de Souza Lima Institute
Bauru, Sao Paulo, Brazil

Kabir Sardana MD, DNB, MNAMS
Professor
Department of Dermatology,
Venereology and Leprosy
Dr Ram Manohar Lohia Hospital and
Postgraduate Institute of Medical Education and
Research, New Delhi

Karthikeyan Govindasamy BOT, MPH
Occupational Therapist
Research Coordinator
The Leprosy Mission Trust India
CNI Bhawan, New Delhi

Krishna Garg MS, PhD, FIMSA, MAMS, FAMS, FASI
Ex-Professor and Head
Department of Anatomy, Lady Hardinge
Medical College, New Delhi

Mallika Lavania BSc, MSc, PhD
Scientist
D National Institute of Virology, Pune
Former Scientist-In-Charge, Stanley Browne
Laboratory, The Leprosy Mission Trust India
New Delhi

Margreet Hogeweg MS
(Reviewer-ocular Leprosy)
Former Ophthalmic Advisor
The Netherlands Leprosy Relief Association
The Netherlands

Neela Shah
Ex-Managing Director
Novartis Comprehensive Leprosy Care
Association, 202 A Wing Rushi Tower
Lokhandwala Complex, Andheri West, Mumbai

Pooja Arora Mrig MD, DNB, MNAMS
Associate Professor
Department of Dermatology,
Venereology and Leprosy
Dr Ram Manohar Lohia Hospital and
Postgraduate Institute of Medical Education and
Research, New Delhi

Premanshu Bhushan MD
Senior Consultant and Faculty
PN Behl Skin Institute and School of Dermatology
GK1, New Delhi

Sarita Sanke MD, DNB, MRCP
Assistant Professor
Department of Dermatology and Venereology
LHMC and Associated Hospitals
New Delhi

Sarita Sasidharanpillai MD
Associate Professor
Department of Dermatology and Venereology
Government Medical College
Kozhikode

SK Malhotra MBBS, MD
Professor
Department of Dermatology, Venereology and
Leprosy, Government Medical College
Amritsar, Punjab

Surabhi Sinha MD, DNB, MNAMS
Specialist and Associate Professor
Department of Dermatology,
Venereology and Leprosy
Dr Ram Manohar Lohia Hospital and
Postgraduate Institute of Medical Education and
Research, New Delhi

Taru Garg MD
Professor
Department of Dermatology and Venereology
LHMC and Associated Hospitals
New Delhi

Tarun Narang MD, MNAMS
Associate Professor
Department of Dermatology,
Venereology and Leprology
PGIMER, Chandigarh, India

Utpal Sengupta MVSC, PhD (Path)
Consultant, Stanley Browne Laboratory
The Leprosy Mission Trust India
New Delhi

Vinita Puri MS
Professor and Head
Department of Plastic Reconstructive
Surgery and Burns
Seth GS Medical College and KEM Hospital
Parel, Mumbai, India

Vishal Thakur MD
Senior Resident
Department of Dermatology,
Venereology and Leprology
PGIMER, Chandigarh, India

Yasim Khan MS
Senior Resident, Orthopedics
Maulana Azad Medical College and Associated
LN Hospital and GIPMER
New Delhi

PHOTOCREDITS

Aastha Aggarwal
Junior Resident, Department of Dermatology,
Venereology and Leprosy
Dr Ram Manohar Lohia Hospital and Postgraduate
Institute of Medical Education and Research, New Delhi

Diksha Agrawal
Junior Resident, Department of Dermatology,
Venereology and Leprosy
Dr Ram Manohar Lohia Hospital and Postgraduate
Institute of Medical Education and Research, New Delhi

Konchok Dorjay DVD, DNB
Senior Resident
Department of Dermatology, Venereology and Leprosy
Dr Ram Manohar Lohia Hospital and Postgraduate
Institute of Medical Education and Research, New Delhi

Purnima Paliwal MD
Specialist, Department of Pathology
Dr Ram Manohar Lohia Hospital and Postgraduate
Institute of Medical Education and Research, New Delhi

Shubhra (*Dedication Image*)
Adviser (Trade)
Ministry of Agriculture and Farmers Welfare
Government of India

Preface to the Revised Sixth Edition

Jopling's Handbook of Leprosy has been read and referred to by generations of dermatologists across the country and outside and is probably one of the most acclaimed texts on leprosy. The revised 6th edition comes after a huge gap of 25 years from the last edition. The 5th edition had been reprinted 14 times from 1996 till 2019, with no additions/changes in text. The aim of this edition was to retain the original concepts and the clinical content of the previous editions and in addition updating the book with the enormous advancements made since, while keeping the text concise and the book handy and easy to read. The reader will note that the original table of contents has been enlarged encompassing the additions to the text.

Most of the classical text on clinical leprosy from the previous editions is retained and a section on special scenarios has been added. The major changes in 6th edition include an updated review on immunopathogenesis of disease which has seen several advancements over past two decades. From a simplified view on involvement of humoral and cell-mediated immunity at the two poles as detailed in the last edition, this edition incorporates the established and proposed immunopathogenetic mechanisms and deals with the complexities of the topic in a simplified manner with representative schematic diagrams. The diagnosis section includes the classical descriptions from the 5th edition with added text on newer methods. The second part of the diagnosis chapter comprehensively covers aspects on histopathology of leprosy in detail. Reactions are covered separately and include recent treatment concepts. Resistance in leprosy is now a reality and a summary of the topic with a section on its clinical relevance has been included. The treatment of leprosy has undergone some significant changes since the last edition and this has been thoroughly updated, even though we feel some changes in treatment have been hasty and could have waited for longer follow-up data. We have added a drug formulary which summarizes the essential aspects of the drugs used not only in treatment of leprosy but also in reactions. The second section under treatment covers the concepts of chemoprophylaxis and immunoprophylaxis in leprosy and provides the reader a review of all important work done on these aspects so far and gives them insight into concerns remaining and future directions. The section ends with a brief segment on immunotherapeutics, the majority of work on which has been done in India.

It is an accepted reality that while MDT has been successful for multiple reasons, a proportion of cases suffers from disability and the management of this domain is largely relegated to ancillary branches. We believe that this is a crucial aspect and we have tried to present a concise summary of diagnosis and management of neural involvement and the consequent deformities. The section on differential diagnosis provides an illustrated review with large portions of original text retained and many photographs added.

We believe a book of leprosy should have contributors who see and manage cases and not just those who interpret data which is a mechanical and abstract way of tackling a disease. This accounts for our contributors who range from dermatologists, physicians, scientists, rehabilitation experts and those who have worked on core aspects of the disease. Some of our contributors have doubled up both as contributors and reviewers and we are grateful to Dr M Hogeweg and Dr Cynthia Butlin for their efforts.

A big thanks to the fabulous team at CBS Publishers & Distributors, especially to Mr YN Arjuna Senior Vice-President—Publishing, Editorial and Publicity, Mrs Ritu Chawla General Manager—Production, Mr SK Verma Vice-President, Marketing and Operations, Mr Vikrant Sharma and Mr Tarun Rajput for the dedicated reformatting, Mrs Baljeet Kaur for the artistic depiction and image balancing, Mr Neeraj Prasad for layout/cover design and to Mr Ananda Mohanty and Mr Khirod Sahoo for the meticulous proof reading; all of whom have been tolerating our efforts and the delays for the last one year!

We hope the updated *Jopling's Handbook of Leprosy* proves to be useful for postgraduates, academicians, practitioners and field workers alike and helps in understanding and tackling this ancient disease.

Kabir Sardana
Ananta Khurana
Joplingleprosy@cbspd.com

Preface to the First Edition

For a long time I have been impressed by the demand for information on leprosy from all sections of the medical and nursing professions, and I have attempted, in this Handbook, to give the basic facts about the disease and its management as clearly and concisely as possible. During my visit to leprosy centres in Africa in 1968, I noted the responsible work undertaken by paramedical workers and their eagerness to do it well; I have particularly in mind the medical assistants in-charge of rural clinics or travelling in Land-Rovers as members of mobile medical teams, and I hope that these workers and their counterparts in other developing regions will find in this volume the help they need.

As regards the medical profession, I hope that this Handbook will give the student and general practitioners a better understanding of leprosy, and will also have an appeal to the specialist on whom the diagnosis of the disease may fall, especially the dermatologist and the neurologist.

I would like to thank my son-in-law, Mr David Dartnall, for the drawings and diagrams, and I am grateful to Dr Colin McDougall and Dr Tin Shwe for helpful criticism and advice.

WH Jopling, 1971

Contents

List of Contributors — vii
Preface to the Revised Sixth Edition — ix
Preface to the First Edition — xi

1. Epidemiology and World Distribution — 1
   Ananta Khurana

2. The Disease — 6
   2.1 Clinical Leprosy 6
      Kabir Sardana, Premanshu Bhushan, Ananta Khurana
   2.2 Relapse, Reactivation, Reaction and Reinfection 59
      C Ruth Butlin
   2.3 Leprosy in Children 73
      Taru Garg, Sarita Sanke
   2.4 Pure Neuritic Leprosy 85
      Tarun Narang, Debajyoti Chatterjee, Vishal Thakur
   2.5 Special Scenarios and Populations 93
      Kabir Sardana, Ananta Khurana

3. Diagnostic Tests and Histopathology — 97
   3.1 Diagnostic Tests 97
      Ananta Khurana
   3.2 Histopathology of Leprosy 116
      Sarita Sasidharanpillai, Aparna Govindan

4. Microbiology and Immunopathogenesis — 147
   4.1 Bacteriology of Leprosy 147
      Ananta Khurana
   4.2 Transmission of Leprosy 155
      Ananta Khurana
   4.3 Immunology of Disease 163
      Ananta Khurana
   4.4 M. leprae and Nerve Injury 175
      Kabir Sardana, David Scollard
   4.5 Immunopathogenesis of Reactions 182
      Ananta Khurana, Kabir Sardana

5. Reactions in Leprosy — 192
   5.1 Overview and Type 1 Reactions 192
      Kabir Sardana, Surabhi Sinha, Premanshu Bhushan
   5.2a Type 2 Lepra Reaction 211
      Tarun Narang, Divya Kamat

5.2b Management of Type 2 Lepra Reaction *217*
  Tarun Narang, Divya Kamat
5.3 Acute Exacerbations and Lucio Reaction *225*
  Kabir Sardana, Premanshu Bhushan

6. Drug Resistance in Leprosy — 228
6.1 Drug Resistance *228*
  Mallika Lavania, Utpal Sengupta
6.2 Clinical Relevance of Resistance *237*
  Kabir Sardana, Ananta Khurana

7. Chemotherapy — 240
7.1 Treatment of Leprosy *240*
  Kabir Sardana, Premanshu Bhushan, Ananta Khurana
7.2 Chemoprophylaxis, Immunoprophylaxis and Immunotherapeutics in Leprosy *281*
  Ananta Khurana, Kabir Sardana

8. Other Aspects of Treatment — 292
8.1 Neural Involvement and its Management *292*
  Kabir Sardana, Premanshu Bhushan
8.2 Ocular Complications and Management *302*
  Kabir Sardana, Ananta Khurana, Margreet Hogeweg
8.3 Deformities in Leprosy and Their Management *306*
  Kabir Sardana, Premanshu Bhushan
  8.3.1 Common Deformities of Hand and Feet and Their Management *322*
    Karthikeyan Govindasamy, Babu Govindan
  8.3.2 Surgical Correction of Common Deformities of Upper and Lower Extremities *331*
    Anil Dhal, Yasim Khan
  8.3.3 Correction of Deformities of Face in Leprosy *342*
    Atul Shah, Vinita Puri
  8.3.4 Physiotherapy and Orthoses *354*
    Atul Shah, Neela Shah
  8.3.5 Self-care, Footwear and Assistive Devices *367*
    Karthikeyan Govindasamy, Babu Govindan
8.4 Other Treatments *378*
  Kabir Sardana, Ananta Khurana

9. Differential Diagnosis — 380
Pooja Arora Mrig, Kabir Sardana

10. Nerve Function Assessment and Muscle Testing — 412
Surabhi Sinha, Krishna Garg

Appendix — *435*
Gaurish R Laad

Index — *443*

CHAPTER

1

Epidemiology and World Distribution

Ananta Khurana

Leprosy is generally believed to have originated in Asia, and the earliest records of a leprosy-like disease come from China and India in the 6th century BC. In China, a disciple of Confucius named Pai-Niu suffered from a disease resembling lepromatous leprosy, which was known at that time as *lai, li* and *Ta Feng*.[1-3]

WORLD DISTRIBUTION, PAST AND PRESENT

Ma Haide gives "Da Feng" as the early name in China.[4] Lowe[5] records that in India, leprosy was first described in the *Sushruta Samhita*, written about 600 BC, and treatment with chaulmoogra oil was described at that time. Rastogi and Rastogi[6] quote the Sanskrit word "*kustha*" as the original name in India for leprosy. Hopes that the skulls and bones of Egyptian mummies might reveal even earlier evidence of leprosy have not been fulfilled; the earliest paleopathological evidence to date is in mummies of the 2nd century BC.[7]

The disease was probably carried from India to Europe in the 4th century BC by returning soldiers and camp followers from the Greek wars of conquest in Asia, led by Alexander the Great, and the earliest description of a disease which was unmistakably leprosy was by Aretaeus, in Greece, about 150 AD. He called the disease elephantiasis. From Greece, leprosy slowly spread throughout Europe, conveyed by infected soldiers, traders and settlers, and in Western and Northern Europe the disease was active between the 10th and 15th centuries. In the present day, leprosy is restricted to a few nations across the world. WHO has identified 23 "Global priority countries" (Table 1.1) based on a composite index using key parameters of the Global Leprosy Programme (such as prevalence, new case detection, proportions of female, child and grade 2 disability cases) applied to the leprosy data.[8] These account for most of the

Table 1.1: WHO global priority countries for leprosy[8]		
Angola	Federated States of Micronesia	Nigeria
Bangladesh	India	Philippines
Brazil	Indonesia	South Sudan
Comoros	Kiribati	Sri Lanka
Côte d'Ivoire	Madagascar	Sudan
Democratic Republic of Congo	Mozambique	Somalia
Egypt	Myanmar	United Republic of Tanzania
Ethiopia	Nepal	

global burden of leprosy. High endemic pockets were reported from other countries also. Somalia has also now been included in this group, as the number of new cases reported increased from 14 in 2014 to 2610 in 2018.

The **Global Leprosy Strategy 2016–2020**, "Accelerating towards a leprosy-free world", was officially launched on 20 April 2016 with a vision towards a leprosy-free world[9] (Table 1.2). The emphasis is not only on reducing the burden of leprosy but also on providing quality leprosy services.

The emphasis on quality leprosy services encompasses the following aspects:
- **Accessible** to all who need diagnosis and treatment without geographical, economic or gender barriers.
- **Prompt in identifying and managing reactions** and other complications.
- **Patient-centered** and observant of patient's rights, including the rights to timely and appropriate treatment and to privacy and confidentiality.
- **Aimed at empowering patients and their families** through appropriate dissemination of information about the disease and its consequences, the patient's role in care and the service provision, including for rehabilitation.
- **Ensuring information provision** to patients and their families on disease and present them various treatment options, inform about possible reactions and rehabilitation services and emphasize the need for contact examination.
- **Addressing each aspect of case management** ensuring:
  - **Diagnosis** is timely and accurate, with supportive counselling;
  - **Treatment** with MDT is timely, free-of charge and user-friendly;
  - **Prevention of disability** interventions are carried out appropriately and timely;
  - Services for complications and **rehabilitation**, including reconstructive surgery, are provided as needed; and
  - Facilitate access to patients and their families to **psychological and socio-economical support**, in order to guarantee the regularity of treatment and cure and to facilitate social inclusion.
- **Consider patients, cured patients and their families as resources** for the health system.
- **Stigma-free** with regard to attitude of healthcare workers towards persons with signs and symptoms of leprosy or persons diagnosed with leprosy.

Table 1.2: Global leprosy strategy 2016–2020[9]			
Vision: A leprosy-free world	Goal	Targets	
		Indicators	2020 target
• Zero disease • Zero transmission of leprosy Infection • Zero disability due to leprosy • Zero stigma and discrimination	Further reduce the global and local leprosy burden	• Number of children diagnosed with leprosy and visible deformities	0
		• Rate of newly diagnosed leprosy patients with visible deformities	<1 per million
		• Number of countries with legislation allowing discrimination on basis of leprosy	0

CURRENT GLOBAL STATUS[8]

As per the updated data published by WHO in 2019, the registered global prevalence at the end of 2018 decreased by 8501 cases from that at the end of 2017 (Fig. 1.1). Thus, the registered prevalence has decreased by 4% globally, but increases were observed in Americas region (AMR), Eastern Mediterranean region (EMR) and Western Pacific region (WPR) (Table 1.3). The South-East Asia region (SEAR) accounted for 71% of the new leprosy cases globally at the end of 2018, with India and Indonesia contributing 92% of the region's case load. Brazil contributed 93% of new leprosy cases in AMR. These 3 countries together accounted for 79.6% of the new case load globally.

Of the 159 countries and territories that provided data, 32 reported zero new cases in 2018, 47 reported 1–10 cases, 24 reported 11–100 cases, 41 reported 101–1000 cases, 12 reported ≥1000 cases, and 3 countries, Brazil, India and Indonesia, reported >10,000 new cases each. Although SEAR and WPR reported significantly fewer new cases in

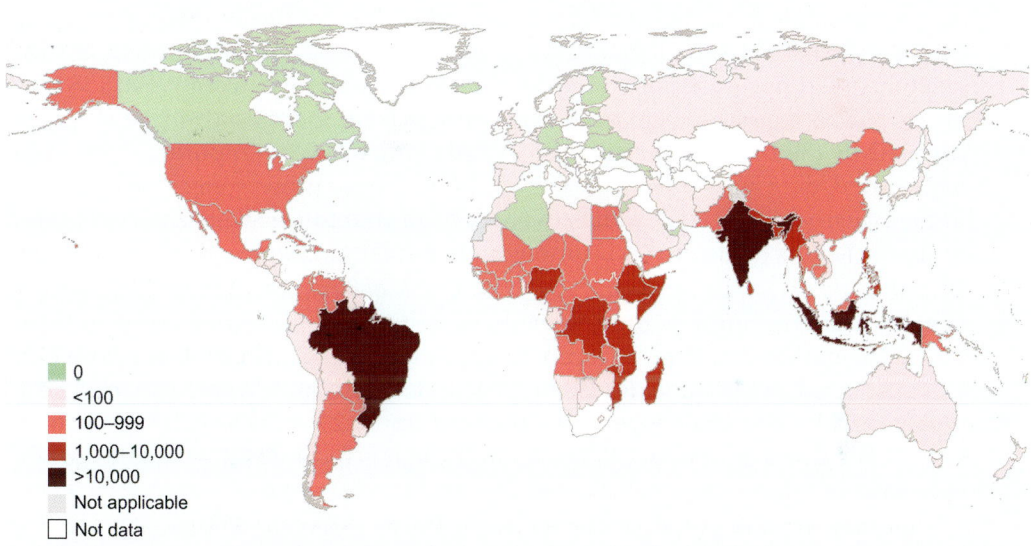

Fig. 1.1: Worldwide prevalence data of leprosy (source WHO 2019)[8]

Table 1.3: Registered prevalence (end of 2018) and new case detection in 2018, by WHO regions		
WHO region	Prevalence/10,000 population	New case detection rate/100,000 population
African region (AFR)	0.21	1.93
Americas (AMR)	0.34	3.08
Eastern Mediterranean region (EMR)	0.07	0.62
European region (EUR)	<0.0	0.01
South-East Asia region (SEAR)	0.58	7.49
Western Pacific region (WPR)	0.04	0.22
World	**0.24**	**2.74**

2018, more new cases were reported from AMR, EMR and European region (EUR). The surge in the number of new cases observed in several countries is due to active case detection campaigns, and especially improved contact screening, in addition to routine leprosy control activities which has influenced trends in new case detection at regional level. SEAR reported 3.2% fewer new cases in 2018 mainly due to reduction in the number of new cases reported by India. India has reported decrease in the numbers of new cases since 2016, by nearly 15,000 cases (135,485 in 2016 to 120,334 in 2017–2018). Globally, the number of new cases detected has decreased by 15% over the past 10 years.

A slight decrease (1.2%) was also observed in the number of new cases detected globally. In all regions and globally, a slight decrease in detection of new pediatric cases has been observed. A total of 16,013 new child cases were reported worldwide in 2018 with a majority being from SEAR (11,793). India alone accounted for 9,227 of these.

As for the targets of WHO global leprosy strategy, the following data was reported for year ending 2018:

1. *Number of children diagnosed with leprosy and visible deformities*: Segregated data was not available from all countries. Overall, 350 new child cases with grade 2 disability (G2D) were reported worldwide. Of these, 9 were from WPR, 138 from SEAR (out of which 84 were from India and 33 from Indonesia), 4 from EMR, 41 from AMR (39 of which were from Brazil) and 158 were reported from AFR. Segregated data was not available for EUR. Thus, more concerted efforts to improve early case detection and coverage of all endemic pockets will be required to reach the target of zero G2D among new pediatric cases.

2. *Rate of newly diagnosed leprosy patients with visible deformities*: A clear decrease was observed in the number of new cases with G2D in all regions and globally indicating earlier detection in recent years. A total of 14,322 new cases with G2D were reported in 2009 and 11,323 in 2018, a decrease of 21% in 10 years. The 23 global priority countries together accounted for 90.2% of new G2D cases in the world. The number of new G2D cases in India has reduced from 5245 in 2017 to 3666 in 2018.

    The data indicates that it may be possible to reach the 2020 G2D target of <1 case per million at global level. The target has already been achieved in EMR (0.45) and WPR (0.14), and the global rate is 1.5 per million. The G2D rates in SEAR (2.88), AFR (2.63) and AMR (2.3) indicate that case detection activities need to be improved.

3. *Number of countries with legislation allowing discrimination on basis of leprosy*: As per the WHO 2019 report, 13 countries still have legislation or laws that permit discrimination on the basis of leprosy. However, a number of national programmes reported that such laws had been repealed. For example, in Nicaragua, leprosy patients are no longer segregated into "homes" since 2015, and all people affected by leprosy are treated in hospital. In India, legislation was amended in 2019 to ensure that leprosy may no longer be ground for divorce. In Thailand, people from other countries who are affected by leprosy are ensured complete treatment. The national leprosy programme in Sri Lanka has issued a technical note to the Government supporting repealing of a law that allows segregation and discrimination of affected people.

WHO has initiated discussions on a post-2020 global leprosy strategy based on the progress achieved in reaching the targets set in the strategy covering 2016–2020 and in consultation with national programmes and partners. The new global leprosy strategy will include prevention of leprosy by mass preventive chemotherapy of contacts and other high-risk groups. Possible indicators and targets for the post-2020 global leprosy strategy discussed with national programmes are zero new cases, zero disability, zero discrimination and coverage of contacts with SDR chemoprophylaxis. However, it must be noted here that the indicator of leprosy "elimination" (prevalence less than 1 per 10,000) was based as the assumption that transmission would stop with such low level of prevalence[10] and not on any scientific evidence.

Leprosy services have been integrated into the general health services in most leprosy endemic countries; much greater emphasis is given here to the need for an effective referral system, as part of an integrated programme. The national programme conducted active case detection campaigns, with high coverage and involvement of female community health volunteers, resulting in sustained new case detection over the past 4 years. The decreasing trend observed in India, which now accounts for <60% of global leprosy, reflects the leprosy situation at regional and global levels.

REFERENCES

1. Skinsnes OK. Leprosy in society. The pattern of concept and reaction to leprosy in oriental antiquity. Leprosy Review 1964;35:10–22.
2. Skinsnes OK. Leprosy in archaeologically recovered bamboo book in China. International Journal of Leprosy 1980;48:333.
3. Skinsnes OK, Chang PHC. Understanding leprosy in ancient China. International Journal of Leprosy, 1985;53:289–307.
4. Haide Ma, Ganyun Ye. Leprosy work in China. Leprosy Review 1982;53:81–4.
5. Lowe J. Comments on the history of leprosy. Leprosy Review 1947;18:54–63.
6. Rastogi N, Rastogi RC. Leprosy in Ancient India. International Journal of Leprosy 1984;52:541–3.
7. Dzierzykray-Rogalski T. Paleopathology of the Ptolemaic inhabitants of Dakhleh Oasis (Egypt). Journal of Human Evolution 1980;9:71–4.
8. WHO weekly epidemiological record 2019,94:389–412 (https://apps.who.int/iris/bitstream/handle/10665/326775/WER9435-36-en-fr.pdf; last accessed 30/11/2019).
9. Global Leprosy Strategy 2016–2020. (http://www.searo.who.int/srilanka/areas/leprosy/global_leprosy_strategy_2016_2020.pdf; last accessed 30/11/2019).
10. WHO Technical Advisory Group on Leprosy report. 16th meeting of TAG on leprosy, 2019.

CHAPTER 2

The Disease

2.1 CLINICAL LEPROSY

Kabir Sardana, Premanshu Bhushan, Ananta Khurana

INTRODUCTION

Mycobacterium leprae was discovered by Hansen in Norway in 1873 and his observations were published in 1874 making it the oldest known bacterium pathogenic to man.[1] Even though *M. lepromatosis* has been discovered, genomic data reveals that *M. lepromatosis* and *M. leprae* diverged from a common ancestor after the massive gene inactivation event described previously for *M. leprae*.[2,3] Shepard was the first to successfully grow *M. leprae* in a laboratory animal. He chose the foot pads of mice because of their cool temperature (as many had done before him) but he succeeded because counting the numbers of bacilli injected, he found that inocula had to contain less than 10^6 bacilli (1 million) for successful establishment of infection and obtained the best multiplication with inoculum of about 10^3 (1000) bacilli.[4] These infections however remained localized to the foot pad, and it was not until 1966 that a disseminated infection was obtained by Rees in immature mice previously treated by thymectomy and whole-body irradiation to depress their immunity.[5]

The transmission of leprosy is discussed in *Chapter 4, Section 4.2*. It is notable that only a proportion of persons infected develop signs of the disease after the usual incubation period of 3–5 years. The majority only develop a subclinical infection with immunological evidence but no clinical manifestations (*see Chapter 4, Section 4.3*).[6] Biopsies from persons who have been in contact with leprosy patients have sometimes shown the presence of a single bacillus in skin, muscle or nerve, yet no signs of leprosy have developed during subsequent follow-up examinations. In the case of a susceptible host, the type of leprosy which will develop is determined by the way in which the defensive cells respond to the challenge once they have 'recognized' the infection. The first resting place for *M. leprae* is likely to be within peripheral nerves, for leprosy bacilli have a predilection for neural tissue and whatever may be the route of entry into nerves, the target organ is the Schwann cell[7] (*see Chapter 4, Section 4.4*). Nerves invaded by leprosy bacilli are either dermal (cutaneous) nerves or nerve trunks, and the two regions which are most vulnerable are where the nerves are most cool and where they are subject to trauma. It has been elegantly shown that route of affliction is via the colonization of epineurial vessels which precedes endoneurial infection. The

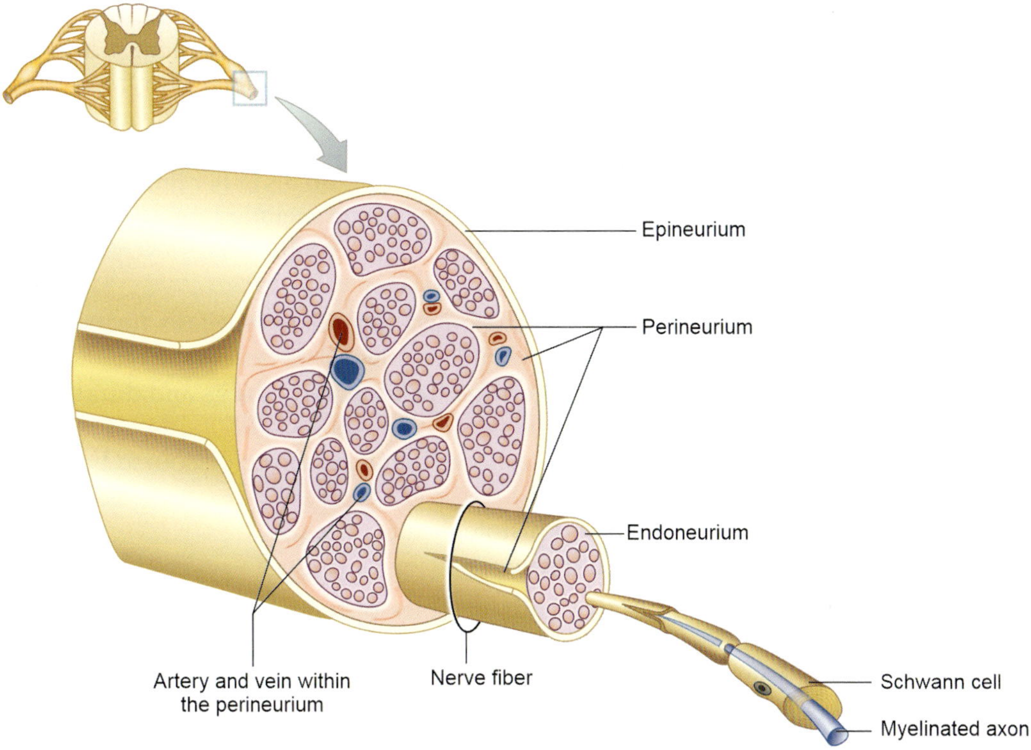

The Disease

Fig. 2.1: A depiction of a nerve with the Schwann cells, the site of tropism of *M. leprae*

endoneurium is the fine layer of tissue enclosing Schwann cells and axons, and a group of these minute structures are enclosed by a multilayered structure known as perineurium to form a nerve fascicle (Fig. 2.1). The epineurium is the outer coat of a nerve and is a loose connective tissue sheath binding the fascicles together.

Once bacilli have been engulfed by Schwann cells, their subsequent fate and the type of leprosy which ensues, depends on the resistance of the infected individual (*see Chapter 4, Section 4.3*). Resistance is highest in tuberculoid leprosy (TT), diminishes through the borderline spectrum, and is lowest in lepromatous leprosy (LL) (Fig. 2.2).

Classification

It is now accepted that clinical manifestations of leprosy reflect the response of host immunity against the *M. leprae* (Fig. 2.2). As with the immune status of the infected individuals, the clinical presentations of leprosy also vary, from inconspicuous to plain obvious. Thus, on one hand patients may have advanced disease and yet may not be recognized by themselves or unsuspecting physicians, while on the other hand, patients may have such easily recognized

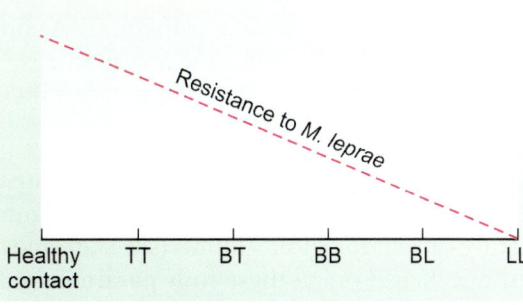

Fig. 2.2: A depiction of the host resistance through the spectrum of leprosy

features that even a lay person can identify as being signs of leprosy. Both settings are highly unfortunate—one leading to delay in treatment and complications while the other leading to social stigmatization. In between these two ends are myriad other presentations. This is akin to the spectrum of light with a series of different wavelengths between two extremes.[8] This spectral nature of clinical leprosy requires classification to understand the nature of an individual patient's disease and his or her immunological resistance. Thus, the reasons leprosy needs to be classified include:

1. To estimate the patient's *immunological* status and stability
2. To know the *infectivity* of the patient
3. To predict the likely *evolution* of disease and formulate *prognosis* for patients including likelihood of complications and reactions
4. To be able to guide the *treatment* regarding the number of drugs and duration of treatment
5. To allow uniform *nomenclature* that allows better scientific discourse between clinicians and researchers
6. To allow *correlation* of clinical and histological features
7. To explain the *host-parasite* relationship.[8]

It is uniformly agreed that the two ends or poles of leprosy are quite distinct.[8,9] However, most confusion and controversies arise in the classification of the intermediate forms. The two polar forms have been variously labelled as nodular and anesthetic (Danielssen and Boeck, 1848)[10] or tuberous and maculoanesthetic (Hansen and Looft, 1895)[11] or cutaneous and neural (Rogers and Muir, 1925). The Manila classification in 1931 introduced term "mixed" for intermediate forms besides the cutaneous (corresponding to nodular) and neural (corresponding to maculo-anesthetic).[12] The Cairo classification (1938) used the term lepromatous for cutaneous (nodular) type besides further subgrouping neural type.[13] The Pan-American classification (1946) retained the term lepromatous, used tuberculoid for neural type and introduced "uncharacteristic" for intermediate forms. Havana classification (1948) replaced uncharacteristic with "indeterminate".[14]

The WHO expert committee (1952) recommended four group classification—lepromatous, borderline, tuberculoid and indeterminate.[15] The Madrid classification (1953) divided leprosy into two stable and mutually exclusive polar types (tuberculoid and lepromatous) and two relatively unstable and indistinctive groups (indeterminate and borderline) with further varieties under each heading.[16] The Indian classification (1955) divided leprosy into 6 types: Tuberculoid (T), borderline (B), lepromatous (L), indeterminate (I), maculoanesthetic (MA) and polyneuritic (P) based on clinical and bacteriological (slit-skin smears) features.[17] The new IAL (Indian Association of Leprologists, 1981) classification merged the MA into tuberculoid group leaving only 5 groups (I, T, B, L, P).

Ridley-Jopling classification: This is the most scientific, widely accepted and research-oriented classification that is based on *four* parameters, namely clinical features, histological features, bacteriological features (slit-skin smears) and immunological features (lepromin testing). Based on all these four parameters, leprosy is divided into five groups:

i. TT: Tuberculoid leprosy
ii. BT: Borderline tuberculoid leprosy

iii. BB: Borderline-borderline leprosy or mid-borderline leprosy
  iv. BL: Borderline-lepromatous leprosy
  v. LL: Lepromatous leprosy

Of these five groups, TT and LL are immunologically stable poles while BT, BB and BL are unstable types. Understandably, these borderline types may up- or downgrade. Thus, we may have a case of LL that started as LL and has remained LL throughout the disease process, and another case of LL that may have downgraded from BL. This downgraded type is referred to as subpolar LL (LLs) and is unstable, while the stable type is called polar LL (LLp). This LLs may also have some lesions of borderline leprosy along with features of polar LL and is immunologically unstable and may undergo reactions. Histologically, LLs is likely to differ from LLp by decreased or absent foamy change and increased lymphocytes, while dermal nerves show slight cellular infiltration and in some cases the peculiar lamination of perineurium known as 'onion-skin' perineurium.[18] If one of the earlier borderline lesions is biopsied, the epithelioid cell granuloma will be found to have given way to a macrophage leproma with many leprosy bacilli. In the absence of reaction, there is little to choose between these two groups as regards prognosis excepting that, as a result of chemotherapy, LLs may become bacteriologically negative sooner than LLp. It should be noted that the term lepromatous leprosy (LL) includes both groups.

Similarly, Ridley in his histological study of about 1500 patients of tuberculoid leprosy observed that TT cases may be of two broad subtypes.[19] These are known as polar tuberculoid (TTp) which is stable throughout and secondary tuberculoid (TTs) which develops as a result of upgrading from BT. TTs is immunologically stable unlike LLs. Thus, we can envisage the extended Ridley-Jopling classification as follows even though there are objections to this straight line classification:

$$TTpTTs \leftarrow BT \leftrightarrow BB \leftrightarrow BL \leftrightarrow LLsLLp$$

Two important types missed by Ridley-Jopling scheme include indeterminate and pure neuritic types. Though, not directly included, pure neuritic type is indirectly referred in this classification as being mostly TT but may be all types except LL. Further, this classification is tedious and not practical in control programmes necessitating a more clinical classification especially for choosing the appropriate treatment and its duration.

WHO classification is accordingly tailored to determine the appropriate therapy for leprosy patients. This has also evolved over years and is adopted with some modifications across the globe. In this scheme, leprosy is classified as paucibacillary (PB) or multibacillary (MB) based on the number of skin lesions, presence of nerve involvement and identification of bacilli on slit-skin smear. The current WHO classification (2017) is as follows:[20]

- PB case: A case of leprosy with 1 to 5 skin lesions without presence of bacilli on skin smear.
- MB case: A case of leprosy with >5 skin lesions; *or* with nerve involvement (pure neuritic or any number of skin lesions and neural involvement) *or* with demonstrated presence of bacilli in a slit skin smear *irrespective* of the number of skin lesions.

It is important to note that WHO has also now used nerves to classify PB or MB leprosy which is a change from the previous classification, which used only skin lesions.

Table 2.1: NLEP classification (India, 2009)		
Characteristic	PB (Paucibacillary)	MB (Multibacillary)*
Skin lesions	1–5 lesions	6 and above
Peripheral nerve	No nerve/only one nerve involvement	More than one nerve
Skin smear	Negative at all sites	Positive at any site

*If a case has any one of the three features suggestive of MB, he/she is classified as MB.

Further, slit-skin smears have not been considered necessary for control programs and WHO has described them as the weakest link in control programs[20,21] (*also see Chapter 3, Section 3.1*). However, if smears are used in conjunction with clinical findings, all smear positive cases would be classified as MB. The current recommendations recognize that "if there is no facility for skin smear examination, some of these cases may be missed".[21] National Leprosy Elimination Programme in India uses a modified version of previous WHO classification (*Table 2.1*).[22]

Thus, NLEP classification is essentially the same as WHO classification except about number of nerves. NLEP classifies two or more nerves as MB, whereas WHO classifies all nerve involvement as MB.

In conclusion, various classification schemes of leprosy highlight the complex, spectral nature of disease and its evolving understanding. While Ridley-Jopling classification is most widely used for research and academic purposes, WHO classification (with its modifications) is most commonly used system in leprosy control programmes.

Clinical Aspects of Leprosy

The most remarkable thing about leprosy is the enormously wide variation in the way the disease affects different persons. In some, the disease involves only one peripheral nerve (a mononeuritis) or causes a single skin blemish which persists indefinitely or disappears of its own accord, while in others it produces countless nodules and other types of skin lesions, together with polyneuritis and damage to vital organs, such as eyes, larynx, testes and bones. Every conceivable variation occurs between these two extremes. The explanation lies in the infected individual's immune status (resistance to infection)[23] (*Figs 2.2 and 2.3*) and the fact that it is *not* a question of bacterial strains of varying pathogenicity has been confirmed by Rees,[24] who has shown that leprosy bacilli from patients with different types of leprosy all behave in the same way when injected into susceptible mice. The clinical manifestations of the new species *M. lepromatosis* are akin to *M. leprae* and contrary to some initial reports, *M. lepromatosis* does not appear to be more ominous than its close relative *M. leprae*[25] (*see Chapter 4, Section 4.1*)

Thus, the spectrum in leprosy depends on the host and without treatment most patients shift (downgrade) towards the low resistant form; while with treatment a *few* will shift (upgrade) towards the high resistant forms. However, these shifts are neither invariable nor irreversible, and they are not always predictable.[26]

M. leprae is believed to enter the human host predominantly through respiratory route while skin may also be important (*see Chapter 4, Section 4.2*). In susceptible individuals, a local lesion may be produced (primary lesion). Early single lesions in children are found mostly on the gluteal region, followed by those on the back and

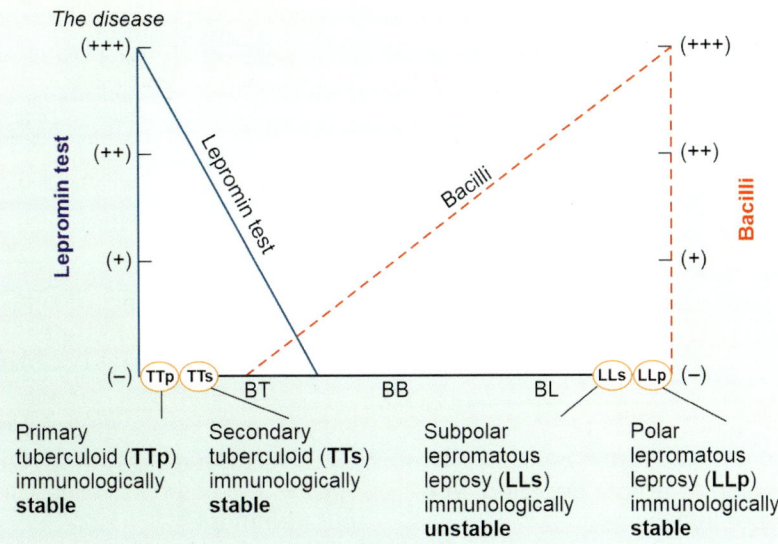

Fig. 2.3: Results of skin smears and lepromin tests according to the position of the patient in the leprosy spectrum

posterior aspects of the arms.[27] In warm climates, children are scantily clad and microtrauma may allow the entry of bacilli. Interestingly, contrary to the Asian experience, in Africa, there is a striking excess of lesions on the face.[28]

Bacilli may stay at the site of entry, they may spread via the lymphatics or there may be a bacillemia. Since the nerves offer a protected site, the bacilli lodging there as a result of the bacteremia escape elimination by the defense mechanisms of the body. This results in the pure neuritic type of leprosy seen in about 18% of cases.[29]

Evolution of the Disease

Most of those exposed to infection (over 95%) appear to be non-susceptible to leprosy in that they do not develop the disease despite close contact with leprosy patients.[30] When clinical symptoms develop, they do so after an incubation period that varies from about two months to ten years and the various ensuing types are mediated both by host immunity and genetic predisposition (*see Chapter 4, Section 4.1*).[31]

Indeterminate phase: The earliest clinically apparent lesions are indeterminate, both clinically and histologically. There is no granuloma present, there are no bacilli found in the lesion and immunological responsiveness has not yet developed.[32] Spontaneous healing may occur in indeterminate lesions and in early TT and BT but the proportion of cases of each sort that heal depends on the manner of classification and the intrinsic immune response.[33]

Development from the indeterminate stage: Non-self-healing early lesions evolve and become histologically classifiable as BT or less often as TTp, BB and BL.[33–35] Primary lepromatous infections appear to be widely disseminated at the first sign of the disease. These relationships and their subsequent development are viewed (on a straightline spectrum) in Fig. 2.4. The evolution of the disease depends on whether treatment is initiated or not and a representative course is depicted in Fig. 2.5.

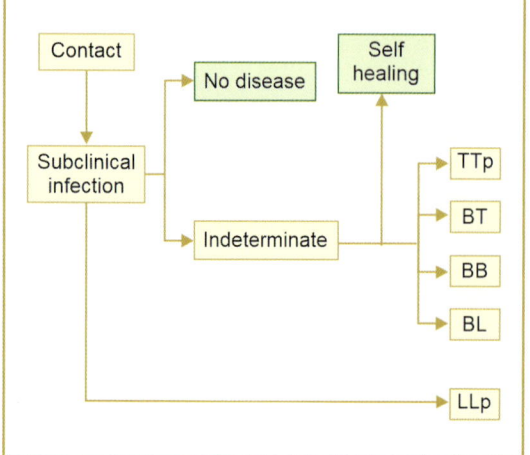

Fig. 2.4: Evolution of leprosy depicted on a straight line spectrum[26]

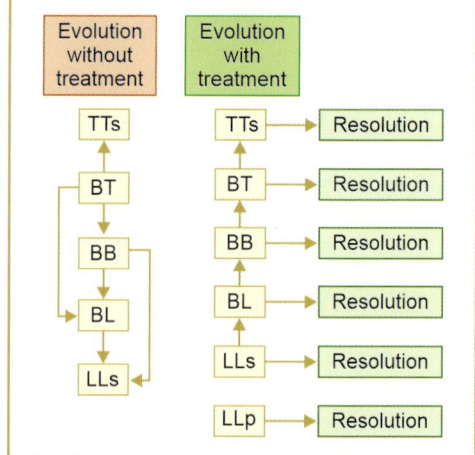

Fig. 2.5: Evolution of disease with and without treatment[26]

In terms of the common types of leprosy seen, it is pertinent to focus on the immunological instability of patients in the mid-spectrum as demonstrated by the distribution curve of types (Fig. 2.6). While the actual distribution might be dependent on the stage of the infection in different endemic areas, the distribution is always bimodal. Tuberculoid patients are rare because they are on the verge of spontaneous healing while BB, because of the rapid transition across the spectrum, is also uncommon. Downgrading leads to the accumulation of cases at LLs. The paucity of LLp patients is more difficult to explain. It suggests that the defect in these patients may be inherent, which would also explain why borderline patients do not downgrade beyond LLs.

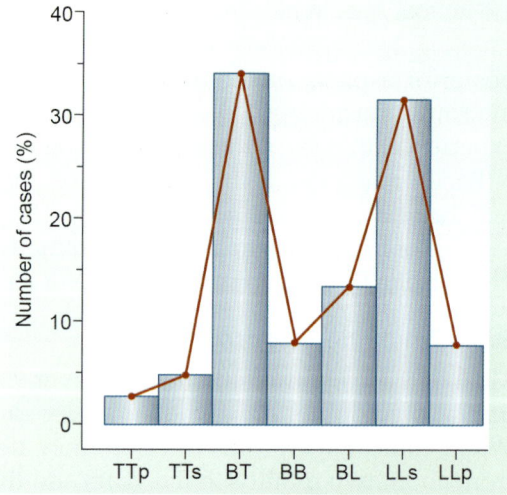

Fig. 2.6: The distribution curve for different spectra of leprosy

Clinical Lesions

In leprosy, earlier the diagnosis, better the ultimate prognosis. Thus, it is pertinent to dwell on the varied presentations of leprosy (Box 2.1).

The commonest early lesion is an area of numbness of the skin or a visible skin lesion. The most common early skin lesion is one or a few hypopigmented macules of indeterminate leprosy. In the tuberculoid spectrum, the lesions are, more or less

 Box 2.1: Early presenting features of leprosy[27]

- Numbness
- Macules and papules
- Anesthesia
- Neuritis
- Reaction

well-defined macules or plaques of hypopigmented, and often erythematous, skin which are usually anesthetic. Early lepromatous macules are hypopigmented and so vague that they are often missed till the infiltration leads to diffuse thickening and formation of papules.

Less commonly, the presenting complaint is anaesthesia of part of a hand or foot or muscular weakness. Rare presenting complaints include tenosynovitis over the dorsa of the hands, edema of the feet, nasal stuffiness and epistaxis or iridocyclitis.[27] Edema of the feet and nasal symptoms (stuffiness, crust formation, and blood-stained discharge) are possibly the earliest signs of a lepromatous disease and may be present for months or years before the skin lesions become apparent.[36] Rarely, uniquely distributed nail changes in an affected nerve distribution may be a clue to early diagnosis of leprosy.[37]

Neuritic pain may also be a presenting symptoms of leprosy. The most common presentation is of localized paresthesias, but pain may be severe especially if hands or feet are accidentally bumped. Shooting pains may occur in the limb, trunk or face. A localized area of hyperalgesia may precede the appearance of a skin lesion. Sometimes reaction is the presenting symptom, especially type 1 downgrading (in patients on no active therapy) or erythema nodosum leprosum (ENL).

The ultimate diagnosis of the various subtypes of leprosy depends on examining and collating various aspects to arrive at a possible clinical diagnosis (as below).

1. *Higher immunity (I, TT and BT)*: There are a few countable lesions which are asymmetrically distributed. Plaques have well-defined and regular borders. Anesthesia, hair loss and hypo-/anhidrosis are seen and asymmetrical—nerve enlargement is seen. As a corollary, AFB are scant and the lepromin test is positive.
2. *Lower immunity (BL and LL)*: There is symmetrical distribution of numerous lesions that are hypo-/normoesthetic and are composed of macules/papules that have ill-defined borders. Many peripheral nerve trunks are symmetrically enlarged. As a corollary, AFB are numerous and the lepromin test is negative.
3. *Mid-immune (BB)*: Features of both the spectrums are present and being immunologically unstable, it is prone to reactions. The instability makes this the rarest type.

While history taking and examination of leprosy case is detailed elsewhere (*see Chapter 10*), the important clinical aspects of the various subtypes are detailed below.

1. INDETERMINATE LEPROSY

This has been described in the Indian classification and refers to a lesion that appears *before* the host mounts a definitive immunological response. It is believed to be the most common type of leprosy seen in India, and is the first sign of the disease in 20–80% of patients and is most commonly seen in children.[38] The patient presents with one or more macules, which are hypopigmented or faintly erythematous (Table 2.2). Outer edges of indeterminate macules vary from ill-defined (hazy) to well-defined, but are usually somewhere between the two. Usually there is a single macule (Fig. 2.7), but if there are several, their distribution is asymmetrical. Indeterminate macules *cannot* be felt by the examining finger; therefore, once the edges become palpable, the lesion is no longer indeterminate.

Table 2.2: Clinical overview of indeterminate leprosy	
Skin	• Site: Lesions are commonly on the extensor surfaces of the limbs or buttocks, or on the face • One or more hypopigmented or faintly erythematous, ill-defined, macules are seen. Infiltration, by definition, is *not* present (lesions *cannot* be felt by the examining finger) • Lesions are normoaesthetic and there are no enlarged nerves
Tests	• Lepromin test: Variable, usually negative • Slit smear for AFB: Variable, usually negative • Histamine test: Reduced or absent wheal and flare may help differentiate it from other hypopigmented macules[41]

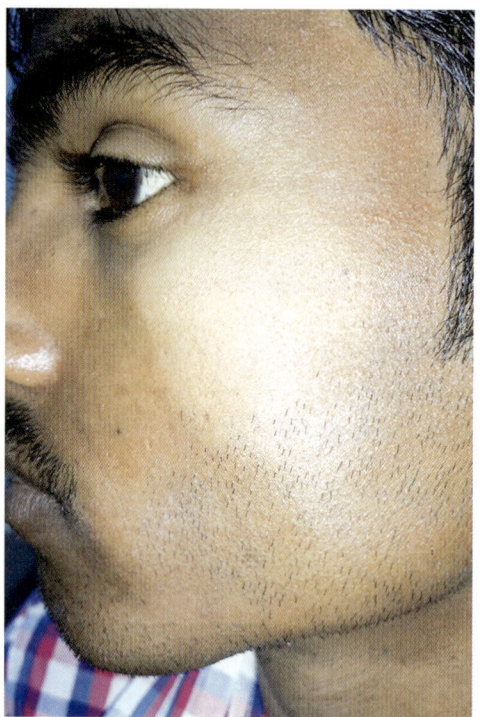

Fig. 2.7: Macular lesion of indeterminate leprosy

The distribution of lesions is variable. While in Africa, forehead is reported as most common site; buttocks, outer aspect of the extremities, scapular areas and face are more commonly involved elsewhere.[39] As it may involve sites that are covered with clothes, it is important to examine entire cutaneous surface to detect these early lesions. Scalp, axillae, groin and lumbar skin tend to be spared.[40] Slight hypoesthesia may be occasionally demonstrable. Smears are negative, but occasionally a bacillus can be demonstrated within a cutaneous nerve in a biopsy. Rarely, a thickened nerve is palpable.

Course and Prognosis

This type of leprosy may heal spontaneously, but about 30% progress to a determinate type, more often towards the lepromatous end of the spectrum.[42] In most leprosy control programs, indeterminate leprosy is grossly overdiagnosed.[43] If lesions are inconclusive, and histology is not available, a useful dictum is to wait for about 3 months, as this allows one to keep the person free of the possible stigma of a diagnosis of leprosy without untoward sequelae.

If the lesions become tuberculoid, there occurs increasing definition, hypopigmentation, anesthesia and marginal infiltration. If there is an increase in the number of lesions, peripheral streaming and central infiltration, this might suggest progression to the lepromatous pole. The prognosis with treatment is excellent; lesions clear with no reaction or neurological sequelae.

2. TUBERCULOID (TT) LEPROSY

In contrast to the lepromatous type, the patient with tuberculoid leprosy is likely to report early for medical examination. Looked at purely from the public health viewpoint this is unfortunate, for the patient is noninfectious (i.e. a 'closed' case), whereas the patient with lepromatous leprosy is infectious (i.e. an 'open' case). However, for the patient with tuberculoid leprosy it is fortunate that he has signs and symptoms which take him to the doctor in good time; his symptoms may be neural or cutaneous, or both.

TT has been divided into two subtypes—TTp and TTs.[19] TTp refers to the stable type of TT that does not downgrade and TTs refers to the type of TT that has upgraded from BT. Sensory loss is a consistent finding *except* in lesions of the face (because of extensive and overlapping nerve supply of face). Common presentations are mentioned in Table 2.3. Less commonly, the lesion is a macule (level with the surrounding skin), erythematous in light skins and hypopigmented (never depigmented) in dark skins, sometimes with a coppery or orange tint (Fig. 2.8a). Here, it must be noted that while testing a lesion for sensory loss, one should *not* rely solely on a wisp of cotton wool, since light touch sensation is likely to be lost in all those skin diseases in which there is

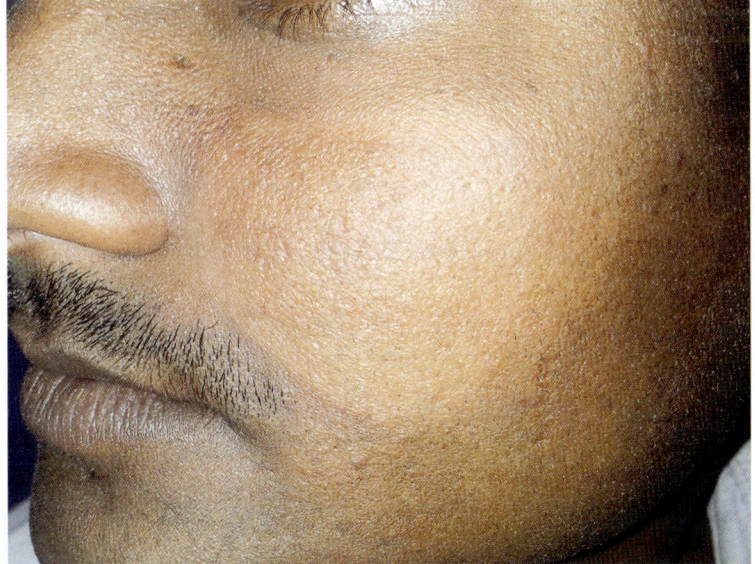

Fig. 2.8a: A TT macule

Table 2.3: Clinical overview of tuberculoid leprosy	
Skin	• Site: Any site may be involved including sometimes the warmer areas: Palms (Fig. 2.8b), soles, scalp, flexures and the midline of the body • Single or few in number, large (up to 10 cm in diameter) Skin lesions are often solitary, particularly in those patients who present as TT *de novo*, unlike those who upgrade to TT from BT, where multiple lesions (usually no more than three) may be found. In both groups, immunity is sufficient to affect cure, thus placing an upper limit of 10 cm on lesion size. • TT plaques are asymmetrical, well-defined, erythematous or copper-colored and can be either homogenously elevated or gradually flatten in the center (representing central healing and peripheral spread) (Fig. 2.8c to e). For this morphology of "a plaque with a sharply defined and elevated border that slopes down to a flattened atrophic center," the term **"saucer right way up"** (Fig. 2.8c and e) has been used.[44] • Macules may also be seen; they are erythematous in light skins and hypopigmented in dark skins with a coppery or orange tint at times; are well demarcated and have a dry, hairless and insensitive surface (Fig. 2.8a and f). • The sensory loss is typically severe and may include all modalities (temperature, pain and touch). The *initial* lesion may be hyperesthetic, but is later replaced by significant loss of sensation. However, it may be difficult or even impossible to demonstrate impaired sensation in a lesion on the face because of the generous supply of sensory nerves. • Hair growth is deficient or absent over the lesion. • Autonomic nerve damage: Dry and scaly, with complete loss of hair and sweating (tested by sitting or exercising the patient in the sun)
Nerve	• Either none or a single nerve may be thickened • A thickened nerve is usually palpable in the vicinity of a tuberculoid lesion (feeding nerve), whether it be a plaque or a macule, e.g. ulnar nerve if the lesion is near the elbow, radial cutaneous nerve if near the wrist, etc., or a thickened nerve may be felt leaving (or entering), the lesion; such a sensory nerve will be missed by the examiner if he does not run his finger lightly all the way around the edge of the lesion, for the thickened nerve is detected by feeling and not by sight.
Tests	• Lepromin test: Strongly positive (+++) • Histamine test: Absence of flare • Slit smear for AFB: Negative

epidermal thickening. A pin is more reliable. Sweating test can demonstrate anhidrosis and a histamine test on a hypopigmented lesion shows absence of flare which confirms that dermal nerves are damaged.

A thickened nerve may be palpable in the vicinity of a tuberculoid lesion and it is a good habit to run fingers lightly all the way around the edge of the lesion, for the thickened nerve is detected by feeling and not by sight. Nerve thickening may be smooth or irregular, and rarely a cystic swelling may be seen and felt in relation to the nerve—a "cold abscess" of nerve. Even more rare is calcification in a nerve which usually involves the ulnar nerve.

Course and Prognosis

True tuberculoid, has a good prognosis and it has been noted[45] in a study, where untreated children were followed for 19 years, that up to 88% of tuberculoid lesions healed spontaneously.[46]

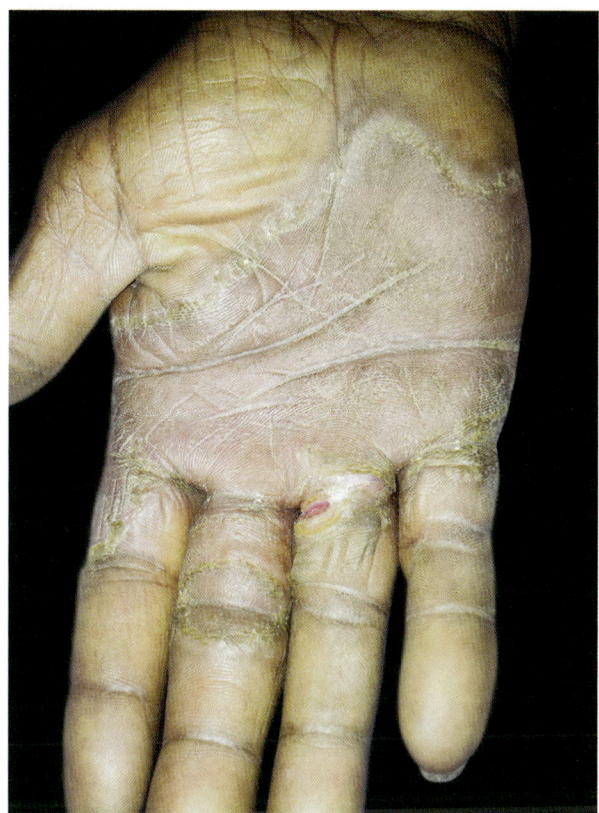

Fig. 2.8b: TT plaque on the palm. An unusual location

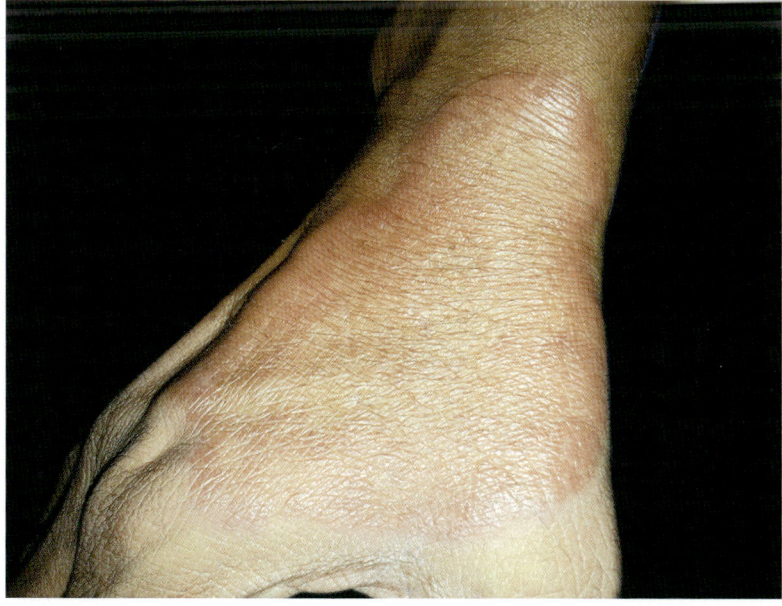

Fig. 2.8c: TT leprosy: Note the well-defined border with peripheral elevation and central flattening (saucer right way up)

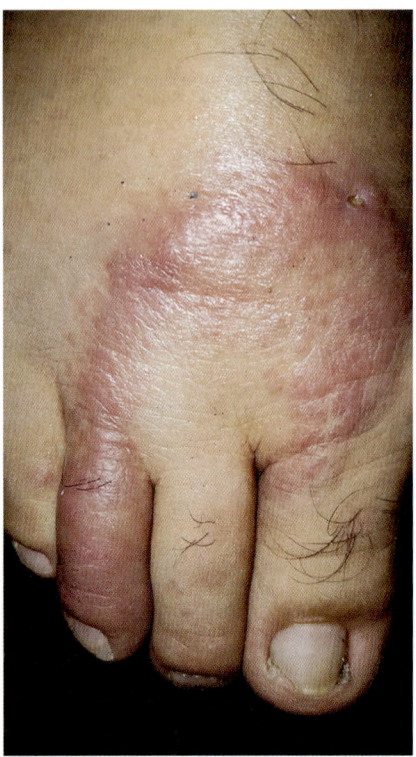

Fig. 2.8d: TT: An annular plaque on the dorsum of foot

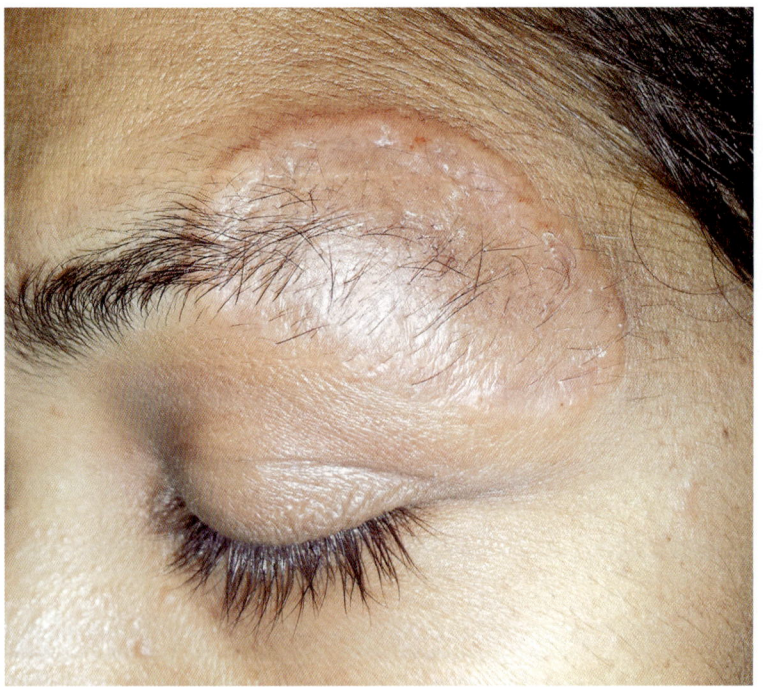

Fig. 2.8e: TT: "Saucer type" lesion with loss of hair on the lesion

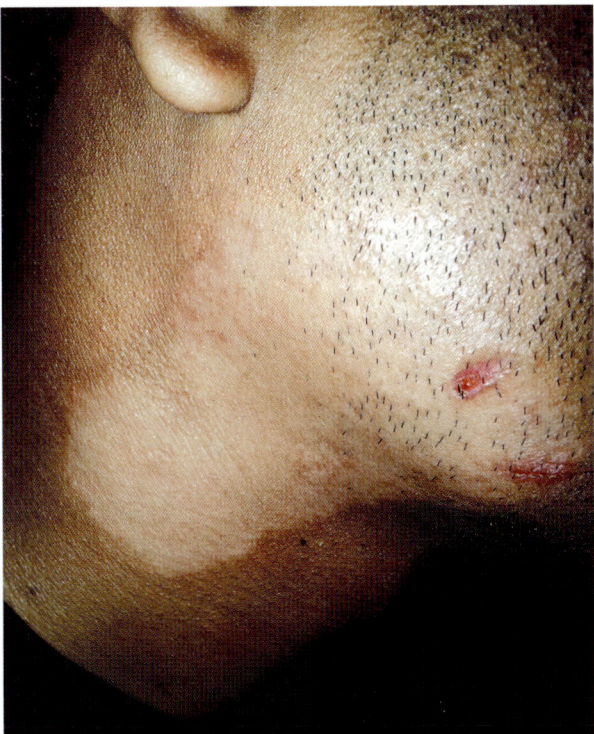

Fig. 2.8f: TT: The macular variant with incidental shaving cuts, consequent to anesthesia

3. BORDERLINE LEPROSY

(Borderline tuberculoid: BT, borderline-borderline: BB and borderline lepromatous: BL)

This type of leprosy occurs in those patients whose degree of resistance lies somewhere in the spectrum between lepromatous and tuberculoid, and therefore the number of lesions and their clinical features vary according to the position in the spectrum. It is not generally appreciated that borderline leprosy is the most *common* type of leprosy to be encountered if we take a global view, and failure to appreciate this fact is due to a failure to recognize the clinical and histological features. The tendency is to classify BT as TT. The slit smear, histopathology and lepromin test result will eventually reveal the exact place of an individual patient in leprosy spectrum, which is typically *lower* than what is clinically obvious. The ratio of BT to BL patients shows an interesting geographical pattern. BT predominates in Africans, while BL predominates in Asians and Europeans and is probably reflective of a genetic difference in the ability to express cell-mediated immunity to *M. leprae*.

The importance of recognizing borderline leprosy and of making a correct classification lies in the fact that this type differs from the two polar types in three principal respects:

1. *Immunological instability* and therefore the tendency to move in either direction along the borderline spectrum; with treatment towards the tuberculoid pole—usually as a result of a 'reversal reaction' (upgrading) *(see Chapter 5, Section 5.1)*,

while the untreated patient tends to move towards the lepromatous pole—a downgrading reaction. Thus, patients may downgrade to LLs or upgrade to TTs and this may be seen on treatment (adequate/inadequate) or without treatment. The downgrading may be silent or is uncommonly associated with reactions.[27]

2. Response to treatment and the length of time required for treatment to be continued in order to eradicate the infection.
3. Tendency to lepra reaction and crippling deformities resulting from nerve damage.

Skin lesions vary in number, surface appearance, presence of anesthesia and of hair growth, and in the definition of the outer edges. Thus, in BL they are more numerous, more shiny and smooth and have more indefinite edges, whereas in BT they are less numerous, less shiny and smooth, and have edges which are better defined or well-defined in parts and poorly in other parts of the same lesion (*see below*).

Reduced sensation and impairment of hair growth are characteristics of all borderline lesions, but are more marked in BT than in BL, and are never as complete as in the tuberculoid type (TT).

One of the important features of borderline leprosy is the frequency with which nerves are damaged; it is not uncommon for a prolonged polyneuritic phase to precede the appearance of skin lesions, and in such cases there is evidence of thickened nerves, with or without muscle paralysis or skin anesthesia, by the time skin lesions appear.[47] Several nerves are likely to be involved asymmetrically, e.g. there may be left-sided facial palsy, right-sided claw hand with ulnar nerve thickening, and a thickened left lateral popliteal nerve with anesthesia of left lower leg and foot.

Bacilli are scanty or absent in BT, are always present in BB, and are numerous in BL lesions; if globi are present in BL, they tend to be small and unlike the large globi seen in LL.

Although in borderline leprosy, granulomas have been found in human tissues, such as lymph nodes, liver and skeletal muscles, there are no clinical symptoms or signs of such tissue invasion.

Skin Lesions in Borderline Leprosy

1. *Macules*

These are erythematous in light skins and hypopigmented in dark skins. Macules of BT leprosy are well-defined and hypoanesthetic, have a dry surface, and bacilli are scanty or absent; this has been previously called 'maculoanesthetic' leprosy in India, while Leiker[48] named it the 'low-resistant tuberculoid leprosy'. The nearer the patient is to the lepromatous end of the spectrum, the more numerous the macules, the less defined and anesthetic they are, the more shiny they appear and the more likely they are to contain leprosy bacilli.

2. *Plaques*

The points described above for macules hold good for the description of plaques excepting that they appear erythematous or coppery on dark skins and hypopigmentation is less obvious. Central flattening is less obvious than in tuberculoid plaques. Differentiation of the infiltrated plaques of tuberculoid leprosy from borderline lesion can be decided by asking oneself, "Where is the most prominent part of the lesion?" If one has to put one's finger towards the center of the lesion rather than at the edge, it cannot be a true tuberculoid lesion.⁴⁹ The definition of the outer border is clinical indicator of host immunity and is sharp towards the tuberculoid pole and vague towards the lepromatous pole. Thus, unlike TT which has a sharply defined regular edge, BT has an edge that may be sharp in some areas and ill-defined (Fig. 2.9) in others and may have finger or pseudopodia like projections with some lesions showing one or more small new lesions (satellites) in the periphery of a larger lesion. A BL plaque, on the other hand, is typically infiltrated in the center and gradually slopes away imperceptibly towards the periphery (Fig. 2.10) (the inverted saucer lesion of Molesworth).[49, 50]

3. Annular Lesions

In leprosy, these are invariably borderline and may assume various sizes and shapes but are predominantly circular or oval. They can be very large. The ring itself is erythematous or coppery and consists of raised tissue with well-defined outer and inner edges (Fig. 2.11). The skin in the center of the lesion is usually of normal skin color and together with the ring itself, shows sensory impairment.

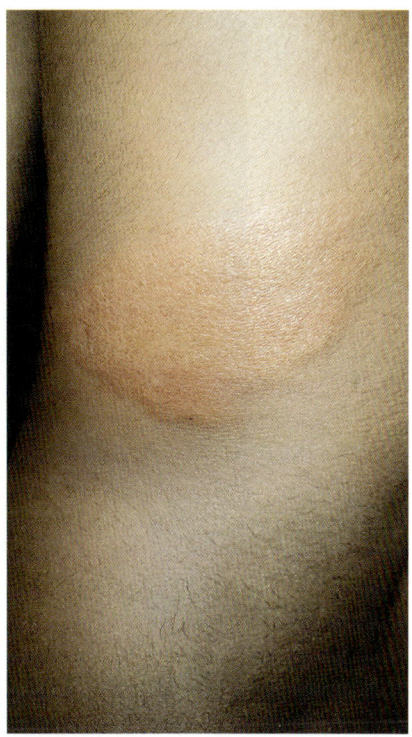

Fig. 2.9: BT plaque with well-defined to ill-defined and regular to irregular borders

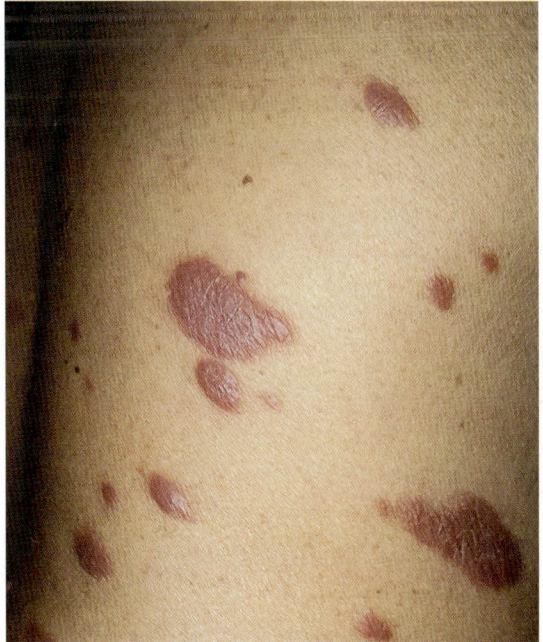

Fig. 2.10: "Inverted saucer" lesions with central infiltration (described in BL leprosy)[49, 50]

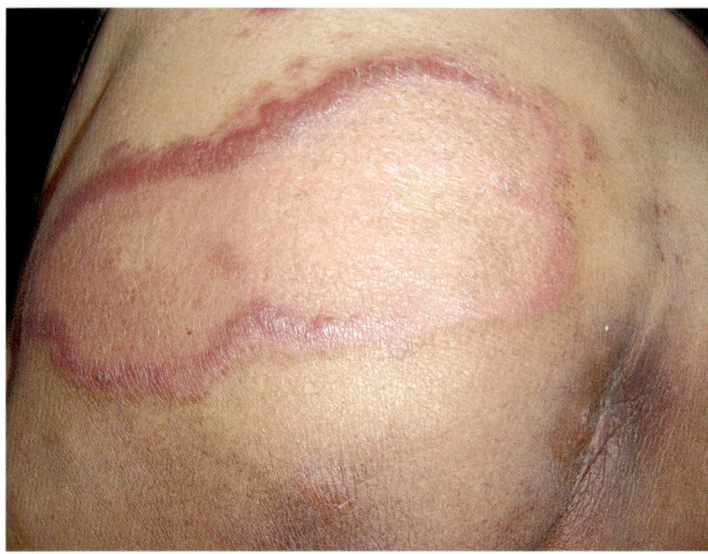

Fig. 2.11: An annular plaque seen in the borderline spectrum of leprosy

4. Punched-out Lesions

These are characteristic of the borderline type and are erythematous plaques with vague outer edges and a punched-out central portion also likened to a "hole-in-cheese" / "Swiss cheese" appearance (Fig. 2.12). The edge of the "punched-out" portion is distinctly palpable and clear cut. Some degree of anesthesia will be found on testing the lesions.

5. Bizarre Lesions

These take the form of raised bands or of geographical lesions (Fig. 2.13) (like the contour of a map). Some degree of anesthesia will be present.

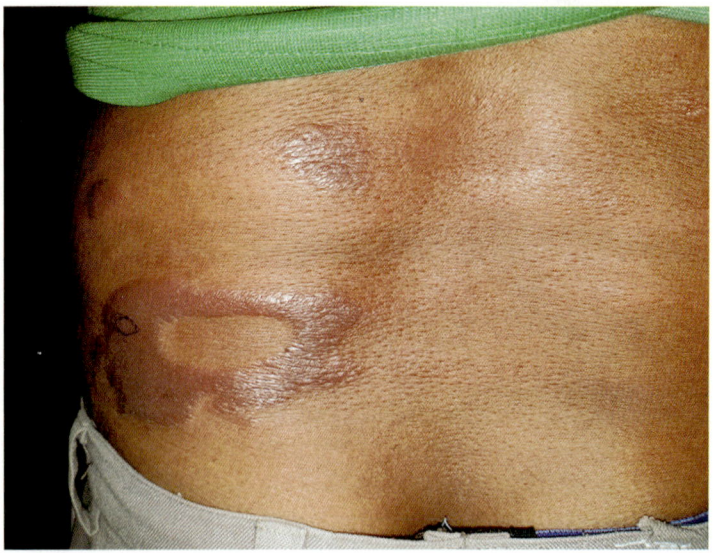

Fig. 2.12: BB Hansen annular plaque with a "Swiss cheese" appearance

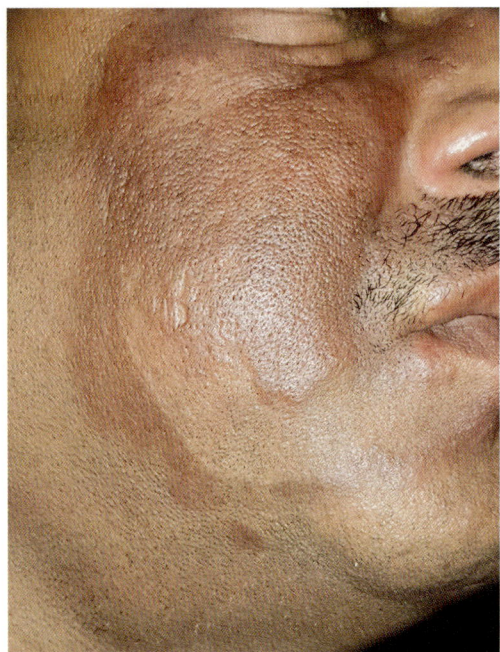

Fig. 2.13: "Bizzare geographical" lesions on the face

6. Nodules

Nodules are not characteristic of borderline leprosy but occur rarely in BL. They differ from lepromatous nodules in that they are scanty, small and asymmetrically distributed.

An overview of the salient features of borderline spectrum leprosy is presented in Tables 2.4 to 2.6.

Table 2.4: Clinical aspects: Borderline tuberculoid (BT) leprosy	
Skin	• Size up to 10 or 20 cm or more (Fig. 2.14a) and may encompass a whole limb • The number of lesions is greater than in true TT, up to 10 or 20 cm or more • The primary skin lesions of BT are plaques and hypopigmentation may be conspicuous in darkly pigmented patients (Fig. 2.14b) • Asymmetrical lesions that are well- to ill-defined, with regular to irregular borders and are hypoaesthetic with moderate loss of hairs • The margins may, at places, stream off gradually into normal skin and satellite lesions are often seen (Fig. 2.14c) • Lesions have less scaling, erythema, induration and elevation (than TT) • BT leprosy with large pale macules and multiple nerve involvement is sometimes called maculoanesthetic or low-resistant tuberculoid leprosy. • There is a propensity for type I reactions that can occur in either skin or nerves or both.
Nerve	• Widespread and asymmetrical nerve enlargement leading to widespread nerve damage is characteristic. • Nerves may be greatly enlarged and "nodulation" on palpation may signify a nerve abscess (Fig. 2.14d)
Tests	• Lepromin test: Weakly positive (+) • Slit smear for AFB: Nil or scanty

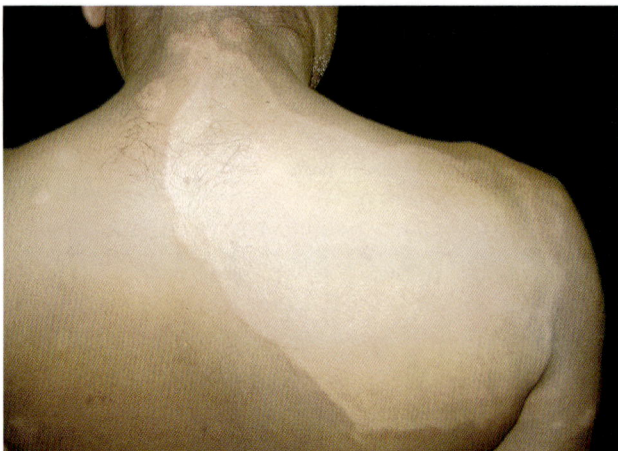

Fig. 2.14a: BT leprosy: A large plaque encompassing the back and upper shoulder with "satellite" lesions

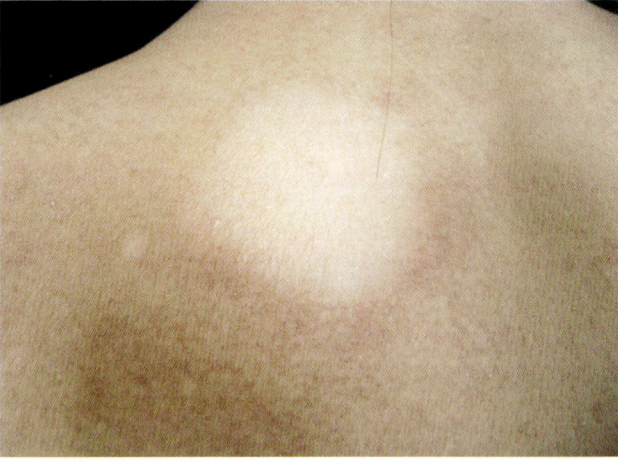

Fig. 2.14b: BT leprosy: The so-called "maculoanesthetic" lesion of leprosy

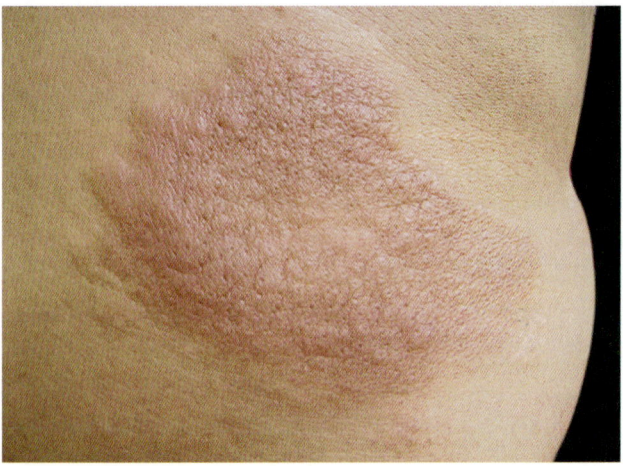

Fig. 2.14c: A plaque of BT leprosy with peripheral streaming

The Disease

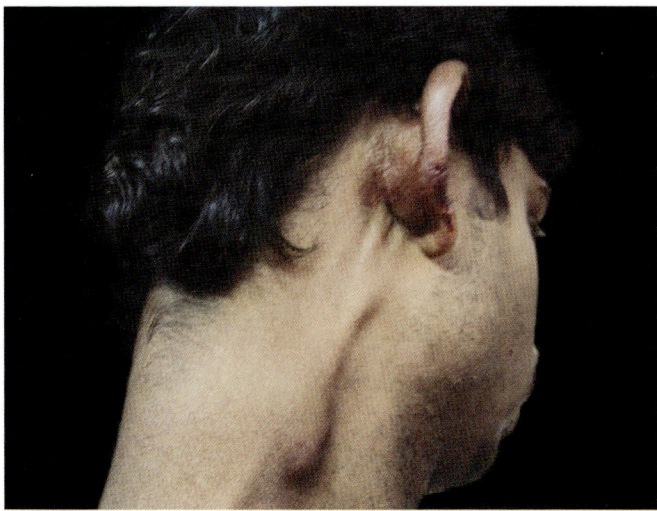

Fig. 2.14d: Greater auricular nerve thickening with abscess

Table 2.5: Clinical aspects: Borderline lepromatous (BL) leprosy	

Skin	• Variable in size, number and morphology.
	• A case of BL can have lesions of BT leprosy as the majority of these patients have downgraded from BT Hansen.
	• Madarosis is absent or less marked than LL
	• Classically, the disease starts with macules. They are more distinct, however, more variable in shape, though still small, and not so perfectly symmetrical in distribution. The earliest infiltration is in "center" of the macules. The signs of nerve damage (such as loss of hair, loss of sensation and decreased sweating and hair growth) start earlier than in LL.
	• Papules and nodules: These lesions have a sloping margin which merges imperceptibly into normal skin (Fig. 2.15a). They are more defined and less symmetrical than those of LL. Some nodules are dimpled in the center. The lepromatous-like nodules, if numerous, are symmetrically arranged.
	• Plaques: Earliest infiltration may take place within the initial macules, sometimes creating a plaque-like appearance
	   – Annular and plaque lesions, although numerous, are asymmetrical
	   – Classic lesion: Poorly marginated outer border (lepromatous-like) but a sharply marginated inner one (tuberculoid-like).
	   – The center is raised and there is sloping towards the periphery, termed **'inverted saucer'** appearance (Fig. 2.15b)
	   – Punched out or "Swiss cheese" appearance *may* also be seen
	• There is mild loss of sensations and hairs

Nerves	• Peripheral nerves become enlarged at the sites of predilection, sooner than in LL, though not so symmetrically and signs of damage occur sooner. • The nerves are less commonly tender than in BT because spontaneous reactions are less common
Sensory loss	• When disease is extensive, BL patients may also develop "gloves and stocking" sensory loss
Tests	• Slit smear for AFB: Many bacilli seen • Lepromin test: Negative

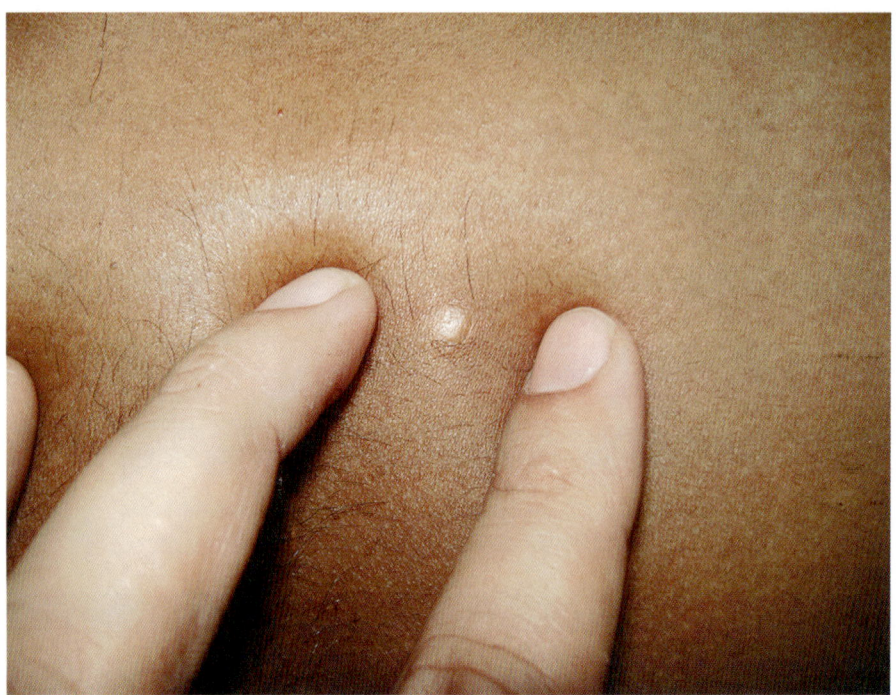

Fig. 2.15a: BL papule on apparently normal skin

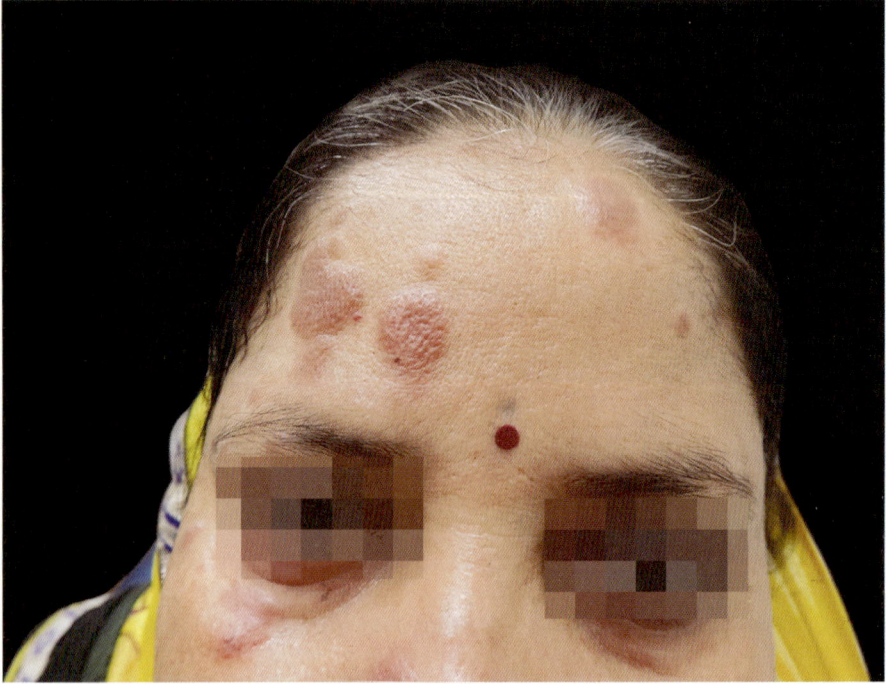

Fig. 2.15b: A case of BT leprosy downgraded to BL (note that the plaques show central elevation, sloping towards the periphery)

The Disease

Table 2.6: Clinical aspects: Borderline-borderline (BB) leprosy	
Skin	• Admixture of tuberculoid and lepromatous type lesions. The lesions may be macules, plaques or papules or a combination of these types. • Asymmetrical, well-demarcated, somewhat shiny lesions are seen • Annular lesions with characteristic, punched-out or **"Swiss cheese"** appearance (the outer border is vague, inner border is clearly defined and well demarcated) is a characteristic lesion of BB leprosy (Figs 2.12 and 2.16a). The border in such lesions has a well-defined 'tuberculoid' interior margin but a poorly defined 'lepromatous' exterior margin. • The presence of both these morphologies is termed 'dimorphic' lesions. • Geographic lesions: The shapes of lesions are characterized by streaming, irregular borders and map-like contours with satellites which represent an infiltration around immune areas (Fig. 2.16b).
Nerve	• Damage is variable • Widespread and asymmetrical nerve enlargement if downgraded from BT (multiple mononeuropathy) and symmetrical nerve enlargement if the patient has upgraded from BL. If there is a reaction, this can present as symmetrical polyneuritis
Sensory loss	• Sensory loss on the extensor surface of the limbs, which characterizes lepromatous leprosy, is unusual.
Tests	• Lepromin test: Negative • Slit smear for AFB: Moderate number of bacilli

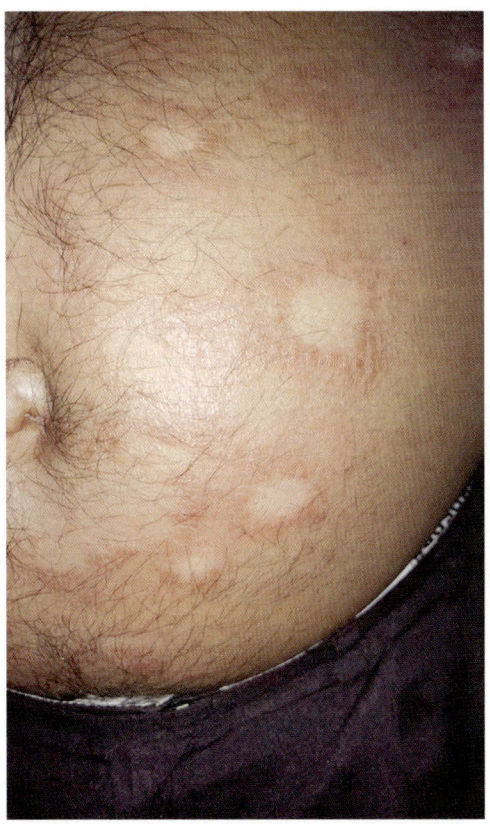

Fig. 2.16a: BB leprosy with the "Swiss cheese" appearance of plaques

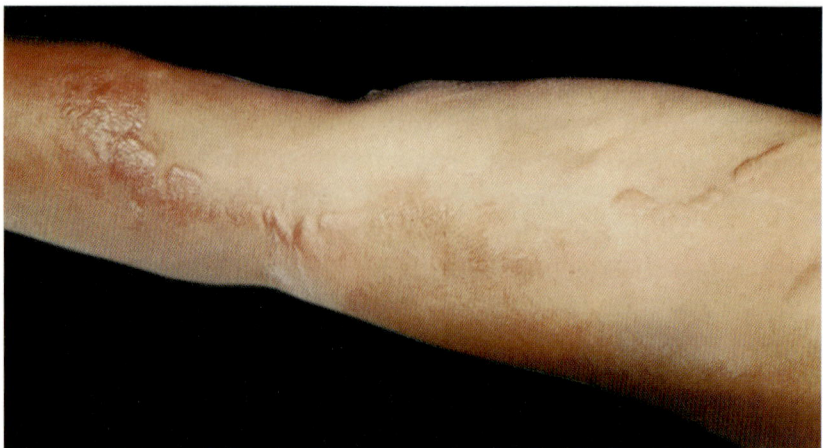

Fig. 2.16b: BB leprosy with peripheral infiltration around a center hyperimmune area—the classic manifestation of a "geographic lesion"

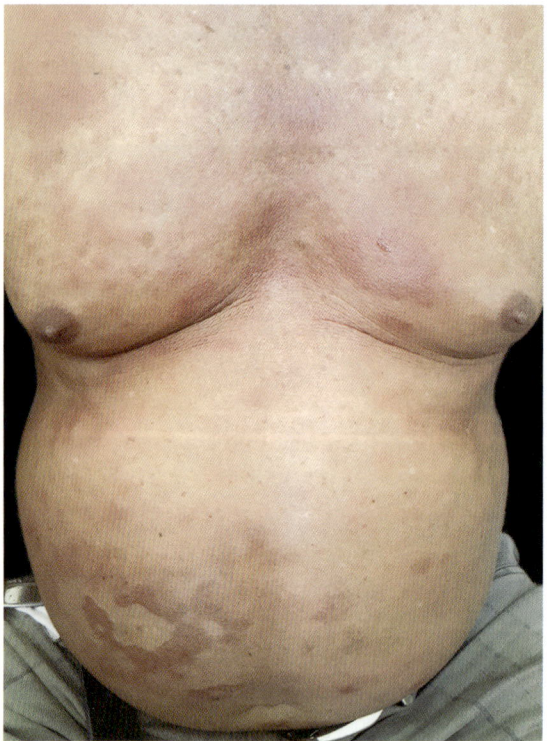

Fig. 2.16c: A case of BB leprosy with macules, papules, plaques and a "geographic" lesion seen on the lower abdomen (*Courtesy:* Dr Jaison A Barreto)

Course

A conspicuous feature of BT leprosy is the frequency and speed with which type 1 reactions can occur in either skin or nerves or both and may be overt or insidious. Because of its intrinsic instability, BB is the rarest form of leprosy. The patients usually stabilize by up- or downgrading with or without a clinical reaction. In BL disease, the resistance is too low to significantly restrain bacillary proliferation, but still sufficient to induce tissue destructive inflammation, especially in nerves. Thus, in BL there is maximum damage due to the twin effect of high bacillary load and inherent immunological instability. If the patients begin with a clinical diagnosis of BL and it is detected early, the prognosis is good. On the contrary, if the patients have downgraded from BT, then there will be nerve damage and further reactions are to be expected. Patients who downgrade to LLs can have additional type 2 reactions besides type 1 reactions. Histologically, those patients can be distinguished from LL, and are known as subpolar, or LLs.[51]

4. LEPROMATOUS LEPROSY (LL)

There are two types of LL:
1. LLp: This refers to the rare polar form of LL that arises *de novo* and is stable.
2. LLs: This refers to the commoner subpolar type that arises after downgrading from BT/BB/BL.

It is unusual to have the opportunity to examine a patient in the early stages of lepromatous leprosy (unless there has been an earlier borderline phase which has attracted attention), as there are no symptoms of nerve involvement and early skin lesions are not likely to be noticed by the patient. This is doubly unfortunate, for not only is the patient infectious and therefore a potential danger to the public health, but an opportunity is missed to have the disease arrested in the shortest possible time and to remain, provided that the treatment is completed, free from the deformities of face and limbs which are the permanent hallmarks of late diagnosis. There are two symptoms which can alert the observant leprosy worker to a possible early diagnosis of lepromatous leprosy, and they may precede the classical skin lesions by months or years. Unfortunately, however, the patient is unlikely to make any mention of them unless specifically asked; these are *nasal symptoms* and *oedema of legs*.

Nasal symptoms consist of stuffiness, crust formation, and blood-stained discharge. Edema of legs and ankles, always bilateral, is likely to be noted towards the end of the day, disappearing after a night's rest and only in the late stages it is persistent, where the legs become "woody hard" on palpation. Edema is due to a combination of gravity and increased capillary permeability, and the latter is probably due to a combination of leprous involvement of capillary endothelium and damage to autonomic fibers within dermal nerves controlling capillaries.[52]

As for skin manifestations, patients may present with macules, papules, nodules, or with all three, but macules are likely to appear first (Table 2.7). When a patient presents with all three types of skin lesions, it will usually be found that the "gross" lesions, such as nodules, are on the face and limbs, while macular lesions are on the trunk. Skin lesions are multiple and have a distribution which is bilateral and symmetrical. Macules in lepromatous leprosy are erythematous on light skins, and on dark skins are coppery or may appear hypopigmented with a faint erythematous or coppery sheen. They have indefinite edges and this indicates the lack of substantial tissue response thus accounting for the lack of contrast from the normal skin. They are best seen in bright sunlight with the rays falling obliquely on the skin.[49] They may become more obvious when the patient becomes heated, e.g. after exercise on a hot day or after a hot bath. Papules and nodules may be of normal skin color or may be pigmented (usually erythematous or coppery), are firm on palpation, are in the skin and not in the subcutis (therefore, the skin cannot be moved over them) and show variation in size (Fig. 2.17a). In light skins, healed lesions sometimes develop a yellow tinge due to the fat liberated by destroyed lepra cells, and xanthelasma palpebrarum is believed to be more common in lepromatous leprosy.

As the untreated disease advances, thickening (infiltration) of the skin of forehead causes deepening of the natural lines (leonine facies), ear lobes are thickened, eyebrows are lost, the nose becomes swollen and broadened and may collapse, eyebrows become thinned (superciliary madarosis) together with eyelashes (ciliary madarosis) (Fig. 2.17b), the voice becomes hoarse, the upper incisor teeth loosen or fall out and bilateral insensitivity of the limbs, known as 'glove and stocking' anesthesia, leads to shortening of fingers and toes due to painless and oft-repeated trauma.[53, 54] Another feature in lepromatous leprosy, both in treated and untreated patients, is ichthyosis which chiefly affects thighs, legs and arms but may also affect the trunk. Alopecia is not a manifestation of leprosy; in fact, a male lepromatous patient without a good head of hair is a rarity. Notwithstanding this, alopecia of the scalp has been rarely reported from Mexico in male patients suffering

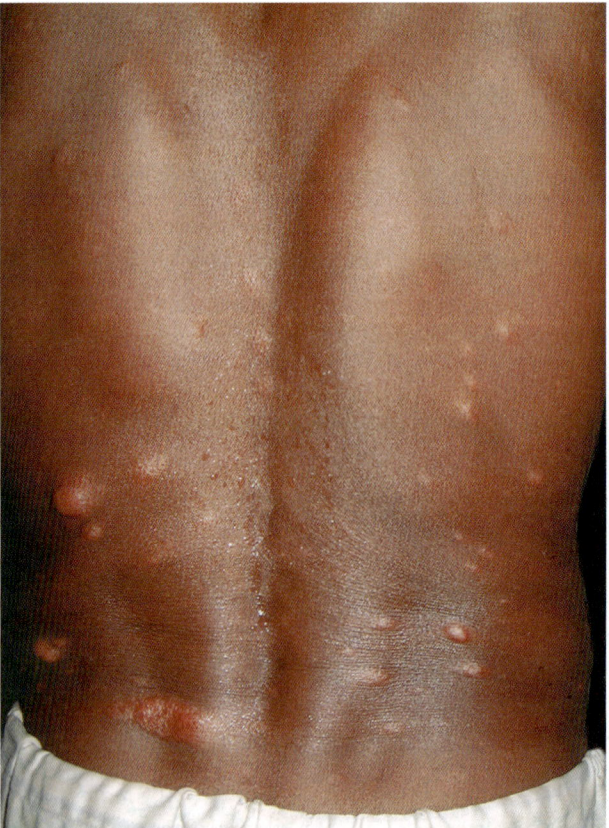

Fig. 2.17a: Papules and nodules in a case of lepromatous leprosy

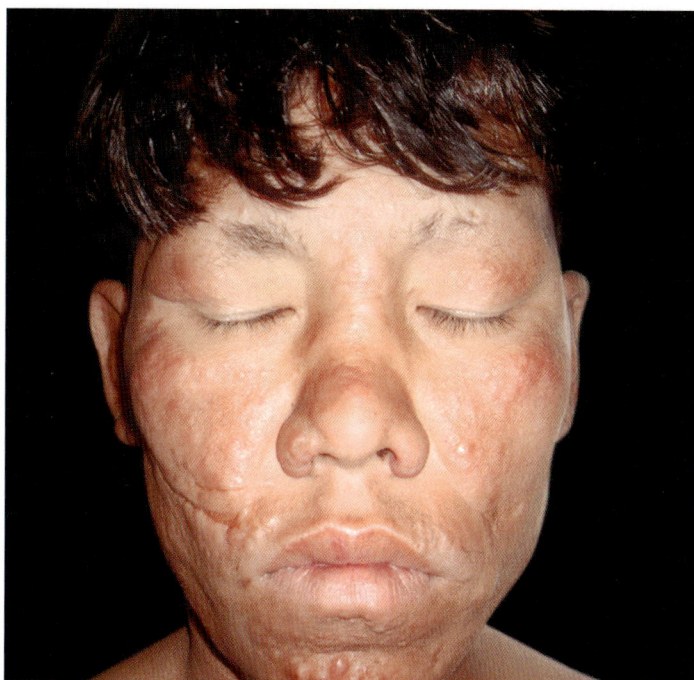

Fig. 2.17b: Lepromatous leprosy: A patient with diffuse infiltration, madarosis and nodules (the so-called "Leonine facies")

from the diffuse non-nodular form of leprosy known as Lucio leprosy and from Spain and India, and is largely restricted to the lepromatous pole.[55, 56] In typical leprous alopecia, hairs are lost over scalp except right over the blood vessels probably as they are warmer.[27]

Evidence of damage to nerves occurs late in lepromatous leprosy and, therefore, skin manifestations are always present when neurological signs and symptoms occur. These consist of nerve thickening and associated sensory or motor dysfunction depending on the type of nerve involved. The thickening of peripheral nerves gradually takes place with the passage of time (in spite of treatment), for there is no nerve thickening in the early stages, whereas in borderline and tuberculoid leprosy, nerve thickening (which is always asymmetrical) occurs early and slowly subsides as treatment is continued over the years. This emphasizes the *importance* of early *diagnosis* of LL, as early diagnosis and treatment can result in perfectly normal sensation in all four limbs with no nerve thickening. Thickened nerves feel firm and smooth, thickening being localized to the portions of nerves which are most superficial (and therefore coolest), e.g. the great auricular nerves in the neck, the supraclavicular nerves as they cross the clavicles, the ulnar nerves just above the elbows, the antebrachial cutaneous nerves in the forearms, the radial and median nerves at the wrists, the femoral cutaneous nerves in the thigh, the lateral popliteal (common peroneal) nerves as they wind round the necks of fibulae, the sural nerves at the back of the legs, the posterior tibial nerves behind the medial malleoli, and the superficial peroneal nerves in front of the ankles and on the dorsa of the feet[57] (Fig. 2.18a to f).

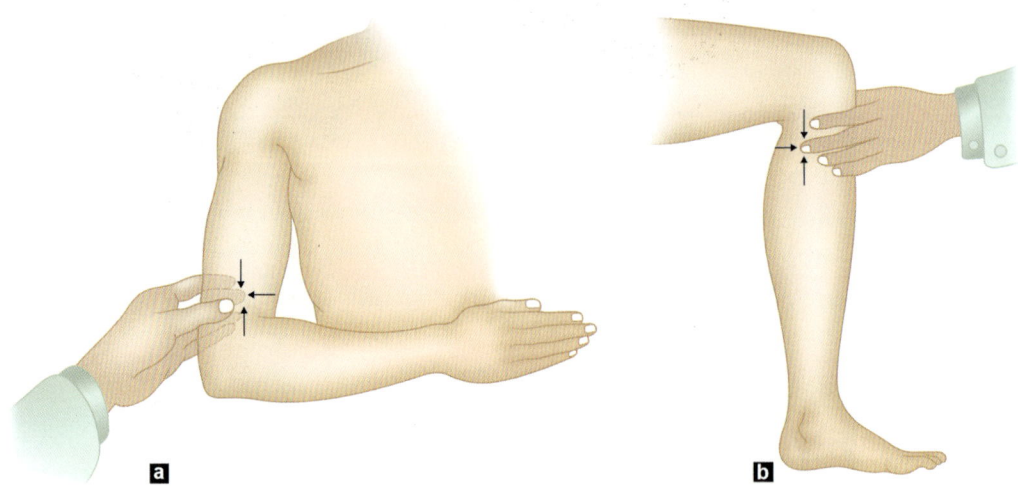

Fig. 2.18: (a) Method of palpating ulnar nerve; (b) Method of palpating common peroneal nerve

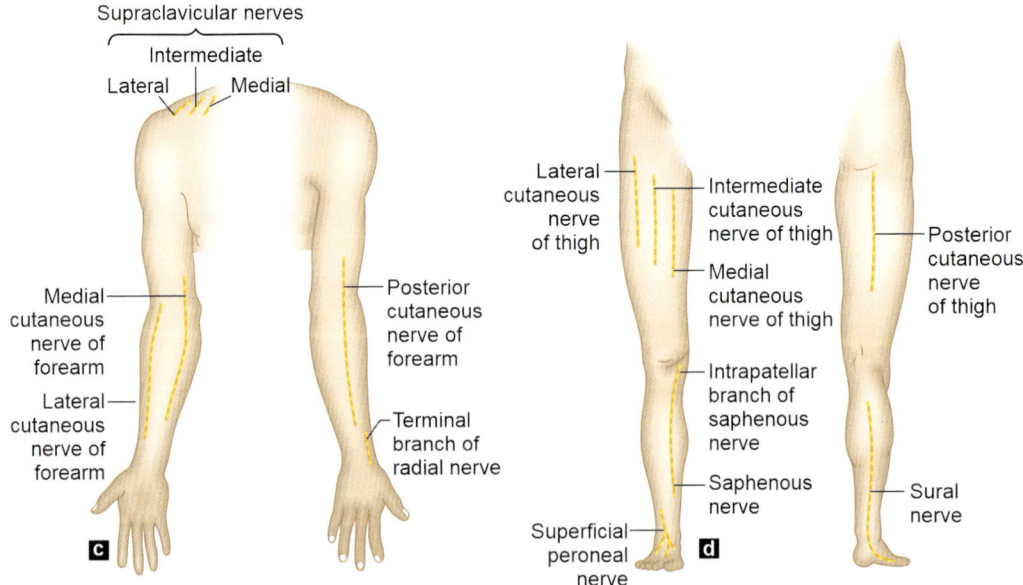

Fig. 2.18: (c) Depiction of cutaneous nerves of upper limb; (d) Depiction of cutaneous nerves of lower limb

Damage to motor nerves is manifested by muscle weakness, the affected muscles later becoming wasted and paralyzed *(also see Chapter 10)*. Muscles typically affected are those supplied by the facial nerve (facial palsy) (Fig. 2.19a), ulnar nerve (claw hand or 'main en griffe') (Fig. 2.19b), median nerve ('main de singe' or ape hand), both ulnar and median nerves (Fig. 2.19c), lateral popliteal nerve (dropped foot), and the posterior tibial nerve (claw toes or hammer toes).

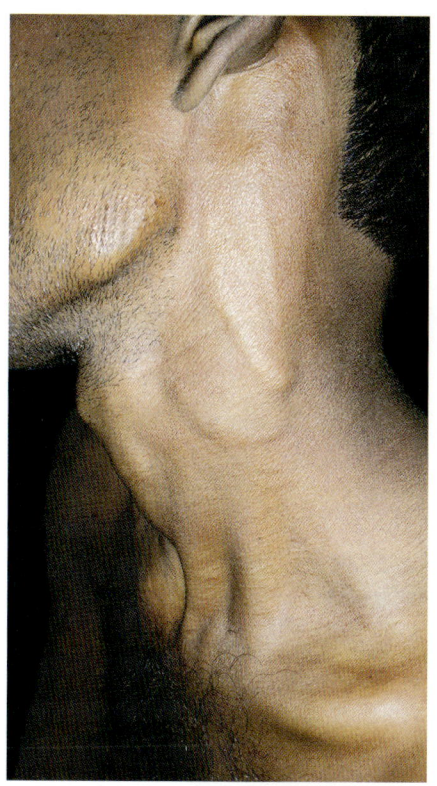

Fig. 2.18e: Enlarged greater auricular nerve

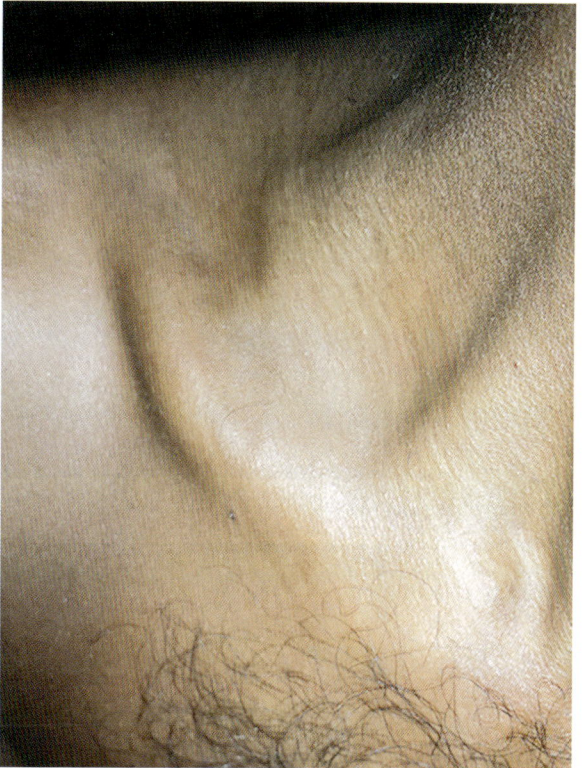

Fig. 2.18f: Enlarged supraclavicular nerves

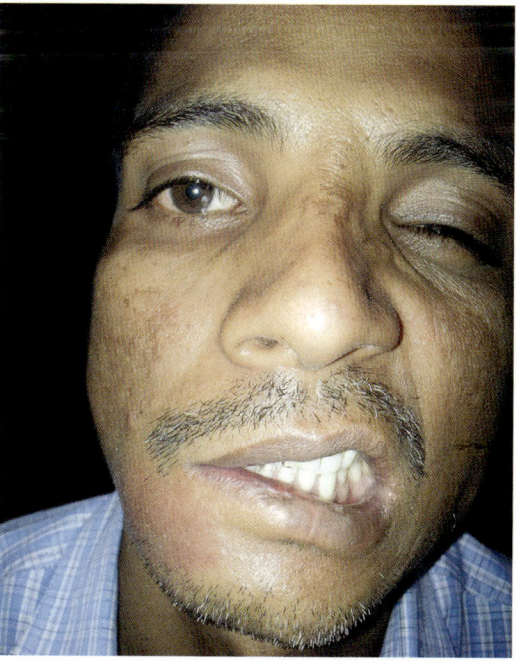

Fig. 2.19a: Right facial palsy

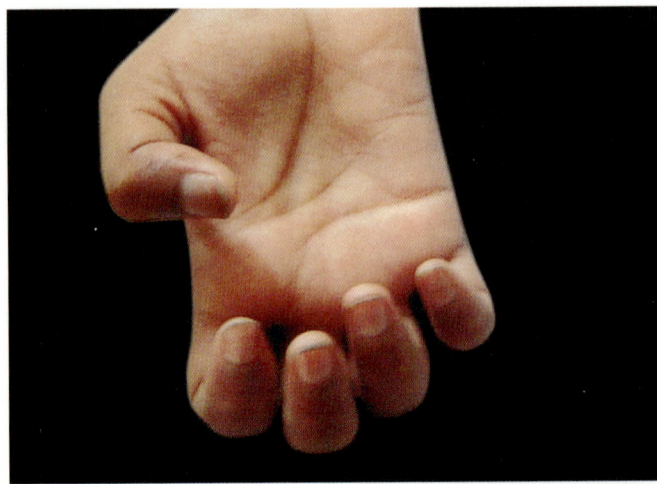

Fig. 2.19b: Claw hand

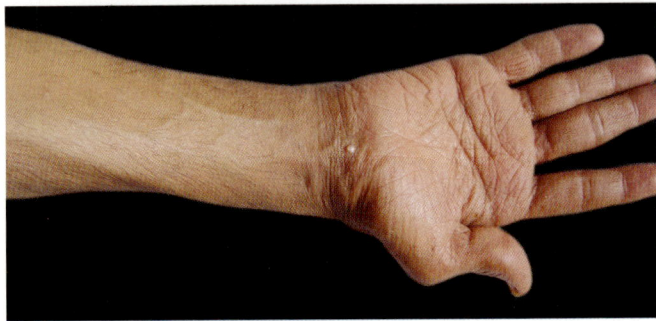

Fig. 2.19c: Ulnar and median nerve palsy showing atrophy of thenar and hypothenar eminences

The earliest stage of damage to the motor fibers of the ulnar nerve manifests as difficulty in approximating the little finger to the ring finger when the fingers are outstretched; while in regard to the lateral popliteal nerve, the earliest sign is weakness in holding the big toe in a dorsiflexed position against light pressure (*also see Chapter 10*). When the facial nerve (7th cranial nerve) is damaged in leprosy, the earliest sign is in the lower lid because of selective involvement of the zygomatic branch which innervates the orbicularis oculi muscles. This can be diagnosed by asking the patient to close his eyes *slowly* and *gently* when it will be seen that faulty closure is due to the lower lid not approximating to the upper lid (*also see Chapter 10*). Likewise, when both lids are involved, the lower one shows a higher degree of paralysis.[58] This differentiates leprous facial palsy from Bell's palsy which is usually a complete lower motor neuron (LMN) palsy. If the patient shuts his eyes in a determined manner, these observations will not be made because of the overaction of the upper lid. Note that in Bell's palsy, which is a complete LMN palsy, there is complete paralysis of all facial muscles on the involved side (brow is smooth, the eye does not close, the nasolabial fold is flat, and that side of the mouth droops).[59] The seventh nerve palsy leading to lagophthalmos is associated with upward rotation of the eyeballs (Bell's phenomenon) which fortunately protects the cornea as it gets raised under upper eyelid. However, eventually there is significant corneal damage (Fig. 2.19d) that may lead to blindness.[60] The corneal reflex may be

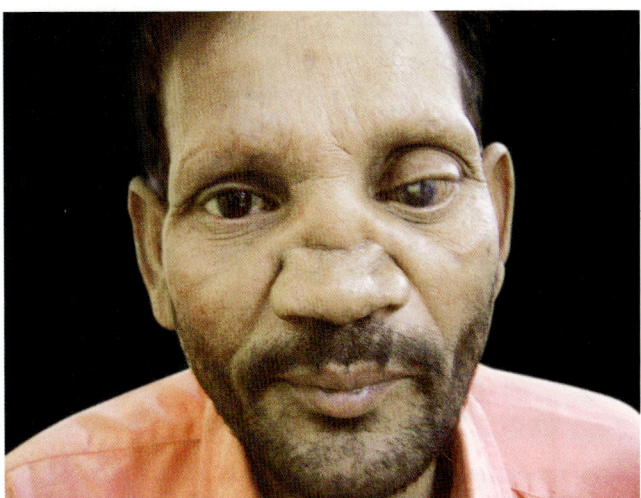

Fig. 2.19d: Corneal opacity (left eye) in a case of LL Hansen along with depressed nasal bridge and madarosis

tested with a wisp of cotton wool; absence of the reflex is indicative of damage to the trigeminal nerve (5th cranial nerve). The corneal reflex is a reliable measure of afferent trigeminal V1 and efferent facial nerve VII fibers (a V–VII reflex) and is present at infancy. Lightly touching the cornea with a tissue or cotton swab induces a rapid bilateral blink reflex. According to traditional teachings, unilateral trigeminal nerve dysfunction (i.e. in the ipsilateral brainstem, V1, or V2 divisions) prevents both eyes from blinking after stimulation of the ipsilateral cornea, whereas unilateral facial nerve dysfunction prevents the ipsilateral eye from blinking when its cornea is stimulated, although the contralateral eye blinks normally.[59] Uncommonly in leprosy, there may be bilateral facial nerve palsy.[60]

The limbs are tested for sensory impairment—light touch, pain and temperature by means of a wisp of cotton wool, a pin and with hot and cold test tubes (one tube containing hot water and the other containing iced water) respectively (*also see Chapter 10*). All three modalities of sensation should be tested as sometimes only one is affected (dissociated anesthesia); in such a case it is usually the ability to differentiate between hot and cold which is lost first. Anesthesia may begin in the feet, or in the hands, but usually affects all four limbs eventually. The area of sensory loss spreads slowly until all the skin is anesthetic except the axillae, groin and scalp.[61] Loss of the warning sensation of pain leads to repeated injuries to hands and feet, and chronic plantar ulceration is one of the chief problems in management. Anesthetic skin is particularly liable to blister when exposed to heat, due to the fact that reflex dilatation of skin capillaries is impaired because of damage to dermal nerves. Although the sensory impairment may begin on one side before the other, it will finally affect both sides symmetrically; hence the expression 'glove and stocking' anesthesia. The reason for this is that all manifestations of lepromatous leprosy are bilateral and symmetrical because of the widespread distribution of leprosy bacilli which, in turn, is due to the absence of a defence mechanism on the part of the host.

The presence of a large numbers of leprosy bacilli in peripheral nerves (the more advanced the disease at time of diagnosis, the more heavily bacillated are the peripheral nerves) leads to fibrosis which very slowly destroys those nerves which have the greatest concentration of bacilli, i.e. those which have a superficial course where they are cool; this applying particularly to limbs. Unfortunately, this slowly-developing fibrosis is likely to occur even if the patient has taken treatment regularly, for leprosy bacilli can be found, albeit in granular form, within peripheral nerves long after they have disappeared from the skin of the treated patient. This fibrosis is a reaction to the presence of dead (granular) bacilli rather than to living ones, for there is no nerve fibrosis in the early stages of the disease when the nerves contain healthy, solid-staining bacilli.

An overview of clinical features of LL leprosy is given in Table 2.7.

Other Systems Involved in LL

Lepromatous leprosy involves tissues beyond the skin and nerves as detailed below in text and in Tables 2.8 and 2.9.

Nails of Fingers and/or Toes

These appear dry, lustreless, shrunken, narrowed and longitudinally ridged. The affected digits become narrowed distally because of bone atrophy and with progressive bone absorption, the shortened digits retain the nail in a shrunken form. Uncommonly, nail dystrophy localized in the distribution of the ulnar nerve may be seen as the presenting feature of leprosy.[62]

Table 2.7: Cutaneous manifestations of LL Hansen's disease	
Skin	• There are numerous, symmetrically distributed, erythematous or copper-colored, shiny macules, papules and nodules • Certain regions of the skin which have the highest temperatures are invariably spared, such as axillae, groins, perineum, and hairy scalp; thus conforming to the general rule that leprosy bacilli favor cooler temperatures. Leprosy lesions may develop on the bald scalp, as the skin temperature of the bald scalp is cooler than that of the hairy scalp[55, 56] • Macules: Ill-defined, slightly hypopigmented, with a shiny or moist surface; erythematous on light skins and coppery or hypopigmented with a faint erythematous or coppery hue in dark skins (Fig. 2.20a) • The papules lie over infiltrated skin (Fig. 2.20b) • Poorly defined nodules are the most common lesions, these are usually up to 2 cm in diameter and are symmetrically distributed, firm on palpation and are in the skin and not in the subcutis. • If and when mixed lesions are seen—nodules usually on face and limbs and macules on trunk • Sensation to touch and pinprick is usually *unimpaired* in early lepromatous macules, but sweating may be *diminished* • If the patient is not treated at this stage, the skin becomes more and more infiltrated, and there is a waxy appearance with infiltration of skin—"leonine facies" with loss of eyebrows.
Hair	Hairs are lost all over except the scalp. Rarely, in advanced lepromatous disease, there may be residual hair growing only in bands over the course of the arterial supply to the scalp, probably where it is warmer. This is called 'leprous alopecia'.
Nerve	Peripheral nerves are affected late in the disease course and first become firm, then enlarged, then hard; at the sites of predilection, symmetrically.
Tests	• Slit smear for AFB: Very many bacilli with many globi • Lepromin test: Negative

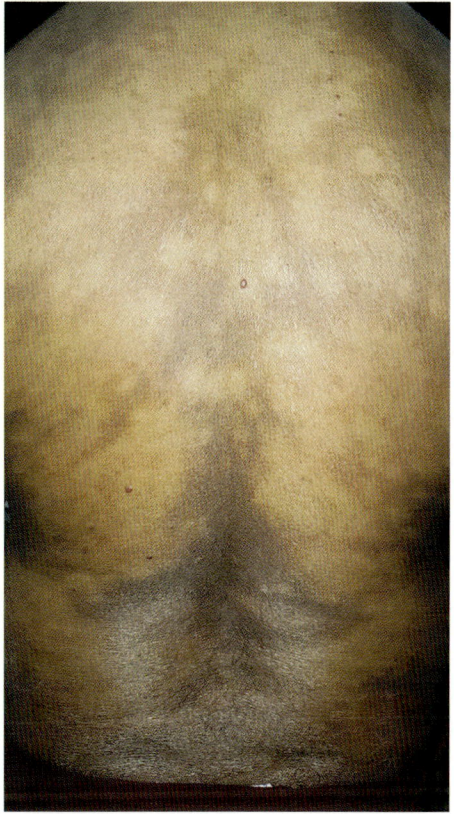

Fig. 2.20a: Lepromatous leprosy: Hypopigmented macules on the back, with occasional papules

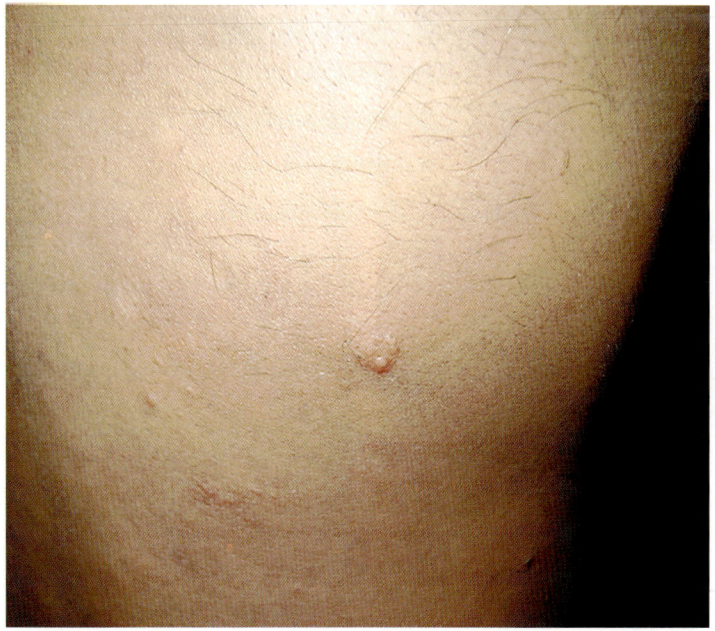

Fig. 2.20b: Lepromatous leprosy: A papule over an infiltrated plaque

Nose

The patient is likely to complain of nasal symptoms long before any skin lesions, and this fact has not been given adequate emphasis in the teaching on leprosy. The history is of nasal stuffiness accompanied by nasal discharge which is at times blood-stained; but the clinician is unlikely to obtain this information unless he specifically asks about nasal symptoms. Involvement of the olfactory nerve (1st cranial nerve) is rarely diagnosed as the patient is unlikely to complain of anosmia, though Barton[63] reported this finding in 44% of patients. On examining nasal mucosa with torch and nasal speculum, one may have to remove crusts before observing a thickened and irregular mucosa bathed in nasal discharge. Mucosa may be insensitive. A later development is perforation of nasal septum (Fig. 2.21a) and increasing destruction of nasal cartilage causing nasal collapse (Fig. 2.21b).[64] These are however a rarity in today's era of widespread MDT coverage.

Mouth, Pharynx and Larynx

Papules may appear on mucosal surface of lips and nodules have been described on tongue, palate and uvula. Palatal nodules are likely to ulcerate and the hard palate may become perforated in advanced disease. The upper incisor teeth may be loose or missing, forming part of the skull changes which Moller-Christensen had named "facies leprosa".[53,54]

Involvement of larynx is a late manifestation and occurs in one of two forms: (1) In the fibrotic form, the vocal cords become immobile and this causes hoarseness of voice; (2) in the ulcerative form, there is thickening, nodulation and ulceration of laryngeal mucosa causing pain and hoarseness of voice. Later, the glottis becomes increasingly narrowed and stridor may have to be relieved by tracheostomy; in both forms the cough has a peculiar hoarse quality.

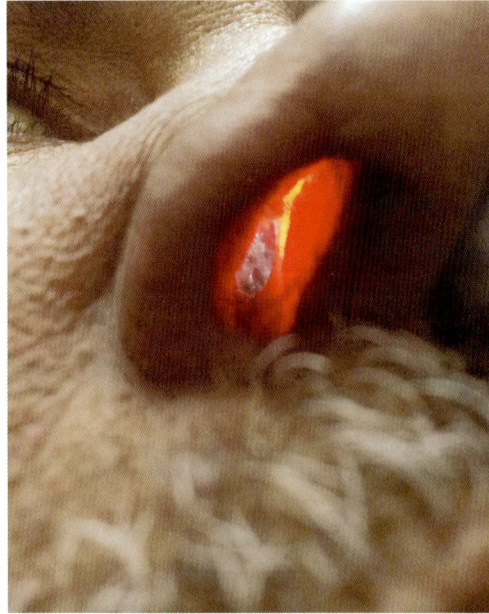

Fig. 2.21a: Nasal perforation

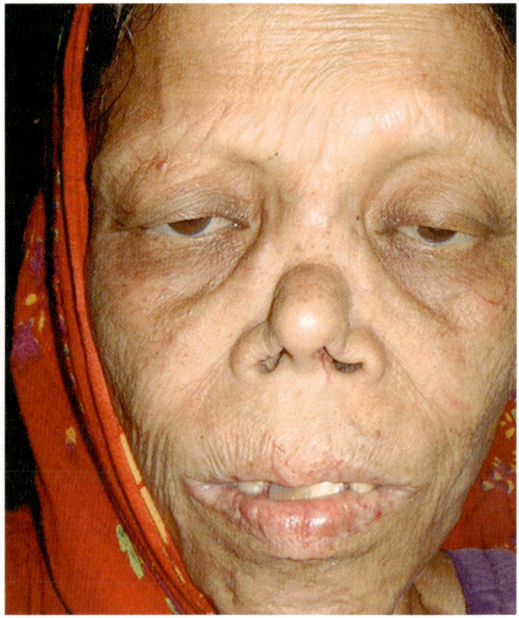

Fig. 2.21b: Depressed nasal bridge

Eyes (also see Chapter 8, Section 8.3.3)

The ocular involvement in leprosy has been classified (Table 2.8) and the potentially "blinding" complications are listed in Box 2.2. A study from India, noted that the most common cause for grade 2 ocular deformity (G2D) was corneal involvement causing ulceration and scarring.[65] Cataract was found to be the most common cause of visual disability (although it is not directly caused by leprosy). In the past, iritis and sclerouveitis with secondary glaucoma were important causes of blindness in leprosy which has decreased in present scenario due to the use of clofazimine in MDT; but chronic uveitis can still be seen in patients with long history of MB leprosy.[66]

The anterior segment of the eye is cooler than the posterior segment, which explains the involvement of nerves in the cornea and iris. The classical finding is the superficial punctate keratitis which is characterized by a milky haze over the upper part of each cornea punctuated by tiny white spots resembling "grains of chalk". These are readily seen with the aid of a torch and corneal loupe (Fig. 2.21c). These white spots are aggregations of leprosy bacilli (miliary lepromata) and are accompanied by pannus formation which commences in the superior lateral limbus (the region where the upper part of the cornea joins the sclera) and spreads all the way round the cornea—in

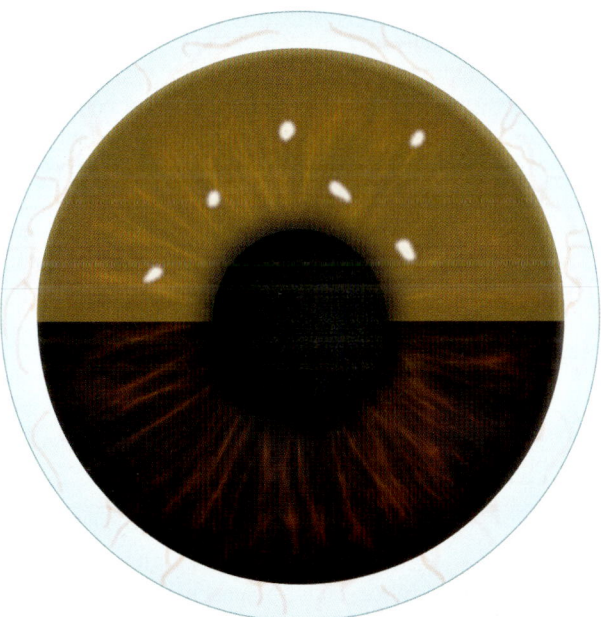

Fig. 2.21c: Depiction of superficial punctate keratitis

 Box 2.2: Important complications of ocular leprosy

1. Lagophthalmos: Whole spectrum
2. Corneal hypoaesthesia: Whole spectrum
3. Acute iritis and scleritis: MB leprosy
4. Chronic iritis and iris atrophy: MB leprosy
5. Cataract (age related and secondary): Whole spectrum

Table 2.8: Eye involvement in leprosy	
How is the eye affected?	1. Due to involvement of the V and VII cranial nerves 2. Infiltration of the eyes (anterior segment) and the surrounding tissues by the leprosy bacillus 3. Inflammation and reactions in ocular tissues 4. Complications of the eyes secondary to involvement of surrounding tissues
1. Cranial nerve involvement	• **Vth nerve**—exposure conjunctivitis and keratitis • **VIIth nerve** (Infranuclear palsy)—lagophthalmos → ectropion → exposure keratitis → corneal ulcer Rare complications of corneal ulcer: Secondary iritis, hypopyon, secondary glaucoma, leukoma adherens, anterior staphyloma, panophthalmitis or phthisis bulbi.[60]

2. Direct involvement	• Eyebrows: Supraciliary madarosis (especially outer third)
	• Eyelids: Nodules, ciliary madarosis, "stern" leprosy stare (mild weakness of orbicularis oculi with slight overaction of deeper fibers of levator palpebrae superioris leading to slight bilateral lid retraction and reduced blinking), ectropion or entropion (ectropion leads to tears flowing on cheek as the puncta does not approximate the eye)[60]
	• Conjunctiva: Mild chronic conjunctivitis
	• Episclera: Episcleritis, episcleral nodules (yellowish gelatinous nodules close to limbus typically at 3 and 9 o'clock)[60]
	• Sclera: Nodules*
	• Cornea[n]: Affected via the myelinated corneal nerves (beaded nerves)
	  a. *Lepromatous pearls*—clumps of globi packed within swollen macrophages
	  b. *Superficial punctate keratitis* (like grains of chalk): Very characteristic of leprosy, grains represent clumps of *M. leprae*
	  c. *Avascular punctate keratitis* most commonly found in the superolateral aspect, interstitial keratitis (usually an extension of an episcleral nodule into substantia propria of the cornea), pannus and perforation of cornea[60]
	• Iris/ciliary body[b]
	  a. Iris pearls
	  b. Nodular lepromata
	  c. Acute and chronic plastic iridocyclitis
	  d. Posterior synechiae can cause occlusio pupillae, secondary glaucoma, complicated cataract and phthisis bulbi.

3. Surrounding Structures	Blockage of NLD—infection, conjunctivitis, corneal ulcers
4. Reactions	Type 2 reactions—iridocyclitis → synechiae → block "Canal of Schlemm" → glaucoma

*Seen in drug-resistant disease and in those who are noncompliant with drug therapy, n: Neural route, b: Blood borne; NLD: Nasolacrimal duct.

contradistinction to the pannus of trachoma which is confined to the upper central region. Pannus eventually leads to sclerosing keratitis which extends right round the cornea. Yellowish gelatinous nodules may appear at the sclerocorneal junction in the 3 and 9 o'clock positions. The eye changes described above are painless and do not affect vision, but if there is a spread of superficial punctate keratitis downwards, which is fortunately rare, vision may become impaired.

Hobbs and Choyce had described a chronic form of iritis called 'insidious iritis' wherein the patient had no ocular discomfort or redness, but if undiagnosed and consequentially untreated, this resulted in increasing iris atrophy and eventual blindness.[67] Another manifestation is the presence of tiny white spots that appear on both irides, miliary lepromata and iris 'pearls', which can be visualized with the aid of a corneal microscope (slit-lamp microscope or slit-lamp). These are deposits of tightly packed bacilli within swollen macrophages, and Ffytche has shown that they are situated in the autonomic nerve plexuses in the iris supplying sphincter and dilator muscles of the pupil and are bloodborne.[68] These "iris pearls" slowly enlarge and coalesce, become pedunculated and drop into the anterior chamber, from which they eventually disappear. Eventually the iris shows progressive signs of atrophy and disintegration, together with a small pupil (miosis) unresponsive to atropine. This is a result of damage to the sympathetic innervation to the dilator pupillae. Further, if the uveitis is not aggressively treated, cataract and hypotony frequently result.

Acute iritis, presenting with red and painful eyes, occurs as one of the manifestations of lepra reaction. While steroids have reduced the complications consequent to iritis, at one time it was the singlemost common cause of blindness in leprosy. In a retrospective study of 531 leprosy patients, 4% had iritis.[69] Another study of 100 patients with leprosy in Brazil, found that 72 had ocular complications, of which 17 had a chronic anterior uveitis, and only two had an acute anterior uveitis.[70] In a study from Nepal, 8% of patients with tuberculoid leprosy had uveitis, whereas 16% of patients with lepromatous leprosy had anterior chamber inflammatory disease.[71] Spaide and colleagues found that uveitis was uncommon in leprosy patients in the United States, which possibly reflects the results of more aggressive treatment with anti-leprosy and anti-inflammatory agents.[72]

An entirely different set of circumstances may cause ocular complications in lepromatous leprosy and in borderline and tuberculoid leprosy and this is consequent to damage to the trigeminal nerve (5th cranial nerve) or to the facial nerve (7th cranial nerve) in their course outside the skull (where they are most cool). In lepromatous leprosy, such neural changes occur late in the course of the disease, whereas in the borderline and tuberculoid types, they occur early and in association with skin lesions on the face, particularly when treatment precipitates lepra reaction. Damage to the 5th cranial nerve leads to corneal anesthesia which renders the eye injury—prone; and lack of prompt treatment produces corneal ulceration. It should be noted that although corneal anesthesia in LL can be due to fibrotic changes in the 5th cranial nerve, it can also be due to damage to corneal nerves. The causes of corneal hypo-/anesthesia are listed in Box 2.3.[73] Involvement of the 7th cranial nerve leads to facial palsy and inability to approximate the eyelids (lagophthalmos), and especially when associated with corneal anesthesia, causes exposure keratitis, a condition in which the cornea becomes vascularized and opaque. If neglected, blindness ensues.

It is pertinent to note that the late complications such as clinically significant corneal pearls, extensive iris atrophy, staphylomas and blindness due to severe iridocyclitis can only found in a few very old and very neglected disabled patients living in remote areas or very disabled old beggars, who never received MDT. Most of them have died already or will die soon thus this is may not be consistently relevant.

Box 2.3: Causes of corneal hypoesthesia

- Reversal reaction in the trigeminal nerve (V cranial nerve).
- Exposure of the cornea in lagophthalmos.
- Severe scleritis and damage to the ciliary nerves (often bilateral).
- Bacterial infiltration and secondary atrophy of ciliary and corneal nerves (often bilateral)

Thus, it is important to appreciate that while variable ocular disease prevalence has been reported, lagophthalmos, vision loss and reaction involving the face should be looked for, especially in newly diagnosed cases above 40 years of age. Interestingly, hand and foot deformities have a 4.1 times higher risk for simultaneous ocular involvement and thus such patients must be closely examined for ocular problems.[74]

Cataract is the leading cause of blindness in patients with leprosy, with age-related cataract being the most common cause. Also common are cataracts developing due to the long-term oral steroid therapy required for managing recurrent lepra reactions. Secondary cataract may also develop in leprosy patients with recurrent or chronic uveitis.[75,76] Pre-existing corneal astigmatism is significantly more severe in leprosy patients than in non-leprosy patients being prepared for cataract surgery. In proper hands, an excellent outcome can be achieved by surgery[77] (*see Chapter 8, Section 8.2*).

Bone

Bone changes do not occur when lepromatous leprosy is diagnosed and treated in the earlier stages. But, when the disease has been neglected over many years, bone changes are bound to occur and are not halted by treatment. The bone changes are detailed in Table 2.9 and Fig. 2.22.

A study from India showed that bone changes were observed radiologically in 90% of cases presenting with disabilities/deformities. *Specific* bone changes were seen largely in the hands and feet, while *non-specific* bone changes were seen in the hands, feet, skull and paranasal sinuses.[78] The common specific bone changes in hands and feet observed were primary periostitis (14%), honeycombing (46%), bone cyst (36%), thinning and irregularity of cortex (28%) and areas of bone destruction (20%); the non-specific bone changes observed were contracted fingers/claw hands/claw toes (64%) and absorption of terminal phalanges (40%). The maxillary sinus and paranasal sinus changes were the most common radiological findings observed in skull.[78]

Apart from the rare development of periostitis of the bones of forearm or lower leg, bone damage is confined to hands, feet and skull. The marrow of the phalanges is replaced with foam cells laden with AFB which invade and destroy the cancellous bones leading to cyst formation.[79] Further, the distal phalanges undergo slow atrophy and absorption, and the fingers shorten (Fig. 2.22); after disappearance of terminal phalanges, middle and proximal phalanges may undergo a similar atrophy in turn, but metacarpals and carpal bones are spared.

In the feet, the atrophic changes occur in phalanges, metatarsal and tarsal bones. Distal phalanges become thinned by rarefying osteitis known as 'concentric bone atrophy', so that eventually only a fine needle of bone is left; this may disappear, in turn causing shortening of the affected toe or toes. In the metatarsals, the first and most pronounced change takes place at the distal ends, usually commencing in the fifth metatarsal, the affected bones becoming thin and pointed—an appearance known

Table 2.9: Skeletal changes in leprosy[‡]	
Specific (direct infiltration or due to reaction)	Less common and includes: **Hands and feet** • Bone cysts or pseudocysts and sequestrae • Honeycomb appearance • Enlarged nutrient foramina (earliest finding) • Subarticular erosions • Concentric cortical erosions (pencilling or sucked candy appearance)[*] • Primary periostitis • Sclerosis: Typically during healing • Subluxation, dislocation or synostosis of joints • Osteoporosis with lepromatous arthritis **Face** • Atrophy of anterior nasal spine • Atrophy of maxillary alveolar process **Lepra reactions** • Terminal tuft dissolution (juxta-articular decalcification) • Destruction/erosion of epiphyseal bone • Sclerosis • Subperiosteal bone erosion • Osteoperiostitis: Severe bone pains over long limb bones during lepra reaction (especially over tibia)
Nonspecific (sensory loss, vascular changes, infection, disuse atrophy or trauma)	More common and includes • Bone erosion • Absent phalanges (resorption of digits) • Osteomyelitis • Charcot type joints • Contracted fingers/claw hand/claw toes • Tarsal disintegration • Disuse osteoporotic changes

[*]May also be caused in part due to nonspecific changes.
[‡]Ankad BS, Hombal A, Rao S, Naidu VM. Radiological changes in the hands and feet of leprosy patients with deformities. J Clin Diagn Res 2011; 5: 703–7; Carayon A, Dharmendra. Bone and joint changes in leprosy. In Dharmendra, Ed. Leprosy. Volume II. Bombay: Samant and Company, 1985:872–85.

as 'pencilling' or the 'sucked candy stick' appearance. Tarsal bone disintegration is an important yet often neglected cause of foot deformity and disability.[80]

The factors responsible for these changes in hands and feet are multiple, and include various combinations of the following:

1. Repeated **trauma** because of absence of pain sensation. In the hands, the terminal phalanges are most exposed to trauma and in the feet, the heads of the metatarsals bear the brunt because of the thrusting action of the rear foot driving the body forward when walking.
2. Impaired **blood supply** to bones due to endarteritis of nutrient vessels during lepra reaction.
3. Impaired **nerve supply** to bones.

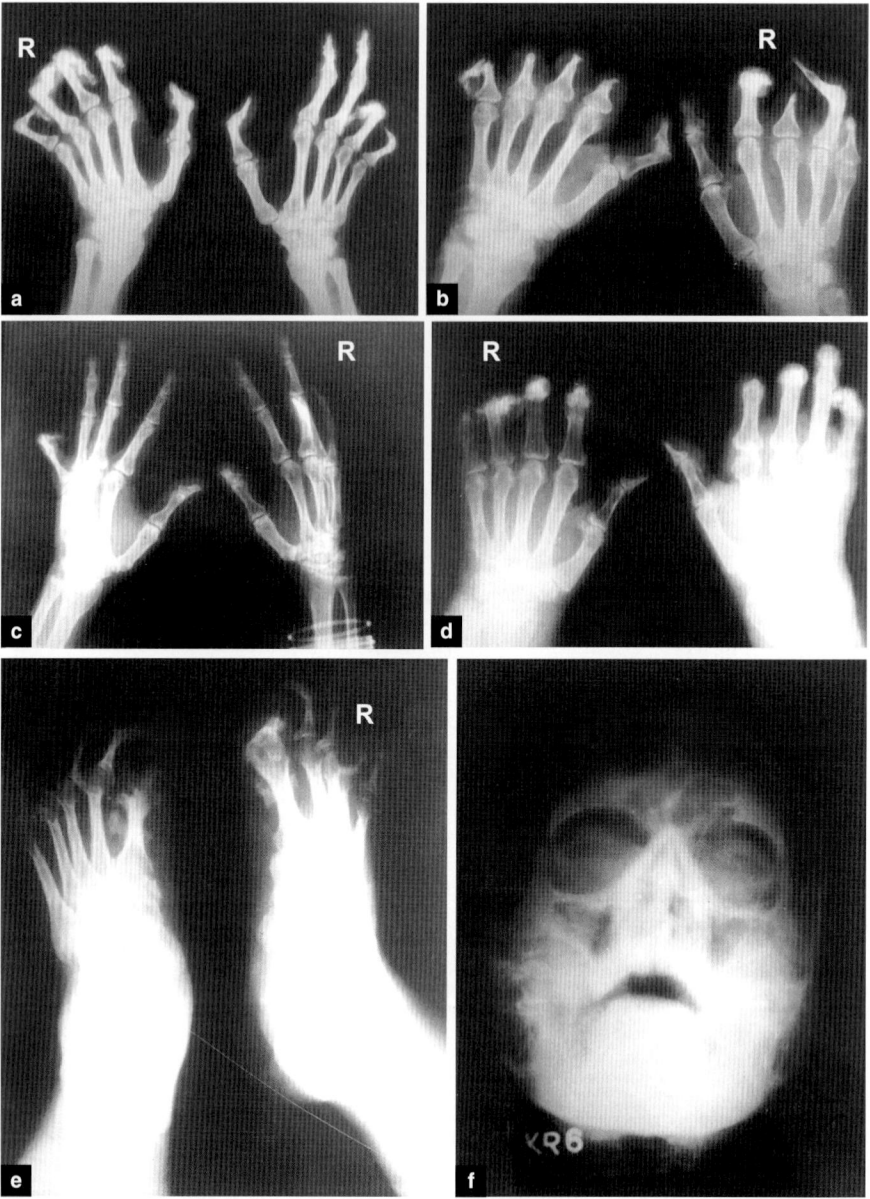

Fig. 2.22: (a) Clawing of the all fingers of both hands. "Licked-socked candy stick" appearance of little finger of left hand; (b) **Left hand** (i) Absorption of middle and distal phalanges of index, middle and ring fingers, (ii) Eccentric absorption of corresponding proximal phalanges, (iii) Clawing of little finger and thumb; **Right hand** (i) Absorption of middle and distal phalanges of middle and little finger, (ii) Eccentric absorption of proximal phalanx of middle finger, (iii) Arthrodesis of proximal and distal interphalangeal joint of ring finger, (iv) Concentric absorption of distal and middle phalanges of finger; (c) Clawing of left little finger; (d) Subluxation at the interphalangeal joint of thumb of right hand; (e) **Left foot** (i) Primary periosteitis of the first metatarsal, (ii) Soft tissue calcification around first metatarsal, (iii) Absorption of distal phalanges of the great toe, (iv) Clawing of the 2nd and 3rd toes; **Right foot** (i) Calcification of soft tissue around first metatarsal, (ii) Absorption of distal phalanx of the great toe, (iii) Eccentric absorption of the proximal phalanx of the great toe, (iv) Clawing of phalanges of the 4th and 5th toes, (v) Honeycombing of the first metatarsal of the right foot, (f) Skiagram showing diffuse opacity and generalized mucosal thickening of both maxillary sinuses (*Courtesy*: Dr SK Malhotra)

4. Deposition of **leprosy bacilli** in bones via the blood stream. (In advanced cases, bacillary deposits cause leprous osteitis, giving phalanges a **cystic** appearance on X-ray).
5. In males, generalized bone **osteoporosis** due to testicular atrophy and defective production of testosterone.
6. **Disuse osteoporosis** may affect hand or foot due to paralysis and/or contractures causing reduced osteoblastic activity.
7. **Osteomyelitis** complicating chronic ulceration of the overlying skin.

It should be noted that whereas all the above-mentioned factors are operative in lepromatous leprosy, only 1, 3, 6 and 7 apply in non-lepromatous leprosy. The main reason why shortened fingers are characteristic of the former is that the hands of lepromatous patients may be insensitive for years before they become weak and therefore they are used in daily work, whereas in non-lepromatous patients, anesthesia and muscle weakness tend to occur together and paralysis of intrinsic muscles is rapid; therefore the affected hand is not used.

In the skull, two pathognomonic changes take place, namely atrophy of the anterior nasal spine and of the maxillary alveolar process. The former contributes to nasal collapse and the latter causes loosening or loss of the upper central incisor teeth or, of all four upper incisors, and these two skull changes have been given the name 'facies leprosa'—wherein there is flattening of cheeks and upper lip.[81,82]

Testes

Testicular atrophy is usually bilateral and may be caused by orchitis due to bacterial infiltration and a type 2 reaction. A positive bacillary index, disability and low testicular volume may be regarded as risk factors for testicular dysfunction in MB leprosy.[83] Leprosy affects the *exocrine* portion first and then the endocrine portion. In the early stage of testicular atrophy, the patient remains sexually potent but his semen is devoid of spermatozoa and therefore he is sterile; impotence and gynecomastia are later developments (Table 2.10).

A study of BL/LL patients noted that decreased libido and testicular volume was commonly seen[84] while another study noted that abnormal semen analysis and/or testicular aspirates are seen.[85] A recent study found that adult onset hypogonadism is seen in cases of leprosy.[86] Here it is important to note that the female reproductive

Table 2.10: Testicular involvement in leprosy*		
Part affected	Effects and consequence	Laboratory abnormality
Exocrine portion (seminiferous tubules)	Spermatozoa (atrophy causes sterility)	Azoospermia ↑FSH
Endocrine portion [interstitial (Leydig) cells]	Testosterone (atrophy causes impotence, osteoporosis, gynecomastia)	↓Testosterone, 17-ketosteroids ↑FSH, LH
Epididymo-orchitis (during reaction)	Severe pain and inflammation	

*Testicular involvement is generally bilateral and azoospermia *precedes* impotence.

organs are *not* significantly affected in leprosy, because of higher temperature at the site.[87]

Kidney

Most of the kidney involvement in leprosy is nonspecific and the different renal lesions described include acute and chronic glomerulonephritis, interstitial nephritis, secondary amyloidosis and pyelonephritis (Fig. 2.23).[88] The exact mechanism that leads to glomerulonephritis in leprosy is not completely understood. Acute glomerulonephritis in lepra reaction may present with oliguria, edema, albuminuria, hematuria or casts, but is typically without hypertension.[89]

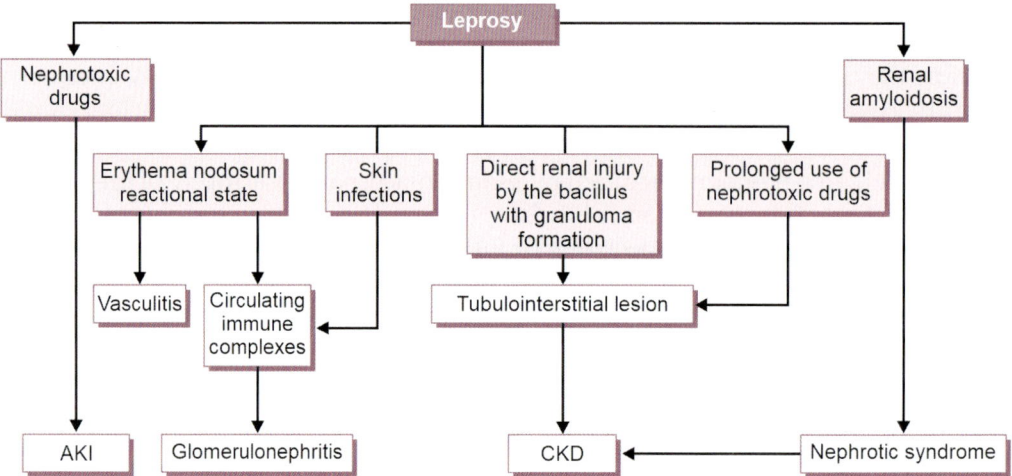

Fig. 2.23: An overview of renal involvement in leprosy (AKI: Acute kidney injury, CKD: Chronic kidney disease)

Muscle

Muscle involvement has been described with symptoms of stiffness and tenderness and occasional nodules. The nodules can show granuloma but no bacilli. Dartos muscle of the scrotum, smooth muscles of blood vessels and arrector pili in the skin are often invaded by the bacilli and these persist even after bacilli have disappeared from the skin following treatment.

Lymph Nodes

The clinical involvement is apparent in reactions when the inguinal and femoral lymph nodes are involved. In lepromatous cases the supratrochlear, axillary, cervical, inguinal and iliac LN are affected. In TT cases, the epitrochlear lymph nodes are affected. Histologically, in LL cases, both the cortex and medulla are involved.

A summary of the involvement of other organs not detailed below is presented in Table 2.11.[90]

CAUSES OF DEATH IN LEPROSY

The causes of death and general mortality rate in the vast majority of leprosy patients are the same as in the general population from which they are drawn, with the *exception*

The Disease

Table 2.11: Systemic involvement in leprosy[90–91a]

Reticuloendothelial system	Unclear, as it is a screening system and presence of bacilli does *not* mean involvement. May act as a source of dormant bacilli *Liver* • LL: Miliary leproma (limited to portal space)[91], but no cirrhosis or LFT dysfunction; no correlation with BI • Type 2 reactions: Jaundice, hepatomegaly, raised transaminases and alkaline phosphatases[91] • Hepatitis B may be an associated finding • Amyloid deposition[91] *Bone marrow* • Miliary granuloma • Hb <9 gm% • Possible source of persisters
Adrenals	• Adrenal infiltration by AFB and granuloma is not uncommon with a reported incidence ranging from 0 to 70% • Adrenals are histologically involved, though no clinical functional deficit is manifested. Subclinical adrenal hypofunction is seen in MB cases • Cortex is affected • Functional insufficiency may be found during reactions, manifesting as hypotension
Autonomic nervous system	• Anhidrosis • Reduced intraocular pressure • Iris dysfunction • Cardiac rhythm disturbances • Decreased response to cough • Abnormal testicular pain • Diminished nocturnal penile tumescence • Neurogenic bladder
Hematology	• Dimorphic picture of hemolytic anemia and megaloblastic anemia (toxic/depressive effect on marrow). • Decreased levels of hemoglobin, serum folate, serum iron, serum albumin are found (more towards lepromatous pole) • ESR is raised • Decreased serum folate levels • Hemolytic anemia may become severe during lepra reactions

of *renal* damage in lepromatous leprosy. These renal complications are mostly self-limiting, but sometimes may result in chronic renal dysfunction leading to death from uremia or from hypertension. A few salient additional comments have been noted as below:

1. It is probable that in leprosy, there is a reduced mortality from malaria because of the protection afforded by regular doses of dapsone.
2. There is a probable increased mortality from the side-effects of antileprosy drugs or from drugs used in the treatment of reactional states.
3. There is an increased mortality from severe lepra reactions, either from toxemia if the reacting lesions are necrotic or from asphyxia resulting from glottic edema. The postmortem study of Desikan and Job found that 21.6% of deaths were from severe reactions.[92]

4. There is also an increased mortality from suicide.
5. Although natural immunity to tetanus occurs and this appears to be higher in leprosy patients than in the general population, it is not completely protective. We would like to draw attention to the report of Desikan and Job,[92] who found that 13% of deaths in their series were due to tetanus, which is consistent with a report of 5 cases of tetanus complicating leprosy.[93] It is prudent to give leprosy patients at least one dose of tetanus toxoid.

A large study from China analyzing 524 deaths in leprosy patients found that the most common causes of death were suicide, cardiovascular disease and organ failure associated with advanced age.[94] The *second month* of MDT was the riskiest for newly treated patients and the cause of death during this period were related to liver failure, dapsone and renal insufficiency. Overall, they found that the first three months seem to be important and newly diagnosed patients should be provided with no more than two months of MDT blister packs—a point that is another good practical reason to avoid the recommendations of accompanied MDT (A-MDT).

NEURITIC HANSEN

Nerves are involved universally in leprosy but when nerve involvement *(see Section 2.4, PNL)* happens without specific cutaneous lesions of leprosy, it is termed pure neuritic leprosy. Neuritic leprosy may further be divided into primary or secondary. Primary neuritic leprosy is when nerves are affected without skin changes, while secondary neuritic leprosy refers to leprosy patients who have skin lesions or had cutaneous lesions before but later present with only nerve involvement.

In Indian classification, only pure or primary neuritic cases are included in polyneuritic leprosy (but it also includes single nerve involvement).[95] It is, nevertheless, important to emphasize that a diagnosis of pure neuritic leprosy based purely on clinical findings should be made with great care and should always be confirmed by a clinician with experience of this disease. A nerve biopsy may be necessary in order to establish the diagnosis, but only after consideration of other cause of palpable nerve thickening *(see Chapter 9)*. But, this should be undertaken only by a qualified doctor with special experience. Sensory nerves supplying areas of lesser functional importance are suitable for biopsy. Motor or mixed motor and sensory nerves are unsuitable, and the procedure should not be considered unless the histopathological findings can be reported competently. The nerve pathology is mostly TT but all types, except LL, have been reported *(see Chapter 3, Section 3.2)*.

Like other leprosy cases, neuritic leprosy also has associated sensory, motor and trophic changes. Sensory involvement is usually earlier and more severe compared to motor involvement and includes sensory loss as well as paresthesias. Temperature and pain sensations are lost before the touch sensation, while the deep touch or pressure sensation remains intact. Motor involvement includes muscle paresis and atrophy. Trophic changes include loss of sweating, glossy skin with loss of hair and idiopathic blisters.[95] The commonest peripheral nerves involved are the ulnar, median, lateral popliteal, posterior tibial, trigeminal and facial nerves. The ulnar nerves are typically involved just above elbows (high ulnar paralysis) and median nerves are involved just above the wrist. Bilateral seventh nerve palsy has been rarely reported as a manifestation of polyneuritic leprosy.[96]

UNCOMMON PRESENTATIONS OF MB LEPROSY

While most MB cases conform to the presentations detailed above, some atypical cutaneous presentations of lepromatous leprosy are reported which may occasionally lead to a diagnostic dilemma (Table 2.12). Of these *four* unusual expressions are detailed below.

The simplest of these is localized lepromatous or borderline lepromatous disease. There is a single nodule or localized area of nodules or papules, while most of the body surface appears normal.[101] The nodules or papules have a very high bacterial index while the rest of the skin is negative, or nearly so, by the standard methods of examination for *M. leprae*.

Table 2.12: Atypical presentations of MB leprosy[97–101]
- Single plaque (Fig. 2.24)
- Single nodule on the face
- Erythema multiforme-like lesion
- Lymphadenopathy masquerading as lymphoma
- Long-standing leg ulcer
- Erythema gyratum repens-like pattern (Fig. 2.25)
- Verrucous lesions of lepromatous leprosy
- Histoid leprosy
- Spontaneous skin ulceration
- Lucio leprosy
- Zosteriform, segmental, dermatomal leprosy (Fig. 2.26a and b)
- Blaschko-like pattern (Fig. 2.27a and b)
- Pigmentary loss
- Anetoderma (Fig. 2.28)

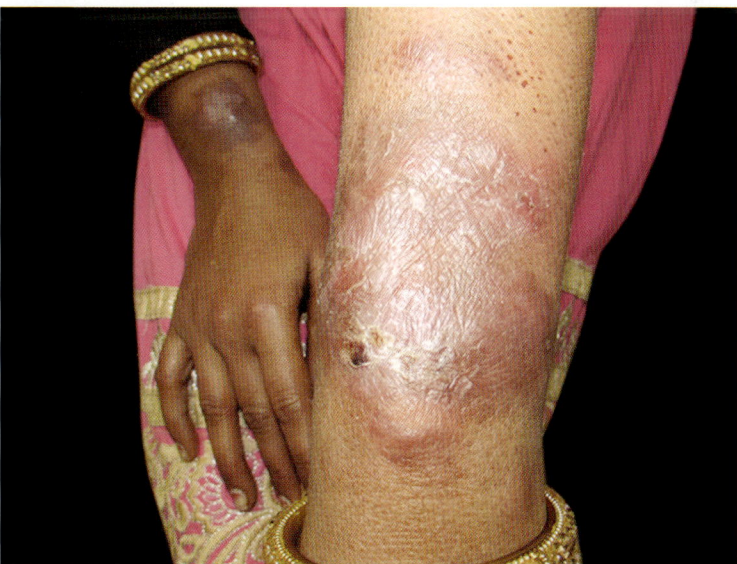

Fig. 2.24: A single plaque of BL leprosy with repeated ENL reactions

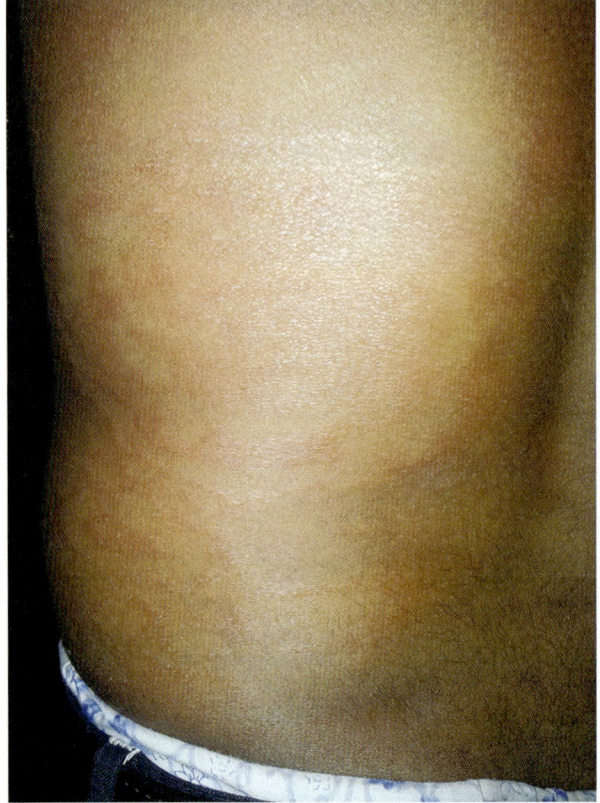

Fig. 2.25: "Erythema gyratum repens"-like lesions in BB leprosy

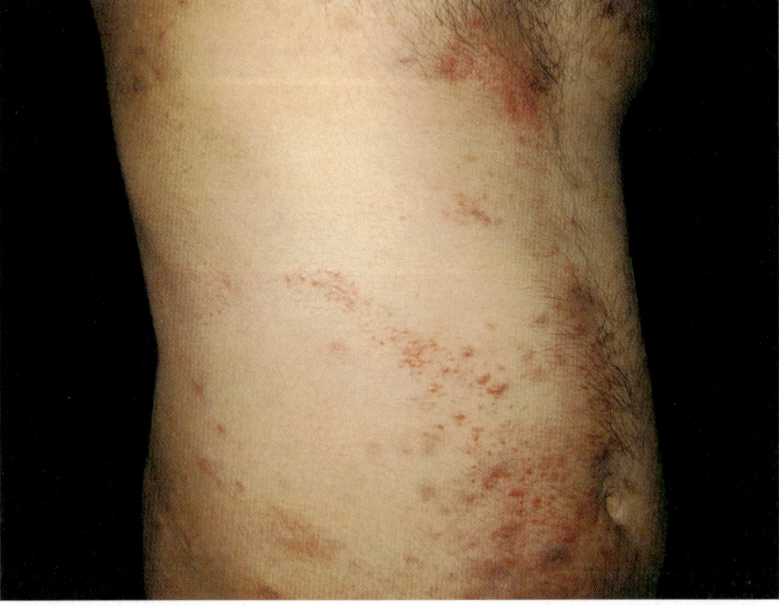

Fig. 2.26a: Lepromatous leprosy with multidermatomal arrangement of papules

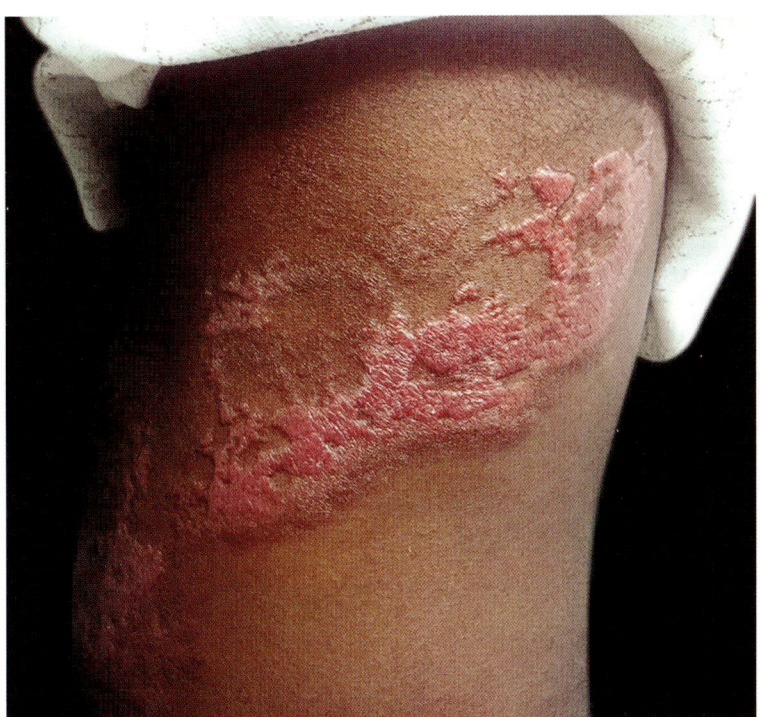

Fig. 2.26b: Zosteriform arrangement of leprosy lesions (*Courtesy*: Dr Surabhi Sinha)

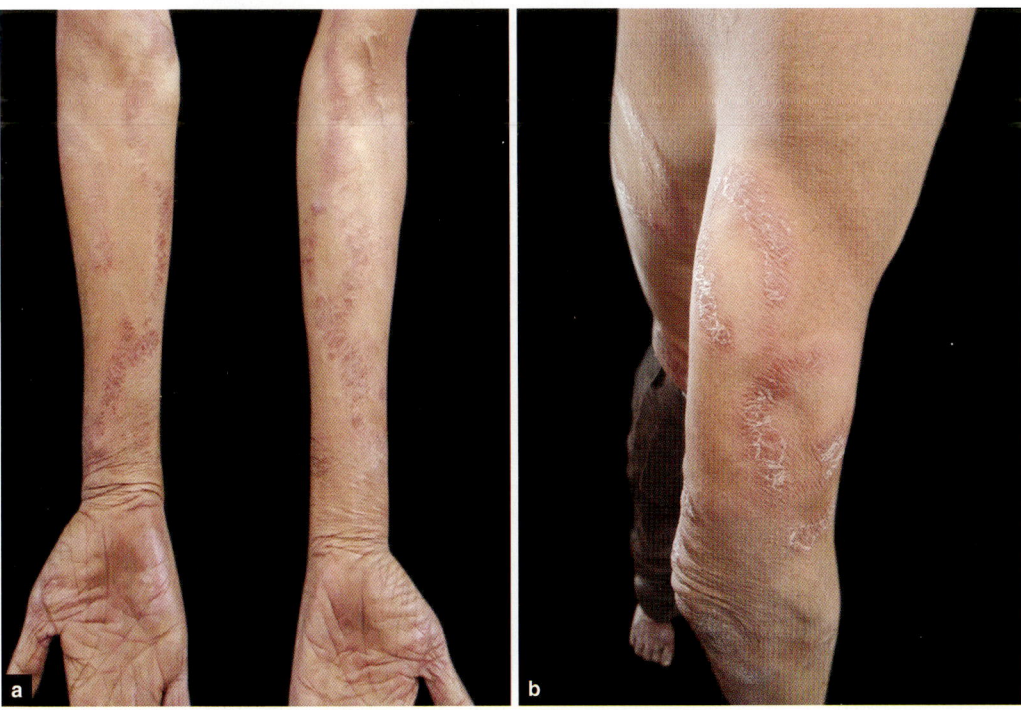

Fig. 2.27a and b: A case of BB leprosy with lesions arranged along the lines of Blaschko (*Courtesy*: Dr Chetan Rajput)

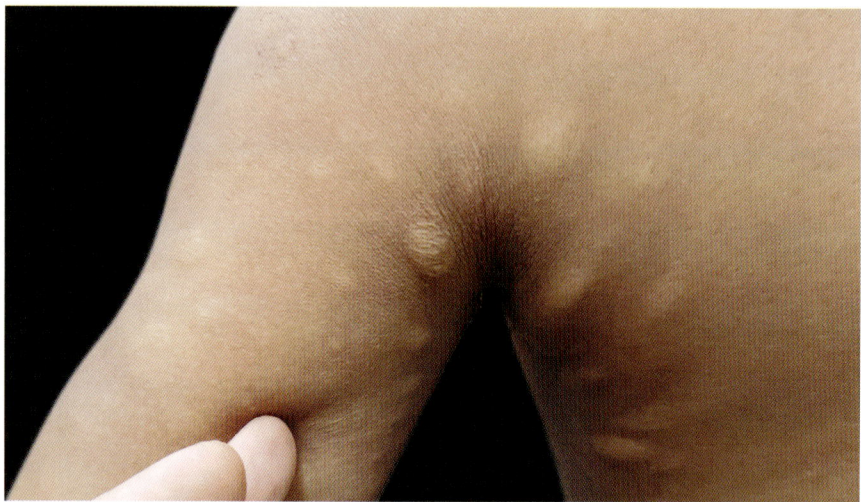

Fig. 2.28: Anetoderma in a case of lepromatous leprosy

The second unusual type of lepromatous disease is more difficult to understand. This is what was termed as **'histoid' leprosy** by Wade (1963).[102] Histoid leprosy is so-called because the microscopic appearance of the nodule shows spindle-shaped cells resembling those that are seen in dermatofibroma.

Clinically, the lesions present as firm papules or nodules (Fig. 2.29). The nodules have a very well-defined edge, are shiny and coppery red in color. The cause is believed to be due to *relapse* in an inactive case of lepromatous leprosy[103] and sometimes the bacilli in these lesions have been shown to be *resistant* to dapsone,[104] especially when the patient is still taking the drug. Less commonly, such nodules may be seen in non-relapsing cases of lepromatous leprosy. Roy-Chaudhari and Srinivasan (1977)[105] reported histoid habitus affecting a superficial radial nerve in a lepromatous patient. Similar cases were reported by Girdhar et al (1990)[106] and thus it is advisable to look for nodular lesions in the course of peripheral nerve trunks and cutaneous nerves in all BL and LL patients. These nodular swellings are firm, nontender and are freely movable. In the modern era of MDT, however, most cases of histoid leprosy appear *de novo*.

Histoid lesions show a very high bacteriological index (BI) and morphological index (MI) as compared to the normal skin. The enormous bacillary population in histoid lesions is suggested to be due to focal loss of immunity (Job et al, 1977).[107] Although some authors have stressed that these histoid nodules contain elongated or spindle-shaped histiocytes and that the bacilli within them are longer than normal, others have found little to differentiate them histologically and bacteriologically from hyperactive lepromatous nodules.

The third unusual manifestation of lepromatous leprosy is spontaneous *skin ulceration* in patients with severe, long-standing, untreated LL. These lesions appear in an area of chronic panniculitis. The skin is fixed to underlying muscle or bone by dense brawny-inflammatory tissue. This is most commonly seen over the anterior thigh, the calf, the triceps area or the dorsum of the forearm. These ulcers are not due to trauma, rather the skin dies and sloughs away leaving irregular, often triangular, defects that look like third degree burns.

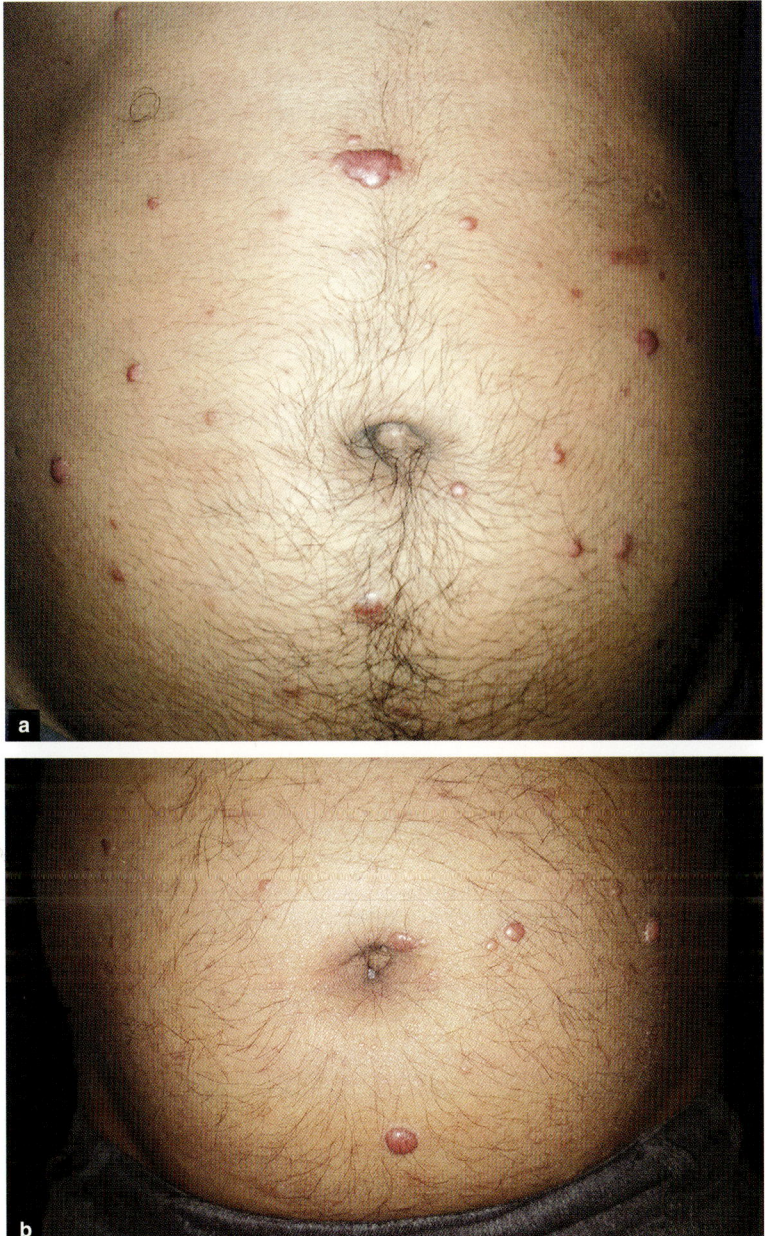

Fig. 2.29a and b: Coppery red nodules of histoid leprosy that arise on a normal looking skin

Lucio-Latapí leprosy and Lazarine leprosy: This term applies to the diffuse nonnodular type of leprosy described by Lucio and Alvarado in Mexico in 1852 and later by Latapi and Zamora in 1948.[108] This form of leprosy has no specific lesions of leprosy on skin and has also been called the 'lepra bonita' (beautiful leprosy). The other name—lazarine leprosy, which is often alluded to in literature, is derived from the name of the Saint Lazaro Hospital (Hospital de San Lázaro) in Mexico City in 1844, where this form of leprosy was first described.

Three presentations of Lazarine leprosy have been described: Tuberous or nodular, anesthetic and spotted. Lucio and Alvarado described the peculiar painful red spots on the skin, which we now know as Lucio's phenomenon (LP) and which by some leprologists is also referred to as ENL necroticans. Latapí and Chévez-Zamora who studied the disorder and recognized the previous description of Lucio and Alvarado, coined the terms Lucio's leprosy and Lucio's phenomenon.[109] Frenken et al have translated the original paper by Lucio and Alvarado and showed that this diffuse type of leprosy is not confined to Mexico as was at one time thought. Some authors believe that this form of leprosy may be caused by *Mycobacterium lepromatosis*[111] though we do not allude to this concept.

Unfortunately, the term lazarine leprosy reaction has been used to describe various conditions in leprosy presenting with acute ulcerations (like a reaction in BT,[91] progressive lepra reaction in lepromatous leprosy[112] or Lucio phenomenon).[113] But on analysis of all the studies and original papers, we are of the opinion that while Lucio-Latapí leprosy refers to the diffuse infiltrative form; the terms "Lucio phenomenon, erythema necroticans, ENL necroticans, spotted leprosy (lepra manchada) and lazarine leprosy" describe the same entity and probably refer to the necrotic ulcerations seen in these patients *(also see Chapter 5, Section 5.3)*.

Diagnosis of Lucio leprosy is easily overlooked unless note is taken of the shiny waxy thickened skin, the loss of body hair, including eyebrows and eyelashes (but not scalp hair), the puffy hands, and the widespread sensory loss due to involvement of dermal nerves, since nodules and other types of skin lesions are absent. Eyes have a shiny appearance but are free from keratitis or iritis and thickening of upper eyelids gives the patient a sleepy or melancholic look. As in LL, a mild-moderate normochromic and normocytic anemia is the rule, chronic edema and chronic ulceration of both legs may develop and ulceration of nasal mucosa may cause nasal symptoms and epistaxis. Unlike LL however, there are no skin lesions or motor palsies and the eyes are not damaged. The fact that the diagnosis is easy to overlook before lepra reaction occurs has been stressed by Donner and Shively, although diagnosis is not difficult once the condition is suspected as skin smears or biopsies from any part of the skin are full of leprosy bacilli.[114]

REFERENCES

1. Hansen GA. Undersogelser angaende spedalskhedens arsager. Norsk Mag Lacgevidensk 1874;4: 1–88. [English translation by Pallamary P, Hansen GA. Causes of leprosy. Int. J. Lepr 1955; 23:307–9."
2. Han XY, Aung FM, Choon SE, Werner B. Analysis of the leprosy agents Mycobacterium leprae and Mycobacterium lepromatosis in four countries. Am J Clin Pathol. 2014;142:524–32.
3. Singh P, Benjak A, Schuenemann VJ, Herbig A, Avanzi C, Busso P, et al. Insight into the evolution and origin of leprosy bacilli from the genome sequence of Mycobacterium lepromatosis. Proc Natl Acad Sci U S A. 2015;112:4459–64.
4. Shepard CC. The experimental disease that follows the injection of human leprosy bacilli into the foot-pads of mice. J Exp Med 1960; 112: 445–54.
5. Rees RJW. Enhanced susceptibility of thymectomised and irradiated mice to infection with Mycobacterium leprae. Nature 1966; 211: 657–8.
6. Godal T, Negassi K. Subclinical infection in leprosy. Br Med J 1973; 3: 557–9.

7. Weddell G, Palmer E, Rees RJW, Jamison DG. In Wolstenholme G EW, O'Conor M Eds The Pathogenesis of Leprosy London1963: J. & A. Churchill Limited: p. 3115.
8. Cochrane RG, Smyly HG. Classification. In: Leprosy in theory and practice. Editors: Cochrane RG, Davey TF. John Wright and sons limited, Bristol 1964:299–309.
9. Dharmendra. Classification of Leprosy. In: Leprosy. Editor: Hastings RC. Churchill Livingstone, Edinburgh 1994:179–90.
10. Danielssen DC, Boeck CW. Traite de la Spedalskedou elephantiasis de grecs. Bailliere, Paris. 1848.
11. Hansen GA, Looft G. Leprosy: in its clinical and pathological aspects. John Wright, Bristol.1895: p67.
12. Leonard Wood Memorial Conference on Leprosy Round table conference in Manila. Philippine Journal of Science 1931;44:449.
13. International Congress of Leprosy, Cairo Report of the sub-committee on classification. International Journal of Leprosy 1938;6:389–97.
14. Pan American Leprosy Conference, Second, Rio de Janeiro Report of the sub-committee on classification. Int J Lepr 1946;15:100–8.
15. World Health Organization Committee on Leprosy. 1st report 1952 World Health Organization Technical Report Series 71:19–22.
16. Lockwood DN, Sarno E, Smith WC. Classifying leprosy patients—searching for the perfect solution? Lepr Rev 2007;78:317–20.
17. Dharmendra. Leprosy Classification. In: Hasting RC Ed. Leprosy, 2nd edn. New York: Churchill-Livingstone, Edinburgh, 1994:p 179–90.
18. Ridley DS. Histological classification and the immunological spectrum of leprosy. Bulletin of the World Health Organization 1974; 51: 451–65.
19. Ridley DS. The pathogenesis and classification of polar tuberculoid leprosy. Lepr Rev 1982; 53: 19–26.
20. Global Leprosy Strategy 2016–2020. Accelerating towards a leprosy-free world. Monitoring and Evaluation Guide. World Health Organization. Available from: http://www.searo.who.int/entity/global_leprosy_programme/documents/sea-glp-2017-1/en/. [Accessed on 29th June,2019]
21. WHO Technical Report Series. Vol. 768. Geneva: World Health Organization; 1988. WHO Expert Committee on Leprosy. Sixth report.
22. National Leprosy Eradication Programme (NLEP). Training Manual for Medical Officer, 2013. Available from: http://nlep.nic.in/pdf/MO%20training%20Manual. pdf. [Accessed on 29th June, 2019]
23. Ridley DS, Jopling WH. Classification of leprosy according to immunity. Int J Lepr 1966;34: 255–73.
24. Rees RJW. Recent bacteriologic, immunologic and pathologic studies on experimental human leprosy in the mouse foot pad. Int J Lepr 1965; 33: 646–55.
25. Scollard DM. Infection with Mycobacterium lepromatosis. Am J Trop Med Hyg. 2016;95:500–1.
26. Ridley DS. Concepts of the spectrum. In. Pathogenesis of leprosy and related diseases. ©Butterworth & Co. (Publishers) Ltd, 1988, p39.
27. Pfaltzgraff RE, Ramu G. Clinical leprosy. In: Hastings RC Ed. Leprosy.2nd edition. New York: Churchill Livingstone; 1994. p. 237–87.
28. Ponnighaus JM, Fine PE, Gruer PJK, Maine N. The anatomical distribution of single leprosy lesions in an African population and its implications in the pathogenesis of leprosy. Lepr Rev 1990; 61: 242–50..
29. Noordeen SK. Epidemiology of (poly) neuritic leprosy. Leprosy in India 1972;44: 90–6.
30. Newell KW. An epidemiologist's view of leprosy. Bull. WHO 1966; 34: 827–57.
31. Cambri G, Mira MT. Genetic Susceptibility to Leprosy: From Classic Immune-related Candidate Genes to Hypothesis-free, Whole Genome Approaches. Front Immunol. 2018;9:1674.
32. Myrvang B, Godal T, Feek CM, Ridley DS, Samuel DR. Immune response to *Mycobacterium leprae* in indeterminate leprosy patients. Acta Pathol. Microbiol. Scand 1973;81:615–20.
33. Scott GC, Russell DA, Boughton CR, Vincin DR. Untreated leprosy: Probability for shifts in Ridley-Jopling classification. Development of 'flares' or disappearance of clinically apparent disease. Int J Lepr 1976;44:110–22.

34. Lara CB, Nolasco JO. Self-healing or abortive and residual forms of childhood leprosy and their possible significance. Int J Lepr 1958;24: 245–63.
35. Ridley DS. The pathogenesis of the early skin lesions in leprosy. J of Pathol. 1973;111:191–206.
36. McDougall AC, Archibald GC. Lepromatous leprosy presenting with swelling of the legs. Br Med J. 1977; 1: 23–4.
37. Bhushan P, Aggarwal A, Yadav R, Baliyan V. Bilateral medial finger nail dystrophy as a presenting feature in a patient with leprosy. Lepr Rev. 2011;82:74–7.
38. Cardama J.E. Early lesions (indeterminate forms) In: Latapi F., Saul A., Rodriguez O., Malacara M., Browne S.G., editors. Leprosy. (Proceedings of the XI Interna-tional Leprosy Congress, Mexico City November 13–18, 1978) ExcerptaMedica; Amsterdam: 1980. pp. 68–74.
39. Cochrane RG. Signs and symptoms. In: Cochrane RG, Davey TF, editor. Leprosy in Theory and Practice. Bristol: John Wright and Sons; 1964. p. 251–79.
40. Browne SG. Self-healing leprosy: report on 2749 patients. Lep Rev. 1974; 45:104–11.
41. Cruz RCDS, Bührer-Sékula S, Penna MLF, Penna GO, Talhari S. Leprosy: current situation, clinical and laboratory aspects, treatment history and perspective of the uniform multidrug therapy for all patients. An Bras Dermatol. 2017;92:761–73.
42. Price JE. BCG vaccination in leprosy Int J Lepr; 1982; 50: 205–12.
43. Pettit] HS. Should indeterminate leprosy ever be diagnosed? Int J Lepr 1981;49: 95–96.
44. Bhushan P, Thatte SS. Saucer lesions in leprosy: Anatomy of the controversy. Indian J Dermatol 2016;61:100–2.
45. Noordeen SK.Evolution of tuberculoid leprosy in a community. Leprosy in India 1975;47: 85–93.
46. Ramanujam K. 1980 Findings of a nineteen year follow-up of children with untreated leprosy. In: Latapi F, Saul A, Rodriguez 0, Malacara M, Browne S G (eds) Leprosy. Proceedings of the XI International Leprosy Congress, Mexico City, 13-18 November1978. Excerpta Medica, Amsterdam, 75–79.
47. Jopling WH. Borderline (dimorphous) leprosy maintaining a polyneuritic form for eight years: a case report. Trans R Soc Trop Med Hyg. 1956;50: 478–80.
48. Leiker DL. Low resistant Tuberculoid leprosy. Int J Lepr 1964; 32:359–67.
49. Cochrane RG. Signs and symptoms. In: Cochrane RG, Davey TF, editor. Leprosy in Theory and Practice. Bristol: John Wright and Sons; 1964. p. 251–79.
50. Bhushan P, Thatte SS. Saucer lesions in leprosy: Anatomy of the controversy. Indian J Dermatol 2016;61:100–2.
51. Ridley DS, Waters MFR. Significance of variation within the lepromatous group. Lepr Rev 1969;40:143–52.
52. McDougall AC, Archibald GC. Lepromatous leprosy presenting with swelling of legs. Br Med J1977;1:23–4.
53. Moller-Christensen V. Bone Changes. Leprosy.Copenhagen: Munksgaard, 1961.
54. Moller-Christensen V. Changes in the anterior nasal spine and the alveolar process of the maxillae in leprosy: a clinical examination. Int J Lepr 1974;42:431–5.
55. Fraguela Rangel JV, FernándezBaquero G, KraftchencoBeoto T, Hernández AnguloM. [Scalp alopecia in leprosy]. Rev Cubana Med Trop. 1977;29:23–31.
56. Abraham S, Ebenezer GJ, Jesudasan K. Diffuse alopecia of the scalp in borderline lepromatous leprosy in an Indian patient. Lepr Rev. 1997;68:336–40.
57. Brand PW. Temperature variation and leprosy deformity. Int J Lepr 1959;27:1–7.
58. Chaco J, Magora A., Zauberman H., Landau Y. An electromyographic study of lagophthalmos in leprosy. Int J Lepr 1968; 36: 288–95.
59. Walker HK. Cranial Nerve VII: The Facial Nerve and Taste. In: Walker HK, Hall WD, Hurst JW, editors.Clinical Methods: The History, Physical, and Laboratory Examinations. 3rd edition. Boston: Butterworths; 1990.
60. Somerset EJ, Dharmendra. Eye lesions in leprosy. In: Leprosy. Volume I. Dharmendra, ed. Bombay: Kothari Medical Publishing House, 1978: 143–64.

61. Sabin TD, Ebner JD 1969 Patterns of sensory loss in Lepromatous leprosy. International Journal of Leprosy 37:239–248.
62. Bhushan P, Aggarwal A, Yadav R, Baliyan V. Bilateral medial fingernail dystrophy as a presenting feature in a patient with leprosy. Lepr Rev 2011:74–7.
63. Barton PE. Olfaction in leprosy. J Laryngol Otol1974; 88:355–61.
64. Bartod RPE. A clinical study of the nose in lepromatous leprosy. Lepr Rev 1974;45:135–44.
65. Singh L, Malhotra R, Bundela RK, et al. Ocular Disability: WHO Grade 2 in persons affected with leprosy. Indian J Lepr 2014;86:1–6.
66. Hogeweg M and Keunen JEE. Prevention of blindness in leprosy and role of the Vision 2020 Programme. Eye 2005;19:1099–105.
67. Hobbs HE, Choyce DP. The blinding lesions of leprosy. Lepr Rev 1977; 42:131–7.
68. Ffytche TJ. The eye and leprosy. Lepr Rev 1981;52:111–19.
69. Sharma N, Koranne RV, Mendiratta V, et al. A study of leprosy reactions in a tertiary hospital in Delhi. J Dermatol 2004;31:898–903.
70. Shields JA, Waring GO III, Monte LG: Ocular findings in leprosy. Am J Ophthalmol 1974; 77:880–90.
71. Brandt F, Malla OK. Ocular findings in leprous patients: a report of a survey in Malunga/Nepal. Albrecht von Graefes Arch Klin Exp Ophthalmol 1981;217:27–34.
72. Spaide R, Nattis R, Lipka A, et al. Ocular findings in leprosy in the United States. Am J Ophthalmol. 1985;100:411–16.
73. Leprosy and the eye: teaching set3rd ed. London: ICEH; 2010.
74. Courtright P, Daniel E, Sundarrao, Ravanes J, Mengistu F, Belachew M, Celloria RV, Ffytche T. Eye disease in multibacillary leprosy patients at the time of their leprosy diagnosis: findings from the Longitudinal Study of Ocular Leprosy (LOSOL) in India, the Philippines and Ethiopia. Lepr Rev 2002;73:225–38.
75. Courtright P, Lewallen S, Tungpakorn N, et al. Cataract in leprosy patients: cataract surgical coverage, barriers to acceptance of surgery, and outcome of surgery in a population based survey in Korea. Br J Ophthalmol 2001;85:643–47.
76. Hogeweg M. Cataract: the main cause of blindness in leprosy. Lepr Rev 2001;72:139–42.
77. Anand S, Neethiodiss P, Xavier JW. Intra and post operative complications and visual outcomes following cataract surgery in leprosy patients. Lepr Rev 2009;80:177.
78. Mohammad W, Malhotra SK, Garg PK. Clinicoradiological Correlation of Bone Changes in Leprosy Patients Presenting with disabilities/Deformities. Indian J Lepr 2016;88:83–95.
79. Carayon A, Dharmendra. Bone and joint changes in leprosy. In Dharmendra, Ed. Leprosy. Volume II. Bombay: Samant and Company 1985;872–85.
80. Warren G. The management of tarsal bone disintegration. Lepr Rev 1972;43:137–47.
81. Moller-Christensen V (1961). Bone Changes. Leprosy. Copenhagen: Munksgaard.
82. Moller-Christensen V. Changes in the anterior nasal spine arid the alveolar process of themaxillae in leprosy: a clinical examination. Int J Leprosy 1974;42:431–5.
83. Quyum F, Hasan M, Atiqur-Rahman M. Risk factors of testicular dysfunction in multibacillary leprosy. Lepr Rev 2019;90:338–43.
84. Abraham A, Sharma VK, Kaur S. Assessment of testicular volume in bacilliferous leprosy: correlation with clinical parameters. Indian J Lepr 1990;62:310–5.
85. Singh N, Arora VK, Jain A, Bhattacharya SN, Bhatia A. Cytology of testicular changes in leprosy. Acta Cytol 2002;46:659–63.
86. Guler H, Kadihasanoglu M, Aydin M, Kendirci M. Erectile dysfunction and adult onset hypogonadism in leprosy: cross-sectional, control group study. Lepr Rev 2019; 90:344–51.
87. Sharma S. C., Kumar B., Dhall K, Kaur S., Malhotra S. Aikat M. Leprosy and female reproductive organs. Int J Lepr 1981;49:177–9.
88. Silva Junior GB, Daher Ede F, Pires NetoRda J, Pereira ED, Meneses GC, Araú-joSM, Barros EJ. Leprosy nephropathy: a review of clinical and histopathological features. Rev Inst Med Trop Sao Paulo 2015;57:15–20.

89. Dharmendra Ramu G. Some systemic manifestations in leprosy. In: Leprosy. Volume I. Dharmendra, ed. Bombay: Kothari Medical Publishing House 1978;180–95
90. Klioze AM, Ramos-Caro FA. Visceral leprosy. Int J Dermatol 2000;39:641–58.
91. Ramu G, Dharmendra. Acute exacerbations (reactions) in leprosy. In: Leprosy. Volume I. Dharmendra, ed. Bombay: Kothari Medical Publishing House 1978: 108–39
91a. Gupta A, Sharma PK, Garga VC, Sharma LK. Adrenal cortical function and adrenal volume in leprosy. A study of 40 cases. Lepr Rev 2018;89(2).148–57.
92. Desikan KV, Job CK. A review of postmortem findings in 37 cases of leprosy. Int J Lepr 1968; 36: 32–44.
93. Hodes RM, Teferedegne B. Tetanus in leprosy patients: report of five cases. Int J Lepr Other Mycobact Dis 1988;56:228–30.
94. Shen J, Liu M, Zhou M, Li W. Causes of death among active leprosy patients in China. Int J Dermatol 2011;50:57–60.
95. Dharmendra. The pure neuritic group. In: Leprosy. Volume I. Dharmendra, ed. Bombay: Kothari Medical Publishing House 1978;94–107.
96. Khan A, Sardana K, Koranne RV, Bhushan P. Bilateral seventh nerve palsy a manifestation of polyneuritic leprosy. Indian J Lepr 2005;77:140–7.
97. Tandon S, Sinha S, Singh J. Bizarre extensive erythematous plaques on the abdomen. Trop Doct. 2019;49:39–42.
98. Chetan R, Shailesh M. Midborderline leprosy in type B. Blaschko linear pattern: A rare phenomenon. Int J Dermatol 2019;58:729–32.
99. Multidermatomal Zosteriform Nodules and Plaques in a Case of Lepromatous Leprosy: An Uncommon Presentation. Trop Doct 2019 (in press).
100. Kumar P, Savant SS, Das A.A curious case of Lepromatous Leprosy Developing Complete loss of Pigmentation, followed by Reappearance of Pigmentation with Multi-drug Therapy (MDT) alone: A Support for Neural Theory of Vitiligo Pathogenesis. IndJ Lepr 2018;90:155–59.
101. Browne S G. Localized bacilliferous skin lesions appearing in patients with quiescent lepromatous leprosy. IntJ Lepr 1966;34:289–93.
102. Wade HW. The histoid variety of lepromatous leprosy. Int J Lepr 1963;31:129–42.
103. Ramanujam K, Arunthathi S, Chacko CJ G, Jacob M. Neural histoid leproma in peripheral nerves—a case report. Lepr Rev 1984;54:63–8.
104. Pearson] MH, Ross WF. Nerve involvement in leprosy: Pathology differential diagnosis and principles of management. Lepr Rev 1975;46:199–212.
105. Roy-Chaudhari SB, Srinivasan H. Nerve abscess in lepromatous leprosy. A case report and discussion of pathogenesis. Lepr India 1977;57:389–92.
106. Girdhar A, Lavanfa RK, Malaviya GN, Girdhar BK. Histoid lesion in nerve of a lepromatous patient. Lepr Rev 1990;61:237–41.
107. Job C K, Chacko CJG, Taylor PM. Electronmicroscopic study ofhistoid leprosy with special reference to histogenesis. Lepr India 1977;49:467–70.
108. Latapi F, Zamora AC. The spotted leprosy of lucio (la lepra manchada' de Lucio): an introduction to its clinical and histological study. Int J Lepr 1948;16:421–30.
109. Latapí F, Chévez-Zamora A. The "spotted" leprosy of Lucio: An introduction to its clinical and histological study. Int J Lepr 1948;16:421–37.
110. Frenken JH. Diffuse leprosy of Lucio and Latapi. Detroit: Blaine Ethridge, 1963.
111. Han Y, Seo YH, Sizer KC, et al. A New Mycobacterium species causing diffuse lepromatous leprosy. Am J Clin Pathol 2008;130:856–64.
112. Cochrane RG. Complicating conditions due to leprosy. In: Cochrane RG, Davey TF, editor. Leprosy in Theory and Practice. Bristol: John Wright and Sons; 1964: p. 331–42.
113. Vargas-Ocampo F. Diffuse leprosy of Lucio and Latapi: A histologic study. Lepr Rev 2007;78: 248–60.
114. Donner RS, Shively JA. The Lucio phenomenon in diffuse leprosy. Ann Intern Med1967;67:831–6.

2.2 RELAPSE, REACTIVATION, REACTION AND REINFECTION

C Ruth Butlin

NATURAL HISTORY OF TREATED LEPROSY

When a person has leprosy, some of the clinical manifestations are a direct result of bacterial multiplication in his body (what one might call "active signs of infection"), but many of the more prominent manifestations are a result of an immunological inflammatory response to the bacterial antigens. The latter can occur in absence of viable bacteria, so may be seen before, during or after effective chemotherapy. These inflammatory phenomena, which we call lepra reactions, include type 1 reactions, type 2 reactions/erythema nodosum leprosum (ENL) and acute neuritis.

Active signs of infection in untreated cases include congestion of nasal mucosa with bleeding, diffuse infiltration, madarosis, lepromatous nodules, hypopigmented or erythematous skin patches with or without impaired sensation, thickening of peripheral nerve trunks and gradual impairment of nerve function in extremities. A positive skin smear does not necessarily indicate active infection since it takes much longer for the bacterial debris to be cleared from the body than it does to kill the bacteria, however, an increasing bacteriological index (BI) in sequential smears from the same area does indicate bacterial multiplication. A reactional episode is not by itself a sign of active infection.

These concepts are difficult for patients to understand and may confuse some clinicians who are unfamiliar with the natural history of leprosy disease.

The normal response to an appropriate course of chemotherapy is a rapid improvement (within weeks) in any nasal symptoms, followed by gradual subsidence of infiltration and lepromatous nodules (over many months), and a slow healing in any skin patches (shown by them becoming flatter and less well-defined, with partial recovery of former pigmentation and sometimes of sensation). If the smear was positive initially, there will be a fall in BI over several years. If serial biopsies were done, histology would show, in lepromatous cases, increasingly foamy cells replacing macrophages stuffed with AFBs, and in borderline or tuberculoid cases, granulomas becoming less well organized and being slowly replaced by fibrous tissue (Job).[1]

Hence, one should not expect to see complete resolution of all signs of infection in every case by the end of a standard MDT course, lasting 6 or 12 (or even 24) months. The clinical appearance cannot be taken as a criterion for "cure" and the decision to stop chemotherapy is taken on the basis of completing a full course within the set time period. Clinical signs of previous infection will continue to subside after cessation of MDT. Reactional episodes may occur months or years after release from treatment and do not signify a need for extending/repeating the chemotherapy course.

Recording and Reporting in Leprosy Control Programmes

In the context of a national programme, one must distinguish and report separately to authorities, "new cases" (never before treated), returned defaulters who are restarting treatment, and relapse cases who need a second course of treatment. However, large numbers in each of these categories have different implications for a control programme: A high proportion of defaulters is suggestive of poor service at clinic level, whereas true relapses may occur despite excellent services. In the WHO guidelines,[3] it is suggested to report "retreatment cases" as one category (which would include both reactivated disease and relapse) as a proportion of all registered new cases (*also see page 257*). This is illogical since these cases belong to cohorts of cases diagnosed in different periods (which may be many years before the cohort of currently registered new cases were diagnosed). It is desirable to report the proportion of those tested whose samples showed drug resistance.[3]

DEFINITION AND CRITERIA FOR RELAPSE

I would recommend use of the definition of relapse given by WHO in 2006[2] which defines relapse as **"the re-occurrence of the disease at any time after the completion of a full course of treatment"**. The emphasis is on a "full" course, implying an appropriate regimen for a suitable duration.

Good clear criteria for diagnosis of relapse are also given in the same document[2] as **"the appearance of new skin lesions and, in the case of an MB relapse, by evidence on a skin smear of an increase in BI of 2 or more units"**, supplemented by the proviso[3] that **"signs and symptoms are not deemed to be due to reaction"** (although this perhaps presupposes that the clinician is an expert in assessing leprosy patients!) and for PB relapse, **relapse is more likely than reaction if it is more than 3 years since treatment ended.**[2]

Other definitions and criteria are sometimes quoted[4,5] but these earlier ones are now superseded by more specific or more practical criteria. Morphological index (MI) is not considered a reliable guide to presence of relapse, as it is subjective and difficult to measure. Most recent authors agree that for MB relapse, there should be an increase of 2 log units in BI[5,6] (not simply a BI of 2+ or more[4]) and the smear should be *repeated* for confirmation. Most authors agree that for PB relapse, there has to be strong evidence, preferably both histological and clinical.[7]

A scoring system to assist in recognition of true relapse has been proposed by Linder,[8] however this needs to be validated in a prospective series. This reliably differentiates relapse from "disease which is still active" or from reactivation of inadequately treated disease.

Etiology of Relapse in Leprosy

As explained above, leprosy can be considered as a syndrome where immunological disturbances (reactions) follow a mycobacterial infection. It is against this background that we need to consider the issue of leprosy relapse, which is a feared but relatively rare event (that is to say, rare compared with reactions or nerve function impairment and its secondary complications). If a patient who has previously completed an effective course of chemotherapy, after a suitable interval (to allow the incubation period of the slow-growing mycobacteria to pass) develops new signs of active infection, then one has to consider whether he has relapsed leprosy and needs a second course of chemotherapy.

This second episode of infection could arise from endogenous "persisters" which remain viable in low numbers in certain sites in the body such as nerves, iris, smooth muscle, lymph nodes, bone marrow or liver. These are "dormant" bacteria which are not killed by antibacterial drugs (although they are drug-sensitive) because of their metabolically-inactive state.[9] Occasionally (after years of dormancy), persisters resume multiplication and eventually reach a critical mass adequate to cause clinical manifestation of disease. It is not known what triggers this "awakening" of persisters, timing and frequency of relapses.

It is impossible to state accurately the probability of relapse after a course of chemotherapy since what evidence is available is not consistent. There have been many attempts to quantify the risk, but published estimates differ widely and cannot easily be compared (because they differ in the measurements reported, in the criteria for classification and for diagnosis of relapse, in the duration of chemotherapy and of follow-up and because local background prevalence may affect results). Commonly quoted figures are 0.1% per annum (p.a.) for PB cases and 0.06% p.a. for MB cases. Several authors have shown that those with initial BI > 3.0 + (or BI of > + 4.0 at end of chemotherapy) are at higher risk of relapse. Some researchers believe that the relapses occur earlier after shorter courses of rifampicin-containing chemotherapy.[10] There have been suggestions (based on case series) that relapse is more likely during pregnancy or in the postpartum period, than in non-pregnant women, though this has not yet been confirmed by any community studies. A selection of the more useful publications from leprosy control programmes and research studies is shown in Table 2.13.

Table 2.13: Relapses after MDT

Reference	Previous chemotherapy	Number of subjects observed	Person years at risk (PYAR)/ maximum duration or mean follow-up period	% subjects relapsed	Relapse rate per thousand (PYAR)	Timing of relapses, if given
WHO 1995[11]		20,000	9 years	0.77%	Not given	
Norman 2004[12]		173	16.4 +/– 1.83 years	2 = 1.16%	0.007/thousand PYAR	At 14 and 15 years after release from treatment (RFT)
Becx-Bleumink 1992 (3)[4]		2379	Mean 4.7 years, (range 2.5–6.0 years)	24 = 1%	2.4/thousand PYAR	
WHO 7th exp-cttee, 1998[13]		Not given	Not given	0.1% each year	Not given	
Ali 2005[14]		356	16 years	3 = 0.84%	0.86/thousand PYAR	
Girdhar 2000[15]	24 months or more MB MDT for MB cases	301	1085 PYAR 2–8 yr follow-up	12 = 4%	0.11/thousand PYAR	
		260	• 980.2 PYAR • 2–8 yr follow-up	20 = 8%	0.20/thousand PYAR	
Gebre 2000[5]		256	• 1091 PYAR • Mean 4.3 years. Max 8 years	None	None	
Cellona 2003[16]		500	• 5368 PYAR • Mean 10.8 years	15 = 3%	0.028/thousand pyar	

(Contd.)

Table 2.13: Relapses after MDT (Contd.)

Reference	Previous chemotherapy	Number of subjects observed	Person years at risk (PYAR)/ maximum duration or mean follow-up period	% subjects relapsed	Relapse rate per thousand (PYAR)	Timing of relapses, if given
Jamet 1995[17]	12 months or more WHO MB MDT	35	• Mean 6 years	7 = 20%	0.33/thousand PYAR	
Marchoux 1992[18]						
Shen 2006[19]		2374	• 19633 PYAR • Mean 8.27 years	5 = 0.21%	0.21/thousand PYAR	
Desikan 2008[20]		660; all highly smear positive	8–12 years	5 = 1%	0.01/thousand PYAR	
Penna 2017[21]		290	2265.8 PYAR	0	0	
Butlin 2016[22]		694	Up to 8 years	0	0	
WHO TAG 2011[23]	UMDT for 6 months-MB	1302	4 years	6 = 0.46%	Not given	At 13–28 months
Penna 2017[21]		323	1568.1 PYAR	7 = 2.17%	2.9–4.5/thousand PYAR	Half at >5 years
Liangbin and Shen 2016[24]		72 all smear positive	8 years	1 =1.3%	0.0035/thousand PYAR	At 13 months after RFT
Butlin 2016[22]		918	up to 8 years	0	Not given	1 relapse at 9 years reported later (0.11%)
WHO 1995[11]		50,000	9 years	1.07%		
Ali 2005[14]		2892	16 years	55 = 1.9%	1.92/thousand PYAR	68% relapses were in first 3 years
Boerrigter 1991[7]		499	4 years	12 = 2.40%	6.5/thousand PYAR	
Becx-Bleumink 1992(3)[4]		3065	Mean 6.1 years after RFT, range 2.5–7.5 years	34 = 1.1%	2.1/thousand PYAR	
Gebre 2009[5]	PB MDT for 6 months	246	1009 pyar, mean 4.1 years, range 0–8.8 years	0	0	

Several authors[4,5] point out that the most common error is to confuse late reaction with relapse. Since reaction is common within 2 years of release from treatment (RFT) from a short course of MDT, and a true relapse is expected to occur only after an interval exceeding the length of the incubation period, it is possible that in some of the reported series where most relapses apparently occurred within 3 years of RFT, a high proportion of these were actually only instances of late reaction.[2,5] It is vital to promptly diagnose a reaction and treat it correctly (usually with corticosteroids) to prevent onset of permanent disability, as well as to relieve suffering. Although there is a small risk of infecting others, restarting chemotherapy for a relapse case is less urgent, and a few days can be taken to assess and investigate the case of a suspected relapse. Hence, in the algorithm (Fig. 2.30), the first question to be addressed is "Is this reaction"? After treating any reaction, one can return to the question of "why is he having a reaction so late: Does he also have evidence of relapse?" (Table 2.14).

REINFECTION

If the person continued to live in an endemic area after RFT, he could be reinfected at any time by exogenous bacteria discharged by another untreated case. In this situation, he could eventually (after the usual incubation period) present with overt manifestations of an active infection. This would be impossible to differentiate clinically from an endogenous relapse (and should be handled in the same way). Relapse due to persisters is thought to be far more common that relapse due to reinfection.[9]

Occasionally, it may be possible to distinguish an endogenous relapse from a new infection by different bacteria, using molecular biology techniques, but only if samples from the time when the person was first diagnosed with leprosy (for example if the case was a subject in a research study with long follow-up) are available for comparison. The bacteria present at the time of relapse may show differences as judged by genomic analysis—one study found that bacteria from 2 of 3 relapse cases investigated had only minor disparities in sequences between first and second episodes of disease (and the same drug sensitivity pattern), consistent with an endogenous relapse. Bacteria from the first and second episodes in the third case were of different strains, suggesting that this was a reinfection.[25]

REACTIVATION OF LEPROSY

Much more *common* than a true relapse is "Reactivated disease" in cases who never completed a full course of adequate chemotherapy.[13] When a person begins chemotherapy, the bacterial load falls rapidly, in a logarithmic fashion, rendering him non-infectious to others within a couple of days. However, premature cessation of therapy would leave some viable bacteria which can immediately recommence replication. After an interval, the bacteria again reach a level at which increasing clinical signs of infection re-occur, and the BI will slowly increase again.

If the bacteria are exposed to a single drug to which they are initially sensitive (for example when a PB patient fails to consume the daily dapsone but receives his monthly rifampicin) there may be natural selection of drug-resistant bacteria which occasionally arise spontaneously in any large mycobacterial population. The patient may have initially responded clinically to the therapy, but after a long interval (during which the drug-resistant bacteria multiply to a critical level) he deteriorates again, developing new active signs of infection.

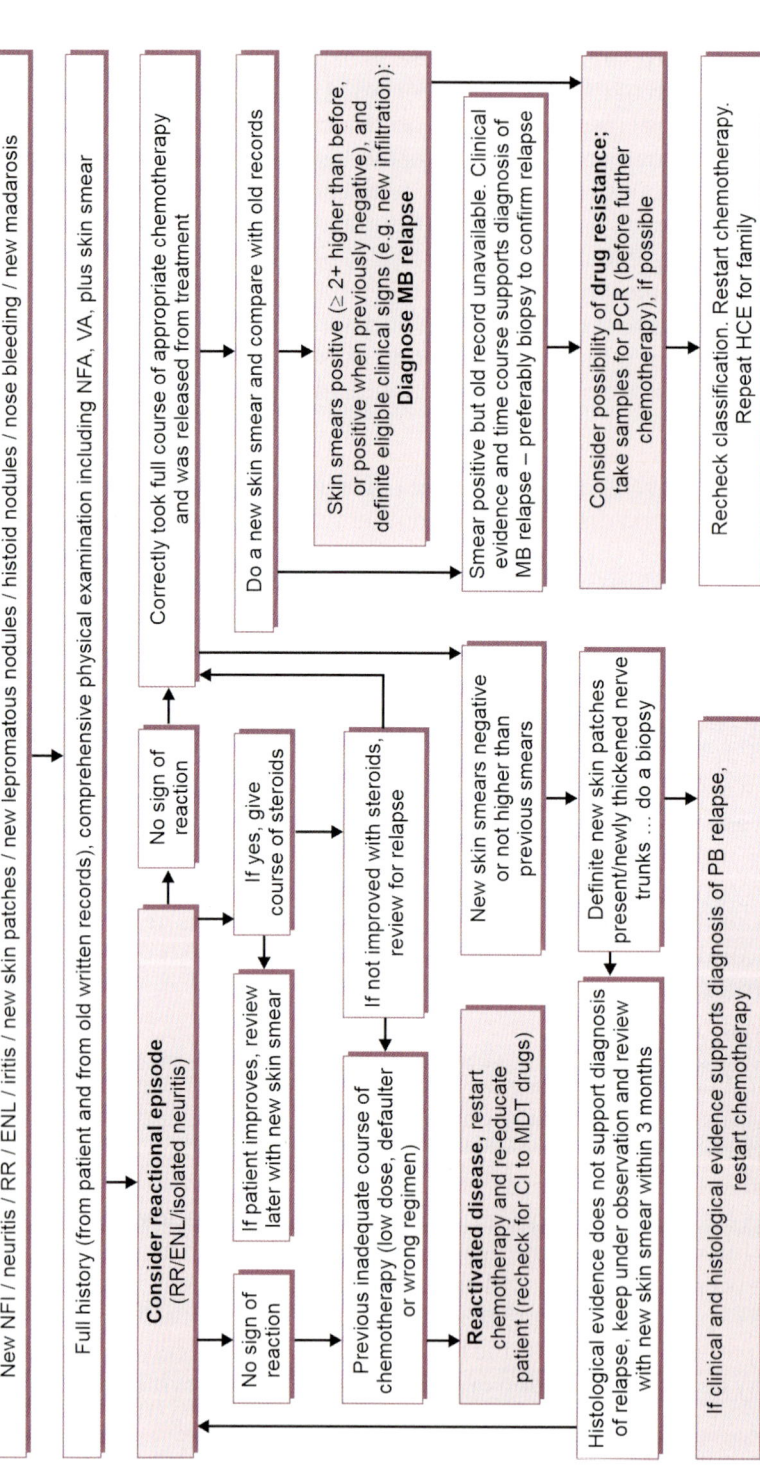

Fig. 2.30: Algorithm of facilitate differentiating relapse from reaction/re-activation in leprosy

NFI: Nerve function impairment; VA: Visual acuity; HCE: Household contact examination; RR: Reversal reaction; CI: Contraindication

Table 2.14: Differentiating reactivated disease from true relapse

	Reactivated disease	Endogenous relapse/reinfection
Timing	Often within a *short time* (months to years) of stopping chemotherapy	Usually long time after completion of chemotherapy (at last 2–5 years)
Onset of new lesions	Gradual worsening	Gradual development of new lesions after an interval following initial improvement during chemotherapy
Character of new lesions	• May be similar to first episode of disease, may be more widespread. • Tendency to downgrade towards LL	Lesions may be typical of different classification, e.g. BL lesions in patient previously classified as LL; or BT in patient previously classified as BL (immunity has "upgraded")
History	• Inadequate chemotherapy • May be due to misclassification of MB cases as PB • May be due to non-compliance on account of adverse effects or misunderstandings • May be due to premature cessation of therapy (defaulting)	Completed a full course of appropriate chemotherapy within recommended time limits
Drug resistance risk	Liable to develop secondary drug resistance, especially if originally had monotherapy	Usually, M. leprae still fully sensitive to all three standard MDT drugs
Pathogenesis	Failure of earlier chemotherapy course to reduce M. leprae to below critical threshold, allowing bacteria to again multiply after cessation of chemotherapy	First course of chemotherapy effective to kill all metabolically active M. leprae, followed by delayed "re-awakening" of persisters, or by new infection from another source, after release from treatment
Management	• Re-educate patient. Recheck for contraindications to MDT drugs • Recheck classification (considering smear results). Collect samples for PCR if feasible • Restart full course of standard MDT and follow-up carefully. Avoid using "Accompanied multi-drug therapy"! • If PCR shows drug resistance, adapt MDT regimen accordingly when receive results • Re-examine all household contacts • If there is evidence of secondary drug resistance, any new cases amongst contacts may have primary resistant infection	• Explain concept of relapse to patient • Recheck for contraindications to MDT drugs. Recheck classification (considering smear results) • Collect samples for PCR if feasible • Restart full course of standard MDT and follow-up carefully. • If PCR shows drug resistance, adapt treatment regimen accordingly • Re-examine all household contacts

Note: Reactivation or relapse may present as a "late reaction" type 1 or type 2, and the significance of the symptoms might be missed if the history of chemotherapy is not reviewed or the skin smear is not done.

With re-activated disease, the patient may present to different clinicians as a new case. But the staff should ensure they question any first-attender about previous chemotherapy elsewhere.

The commonest reason for re-activation of disease is *non-compliance* which does not only refer to "defaulting" (when the patient fails to collect his medication from clinic) but also non-consumption of medicines at home. This may not be suspected by the clinic staff; and it is often due to a patient believing he/she suffers adverse effects from the medication… and he/she may be right! (*Case Scenario 1*).

Case Scenario 1: Relapse *vs* re-activation

A patient presented to a referral centre with new skin lesions and a positive skin smear (BI 5+), about 6 years after being officially "released from treatment" at a village clinic. Old records showed his diagnosis as a BL case, with smear still positive (BI 3+) after being given 12 months MB MDT in blister calendar packs. However, the clinic notes revealed that on most occasions the patient himself was not seen at clinic, and his MDT was handed to a proxy. On questioning the patient, we found that because he had felt ill after taking his MDT, he had discontinued it without telling the staff. When MDT was restarted in hospital, he immediately suffered severe hemolysis and needed a blood transfusion. After withdrawal of dapsone, he was able to continue MDT for up to 24 months without further adverse effects. There was a good clinical improvement in his leprosy.

We believe that when first given MDT including dapsone, at the village clinic where hemoglobin estimation was not available, he had suffered hemolytic anemia, which was undetected by staff. Hence, he had never taken an adequate course of chemotherapy, and was suffering from re-activated disease. But he had to be reported to NLEP as a "relapse case" since he had previously been reported as "RFT".

In some instances, the inadequate chemotherapy is the fault of staff who have *misclassified* an MB patient as PB (e.g. because smear was not done), or who had prescribed a *non-standard* course, or have inappropriately advised *discontinuing* MDT (e.g. during pregnancy/breast feeding). In the past, some LL cases on dapsone monotherapy had their treatment wrongly stopped after 2 years negativity (also *see* Table 2.14, differentiating reactivated disease from true relapse).

MANAGEMENT OF SUSPECTED RELAPSE CASES

One must remember, when taking a history of previous chemotherapy, that regimens differed in the past. According to when he was first diagnosed (and prevailing local policies at that time), the patient may have been started with dapsone monotherapy (any case detected before 1982, and some first registered as late as 1995), may have had MDT with 2 or 3 drugs for 6/12/24 months, or until smear negativity, or may even have had single dose multi-drug therapy for single lesion leprosy (rifampicin, ofloxacin and minocycline) which was in use for several years from 1998.[13] It often helps to show samples of the individual drugs or of blister calendar packs (which only became common about 10 years after MDT was introduced).

There are still many people alive, and at risk of relapse, who were first diagnosed with leprosy before 1982, and who could only have received dapsone monotherapy. In 2019, some of these may be only 40 years old, so this will be a continuing problem for several decades! (*Case Scenario 2*).

Case Scenario 2: Inadequate treatment

An elderly man presented at a clinic with trophic ulcers, giving a vague history of anti-leprosy treatment elsewhere in the past. His smear was negative, and he had then no active signs of infection. So it was assumed he had a full course of chemotherapy and his chart was labelled "old case". Over the next few years, he often received disability care from that clinic.

One day he presented with ENL reaction and was found to have a highly positive smear. New inquiries into his original treatment revealed he had only a short course of dapsone monotherapy, and stopped dapsone when his smear first became negative. It was unclear whether the treatment cessation was his decision or after (inappropriate) advice of staff.

When reviewing past classification, remember that criteria have also changed over the years. A borderline tuberculoid patient with 6 patches, 2 nerves affected and one smear site having BI 1+ could have been correctly given PB MDT in 1983.[26]

History and Background Information

In addition to a thorough physical examination, it is wise to examine any old records available (patient-held cards, old clinic registers, laboratory reports, hospital discharge slips or referral letters) for background information on the relapse suspect, since the patient may not be able to clearly articulate all the information you need—especially if he was a child when first treated. Some relapse cases may not have been told their diagnosis of leprosy when they first received chemotherapy (Fig. 2.30, algorithm).

Clinical Assessment

Having completed a full physical examination (including nerve function assessment and visual acuity) and compared the findings with any old records available, one will be in a position to decide whether a reactional episode is present. A summary of clinical features of relapse cases is given in Boxes 2.4 and 2.5. Should there be clear evidence of reversal reaction or of ENL or of acute neuritis with new nerve function impairment, a course of corticosteroids should usually be prescribed (starting at 1 mg/kg/day of prednisolone for at least 8 weeks) *(also see Chapter 5)*. The case will need to be re-assessed, during and after the anti-reaction treatment (Tables 2.15 and 2.16).

Box 2.4: Clinical features of relapse in PB cases

- Previously subsided skin lesions become active once more.
- Extension of the lesions in size and infiltration or thickening of the lesions
- Lesions are hypopigmented OR have varying shades of erythema.
- Often an increase in the number of lesions
- In macular lesions, there is an increase in the extent of lesions and they become infiltrated
- Appearance of satellite lesions
- Fresh nerve thickening and tenderness
- An increase in the extent of sensory loss in distribution of affected peripheral nerves with insidious onset of motor deficit.

Box 2.5: Clinical features of relapse in MB cases

- The occurrence of bacteriological positivity in patients who had become bacteriologically negative
- An increase of BI higher than 2+ over the previous value in BI +ve patients
- In patients with resolved infiltration, localized areas of new infiltration may appear. The common sites are forehead, the lower part of the back, the dorsum of the hands and feet and the upper part of the buttocks
- Histoid lesions: A soft pink papule or nodule or several such lesions with or without a background of infiltration may be found at these sites. The papules may enlarge and become plaques of BL leprosy-Hypodermal nodules which feel like peas in size and consistency. The common sites are posterior aspects of arms and anterolateral aspects of thighs
- Mucosal lesions: Papular or nodular lesions in the center of hard palate, inner aspects of lips or glans penis. Nasal congestion and slight bleeding
- Ocular lesions: Iris pearls or rarely leproma (in cases which have had lesions in iris)
- Peripheral nerve lesions: Fresh nerve thickening and tenderness, with insidious loss of function.

Table 2.15: Differentiating late reactions (reversal reaction) from relapse in treated leprosy cases

	Reversal reaction (RR)	Relapse
Which patients (original classification)	BT, BB, BL cases (PB and MB) Unusual in LL cases	Any classification
Timing	Predominantly within 2 years of diagnosis	Usually >2 years after completing chemotherapy
Onset of new lesions	Rapid	Gradual
Old skin lesions	Inflamed (swelling and erythema), may be ulceration	No change in residual lesions, or extension of lesions
Course	• New lesions may spontaneously subside after an interval • Desquamation is a feature of subsiding skin lesions in RR	• Persist and enlarge/increase • Desquamation not a feature
Sites of new lesions	Predominantly at previously affected locations	Found in new locations
Character of new skin lesions	Inflamed lesions	Infiltrated lesions
New nerve lesions	Tender thickening of nerves/spontaneous nerve pain, acute nerve function impairment, nerve abscess	Non-painful thickening of nerves, which were previously not thick; gradually progressive neural impairment
Constitutional symptoms	May be malaise, peripheral edema, low fever	No constitutional symptoms
Response to steroids	Usually improvement within a few days	If improves, it is only temporary
Skin smear	BI same as previous one or less	BI may be increased, or positive when previously negative

Table 2.16: Differentiating late reactions (ENL) from relapse in treated leprosy cases*

	Type 2 reaction	Relapse
Which patients (original classification)	• BB, BL or LLs • Only smear positive MB cases	• BT, BB, BL or LL • Cases who were originally • PB may downgrade to MB forms on relapsing (e.g. BT to BL)
Timing	• Whilst still smear positive • Predominantly within 5 years of diagnosis • Episodic	• Usually >2 years after completing chemotherapy • Progressive
Onset of new lesions	Rapid	Gradual
Old skin lesions	No change in diffuse infiltration	Increased area, more nodular
Course	• Recurrent "crops" of new erythematous skin nodules which spontaneously subside in 2–3 days leaving a "bruise-like" mark or may "blister" leaving a shallow erosion. • Each episode may subside after a few days/weeks.	Skin nodules persist and increase, infiltration extends
Sites of new lesions	Many parts of body can be affected by inflammation, but rarely see epistaxis due to ENL reaction.	Infiltration predominantly on face/ears, extensor surfaces, back. Lepromatous nodules predominantly around ears, on face, near elbows, wrists, knees and ankles; also, on palate.
Character of new lesions	• Inflamed subcutaneous nodules, or tender thickening of nerves/spontaneous nerve pain/acute nerve function impairment. • Circumcorneal inflammation and eye pain. Acute orchitis. • Pain in bones and joints.	• Diffuse infiltration, superficial firm non-tender nodules which do not blanch on pressure, non-painful thickening of nerves, gradually progressive neural impairment. • Lepromatous pannus/pearls in painless eye. • Stuffiness of nose and bleeding.
Constitutional symptoms	• Usually malaise, peripheral edema, high fever, anorexia. • Often neutrophil leukocytosis. • High ESR/CRP	• No constitutional symptoms • May be mild anemia, otherwise blood picture normal
Response to steroids	Usually improvement within a few days	If improves, it is only temporary
Skin smear	• BI same as previous one or less. • Bacteria appear fragmented	• BI higher than previous smear. • May see solid-staining rods.

*Based on table in a guide to leprosy control, WHO, 1988 **(p. 42)**.

Smear Examination

Having excluded reaction as the reason for the new signs and symptoms, one should review smear results (Fig. 2.30). A patient who was previously smear positive and became negative during or after a full course of chemotherapy, and who returns with a positive smear, is probably a relapse case. The smear should be *repeated* and read by a second trained person for confirmation. If a patient who was originally smear positive, and has no record of becoming negative, has a smear result definitely higher than the most recent one available (new BI at least 2+ higher than last one), he is likely to be a relapse case. However, it is often not possible to obtain previous smear results (e.g. when the patient with suspected relapse presenting to a dermatologist at a medical college hospital or in private practice, was previously treated for leprosy at a primary health center in another area). In this situation, a smear positive case should be evaluated by an expert leprologist, taking into account all other features, including timing of the presentation in relation to time of release from treatment[8] (Table 2.17). A biopsy might add useful information, including showing an influx of immature macrophages packed with acid-fast bacteria, rather than only old foamy cells.[1]

If the new smear is negative (or not higher than the most recent one available in records), but there are clinical signs such as definite new skin patches (having features consistent with leprosy), a biopsy is necessary (Fig. 2.30) and needs to be examined by a pathologist familiar with leprosy histology. The person sending it should give as much clinical information as possible and specifically ask the pathologist to look for both signs of reaction and signs of relapse (such as well-organized granulomas) and

Table 2.17: Linder's proposed diagnostic scoring system for MB relapse in leprosy[8]

	Factors	Criteria	Score
I	Time factor	Time after release from treatment (months)	
		≤12	0
		13–24	1
		25–60	2
		>60	3
II	Risk factor	If the initial BI is >3+	1
III	Clinical presentation at relapse	1. If the BI in a single lesion is ≥2+ higher than the expected BI[a]	1
		2. If the average BI is ≥2+ higher than the expected BI[a]	1
		3. If no signs of a reaction are present[b]	1
		Maximum score	7

MB: Multibacillary; BI: Bacterial index.
[a]Expected BI = calculated BI with an assumed fall of 1 log-unit/year; if the initial BI was negative, a positive BI at relapse is sufficient to score 1.
[b]Clinical signs of inflammation of the nerve or the skin or erythema nodosum leprosum.
Relapses are diagnosed with a score of ≥3.
The 'Linder score' includes primary PB cases (negative BI at first diagnosis) relapsing into MB leprosy (positive BI at relapse). In these cases, a positive BI (instead of an increase of the BI of ≥ 2+) at relapse is sufficient to score for clinical presentation at relapse.

also to do a suitable stain to search for small number of AFBs in the tissue *(also see Chapter 3, Section 3.2)*. After seeing a histology report as well as all other information, if there is still doubt, one must rely on keeping the patient under regular review to observe his progress. In a paucibacillary relapse, there is no danger of him infecting others if chemotherapy is delayed by a few weeks. The difficulty with suspected relapse cases who have negative smears has long been recognized:[2] "The diagnosis of a PB relapse can never be absolutely certain and the evidence for either a relapse or a reaction must be weighed up and a decision made".

Once a diagnosis of relapse has been confirmed, it is essential to advise the patient to have his household contacts examined for leprosy. Preferably this will be done at a home visit by a trained staff, but otherwise household members can be requested to report to the clinic for examination.

In many countries, it is now possible to have samples from relapse cases checked for drug resistance.[2,3,27] If this service is available, it should be used. However, restarting chemotherapy should not be delayed while awaiting results *(see Chapter 6)*.

Chemotherapy of Relapsed Cases

In the vast majority of relapse cases, the bacteria are still *sensitive* to standard MDT drugs and do not need second line drugs nor a specially-tailored chemotherapy course. Only if the results of drug resistance testing *(refer to Chapter 6, Section 6.1)* indicate rifampicin resistance or multidrug resistance does one need to give a different regimen, where it is wise to follow published expert advice.[27]

REFERENCES

1. Job CK. Histopathological features of relapsed leprosy. Ind J Lep 1995;67:69 80.
2. WHO, Operational Guidelines for the implementation of the Global Strategy for Further Reducing the Leprosy Burden and Sustaining Leprosy Control Activities 2006–2010, WHO, SEARO, 2006.
3. WHO, Global Leprosy Strategy 2016–2020 "Accelerating towards a leprosy-free world": Monitoring and Evaluation Guide. New Delhi: World Health Organization Regional Office for South-East Asia; 2017.
4. Becx-Bleumink M. Relapses amongst leprosy patients treated with multi-drug therapy: Experiences in the leprosy control programme of the all Africa leprosy research and training centre in Ethiopia; practical difficulties with diagnosing relapses, operational procedures and criteria for diagnosing relapses. Int J Lep 1992b;60:421–35.
5. Gebre S, Saunderson P, Bypass P. Relapses after fixed duration multiple drug therapy: The AMFES cohort. Lep Rev 2000;71:325–31.
6. Becx-Bleumink M 1992 (2). Relapses in leprosy patients after dapsone monotherapy: Experiences in leprosy control programme of all Africa leprosy, rehabilitation and training centre (ALERT) in Ethiopia. Int J Lep 1992;60:161–72.
7. Boerrigter G, Ponninghaus JM, Fine PEM, et al. Four-year follow-up results of a WHO-recommended multi-drug regimen in paucibacillary patients in Malawi. Int J Lep 1991;59:255–61.
8. LindersKatharina, Zia Mutaher, Kern Winfried V, Pfau Ruth KM, Wagner Dirk. Relapses vs. reactions in multibacillary leprosy: Proposal of new relapse criteria. Tropical Medicine and International Health 2008;13:295–309.
9. WHO Expert Committee on leprosy: Eighth report, 2012. WHO technical report series no. 968.
10. Gonçalves, et al. Underlying mechanisms of leprosy recurrence in the Western Amazon: A retrospective cohort study. Gonçalves Franciely Gomes, BeloneAn-dréa de Faria Fernandes, RosaPatríciaSammarco and LaportaGabrielZorello. BMC Infectious Diseases 2019;19:460 https://doi.org/10.1186/s12879-019-4100.

11. WHO 1995, The Leprosy Unit, WHO. Risk of relapse in leprosy. Ind J Lep 1995;67:13–26.
12. Norman G, Joseph G, Richard J. Relapses in multibacillary patients treated with multi-drug therapy until smear negativity: Findings after twenty years. International Journal of Leprosy, 2004; 72: 1–7.
13. WHO Expert cttee on leprosy: 7th report, 1998, WHO tech rep series number 874.
14. Ali MK, Thorat DM, Subramanian M, et al. A study on trend of relapse and factors influencing relapse. Ind J Lep 2005;77:105–15.
15. Girdhar BK, Girdhar A, Kumar A. Relapses in multibacillary leprosy patients: Effects of length of therapy. Leprosy Review 2000; 71: 144–53.
16. Cellona, RV Balagon MVF, Dela Cruz EC, Burgos JA, Abalos RM Walsh GP, Topolski R, Gelber RH, Walsh DS. Long-term efficacy of 2-year WHO multiple-drug therapy (MDT) in multibacillary (MB) leprosy patients. International Journal of Leprosy 2003; 71: 308–19.
17. Jamet P, Ji B. The Marchoux Chemotherapy Study Group. Relapse after long-term follow-up of multibacillary patients treated with WHO multidrug regimen. International Journal of Leprosy 1995;63:195–201.
18. Marchoux Chemotherapy Study Group (prepared by Jamet and Ji). Relapse in multibacillary leprosy patients after stopping treatment with rifampicin-containing combined regimens. International Journal of Leprosy 1992; 60: 525–35.
19. Shen J, Liu M, Zhang J, Su W, Ding G. Relapse in MB leprosy patients treated with 24 months of MDT in SW China: A short report. Lep Rev 2006; 77:219–24.
20. Desikan KV, Dundaresh P, Tulasisdas I, Ranganadha Rao Pv. An 8–12 year follow-up of highly bacillated Indian leprosy patients treated with WHO multi-drug therapy. Leprosy Review 2008;79: 303–10.
21. Penna GO, Buèhrer-SeÂkula S, Kerr LRS, Stefani MMdA, Rodrigues LC, de ArauÂjo MG, et al. Uniform multi-drug therapy for leprosy patients in Brazil (U-MDT/CT-BR): Results of an open label, randomized and controlled clinical trial, among multibacillary patients. PLoSNegl Trop Dis 2017;11(7): e0005725.
22. Butlin CR, Pahan D, Aung Kya Jai Maug, Withington S, Nicholls P, Alam K, Salim MAH. Outcome of 6 months MB MDT in MB patients in Bangladesh preliminary results. Leprosy Review 2016;87: 171–82.
23. WHO, 2011, Technical Advisory Group on Leprosy,Report of the 11th meeting, 2011.
24. Liangbin, 2016. Yan Liangbin, Shen Jianping, Yu Meiwen, Zhang Guocheng, Li Jinlan & YuXiufeng. Results of 8 years follow-up among multibacillary patients treated with uniform multi-drug therapy in China. Lepr Rev 2016;87:314–21.
25. Stefani MMA, Avanzi C, Bührer-Sékula S, Benjak A, Loiseau C, Singh P, et al. Whole genome sequencing distinguishes between relapse and reinfection in recurrent leprosy cases. PLoSNegl Trop Dis 2017; 11: e0005598.
26. WHO, chemotherapy of leprosy for control programmes. Report of a WHO study group, 1982. WHO Tech rep series number 675.
27. WHO, a guide for surveillance of antimicrobial resistance in leprosy. 2017 update. WHO, Geneva.

2.3 LEPROSY IN CHILDREN

Taru Garg, Sarita Sanke

INTRODUCTION

"Childhood leprosy" refers to leprosy in the age group of 0–14 years. "Child rate" is an important parameter in leprosy control programmes and refers to the percentage of children (less than 15 years of age) among all new cases of leprosy detected.[1]

The importance of this group is that children are considered to be the most vulnerable group to infection due to their naive immunity and close family contacts. Leprosy in this age group serves as a marker of ongoing recent transmission of the disease in the community. Also, early diagnosis and treatment of childhood leprosy is necessary to prevent deformities and to reduce the psychosocial and economic burden of the disease. The new case detection rate in children helps to determine the burden of the disease in a community. The Global Leprosy Strategy 2016–2020 has set a target of zero new pediatric cases with grade 2 deformity (G2D) by 2020.[1]

EPIDEMIOLOGY

A total of 16,013 new child cases were reported worldwide in 2018 with a majority being from South East Asian Region (11,793).[2] India alone accounted for 9227 of these. Overall however, there has been a small decline in new child cases since 2014. G2D was reported in 350 new pediatric cases globally in 2018 *(also see Chapter 1)*.[2]

Leprosy is more common in the age group of 10–14 years, than in younger children. Higher frequency in older children may be due to the long incubation period of leprosy, delay in diagnosis of early lesions and difficulty in assessing the sensory loss in younger children.[3] However, the disease may not be as rare in younger children and infants. Brubaker et al reported 91 infants with leprosy, of which biopsy confirmation was available on 19 infants, and, in an additional 32 patients, the diagnosis of leprosy was considered clinically certain.[4] The mother was the most common source of infection (29 infants).[4] But interestingly, in 43% of cases, the source was the father, another relative or an unknown contact.[4] The youngest infant with leprosy has been reported at 3 weeks from Martinique.[5] The youngest case of tuberculoid leprosy confirmed by histopathology was a 2.5 months old infant.[5] A study from a tertiary pediatric referral hospital found that the youngest age for borderline (BB) leprosy was 6 months.[6] A recent study from Colombia has used circulating antibodies against NDO-LID *(also see Chapter 3, Section 3.1)* and opined that a poor socioeconomic and environmental conditions may predispose to childhood leprosy.[7]

ROUTES OF TRANSMISSION

The importance of physical and genetic closeness in transmission and the various possible routes of transmission of leprosy are dealt with in detail in *Chapter 4, Section 4.2*. Children with leprosy are often first identified during household contact screening, and acquire infection via family members. The risk of leprosy transmission is estimated to be 9 times from a family member contact, 4 times from a neighborhood contact and 14 times if the index case is a mother or a multibacillary (MB) patient.[8] Various series have showed presence of a household contact in 10–36% of childhood cases.[9–17]

Case reports of leprosy in young infants[5] suggest a vertical mode of transmission from mothers to fetus via placenta or via breastfeeding, although it is uncommon. In infants, the most likely route of transmission are skin-to-skin contact with mother and through nasal droplets if the mother has not yet had chemotherapy. The chances of air-borne infection due to close proximity during breastfeeding is low if the mother is on treatment or has already completed multidrug therapy (MDT).[18] Acid-fast bacilli resembling *Mycobacterium leprae* have been detected in the breast milk, but the viability is uncertain.[19] Also, there is no evidence that orally ingested *Mycobacterium leprae* can cause leprosy. Thus, breastfeeding by women who are on MDT is safe for infants.[18]

CLINICAL PRESENTATION AND DIAGNOSIS

There are certain differences between adult and childhood leprosy (enumerated in Table 2.18). When a child is infected with *Mycobacterium leprae*, he/she will either *not* develop leprosy, or *will* develop indeterminate leprosy. This can either self-resolve, remain stationary or may progress to a determinate type. In a leprosarium in the Philippines, of the total 2000 children examined, 470 had symptoms of leprosy and were treated. Amongst those who had doubtful leprosy (and were untreated) and

Table 2.18: Differences between childhood and adult leprosy		
	Adult leprosy	Childhood leprosy
Age	15 years and above	0–14 years, most commonly involved is 9–14 years
Incubation period	Long (12–13 years)	Short. Few weeks to 10–12 years
Bacillary load	Usually multibacillary	Usually paucibacillary
Most common type of leprosy	Can be borderline or lepromatous	Usually indeterminate Single skin lesion is more common followed by 2 to 3; more than 4 skin lesions are rare
Self-resolving skin lesions	Uncommon	Common in children. With the development of immunity as the child grows, the skin lesions can self-resolve
Pure neuritic, histoid and Lazarine leprosy	Can be the presentation in adults	Rarely reported
Reactions and relapses	Both type 1 and type 2 lepra reactions are common. Relapses too can occur	Reactions are usually rare, and more common in older children with multibacillary disease. ENL and relapses are uncommon
Deformities	Common	Rare
Histology	Granuloma formation is an indication of effective build-up of cell-mediated immunity, commonly observed in adult skin and nerve biopsies	Well defined granulomas are usually rare

were followed up for 6 years or more, 75% self-resolved.[20] Similar results were reported by Keeler et al as well.[21] But contrary to this, a study on the natural history of leprosy from Africa revealed that, if observed over 2 years, a proportion of untreated lesions apparently self-healed with overall self-healing being seen in 33% of cases but only in 12% cases in the 0–19 years age group.[22]

Leprosy in children presents mostly as paucibacillary (PB) disease and MB disease is less common. About 60–80% patients show nerve thickening.[13,23–26] The most common presentation described from most series is a single hypopigmented patch predominantly on the exposed body parts with normal or impaired sensations.[3,9,11–13,15]

Amongst the determinate type, borderline tuberculoid (BT) leprosy is the commonest form, reported in several studies (Figs 2.31 and 2.32).[6]

While the details of each type are given below some general principles apply to the clinical presentation of leprosy in children, including affliction of the exposed parts, high rates of nerve involvement, low rate of deformities and reaction and low clinico-histopathological correlation (varies from 45 to 63%).[6]

Diagnosis may be hampered by the inability of the child to co-operate with sensory testing. A method that can be adopted is stroking the skin of the child with a feather and asking him where he felt the tickle. This can then be repeated with his eyes closed.[27] Another technique is to demonstrate on the mother's skin as the child watches, then asking the child to copy his mother. It is crucial to understand that slit skin smear should be the *last* test attempted as it is frequently traumatic to the patient.[27] The frequent differential diagnosis that can be considered in a case of childhood leprosy is enumerated in Table 2.19 (*also see Chapter 9*).

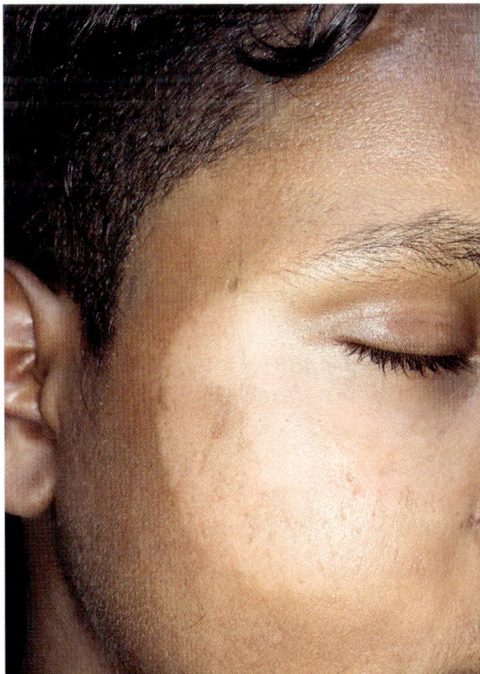
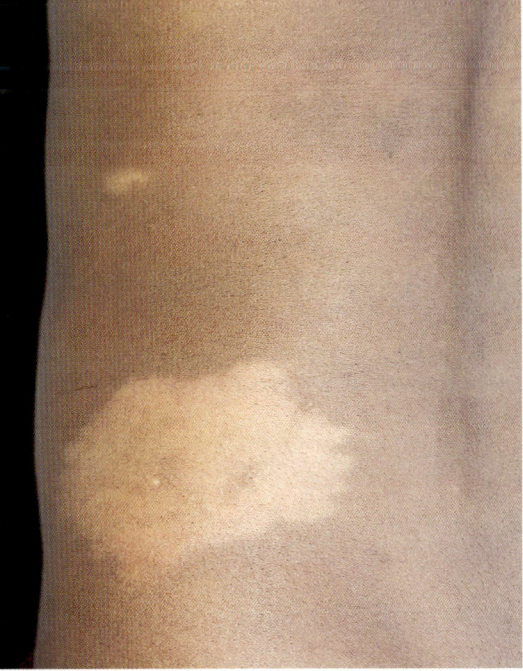

Fig. 2.31: Hypopigmented plaque of BT leprosy over the face in a child

Fig. 2.32: Hypopigmented macules over the trunk in a childhood case of BT leprosy

Table 2.19: Differential diagnosis of leprosy in children *(also see Chapter 9)*	
Hypopigmented patches	Pityriasis alba, vitiligo, pityriasis versicolor, nevus depigmentosus
Erythematous to skin colored plaques	Tinea corporis, histiocytosis, leishmaniasis, lupus vulgaris
Sensory/motor neuropathy	Congenital insensitivity to pain, hereditary sensory motor neuropathy, neuropathy associated with spinal deformity, neurofibromatosis

Indeterminate Leprosy

This presents as a barely palpable hypochromic or erythematous plaque (usually single, but can be up to 5 in number) with ill-defined borders. The sensation can be intact or slight loss is present with loss of hair and sweating. It is commonly present over the exposed areas of the body. Nerves are generally not involved. The indeterminate lesions can self-resolve in 2 to 5 years or may progress to a determinate type. Slit skin smear is negative. Histopathology from the plaque reveals lymphohistiocytic inflammatory infiltrate in perineural, intraneural and periadnexal areas and in the subepidermal zone. Molecular diagnostic tests like multiplex PCR can help in the diagnosis of leprosy with limited clinical manifestations.[28]

Tuberculoid Leprosy

Children with good immunity will confine the bacillus in a localized area with the consequential development of TT leprosy. These lesions, in comparison to indeterminate type, are usually single, more well defined and raised with usually complete loss of sensation. Asymmetrical thickened nerves are usually present. Slit skin smear does not show any bacilli.

Nodular Leprosy of Childhood

Nodular leprosy (NL) or Souza-Campos nodule of leprosy is a benign variant of tuberculoid leprosy commonly found in children. It presents as indurated papulo-nodules, wheal-like lesions, solitary infiltration and lichenoid skin lesions over the limbs, face and buttocks. On histopathology, NL lesions are characterized by dense granulomas with a greater number of confluent tubercles in comparison to the classical tuberculoid lesions.[29] These nodules remain stable for a few years and then self-resolve leaving quite a characteristic scar. There is no peripheral neural involvement or deformity. Acid-fast bacilli are usually not demonstrated in the skin lesions.

Borderline and Lepromatous Leprosy

BT leprosy (Fig. 2.33) is the most common determinate type of leprosy with the prevalence ranging from 42 to 78% of all childhood cases. The presentation in children is similar to that in adults. Borderline-borderline (Fig. 2.34), Borderline lepromatous (Figs 2.35 to 2.38) and lepromatous leprosy (Fig. 2.39) can also be seen in children. However, these are generally not seen in the early stages.

Other variants of leprosy like pure neuritic, histoid and Lazarine leprosy are very rare in children.

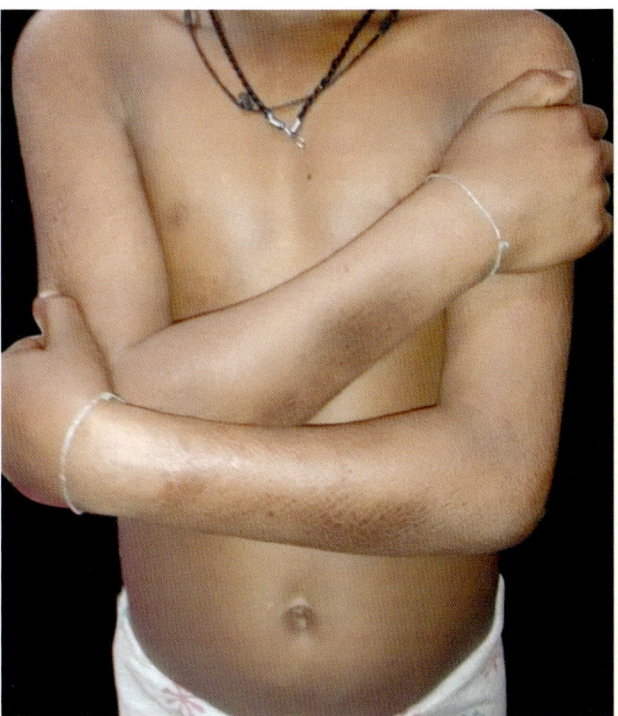

Fig. 2.33: Large dry "ichthyotic" patches of BT leprosy over upper limbs

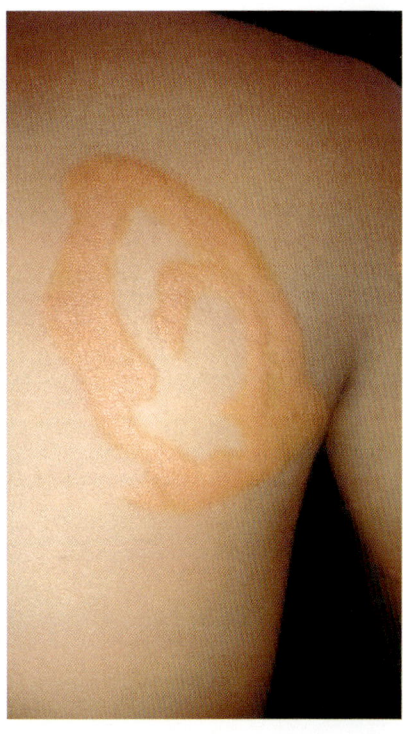

Fig. 2.34: Classic annular skin lesion of mid-borderline (BB) leprosy

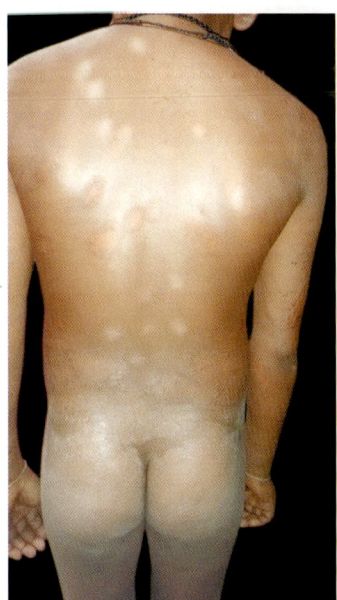

Fig. 2.35: Multiple hypopigmented skin lesions (tending to be symmetrical) of BL leprosy in a child

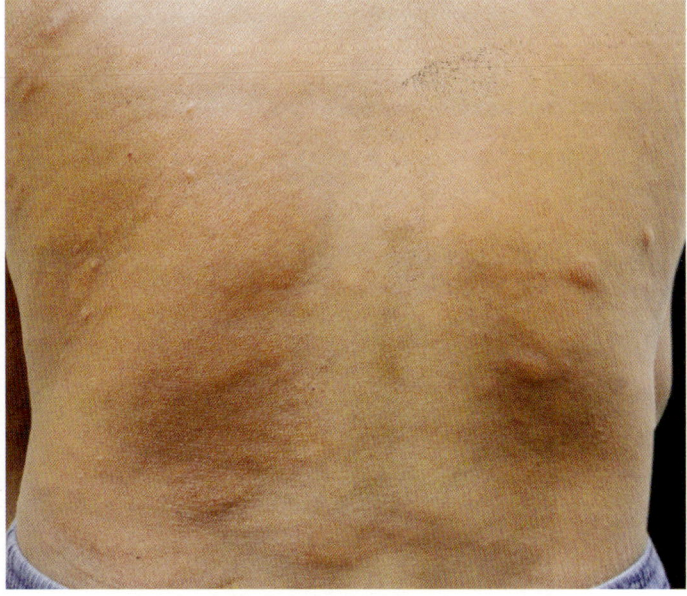

Fig. 2.36: Borderline lepromatous leprosy in an adolescent

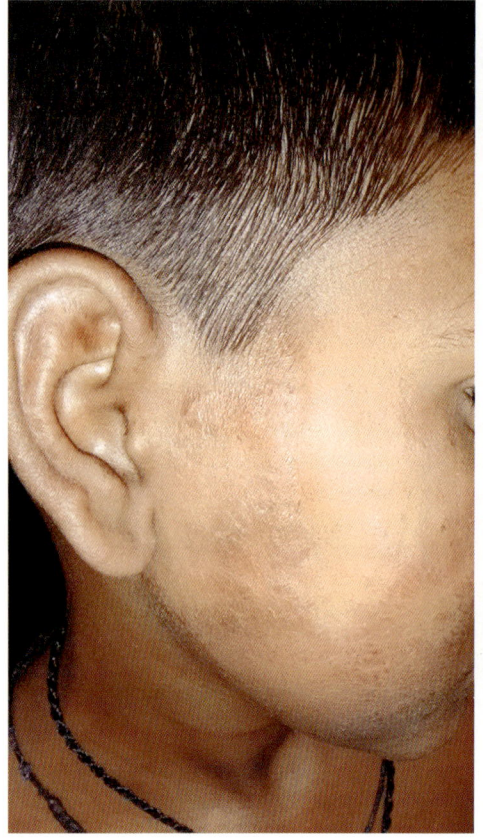

Fig. 2.37: Plaques over the face in borderline lepromatous leprosy

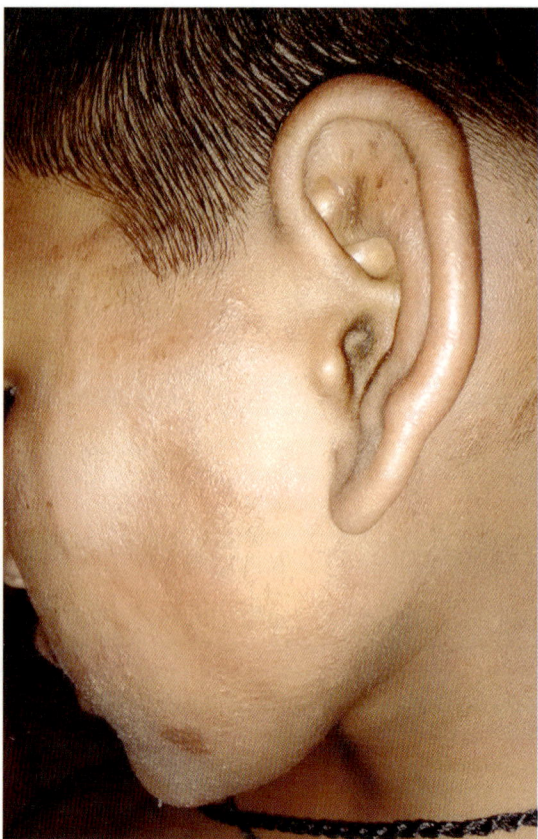

Fig. 2.38: Ear lobe infiltration in a borderline lepromatous case

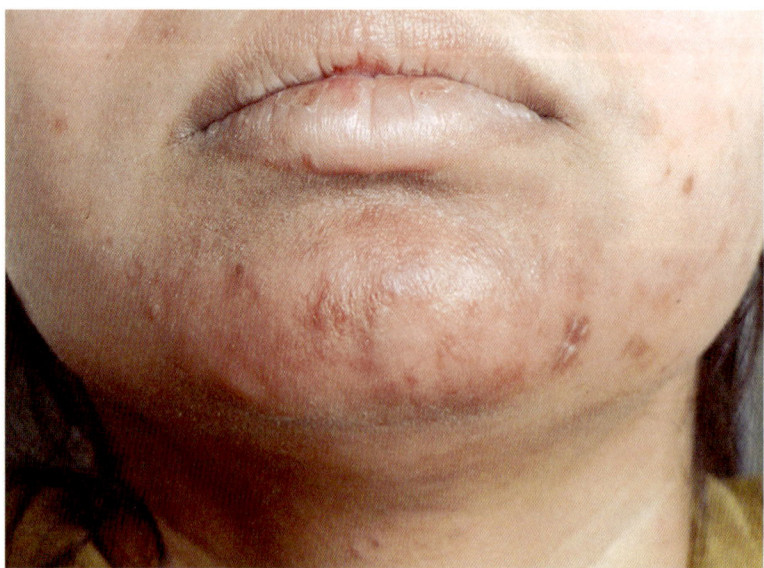

Fig. 2.39: Infiltration over the chin in lepromatous leprosy

Reactions in Childhood Leprosy

Reactions in children are not as common as in adults, possibly due to the high PB proportion amongst children and relatively weak immunity. The occurrence of reactions or neuritis is reported in 20–30% of child cases but little has been published on the frequency, management or outcome of treatment of reaction or neuritis in children.[27] Older children and children with borderline disease are at higher risk. A review of Indian literature from the last two decades, revealed that reactions occurred in 1.36–29.7% of pediatric cases and this included both type 1 (1.16–28.10%) and type 2 (0.12–5.81%) reactions.[30] This is low as compared to adults where more than 50% of the patients develop reactions.

Type 1 reactions have been reported in children with BT leprosy and the implicated triggering factors include MDT, infections, parasite infestations, immunization and stress. Type 2 reaction/erythema nodosum leprosum (ENL) however is rare in children (Figs 2.40 and 2.41). Lepra reactions are the main cause of neural damage and deformities, and also cause considerable suffering to children. Nerve function assessment should be done regularly, especially in children with MB leprosy, as a child may not self-report new impairment.

Deformities in Children

Deformities hinder the physical, social and academic development of a child. Though rare in children, deformities can be found in older children with MB disease, or those who have neuritis at presentation. This is dependent on varied factors including increasing age, delay in accessing health care, multiple skin lesions, MB disease, smear positivity, multiple nerve involvement, and reaction at the time of presentation to the hospital. Children with thickened nerve trunks have 6.1 times higher risk of developing deformities compared to those who do not have nerve enlargement.[31] A study from a

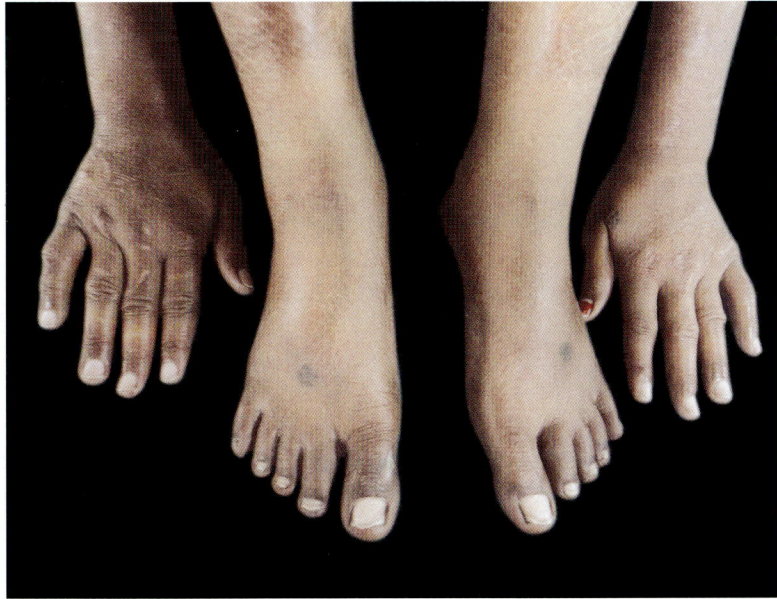

Fig. 2.40: Type 2 reaction in a child with edema of hands and feet

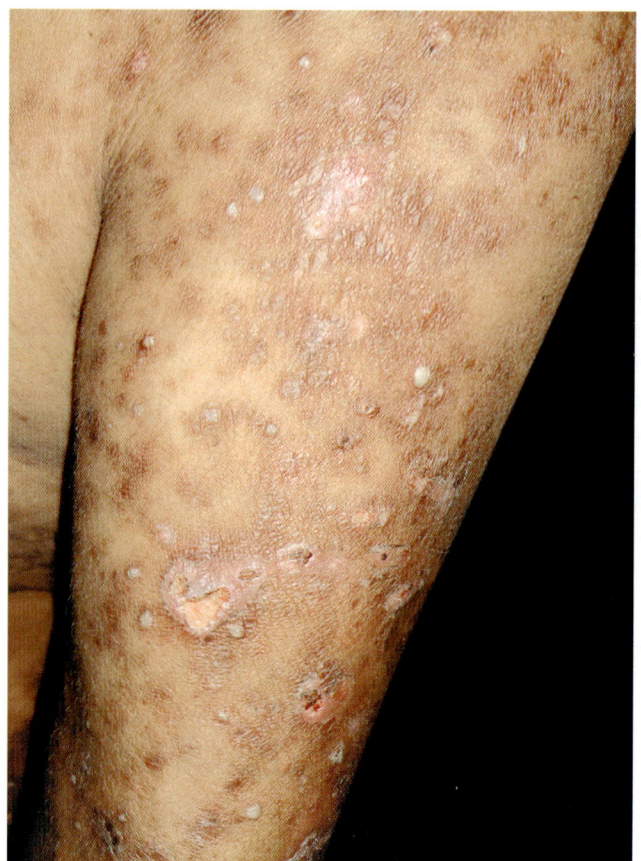

Fig. 2.41: "Pustular" erythema nodosum leprosum in an adolescent

pediatric hospital from India showed that claw hand was the commonest deformity, followed by trophic ulcer, foot drop, and wrist drop in that order.[6]

CHEMOTHERAPY

Treatment in Children (also see Chapter 7)

In children with diagnostic signs, it is usual to treat immediately with MDT (Figs 2.42 and 2.43) rather than to wait and observe. If there is a doubt about the diagnosis (and there is no new nerve function impairment/reaction requiring urgent intervention), it is usually safe and acceptable to keep the child under observation (untreated) for some period of time. When the lesion is re-examined after an interval, it may show more definitive features.[27]

The patient's weight should always be recorded and used to determine the correct dosage of MDT, bearing in mind that in some endemic countries the standard 'child pack' contains doses (Table 2.20) too high for the majority of child cases. Thus, the aim should be for doses close to 10 mg/kg of rifampicin, 2 mg/kg/day of dapsone and 1 mg/kg (daily) and 6 mg/kg (monthly supervised dose) of clofazimine. Ingestion of capsules and tablets may become a reason for noncompliance but unfortunately appropriate syrup preparations are not available.

The Disease

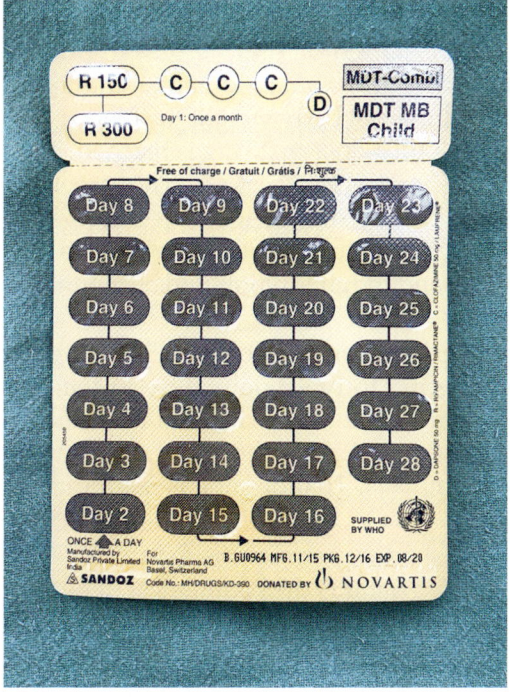

Fig. 2.42: MB MDT blister pack for children (yellow kit)

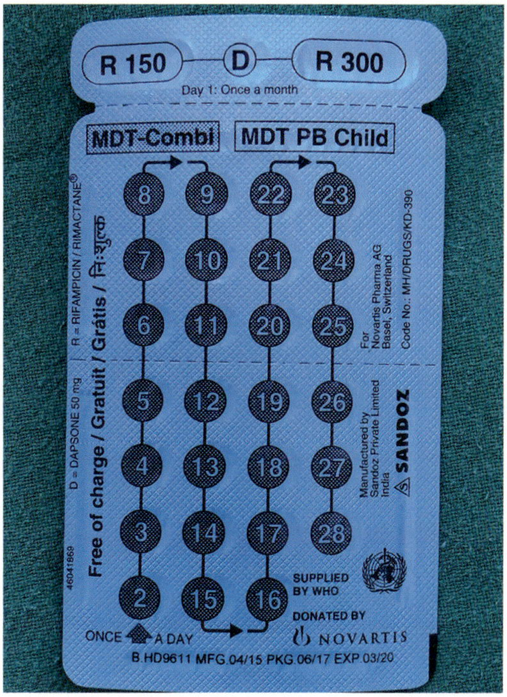

Fig. 2.43: PB MDT blister pack for children (blue kit)

Table 2.20: Treatment of leprosy in children		
	Paucibacillary MDT (6 months)	*Multibacillary MDT (12 months)*
0–9 years	Rifampicin 10 mg/kg monthly, supervised	Rifampicin 10 mg/kg monthly, supervised
	Dapsone 2 mg/kg daily	Dapsone 2 mg/kg daily
		Clofazimine 6 mg/kg monthly supervised and 1 mg/kg daily
10–14 years (<40 kg)	Rifampicin 450 mg monthly, supervised	Rifampicin 450 mg monthly supervised
	Dapsone 50 mg daily	Dapsone 50 mg daily
		Clofazimine 150 mg monthly, supervised and 50 mg every other day
Blister pack	Blue kit (Fig. 2.43)	Yellow kit (Fig. 2.42)
>14 years	Rifampicin 600 mg monthly, supervised	Rifampicin 600 mg monthly, supervised
	Dapsone 100 mg daily	Dapsone 100 mg daily
		Clofazimine 300 mg monthly supervised and 50 mg daily
Blister pack	Green	Red

Treatment of Reactions and Management of Deformities

The children with severe reaction/neuritis can be started on oral steroids to prevent deformities. Steroids are prescribed similar to that in adults but modified for the child's weight. Prednisolone can be started at a dose of 1 mg/kg body weight for 1 week, and then slowly tapered by 5 mg in subsequent weeks till a dose of 20 mg is reached. Then the dose can be slowly tapered by 5 mg every 2–4 weeks (*see Chapter 5*). The associated risks with steroids including immunosuppression interfering with the vaccination schedule, effect on skeletal growth and puberty, osteoporosis, hyperglycemia and adrenal suppression must always be kept in mind and the children should be monitored frequently for these side effects.

For type 2 (ENL) reaction, clofazimine can also be given at a dose of 1.5 to 2 mg/kg three times daily for 1 month, followed by tapering to twice daily dose in the next month and then to once daily dose in the subsequent month.[32] The total dose should not exceed 300 mg/day. The parents should be counseled about the risk of clofazimine-induced pigmentation and gastrointestinal side effects. Thalidomide is *not* indicated in children <12 years of age.

Reconstructive surgery for those with established impairment is feasible even in young patients. A study has shown that ulnar claw hand is the commonest deformity in children and early intervention in the form of tendon transfer surgery is a useful modality.[33] Tendon transfer corrects established clawing of fingers and yields good results thereby facilitating hand functions to complete daily routine and academic activities. Lasso surgery for intrinsic replacement, using the flexor digitorum sublimus (FDS) of the middle or ring finger, the palmaris longus or extensor carpi radialis longus with fascia lata graft, has been a standard procedure for correcting clawed fingers in leprosy affected children.[33] For trophic ulcers, off-loading options such as the use of plaster of Paris (a double rocker shoe/BK cast with Bohler iron) should be considered. Microcellular rubber footwear (MCR) has been found to be helpful in healing plantar ulcers as well as in the prevention of recurrences. It has a soft insole, which reduces pressure over the plantar surface.[34] Also importance needs to be given on adequate nutrition for wound healing in a growing child.

Vaccination and Chemoprophylaxis

BCG vaccination, an inexpensive measure may provide protection (although partial) against leprosy and may halt the progression of the disease (*also see Chapter 7, Section 7.2*). BCG at birth is effective at reducing the risk of leprosy; therefore, its use should be maintained at least in all leprosy high-burden countries or settings (good quality of evidence).[35]

Chemoprophylaxis has been suggested by WHO in high risk contacts like children (more than 2 years of age) with MB patients. Single dose rifampicin (SDR) is given at a dose of 450 mg for children 10–14 years of age, 300 mg for children 6–9 years (or >20 kg) and 10–15 mg/kg for children <20 kg (>2 years) as a chemoprophylactic agent[30] (*also see Chapter 7, Section 7.2*).

CONCLUSION

In a study done to evaluate the attitude of children and adolescents with leprosy using the Child Attitude Towards Illness Scale (CATIS), one-third reported experiencing internalized stigma.[36] Srinivas et al[37] found that the most common initial symptom in childhood leprosy is a white patch and the median duration between recognition of the symptom and care-seeking was 6 months. The most commonly reported side effect was clofazimine-induced discoloration which leads to non-adherence as well as school absenteeism. Also none of the parents had any knowledge of reactions. Thus, it is essential to counsel and educate the parents to ensure proper therapy, as they would directly administer the therapy to the children, and to explain to the child as much as he/she can understand.

The high incidence of childhood leprosy has an epidemiological significance and there is a need for a community survey to detect hidden cases of leprosy. Regular school surveys and annual household contact surveys for early detection of cases is also an important tool in achieving the goal of elimination of leprosy and both WHO and governments advise at least one household contact survey. Early detection and treatment will decrease the burden of leprosy related complications thereby preventing school dropouts due to the disease and lifelong disability due to childhood leprosy. Directly Observed Treatment (DOT) centers have been proposed by WHO for ensuring compliance of treatment at least in pediatric cases.[30]

REFERENCES

1. World Health Organization. Global Leprosy Strategy 2016–2020: accelerating towards a leprosy-free world—operational manual.
2. WHO. Weekly epidemiological record 2019; 94: 389–412 (https://apps.who.int/iris/bit-stream/handle/10665/326775/WER9435-36-en-fr.pdf)
3. Singal A, Sonthalia S, Pandhi D. Childhood leprosy in a tertiary-care hospital in Delhi, India: A reappraisal in the post-elimination era. Lepr Rev 2011;82:259–69.
4. Brubaker ML, Meyers WM, Bourland J. Leprosy in children one year of age and under. Int J Lepr Other Mycobact Dis. 1985;53:517–23.
5. Montestruc E, Berdonneau R. 2 New cases of leprosy in infants in Martinique. Bull Soc Pathol Exot Filiales 1954;47:781–3.
6. Mahajan S, Sardana K, Bhushan P, Koranne RV, Mendiratta V. A study of leprosy in children, from a tertiary pediatric hospital in India. Lepr Rev 2006;77:160–2.
7. Serrano-Coll H, Mora HR, Beltrán JC, Duthie MS, Cardona-Castro N. Social and environmental conditions related to *Mycobacterium leprae* infection in children and adolescents from three leprosy endemic regions of Colombia. BMC Infect Dis 2019;19:520.
8. Oliveira MB, Diniz LM. Leprosy among children under 15 years of age: Literature review. An Bras Dermatol 2016;91:196–203.
9. Naik S. Repeat leprosy survey after 7 years in night high schools in greater Bombay. Indian J Lepr 1996;68:377–8.
10. Burman KD, Rijall A, Agrawal S, Agarwalla A, Verma KK. Childhood leprosy in Eastern Nepal: A hospital-based study. Indian J Lepr 2003;75:47–52.
11. Selvasekar A, Geetha J, Nisha K, Manimozhi N, Jesudasan K, Rao PS, et al. Childhood leprosy in an endemic area. Lepr Rev 1999;70:21–7.
12. Shetty VP, Ghate SD, Wakade AV, Thakar UH, Thakur DV, D'souza E, et al. Clinical, bacteriological, and histopathological characteristics of newly detected children with leprosy: A population-based study in a defined rural and urban area of Maharashtra, Western India. Indian J Dermatol Venereol Leprol 2013; 79:512–7.
13. Dogra S, Narang T, Khullar G, Kumar R, Saikia UN. Childhood leprosy through the post-leprosy-elimination era: a retrospective analysis of epidemiological and clinical characteristics of disease over eleven years from a tertiary care hospital in North India. Lepr Rev 2014;85:296–310.

14. Sehgal VN, Rege VL, Mascarenhas MF, Reys M. The prevalence and pattern of leprosy in a school survey. Int J Lepr Other Mycobact Dis 1977;45:360–3.
15. Palit A, Inamadar AC. Childhood leprosy in India over the past two decades. Lepr Rev 2014; 85:93–9.
16. Van Beers SM, Hatta M, Klatser PR. Patient contact is the major determinant in incident leprosy: implications for future control. Int J Lepr Other Mycobact Dis 1999;67:119–28.
17. Dave DS, Agrawal SK. Prevalence of leprosy in children of leprosy parents. Indian J Lepr1984; 56:615–21.
18. World Health Organization. The final push strategy to eliminate leprosy as a public health problem: Questions and answers. Geneva: World Health Organization; 2003.
19. Girdhar A, Girdhar BK, Ramu G, Desikan KV. Discharge of *M. Leprae* in milk of leprosy patients. Lepr India 1981; 53:390–4.
20. Lara CB, Nolasco JO. Self-healing or abortive, and residual forms of childhood leprosy and their probable signifiicance. Int J Lepr 1956;24:245–63.
21. Keeler R, Deen RD. Leprosy in children aged 0–14 years: report of an 11-year-control programme. Lepr Rev 1985;56:239–48.
22. Browne SG. Self-healing leprosy: Report on 2749 patients. Lepr Rev 1974;45:104–11.
23. Kumar B, Rani R, Kaur I. Childhood leprosy in Chandigarh; clinico-histopathological correlation. Int J Lepr Other Mycobact Dis 2000;68:330–1.
24. Sehgal VN, Chaudhry AK. Leprosy in children: a prospective study. Int J Dermatol 1993; 32:194–7.
25. Jain S, Reddy RG, Osmani SN, Lockwood DN, Suneetha S. Childhood leprosy in an Urban Clinic, Hyderabad, India: clinical presentation and the role of household contacts. Lepr Rev 2002;73:248–53.
26. Grover C, Nanda S, Garg VK, Reddy BS. An epidemiologic study of childhood leprosy from Delhi. Pediatr Dermatol 2005; 22: 489–90.
27. Butlin CR, Saunderson P. Children with leprosy. Lepr Rev 2014;85:69–73.
28. Chaitanya VS, Cuello L, Das M, Sudharsan A, Ganesan P, Kanmani K, et al. Analysis of a novel multiplex polymerase chain reaction assay as a sensitive tool for the diagnosis of indeterminate and tuberculoid forms of leprosy. Int J Mycobacteriol 2017;6:1–8.
29. Fakhouri R, Sotto MN, Manini MI, Margarido LC. Nodular leprosy of childhood and tuberculoid leprosy: A comparative, morphologic, immunopathologic and quantitative study of skin tissue reaction. Int J Lepr Other Mycobact Dis. 2003;71:218–26.
30. Guidelines for the diagnosis, treatment and prevention of leprosy. New Delhi: World Health Organization, Regional Office for South-East Asia; 2017. Licence: CC BY-NC-SA 3.0 IGO.
31. Kar BR, Job CK. Visible deformity in childhood leprosy—a 10-year study. Int J Lepr Other Mycobact Dis. 2005;73:243–8.
32. Yawalkar SJ. 1993. Lamprene in leprosy. Basic information (4th ed). Ciba-Geigy, Basle, Switzerland.
33. Manivannan G, Das P, Karthikeyan G, John AS. Reconstructive surgery in children to correct ulnar claw hand deformity due to leprosy. Lepr Rev 2014;85:74–80.
34. Lal V, Sarkar D, Das S, Mahato M, Srinivas G. A study to assess the usage of MCR footwear in West Bengal, India. Lepr Rev 2015;86:273–7.
35. World Health Organization. BCG vaccines: WHO position paper—February 2018. Wkly Epidemiol Rec 2018;93:73–96.
36. Govindharaj P, Darlong J, John AS, Mani S. Children and adolescents' attitude towards having leprosy in a high endemic district of India. Lepr Rev 2016;87:42–52.
37. Srinivas GO. What parents should know while their child is on MDT? Insights from a qualitative study in Eastern India. Lepr Rev 2014;85:81–4.

2.4 PURE NEURITIC LEPROSY

Tarun Narang, Debajyoti Chatterjee, Vishal Thakur

Pure neuritic leprosy (PNL) is defined as exclusive nerve involvement in the form of nerve thickening or neural deficit without any skin lesions, a negative slit skin smear, in the absence of other causes of nerve involvement.[1] Although, exclusive neural involvement is needed for defining PNL, subclinical cutaneous involvement surrounding involved nerves has been noted histopathologically, which consequentially leads to development of cutaneous lesions. The prevalence of PNL in India ranges from 4.7 to 17%,[2] with higher prevalence in Southern part of India. PNL is less prevalent outside Indian subcontinent, but significant number of cases are reported from Africa and South America.[3] PNL is more common in males with 15–30 years of age group being most commonly affected.[2, 4]

The pathogenesis of neural involvement has been discussed in *Chapter 4, Section 4.4* and a similar process has been implicated in PNL, with selective localization of *M. leprae* to Schwann cells,[5,6] antigen presentation by Schwann cells,[7] presence of pro-inflammatory cytokines such as TNF-α[8] and resultant loss of myelination.

Clinical Features

PNL may present with one or more of the following features: Area of sensory loss, weakness of a limb (with or without deformities), ulcers and other secondary changes over skin (xerosis, ichthyosis, decreased or absent sweating, loss of appendages), thickened nerve trunks (regular, irregular, beaded or nodular), nerve tenderness, neuropathic pain and occasionally nerve abscesses.

Nerves of upper extremities, especially ulnar nerve, is the most commonly affected in PNL followed by lower limbs (common peroneal nerve and posterior tibial nerve). Other nerve trunks are less commonly affected. Nerve involvement is mostly in the form of mononeuritis (approximately 60%).[9] However, mononeuritis multiplex and polyneuritic form, also called 'mononeuritis multiplex summation', are also not uncommon[10] and if present, should lead to thorough evaluation to rule out lepromatous leprosy.[3]

While low grade inflammation of nerves leading to silent neuritis is always present in PNL, type 1 reaction may produce intermittent episodes of acute severe neuritis and new nerve function impairments *(also see Chapter 5, Section 5.1)*.

There are *no* specific clinical features of PNL and thus a high index of *suspicion* is required to make a clinical diagnosis of PNL. A diagnostic criteria of PNL has been proposed and is listed in *Table 2.21*.[2] Other causes which should be excluded are metabolic (diabetes, amyloidosis), infections (syphilis, HIV neuropathy, poliomyelitis), sarcoidosis, hereditary causes (Charcot-Marie-Tooth disease, syringomyelia, hereditary neuropathy) and tumors *(also see Chapter 9)*.[1]

Investigations *(also see Chapter 3)*

A slit skin smear (SSS) should be done in all suspected cases of PNL to rule out early cases of lepromatous leprosy in patients with symmetrical polyneuropathy.

Table 2.21: Diagnostic criteria of PNL[2]	

A. Essential criteria
  i. *Epidemiological features*
    • Residence in an endemic area or a history of contact with cases of leprosy
  ii. *Clinical features*
    • Thickened peripheral nerve(s) with definitive sensory impairment[*] with or without motor impairment[#] or loss of function
    • Absence of any skin lesion
  iii. *Laboratory features*
    • SSS from 3 different sites including the anesthetic area should be negative.
    • No definitive histological features of leprosy in skin biopsy from area of sensory impairment
	B. Auxiliary criteria
	• Nerve biopsy/fine needle aspiration cytology when done shows *definitive* (AFB or caseous necrosis) or *suggestive* (perineural or endoneural infiltrate and perineural fibrosis) features of leprosy neuritis
	• Nerve conduction studies showing decline in amplitude and nerve conduction velocities or increase in latency

[*]Assessed by Semmes-Weinstein monofilaments. [#]Assessed by British Medical Research Council grading system.

Nerve biopsy is the gold standard for the diagnosis of PNL *(also see Chapter 3, Section 3.1)*. Nerve biopsy should only be taken from a sensory branch. However, it is associated with certain risks such as nerve damage, inappropriate site selection, permanent functional deficit of area supplied by the nerve and low sensitivity.[11–13] The histopathology from nerve biopsy in PNL ranges from the tuberculoid pole to lepromatous pole *(Figs 2.44 to 2.50)*.

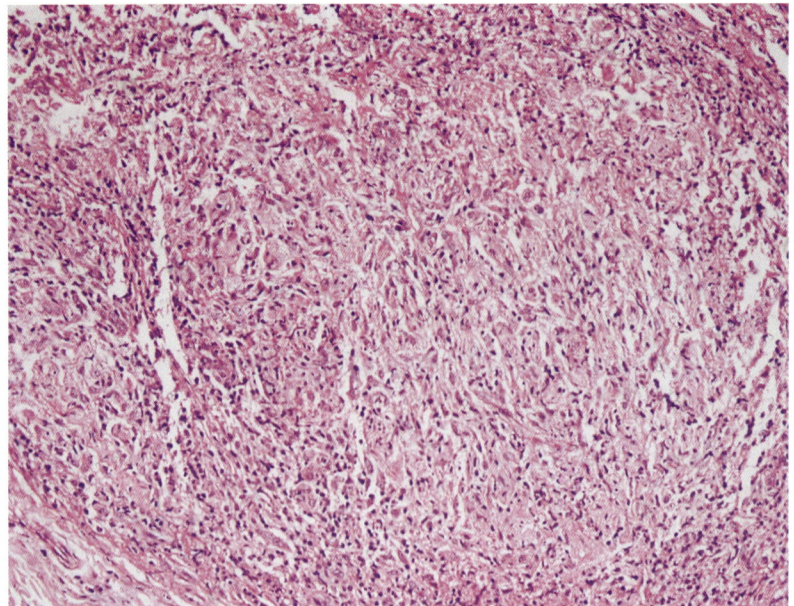

Fig. 2.44: Lepromatous leprosy. Transverse section of nerve biopsy shows expanded nerve fascicle, with endoneural infiltration by foamy macrophages

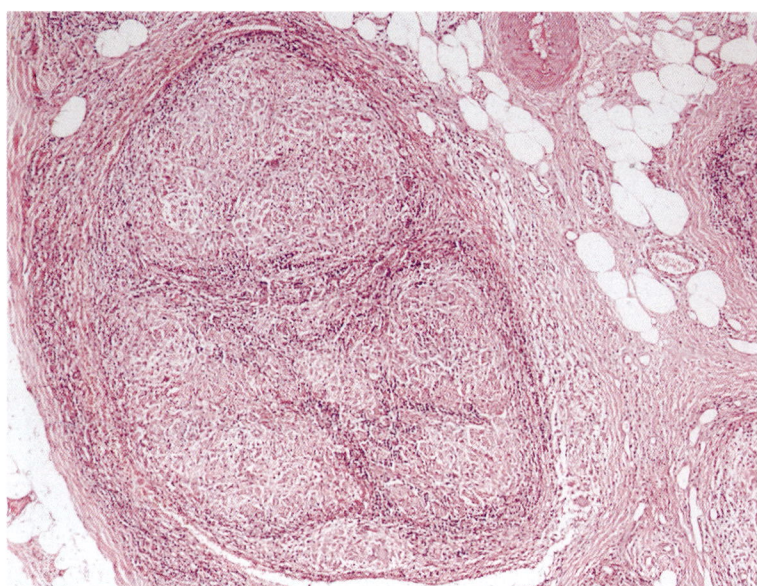

Fig. 2.45: Borderline lepromatous leprosy. Transverse section of nerve biopsy shows expanded nerve fascicles, with endoneural infiltration by foamy macrophages, admixed with few epithelioid cells and lymphocytes. Mild perineural inflammation is also noted

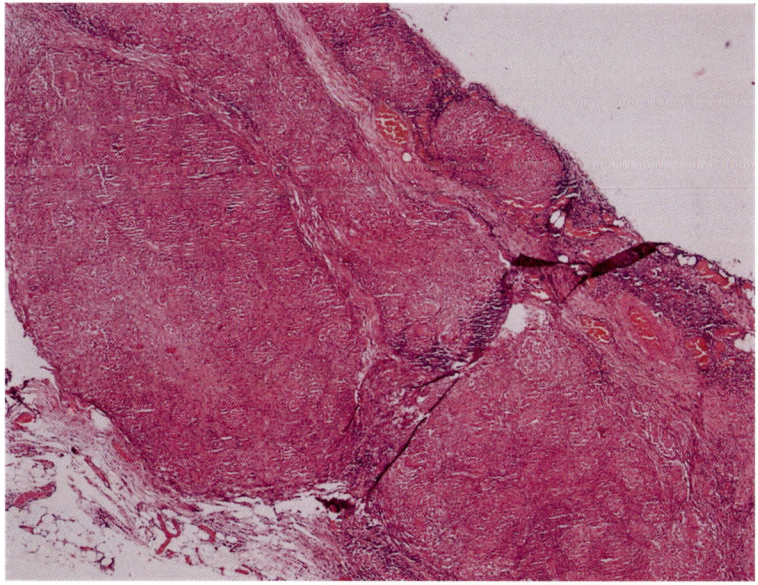

Fig. 2.46: Borderline tuberculoid leprosy. Longitudinal section of nerve biopsy shows multiple expanded nerve fascicles, due to multiple well-formed epithelioid cell granulomas in the endoneural location, along with mild lymphomononuclear cuffing

Auxiliary investigations that may have a potential role in diagnosing PNL include skin biopsy (from area of sensory loss or even normal appearing skin),[14,15] biopsy from nasal mucosa,[16] immunohistochemistry with phenolic glycolipid 1 (PGL-1) or lipoarabinomannan, fine needle aspiration cytology (FNAC) of the affected nerves

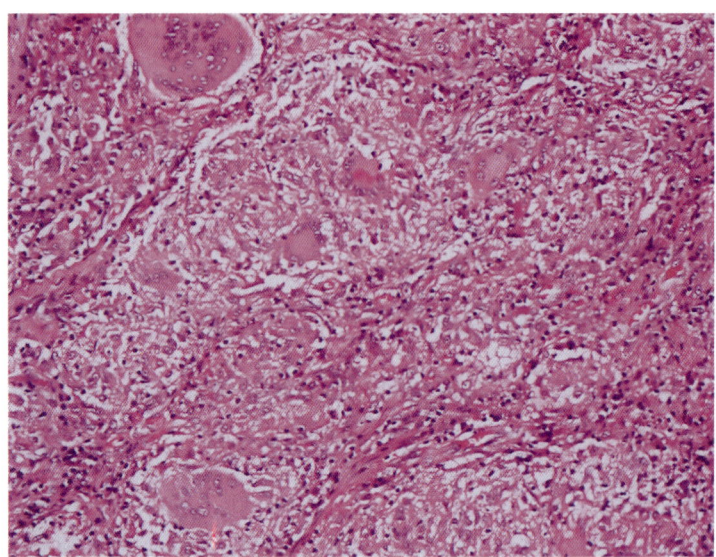

Fig. 2.47: Borderline tuberculoid leprosy. Higher magnification of the same case showing multiple, compact, epithelioid cell granulomas along with Langhans' giant cells

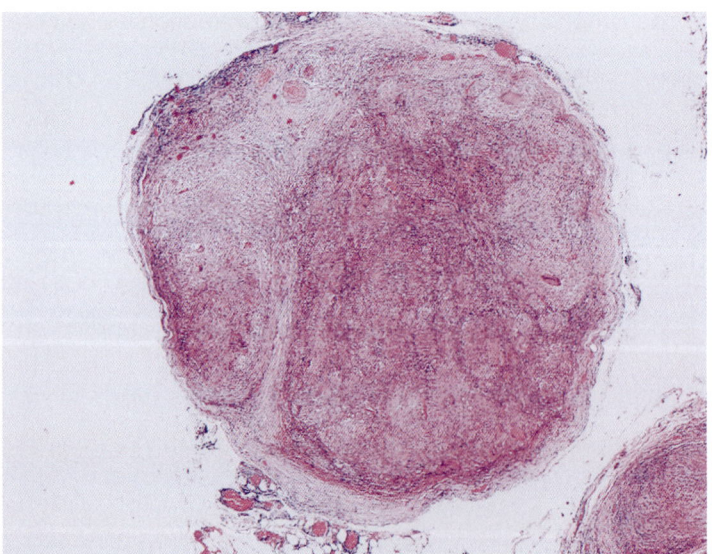

Fig. 2.48: Tuberculoid leprosy (TT). Transverse section of nerve biopsy showing multiple, varying size, endoneural epithelioid cell granulomas. Perineural fibrosis and mild epineural lymphoid infiltrate are also noted

(safe, easy, less invasive procedure and results comparable with nerve biopsy) and *M. leprae* DNA polymerase chain reaction (PCR) analysis from nerve aspirate[17, 18] (*also see Chapter 3*).

Electrophysiological studies such as nerve conduction study (NCS) also serve as a diagnostic as well as monitoring tool. Findings commonly seen in NCS are reduced amplitude of sensory and motor nerve action potentials (SNAP and compound muscle action potential or CMAP) which is indicative of axonal damage, decreased nerve

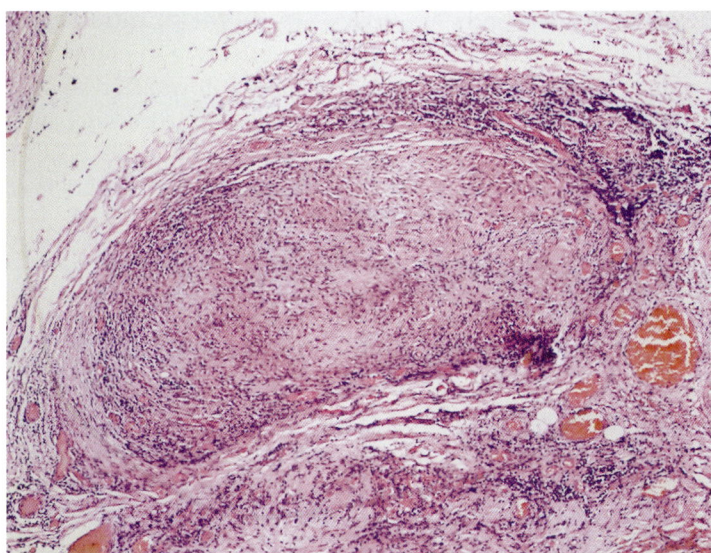

Fig. 2.49: Chronic tubercular leprosy. Transverse section of nerve biopsy showing a nerve fascicle showing marked endoneural fibrosis, along with few vague epithelioid cell granulomas and mild endoneural lymphocytic infiltrate. Epineural lymphoid infiltrate is also present

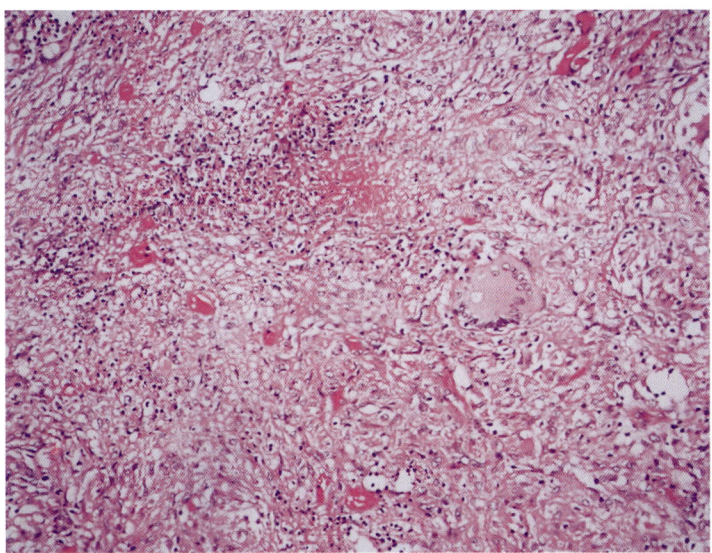

Fig. 2.50: Borderline lepromatous leprosy in type 2 lepra reaction. Nerve biopsy showing endoneural infiltration by foamy macrophages, along with few epithelioid cells and a few giant cells. Features of type 2 reaction such as focus of necrosis, nuclear debris and neutrophilic infiltrate are also identified

conduction velocity and increased latency.[1] These findings usually precede the clinically apparent nerve function impairment (NFI) and can detect subclinical neural involvement. However, a study comparing combination of nerve palpation with Semmes-Weinstein (SW) monofilament testing and voluntary muscle testing (VMT) showed comparable efficacy to NCS in detecting nerve damage.[19]

Recently, development of high frequency (15–20 MHz) ultrasonography (HRUS) has made visualization of nerves easier and cost-effective in comparison to magnetic resonance imaging (MRI). This technique provides information about exact site and size of nerve thickness, morphological variations in nerve trunk such as texture, pattern of fascicles and vascularity.[20, 21] This is very important in diagnosis of PNL and also in identifying reactions in PNL as increased vascularity and edema of nerve trunk signifies neuritis. A diagnostic algorithm has been illustrated in Fig. 2.51.

Complications and Sequelae

As with other types of leprosy nerve involvement, PNL may also produce complications like sensory and motor impairments, trophic changes and ulcerations and deformities such as claw hand or foot drop (which may be the initial presentation of PNL in neglected cases).[4, 22] Another significant complication of PNL includes nerve abscess which may be single or multiple in same or different nerve trunks.[23, 24] Another rarely reported entity in PNL is segmental necrotizing granulomatous neuritis (SNGN) which presents as nodular lesions of varying sizes along the nerve trunk.[25]

Over time, PNL can progress to the other clinical forms of leprosy including indeterminate, BT and BL spectrum.[26] This has been noted in approximately 15–35% of patients within 2 years of diagnosis of PNL,[27] while a few of them may develop cutaneous lesions during the multi-drug therapy (MDT). Moreover, cutaneous lesions

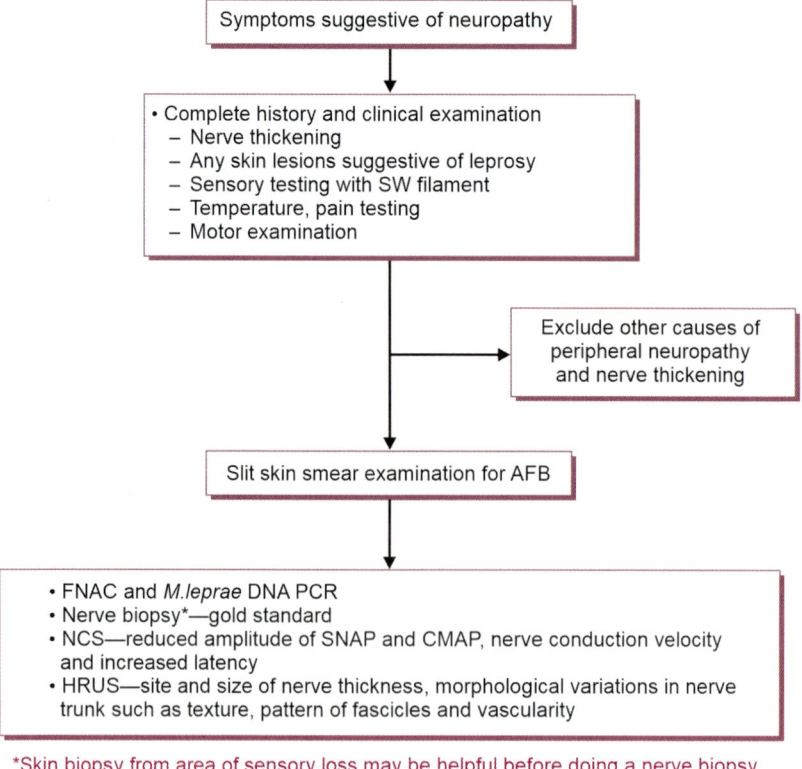

*Skin biopsy from area of sensory loss may be helpful before doing a nerve biopsy

Fig. 2.51: An algorithm depicting diagnostic approach for pure neuritic leprosy
NCS: Nerve conduction study, HRUS: High-resolution ultrasound

in PNL may appear first time during the episodes of reactions.[28] Thus, these patients require a close follow-up even after completion of treatment. If not treated early, the chronic inflammation of nerves associated with PNL leads to nerve destruction and later on fibrosis.

Treatment

Earlier, single nerve involvement was classified as paucibacillary and two or more nerve involvements as multibacillary leprosy. However, according to the latest WHO guidelines, even a single nerve involvement qualifies as multibacillary (MB) and should be treated with 12 months of 3 drugs regimen, i.e. rifampicin, clofazimine and dapsone.[29] A paradoxical aspect is that MDT does *not* halt the progression of nerve damage, rather nerve damage may occur during MDT and reactions. Thus, nerve damage needs to be treated aggressively with systemic corticosteroids. Moreover, there are no guidelines for the management of chronic low grade inflammation and silent neuritis in PNL, with the prophylactic role of steroids in prevention of NFI being controversial.

Recently, a study demonstrated efficacy of minocycline 100 mg/day in recent onset NFI in leprosy patients.[30] Minocycline possesses antiapoptotic and immunomodulatory properties along with anti-nociceptive effects.[31] Also, minocycline helps in controlling neuropathic pain which is another key management issue in PNL. Tricyclic antidepressants such as amitriptyline and anticonvulsants like pregabalin and gabapentin are the commonly used drugs for management of neuropathic pain.[32] Other aspects in management of PNL include education about self-care of hands and feet, physiotherapy and rehabilitation surgeries (*see Chapter 8, Sections 8.1 to 8.4*).

REFERENCES

1. Kumar B. Pure or primary neuritic leprosy (PNL). Lepr Rev 2016;87:450–55.
2. Narang T, Vinay K, Kumar S, Dogra S. A critical appraisal on pure neuritic leprosy from India after achieving WHO global target of leprosy elimination. Lepr Rev 2016;87:456–63.
3. Rao PN, Suneetha S. Pure neuritic leprosy: Current status and relevance. Indian J Dermatol Venereol Leprol 2016;82:252–61.
4. Mendiratta V, Khan A, Jain A. Primary neuritic leprosy: A reappraisal at a tertiary care hospital. Indian J Lepr 2006;78:261–7.
5. Rambukkana A, Salzer JL, Yurchenco PD, Tuomanen EI. Neural targeting of *Mycobacterium leprae* mediated by the G domain of the laminin-α_2 chain. Cell 1997;88:811–21.
6. Ng V, Zanazzi G, Timpl R, Talts JF, Salzer JL, Brennan PJ, et al. Role of the cell wall phenolic glycolipid 1 in the peripheral nerve predilection of *Mycobacterium leprae*. Cell 2000;103: 511–24.
7. Steinhoff U, Wand-Wurttenberger A, Bremerich A, Kaufmann SH. *Mycobacterium leprae* renders Schwann cells and mononuclear phagocytes susceptible or resistant to killer cells. Infect Immun. 1991;59:684–8.
8. Skoff AM, Lisak RP, Bealmear B, Benjamins JA. TNF-α and TGF-β act synergistically to kill Schwann cells. J Neurosci Res. 1998;53:747–56.
9. Nascimento OJ. Leprosy neuropathy: Clinical presentations. Arq Neuropsiquiatr 2013;71:661–6.
10. Jardim MR, Chimelli L, Faria SC, Fernandes PV, Da Costa Neri JA, Sales AM, et al. Clinical, electroneuromyographic and morphological studies of pure neural leprosy in a Brazilian referral centre. Lepr Rev 2004;75:242–53.
11. Jardim MR, Antunes SL, Santos AR, Nascimento OJ, Nery JA, Sales AM, et al. Criteria for diagnosis of pure neural leprosy. J Neurol 2003;250:806–9.

12. Pannikar VK, Arunthathi S, Chacko CJ, Fritschi EP. A clinicopathological study of primary neuritic leprosy. Lepr India 1983;55:212–21.
13. Kaur G, Girdhar BK, Girdhar A, Malaviya GN, Mukherjee A, Sengupta U, et al. A clinical, immunological, and histological study of neuritic leprosy patients. Int J Lepr Other Mycobact Dis 1991;59:385–91.
14. Suneetha S, Arunthathi S, Chandi S, Kurian N, Chacko CJ. Histological studies in primary neuritic leprosy: Changes in the apparently normal skin. Lepr Rev 1998;69:351–7.
15. Kumar B, Kaur I, Dogra S, Kumaran MS. Pure neuritic leprosy in India: An appraisal. Int J Lepr Other Mycobact Dis 2004;72:284–90.
16. Suneetha S, Arunthathi S, Job A, Date A, Kurian N, Chacko CJ. Histological studies in primary neuritic leprosy: changes in the nasal mucosa. Lepr Rev 1998;69:358–66.
17. De A, Hasanoor Reja AH, Aggarwal I, Sen S, Sil A, Bhattacharya B, et al. Use of Fine Needle Aspirate from Peripheral Nerves of Pure Neural Leprosy for Cytology and Polymerase Chain Reaction to Confirm the Diagnosis: A Follow-up Study of Years. Indian J Dermatol 2017;62:635–43.
18. Reja AH, De A, Biswas S, Chattopadhyay A, Chatterjee G, Bhattacharya B, et al. Use of fine needle aspirate from peripheral nerves of pure neural leprosy for cytology and PCR to confirm the diagnosis: a pilot study. Indian J Dermatol Venereol Leprol 2013;79:789–94.
19. Khambati FA, Shetty VP, Ghate SD, Capadia GD. Sensitivity and specificity of nerve palpation, monofilament testing and voluntary muscle testing in detecting peripheral nerve abnormality, using nerve conduction studies as gold standard; a study in 357 patients. Lepr Rev 2009; 80:34–50.
20. Jain S, Visser LH, Praveen TL, Rao PN, Surekha T, Ellanti R, et al. High-resolution sonography: A new technique to detect nerve damage in leprosy. PLoS Negl Trop Dis 2009;3:e498.
21. Bathala L, Kumar K, Pathapati R, Jain S, Visser LH. Ulnar neuropathy in Hansen disease: Clinical, high-resolution ultrasound and electrophysiologic correlations. J Clin Neurophysiol. 2012;29:190–3.
22. Mahajan PM, Jogaikar DG, Mehta JM. A study of pure neuritic leprosy: Clinical experience. Indian J Lepr 1996;68:137–41.
23. Laxmisha C, Thappa DM, Kumar MS, Joseph LC, Jayanthi S. Pure neural leprosy presenting with multiple nerve abscesses. Indian J Lepr 2004;76:343–50.
24. Rai D, Malhotra HS, Garg RK, Goel MM, Malhotra KP, Kumar V, et al. Nerve abscess in primary neuritic leprosy. Lepr Rev 2013;84:136–40.
25. Jayalakshmy PS, Prasad PH, Kamala VV, Aswathy R, Pratap P. "Segmental necrotizing granulomatous neuritis": A rare manifestation of Hansen disease—report of 2 cases. Case Rep Dermatol Med 2012;2012:758093.
26. Mishra B, Mukherjee A, Girdhar A, Husain S, Malaviya GN, Girdhar BK. Neuritic leprosy: Further progression and significance. Acta Leprol 1995;9:187–94.
27. Suneetha S, Sigamoni A, Kurian N, Chacko CJ. The development of cutaneous lesions during follow-up of patients with primary neuritic leprosy. Int J Dermatol. 2005;44:224–9.
28. Guilloton L, Drouet A, Combemale P, Cruel T, Dupin M, Ribot C [neuritic leprosy disclosed by reversal reaction]. Rev Neurol (Paris) 2002;158:84–6.
29. Global Leprosy Strategy 2016–2020. Accelrating towards a leprosy-free world. Monitoring and Evaluation Guide. World Health Organization. Avaialbale from: http://www.searo.who.int/entity/global_leprosy_programme/documents/sea-glp-2017-1/en/. [Accessed on 29th June, 2019]
30. Narang T, Arshdeep, Dogra S. Minocycline in leprosy patients with recent onset clinical nerve function impairment. Dermatol Ther 2017;30:e12404.
31. Rojewska E, Popiolek-Barczyk K, Jurga AM, Makuch W, Przewlocka B, Mika J. Involvement of pro- and antinociceptive factors in minocycline analgesia in rat neuropathic pain model. J Neuroimmunol 2014;277:57–66.
32. Haanpaa M, Lockwood DN, Hietaharju A. Neuropathic pain in leprosy. Lepr Rev 2004;75: 7–18.

2.5 SPECIAL SCENARIOS AND POPULATIONS

Kabir Sardana, Ananta Khurana

PREGNANCY AND LEPROSY

Sixty years ago, Ryrie wrote "In the interaction of pregnancy and associated pathological conditions, leprosy must be one of the few systemic diseases where such action is totally one sided. Leprosy does not have the slightest effect on the course of pregnancy; pregnancy has a marked effect on leprosy".[1]

Part of the normal physiology of pregnancy is a relative *immunosuppression* with the maternal immune response being directed away from cell-mediated immunity and towards humoral immunity. Following parturition, there is a recovery of cell-mediated immunity (CMI) in the mother, and this puts women at risk of developing immune-mediated complications.[2] A seminal paper has opined on the association between pregnancy and leprosy and the salient points listed include:[3]

1. Worsening of leprosy status (third trimester particularly)
2. Type 1 reaction (especially during the first 6 months of lactation, probably related to the regaining of CMI suppressed during pregnancy)
3. Type 2 reaction (particularly in the third trimester and the first 6 months of lactation).

Dr Elizabeth Duncan and colleagues have noted that pregnancy is associated with the appearance of new lesions, with relapse of 'cured' patients and with downgrading of the disease.

Two factors are known to precipitate type 2 reaction. In the puerperium, type 2 reactions may be triggered by the physical stress of parturition and a reverting to normal of the increased plasma ACTH and cortisol of the second and third trimesters. In third trimester, infections may trigger ENL.

The initial studies have also studied neuritis in pregnancy and lactation, and showed that nearly 50% suffered deterioration of nerve function; they stressed that insidious silent neuritis was a dangerous and hitherto undescribed risk in pregnancy.[4] On the question of the health of babies born to mothers with leprosy, Duncan found that they weighed less than babies of healthy mothers and grew more slowly. An overview of the literature on pregnancy and leprosy is given in *Table 2.22*.[5]

The treatment of leprosy in pregnancy is discussed in *Chapter 7, Section 7.1*. Among the anti-reactional drugs, oral steroids are preferred and thalidomide and methotrexate are obviously contraindicated.

HIV AND LEPROSY

Despite the importance of CD4+ T cells and the role of the cellular immune response in control of *M. leprae*, current evidence indicates that human immunodeficiency virus (HIV)-associated immunodeficiency has little effect on the course of leprosy.

Unlike the well-documented increased risk for infection with *M. tuberculosis* in HIV-infected individuals, HIV infection is neither thought to be a risk factor for acquisition of leprosy, nor it is associated with increased disease severity, rapidity of onset of disease, or a delayed response to treatment. In addition, HIV infection has not been found to affect the clinical form of leprosy (i.e. lepromatous disease is not more common

Table 2.22: Pregnancy and leprosy	
Effects of pregnancy on the woman with leprosy	
Worsening of the leprosy	Women already infected with *M. leprae* and incubating leprosy are likely to show overt *signs* of the disease in pregnancy and early in the puerperium.
	With established leprosy, the disease worsens during pregnancy and the puerperium and this worsening is particularly associated with deterioration of *nerve function*.
Increased incidence of lepra reactions occur	**Type 1 reaction** In borderline leprosy, upgrading (reversal) reaction is most likely to develop during the *puerperium* when there is a rapid regaining of CMI which was depressed during pregnancy. During pregnancy, *downgrading* reaction may occur because of decreased CMI, and is most likely to be manifested in the *third trimester*.
	Type 2 reaction (ENL reaction) In LL, this type of reaction is most likely to occur in the *third trimester* and the *puerperium*, but may complicate *early pregnancy* because of mental stress, and any stage of pregnancy because of increased incidence of intercurrent infections.
Effects on the infant	
	Babies of mothers with leprosy weigh *less* than those of healthy mothers and grow more slowly. Infant runs a high risk of contracting leprosy from the mother if she is an 'open' case (i.e. has untreated LL)

or tuberculoid disease less common than in HIV negative control subjects).[6,7] HIV infection also does not appear to affect the histopathologic appearance of leprosy lesions. The possible reason for this could be that *M. leprae* may grow too slowly to affect the clinical form of leprosy in people with HIV infection in developing countries, because other complications of HIV infection may dominate. An interesting observation is the granuloma paradox[8] wherein histopathological features of leprosy seem to be maintained in co-infected patients, indicating an apparent preservation of the ability to form granulomas that contrasts with what is observed in *Mycobacterium tuberculosis* and HIV co-infected individuals.

A study noted that the most common type of leprosy among HIV patients was BT leprosy and there was a history of early loss of sensation, and in some cases, a possibility of relapse was also considered. Besides typical cutaneous and neurological manifestations of leprosy, co-infected patients may present with hyperkeratotic eczematous and ulcerated lesions.[9] HIV infection is also believed to "unmask" subclinical leprosy in some patients, and, in addition, individuals with HIV and *M. leprae* coinfection frequently exhibit reversal reactions as a manifestation of immune reconstitution after antiretroviral therapy.[10,11] According to published data, *M. leprae* and HIV co-infected patients respond to MDT as well as immunocompetent individuals, without the need for prolonged treatment courses.[12]

LEPROSY IN OTHER IMMUNOCOMPROMISED HOSTS

There are other related, though uncommon, situations of immunosuppression which may have significance in relation to leprosy and its treatment. Leprosy has been reported in solid-organ (renal, heart, liver) and hematopoietic stem cell transplant recipients, with the majority of cases reported in renal transplant recipients living in leprosy-endemic areas.[13,14] Two cases reported an indirect contact with infected armadillos through dogs.[15,16] Six cases have been reported in HLA-identical allogeneic hematopoietic stem cell transplant recipients.[17] One challenge in treating transplant recipients with leprosy is the potential for adverse medication interactions, particularly between rifampin and cyclosporine; for this reason, leprosy in this patient group may require the use of *alternative* antimycobacterial agents (e.g. minocycline, clarithromycin, ofloxacin). In addition, the duration of therapy in these patients is debatable, because it is unclear if this group should receive a prolonged treatment course in light of their immunocompromised state.

A second common scenario of immunosuppression is patients who receive TNF-blocking agents (e.g. adalimumab, infliximab, etanercept). There are several documented cases of newly diagnosed leprosy in patients receiving infliximab and etanercept.[18–20] In one case (Scollard et al)[19] treatment with infliximab resulted in rapid development of borderline lepromatous lesions in the first 2 years after infliximab treatment; their disease was most likely due to reactivation of subclinical disease. A similar type 1 reaction has been seen with the use of adalimumab.[21] Both patients developed reversal reactions after infliximab was discontinued and multi-drug therapy was initiated; presumably, the reactions developed when host immunity was restored after the discontinuation of the TNF-α antagonist. This pathophysiology may be similar to the HIV-associated immune reconstitution syndrome, in which patients develop manifestations of leprosy after immune restoration while on antiretroviral therapy. Interestingly, although TNF-α inhibitors are associated with reactivation of subclinical leprosy, these agents have occasionally been used in the treatment of reactions, specifically ENL.[22,23]

REFERENCES

1. Ryrie GA. Pregnancy and leprosy. Br Med 2 1938;39–40.
2. Lockwood DN, Sinha HH. Pregnancy and leprosy: a comprehensive literature review. Int J Lepr Other Mycobact Dis 1999;67:6–12.
3. Duncan ME, Pearson JM, Ridley DS, Melsom R, Bjune G. Pregnancy and leprosy: The consequences of alterations of cell-mediated and humoral immunity during pregnancy and lactation. International Journal of Leprosy 1982;50:425–35.
4. Duncan ME, Pearson JMH. Neuritis in pregnancy and lactation. International Journal of Leprosy1982;50:31–8.
5. Duncan ME. Babies of mothers with leprosy have small placentae, low birth weights and grow slowly. British Journal of Obstetrics & Gynaecology 1980;87:471–9.
6. Gebre S, Saunderson P, Messele T, Byass P. The effect of HIV status on the clinical picture of leprosy: A prospective study in Ethiopia. Lepr Rev 2000;71:338–43.
7. van den Broek J, Chum HJ, Swai R, ÔBrien RJ. Association between leprosy and HIV infection in Tanzania. Int J Lepr Other Mycobact Dis 1997;65:203–10.
8. Ustianowski AP, Lawn SD, Lockwood DNJ. Interactions between HIV infection and leprosy: A paradox. Lancet Infect Dis 2006;6:350–60.

9. Talhari C, Mira MT, Massone C, Braga A, Chrusciak-Talhari A, Santos M, Orsiat, et al. Leprosy and HIV coinfection: A clinical, pathological, immunological, and therapeutic study of a cohort from a Brazilian referral center for infectious diseases. J Infect Dis 2010;202:345–54.
10. Batista MD, Porro AM, Maeda SM, Gomes EE, Yoshioka MC, Enokihara MM, et al. Leprosy reversal reaction as immune reconstitution inflammatory syndrome in patients with AIDS. Clin Infect Dis 2008; 46:e56–e60.
11. Talhari C, Ferreira LC, Araújo JR, Talhari AC. Immune reconstitution inflammatory syndrome or upgrading type 1 reaction. Report of two AIDS patients presenting a shifting from borderline lepromatous leprosy to borderline tuberculoid leprosy. Lepr Rev 2008;79:429–35.
12. Pereira GA, Stefani MM, Araújo Filho JA, Souza LC, Stefani GP, Martelli CM. Human immunodeficiency virus type 1 (HIV-1) and *Mycobacterium leprae* co-infection: HIV-1 subtypes and clinical, immunologic, and histopathologic profiles in a Brazilian cohort. Am J Trop Med Hyg 2004;71:679–84.
13. Shih HC, Hung TW, Lian JD, et al. Leprosy in a renal transplant recipient: A case report and literature review. J Dermatol 2005;32:661–6.
14. Trindade MA, Palermo ML, Pagliari C, et al. Leprosy in transplant recipients: Report of a case after liver transplantation and review of the literature. Transplant Infect Dis 2011;13:63–69.
15. Launius BK, Brown PA, Cush E, et al. A case study in Hansen's disease acquired after heart transplant. Crit Care Nurs Q 2004;27:87–91.
16. Modi K, Mancini M, Joyce MP. Lepromatous leprosy in a heart transplant recipient. Am J Transplant 2003;3:1600–3.
17. Pieroni F, Stracieri AB, Moraes DA, et al. Six cases of leprosy associated with allogeneic hematopoietic SCT. Bone Marrow Transplant 2007;40:859–63.
18. Vilela Lopes R, Barros Ohashi C, Helena Cavaleiro L, et al. Development of leprosy in a patient with ankylosing spondylitis during the infliximab treatment: Reactivation of a latent infection. Clin Rheumatol 2009;28:615–17.
19. Scollard DM, Joyce MP, Gillis TP. Development of leprosy and type 1 leprosy reactions after treatment with infliximab: A report of 2 cases. Clin Infect Dis 2006;43:e19–e22.
20. Lluch P, Urruticoechea A, Lluch J, et al. Development of leprosy in a patient with rheumatoid arthritis during treatment with etanercept: A case report. Semin Arthritis Rheum 2012; 42:127–30.
21. Camacho ID, Valencia I, Rivas MP, Burdick AE. Type 1 leprosy reaction manifesting after discontinuation of adalimumab therapy. Arch Dermatol 2009;145:349–51.
22. Ramien ML, Wong A, Keystone JS. Severe refractory erythema nodosum leprosum successfully treated with the tumor necrosis factor inhibitor etanercept. Clin Infect Dis 2011; 52:e133–35.
23. Faber WR, Jensema AJ, Goldschmidt WF. Treatment of recurrent erythema nodosum leprosum with infliximab. N Engl J Med 2006;355:739.

CHAPTER 3

Diagnostic Tests and Histopathology

3.1 DIAGNOSTIC TESTS

Ananta Khurana

The diagnosis of leprosy relies largely on clinical presentation, especially in field conditions. The most useful and commonly utilized laboratory diagnostic methods remain the slit skin smears and histopathology. Histopathology helps in determining the position of a patient in the spectrum of leprosy. It also is useful to differentiate between leprosy and other cutaneous/neurological conditions presenting in a similar pattern *(see Chapter 9)*.

While most clinicians rely on smear examination and histopathology, it is necessary to dwell on the novel aspects of diagnosis for which the concepts and utility of serology, PCR and cytology will be detailed.

Skin Smears

All universal precautions must be followed while making the slit skin smears. The site is first cleaned with ether and a portion of it is gripped between thumb and forefinger of the left hand to drive out the blood. With a small-bladed scalpel (e.g. size 15 Bard-Parker blade), an incision is made between the fingers of the left hand about 5 mm long and 3 mm deep, pressure of the fingers being maintained. The blade is then turned at right angles to the cut and the wound is scraped several times in the same direction so that tissue fluid and pulp (not blood) collects on one side of the blade; this is gently smeared on a glass slide. The smear is fixed over a flame before being sent for staining. Two or more smears can be made on one slide, each being numbered with a marking pencil.

The sites of the smears are recorded, so that the same sites can be used for successive sets of smears during the course of treatment. Slides with smears on them should not be exposed to sunlight, dust, extremes of temperature and humidity, since these factors may interfere with the capacity of bacilli to take up carbol fuchsin in the Ziehl-Neelsen staining method. Another factor interfering with good staining is long storage of fixed slides.[1] Faulty results will be obtained if the incision is not sufficient to include the deepest portion of the dermis, for it is useless to examine a smear consisting of epidermal cells.

Ziehl-Neelsen Method of Staining M. leprae in Smears

The term 'acid-fast' refers to the capacity of the bacillus, when stained with a red dye (carbol fuchsin), to retain its red color when treated with acid. Tubercle and leprosy bacilli are alcohol-fast as well as acid-fast, and a mixture of acid and alcohol is used in the standard method of staining—the Ziehl-Neelsen method. However *M. leprae* is less acid- and alcohol-fast than *M. tuberculosis* is and this fact is of practical importance when it comes to applying the Ziehl-Neelsen method of staining, for if it is used in leprosy in the same manner as in tuberculosis, it is likely that bacilli will not be found for the simple reason that the leprosy bacilli will have been decolorized and therefore will not be identifiable under the microscope. This problem is overcome by having a weaker acid-alcohol mixture and by leaving it in contact with the slide for a shorter time. In a properly stained skin smear, the leprosy bacilli appear bright red and everything else takes the color of the counterstain used. If stained smears are treated with pyridine, the bacilli lose their red color; this is known as pyridine extractability,[2] and distinguishes *M. leprae* from all other pathogenic mycobacteria (*M. vaccae* and *M. phlei* have been shown to lose their acid-fastness when extracted with pyridine,[3] but these are nonpathogenic mycobacteria). There are many minor modifications of this method, each as good as another in the hands of an experienced technician, and the method described here is a reliable guide (Fig. 3.1a to d):

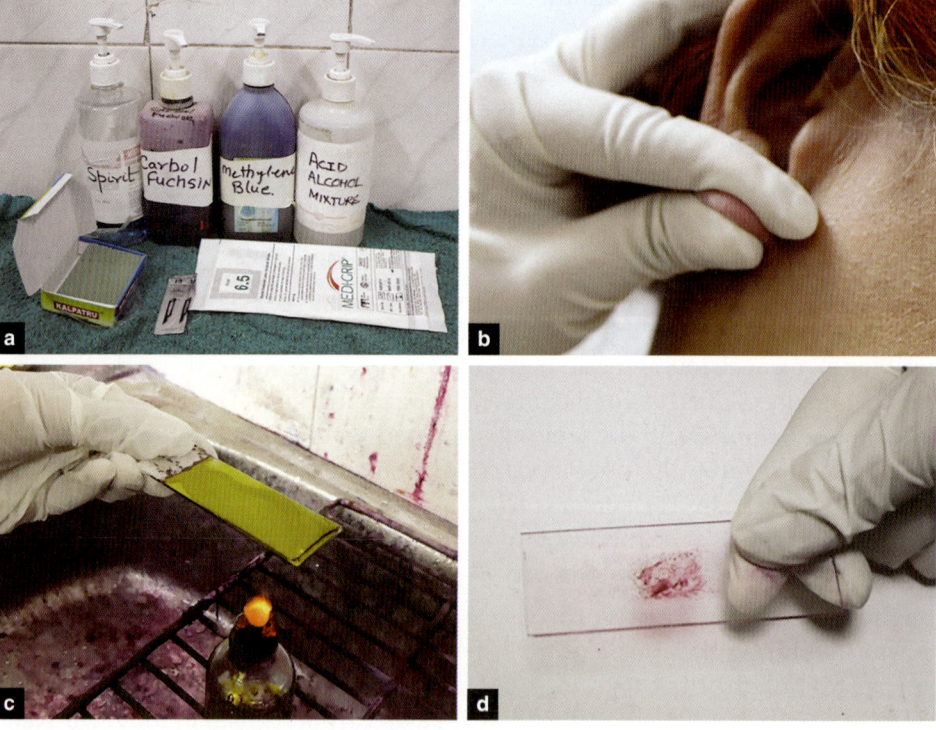

Fig. 3.1a to d: Procedure of slit skin smear making and Ziehl-Neelson staining. (a) Materials required beforehand to perform the procedure; (b) Hold the skin firmly between the thumb and index finger to drive out the blood; (c) Heat the carbol fuchsin (while avoiding boiling the solution) until a greenish yellow sheen is achieved; (d) The stained smear after rinsing off the carbol fuchsin with water (*Courtesy:* Dr Aastha Aggarwal, Dr Diksha Agrawal)

1. The slide with the smear on it should be covered with carbol fuchsin (freshly made or filtered) and heat applied beneath it, either with a gas flame (Bunsen burner) or with a spirit lamp. Heating should be sufficient to cause steam to rise from all parts of the slide, but boiling is avoided. The slide should be left for 15 minutes without any further heating.
2. The stain is tipped away and the slide is held under a gentle stream of water.
3. Pour acid-alcohol mixture onto the slide and leave for 3 seconds if the smear is thin or for 5 seconds if the smear is thick, then wash it away with running water. The acid-alcohol mixture consists of 1% hydrochloric acid in 70% alcohol. The slide is inspected to see the degree of pinkness; if faintly pink, proceed to the next stage, but if deeply pink, treat again with acid-alcohol for 2 seconds and wash with running water.
4. Cover the slide with counterstain such as 1% methylene blue for about 10 seconds.
5. Wash in running water and allow to dry.

Interpretation of Smears

It is to be noted that *M. leprae*, similar to other mycobacteria, retains the property of staining with carbol fuchsin when no longer alive. Therefore, a technician examining skin smears during treatment will get the impression that the patient is making no progress unless he can differentiate living from dead bacilli. The morphology or structure of the bacilli seen after Ziehl-Neelsen staining is all-important, since living bacilli appear as uniformly stained rods (solid-staining) and dead bacilli appear irregularly stained (fragmented bacilli) or as granules (granular bacilli) (Fig. 3.1). The density of bacilli in smears is known as the bacterial (bacteriological) index (BI) and includes both living and dead bacilli. Ridley's logarithmic scale is recommended to be used to express this (Table 3.1 and Fig. 3.2). This is based on the number of bacilli seen in an average microscopic field using an oil-immersion objective (1/2 in or 2 mm).

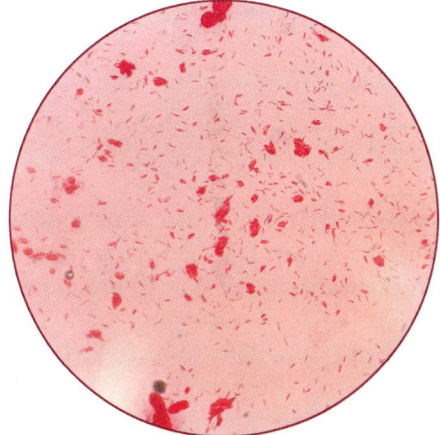

Fig. 3.1e: A smear examination in a suspected case of LL Hansen's with numerous bacilli and globi (BI- 6+)

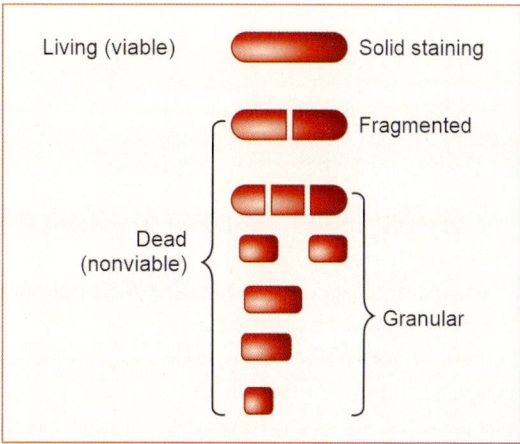

Fig. 3.1f: Diagrammatic representation of various forms of *Mycobacterium leprae* stained by modified Ziehl-Neelsen method

Table 3.1: Bacteriological index (BI) calculated as per Ridley's logarithmic scale

Bacteriological index (BI)	No. of bacilli seen
0	0 bacilli in 100 fields
1+	1–10 bacilli in 100 fields
2+	1–10 bacilli in 10 fields
3+	1–10 bacilli, on average, in each field
4+	10–100 bacilli, on average, in each field
5+	100–1000 bacilli, on average, in each field
6+	Many clumps of bacilli in an average field (over 1000)

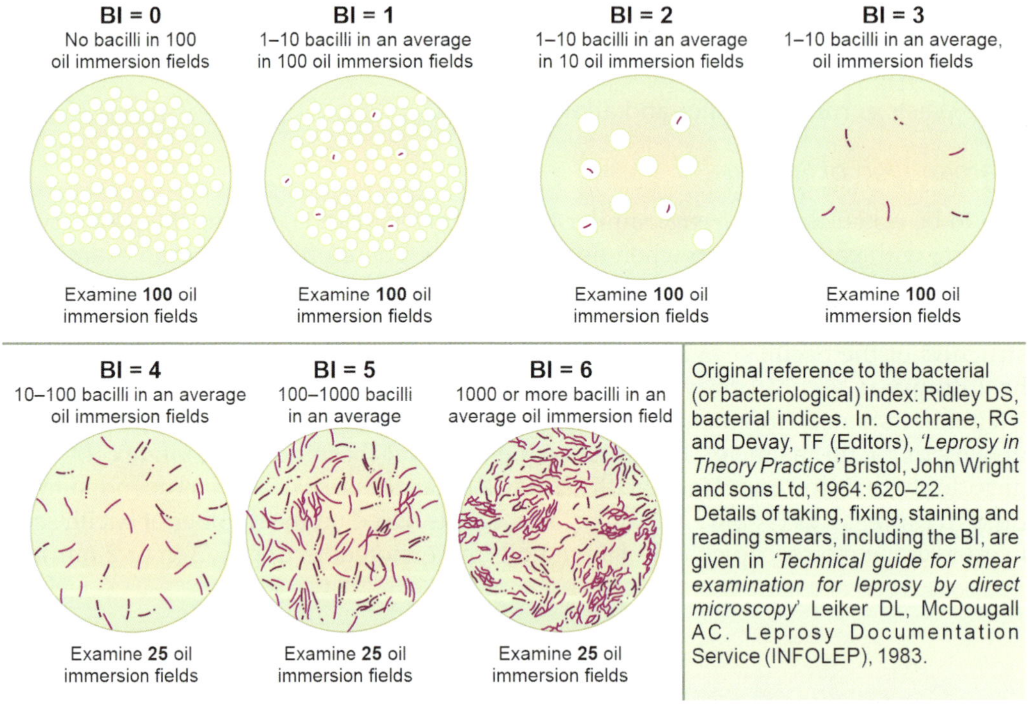

BI = 0 — No bacilli in 100 oil immersion fields — Examine **100** oil immersion fields

BI = 1 — 1–10 bacilli in an average in 100 oil immersion fields — Examine **100** oil immersion fields

BI = 2 — 1–10 bacilli in an average in 10 oil immersion fields — Examine **100** oil immersion fields

BI = 3 — 1–10 bacilli in an average, oil immersion fields — Examine **100** oil immersion fields

BI = 4 — 10–100 bacilli in an average oil immersion fields — Examine **25** oil immersion fields

BI = 5 — 100–1000 bacilli in an average — Examine **25** oil immersion fields

BI = 6 — 1000 or more bacilli in an average oil immersion field — Examine **25** oil immersion fields

Original reference to the bacterial (or bacteriological) index: Ridley DS, bacterial indices. In. Cochrane, RG and Devay, TF (Editors), 'Leprosy in Theory Practice' Bristol, John Wright and sons Ltd, 1964: 620–22. Details of taking, fixing, staining and reading smears, including the BI, are given in 'Technical guide for smear examination for leprosy by direct microscopy' Leiker DL, McDougall AC. Leprosy Documentation Service (INFOLEP), 1983.

Fig. 3.2: Leprosy smears: Bacterial (bacteriological) index (BI)—Ziehl-Neelsen stain. (*Courtesy*: A. Colin McDougall, Department of Dermatology and David Webster, Department of Medical Education, John Radcliffe Hospital, Oxford, UK, July 1985 (Revised))

If several smears are taken, the *mean index* is calculated. In lepromatous patients under treatment, it will be found that there will be no fall in the BI during the first 12 months because dead and living bacilli are being counted, since both are stained red by carbol fuchsin, but after this a steady fall takes place over the next 5–10 years. Clearly, a more sensitive index of bacteriological improvement is required for such patients; hence the introduction of a system of classifying the bacilli in smears into two groups, solid stained (living) and irregularly-stained (dead) (Fig. 3.1f).

The view that granular bacilli are nonviable was first put forward by Hansen in 1895.[4] Later Waters and Rees (1962) reported rapid fall in percentage of uniformly stained bacilli on serial smears taken at intervals of 3 months and suggested this as a measure of viability of bacilli.[5] Morphological index (MI) is a tedious but useful measure of viability of bacilli in smears based on the above mentioned premise. This involves measuring the proportion or percentage of solid stained (uniformly and brightly stained down their length) bacilli, calculated after examining preferably 200 red staining elements, lying singly (not superimposed). A knowledge of this index will tell if a patient's leprosy is active or not, will give valuable information as to response to treatment, and will give early intimation of bacterial resistance to chemotherapy or of defaulting on treatment. That is to say, an increase in MI indicates a worsening of the patient's condition, and a decrease indicates improvement. In general, it can be said that the MI of lepromatous patients, commencing treatment, will be somewhere between 25 and 75% and there is a steady fall in MI to zero in 4–6 months of dapsone monotherapy and considerably faster with multi-drug therapy. Rifampicin given alone in a daily dose of 450 mg/day reduced MI of six lepromatous patients from 32 at baseline to 0 at 6 weeks.[6] It is important to note that MI may show considerable differences between different sites examined, with smears from nasal mucosa of LL patients often revealing higher index than those from skin and ear lobes.[7] Further, the higher index may persist for longer in nasal mucosa and normal bacilli may reappear here but not elsewhere.[7] There is little correlation between the initial value of MI with initial height of BI in general. Also, fall in MI bears no relation to the initial MI[7] (Fig. 3.3).

There are some contradictions to the accuracy of MI in determining viability with reports of successful foot pad cultivation of *M. leprae* obtained from patients with zero MI and nonconcordance with viability results obtained using fluorescent vital dyes and biochemical tests.[8–11] Thus, MI is significantly dependent on the staining methods, including the extent of heat treatment and drying of the specimen and there is subjective variation in determining non-solid staining bacilli.[12,13]

The SFG index divides bacilli further into 3 classes: "Solid" (S), i.e. solid-staining unbroken rods; "fragmented" (F), i.e. bacilli in which the acid-fast substance is interrupted at one or more points, but at least one fragment displays an elongated form; also single very short rods; and "granular" (G), i.e. round granules either in line

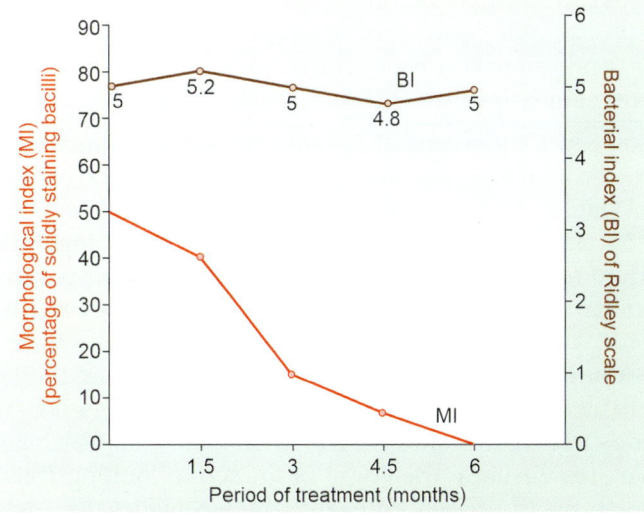

Fig. 3.3: Effect of treatment on BI and MI

or in clumps.[14] But it is difficult to estimate the exact percentage of bacilli in each class and the index seems not to provide any further advantage over MI and thus has not come into wider use.

Certain sites have been shown to have higher probability of demonstrating AFB including ear lobes, forehead, chin, extensor surface of the forearms, dorsal surface of the fingers, buttocks and extensor surface of knees. Thus, the ear lobe has been recommended and used as a site for making SSS by WHO, ILEP and various authors over the years. Some authors have observed that in long-treated lepromatous patients, the skin sites where bacilli are most frequently detected, whether granular or solid-staining, are the dorsa of fingers[15,16] and smears from fingers give the earliest indication of an impending relapse.[16] In a follow-up of 116 multibacillary patients who had received multi-drug therapy in the Malta-Project, skin smears from six sites (two from fingers) revealed scanty solid-staining bacilli in 10 patients; one or other finger was positive for 'solids' in 8 of these 10 patients, but in 7 of them the fingers were the only positive sites.[18] But making smears from fingers have inherent practical difficulties which account for its restricted use. Macrery et al (1988) reported contrary findings wherein BI of the finger site was actually the lowest or equal to the lowest routine site used by authors.[19]

The recommendations on use of SSS in leprosy programs have been changing. In 1982, the WHO study group on chemotherapy of leprosy for control programmes classified leprosy as multibacillary (MB) and paucibacillary (PB) according to the degree of skin smear positivity.[20] MB leprosy included polar lepromatous (LL), borderline lepromatous (BL), and midborderline (BB) cases with a BI of 2+ or more at any site in the initial skin smears. PB leprosy included indeterminate (I), polar tuberculoid (TT) and borderline tuberculoid (BT) cases in the Ridley-Jopling classification, with a bacteriological index of <2 at all sites in initial slit smears. At its sixth meeting in 1988, the Expert Committee on leprosy specified that all smear positive cases should be classified as MB leprosy for the purposes of MDT programmes.[21] In 1994, the second WHO study group on chemotherapy of leprosy concluded that where skin smears are not available, cases can be classified on the basis of clinical examination alone as either PB leprosy (one to five skin lesions) or MB leprosy (six or more skin lesions).[22] This clinical classification system has been shown to be about 89% sensitive and 86–88% specific at detecting smear positive MB cases.[23,24]

There has also been a difference of opinion regarding number of skin smear sites from time to time. From 6 to 8 sites during 1960s,[25] 7 sites (two ear lobes, nasal smear, 4 lesions) as per WHO Expert Committee on leprosy in 1980[26] to 6 sites (both ear lobes and 4 lesions),[27] 5 sites (two ear lobes, right elbow, left hand finger, right toe),[28] 4 sites (right ear lobe, right forehead, chin, left buttock in males or upper thigh in females or any 2 sites (Poricha et al 2011) have been suggested by several workers over the years.[29,30] WHO in 1988 recommended a minimum of *three* sites (one ear lobe and two active lesions) for smears. In the case of single leprosy lesion the two smears taken from diametrically opposite active edge of the lesion was advised. ILEP, on the other hand, recommends use of two sites for initial smears—one ear lobe and the second from most active area (usually the edge) of an active looking (raised and reddish) lesion.[31] Here, when the BI varies significantly between sites, the highest BI should be taken in labeling and classifying the disease.

The Significance of Positive or Negative Smears on Skin Smear Examination

It is important to appreciate that the results of routine skin smear examinations, particularly when performed by inexperienced and untrained staff under difficult conditions, may be misleading. Many mistakes in diagnosis and classification have been made (and continue) because of over-dependence on a laboratory report of doubtful accuracy. The following points may help the clinician or field worker to use the results of skin smears to best advantage:

1. **'Cardinal' signs** *of leprosy. It is traditional to list these as*:
   a. Diminution or loss of sensation in a typical skin lesion, or in an area supplied by one of the peripheral nerves typically affected in leprosy
   b. Enlargement and/or tenderness in a peripheral nerve typically affected in leprosy, and
   c. The finding of acid-fast bacilli in smears.

   However, even with the proviso that two out of these three signs must be present for a diagnosis of leprosy, all three call for qualification before acceptance at face value. In the case of point c), for instance, the finding of acid-fast bacilli in smear (or smears) in a patient with absolutely no clinical evidence of leprosy is by itself unacceptable as a basis for the diagnosis of leprosy, and should, at the very least, call for repeat examination of the smears by an expert. If there is doubt in such cases, it is prudent to depend or the clinical findings.

2. *The expected correlation between clinical and bacteriological findings*: As already indicated above quite clearly, acid-fast bacilli are absent in a typical tuberculoid (TT) lesion and either absent or scanty in borderline tuberculoid (BT) lesions. This is because it requires about 10^4 bacilli/gm of tissue for reliable detection by Ziehl-Neelsen staining.[32,33]

   Thus, laboratory reports recording 'many' bacilli in such cases are very likely to be wrong, provided the clinical classification is reasonably confident. Similarly, in a totally untreated lepromatous (LL) or borderline lepromatous (BL) patient a negative result from properly taken smears is impossible, and a low BI reading (for instance of 1 or 2) exceedingly unlikely. A study from India reported a SSS positivity of 100% in LL and histoid cases, 86.4% in BL, 38.8% in BT and none in clinico-pathologically diagnosed TT, indeterminate and neuritic leprosy.[32] The overall sensitivity of SS was 59.8% in MB versus only 1.8% in PB leprosy.[32] The specificity of SSS is 100% as it directly demonstrates the lepra bacilli.

3. *The influence of treatment*: Even in the BL and LL cases mentioned above, which are invariably positive on smears at the outset, smears will become negative at various times after, or during, successful chemotherapy. In such patients, negative smears or low BI figures are the expected result and should be interpreted in relation to the history and clinical findings, bearing in mind that patients frequently conceal the truth with regard to previous treatment, including the taking of rapidly bactericidal drugs such as rifampicin. Smears will *never* become negative in a new LL patient during MDT but will become granular (dead) after a relatively short time; thereafter granular bacilli decrease in numbers at a rate of about 1 log per year and disappear 5 or 6 years after stopping MDT.

Nasal Smears and Nose-blows

Nasal smears or scrapings were used in the past, in some circumstances almost routinely, but it is an unpleasant and often painful procedure and has now been virtually abandoned. Of late, however, nasal smears have been used for research related to transmission routes of leprosy and this has yielded useful results as discussed in *Chapter 4, Section 4.2*.

Nerve Biopsy

This is essential in pure neural leprosy and will show typical tuberculoid or borderline histology as the case may be, together with bacilli in most borderline cases. But nerve biopsy will not be required if a skin lesion is present. A thickened sensory nerve is suitable such as a supraorbital branch of the 5th cranial nerve, a supraclavicular nerve, the great auricular nerve in the neck, the radial nerve at the wrist, a cutaneous nerve of forearm or thigh, the sural nerve at the back of the leg or at the lateral border of the foot, or a superficial peroneal nerve on the dorsum of the foot. These nerves do not contain motor fibers and therefore there is no risk of motor damage.

Molecular Diagnosis and Serology

The novel diagnostic tests can be divided into two main subheads (Box 3.1).

The need for additional tests for diagnosis of leprosy mainly lies in early leprosy, indeterminate, PB and pure neural leprosy. Also novel laboratory diagnostic tests have been explored for early diagnosis of reactions and diagnosis in asymptomatic contacts.

From the sophisticated laboratory based testing of host immune markers and the pathogen DNA/RNA, there is now an attempt to develop minimally invasive point-of-care (POC) tests that can be utilized in field conditions. Though anti-*M. leprae* antibody detection has limitations for routine clinical use, a combined detection of humoral (antibodies) and cellular (cytokines) biomarkers may significantly improve the diagnostic potential, for both MB and PB leprosy. Polymerase chain reaction (PCR) can in principle improve identification of PB leprosy as complementary to histological analysis and has also found an important use in drug resistance monitoring.

Molecular diagnosis: In the last two decades, studies have demonstrated the potential of PCR for the rapid detection and identification of leprosy in clinical specimens.[34–38] RLEP and groEL are the most sensitive genes for detecting *M. leprae* and RLEP is the most commonly used.[39–41] Other genes which have been used include *16SrRNA, esxA, Ag85B, sodA, pra, rpoT, ML2179, ML1545, ML0098, ML0024, MntH, AT repeats, AGT repeats* and *TTC repeats*.[42–55]

 Box 3.1: Novel diagnostic procedures in leprosy

Markers of early host responses to *M. leprae*	• Tests for antibodies to *M. leprae* • Tests for cytokines produced in response to *M. leprae* infection • Changes in metabolites like fatty acids that may accompany *M. leprae* infection
Detection of *M. leprae* in biopsies or skin smears	• PCR methods to detect *M. leprae* • *M. leprae* genotyping and related efforts

More recently, real-time PCR (quantitative polymerase chain reaction or qPCR) has improved the rate of disease detection by facilitating the direct quantification of the bacterial DNA content in clinical samples, thereby increasing the reliability of the results.[56–58] qPCR is probably the best molecular method to confirm disease among PB patients. However, there are two main issues that need to be addressed to validate its use for disease confirmation: Firstly that several different targets are available and secondly most of the published data on qPCR use research reagents and not GMP products, which are designed for diagnostic purposes.[59]

qPCR has also proved to be particularly useful for the identification of drug-resistant bacilli and distinguishing between reaction and relapse by viability analyses of the bacillus, apart from facilitation of diagnosis in difficult cases and a possible role in monitoring treatment response.[39,60–63] Recently, a duplex-droplet digital PCR (ddPCR) has been tested for MB and PB leprosy.[64] The authors reported a greater sensitivity of ddPCR in detecting *M. leprae* DNA in PB patients compared with qPCR (79.5% *vs* 36.4%), while both assays had a 100% sensitivity in MB patients.

Molecular genotyping techniques such as typing selected single nucleotide polymorphisms (SNP) or counting variable number tandem repeats (VNTR) have also been used to differentiate reinfection from relapse.[65–69] The resolution of such techniques is however limited because of the exceptional level of genome conservation in *M. leprae* and the limited sequence diversity between strains from the same geographical area in particular. As a means to counter this limitation, Stefani et al performed whole genome sequencing analysis of *M. leprae* collected from skin lesions of patients with recurrent signs of disease after treatment completion.[70] The samples collected at the initial diagnosis and during the recurrence of disease were compared. None of the patients harboured mutations responsible for resistance to rifampicin, dapsone and ofloxacin. However, sequence differences were detected between the strains from the first and second disease episodes in all three patients. In one case, clear evidence was obtained for reinfection with an unrelated strain, whereas in the other two cases, relapse appeared more probable.

Thus, the use of molecular testing in leprosy is expanding and the PCR technology is becoming accessible, faster, and cheaper. The use of PCR in furthering our knowledge on transmission of leprosy and positivity in contacts has been discussed in *Chapter 4, Section 4.2*. Of note, the use of molecular-based techniques in finding mutations in drug-resistant determining region (DRDR) of *M. leprae* is increasing with the access to WHO recognized reference laboratories in endemic regions.

However, the infrastructure such as equipment and trained professionals, is still a barrier to implementing use in most resource limited settings. Further, heterogeneity in methodology and in the reported results (Table 3.2) among different studies available so far also impedes the inclusion of PCR in diagnostic recommendations as yet.

Serology: Phenolic glycolipid 1 (PGL-1) was the first, and is the most widely used antigen for serological assays in leprosy.[71] The increase of anti-PGL-1 antibody levels from the TT to the LL pole shows the activation of the humoral immune response and relates to the bacillary load.[72,73] Later, specific epitopes of PGL-1 were found to be the components which react specifically with IgM antibodies in patients' sera. Thus, the synthetic sugars—natural trisaccharide (NT) and natural disaccharide (ND) were synthesized individually and conjugated with either bovine serum albumin (BSA) or

Table 3.2: Sensitivity of serological methods and PCR for diagnosing leprosy[88]

Test	Sensitivity*	Specificity*
ELISA	63.8%	91%
Lateral flow	67.9%	86.7%
Agglutination	72.8%	90.1%
Conventional PCR	75.3%	94.5%
qPCR	78.5%	89.3%

*Results as per a systematic review and meta-analysis done by Gurung et al[88] (2019) qPCR: Real time PCR. The sensitivity and specificity of serological tests did not vary significantly with the antigen used for ELISA.

human serum albumin (HSA) using either octyl (O) or phenyl (P) linker arms (ND-O-BSA/HSA or NT-O-BSA/NT-P-BSA). These showed higher affinity for IgM antibody than PGL-1. Recombinant 35kD protein, LID-1 (Leprosy Infectious Disease Research Institute Diagnostic 1; a fusion construct of ML0405 and ML2331 proteins), NDO-LID (synthetically conjugated LID-1 and ND-O-BSA) and the major membrane proteins-I and II are the other antigens which have been used.[74-78] *M. leprae* dipstick assay and particle agglutination assay are further modifications utilizing the above antigens.[78] An immunochromatographic strip test (ML flow test) is a quick output lateral flow assay for the detection of antibodies in field conditions and takes only 10 min to perform.[72] Large scale (population-based) studies using rapid test to detect anti-*M. leprae* antibodies are currently ongoing.

The sensitivity of various serological methods in diagnosing leprosy is mentioned in Table 3.2. Broadly, while anti-PGL-1 IgM or NDO-LID may be useful in diagnosis of MB leprosy, serological methods are not sensitive enough to aid diagnosis of PB leprosy and the presence of anti-*M. leprae* antibodies is not predictive for disease.

Serology has also been studied for potential use in predicting reactions by a few authors. Mizoguti et al (2015) found higher anti-LID-1 levels in patients with type 2 reaction (T2R) at diagnosis (*vs* patients with type 1 reaction at diagnosis, $p = 0.008$; *vs* non-reactional patients, $p = 0.020$) and in patients with T2R during MDT (*vs* non-reactional MB, $p = 0.020$), and concluded that in MB patients, high and persistent anti-LID-1 antibody levels might be a useful tool for clinicians to predict which patients are more susceptible to develop T2R.[79] Similar findings were later reported by Devides et al using anti-PGL-1 and anti-NDO-LID-1.[80] However, Hungria et al noted that ML Flow test at baseline had limited sensitivity and specificity to predict whether patients will develop leprosy reactions during follow-up.[81,82] High ML flow seropositivity was not always associated with leprosy reactions as high positivity was also observed in reaction-free patients.

The utility of serology for household contacts is also not established as yet. Although several studies described that positive anti-PGL-I titers in household contacts of leprosy patients were related to a higher risk of developing leprosy later and thus could be used to identify the disease in preclinical stage, seropositivity in endemic areas can be found in numerous individuals who will never develop leprosy. It is clear that more than half of the individuals with antibodies against PGL-1 will never develop leprosy.[83-86] A recent meta-analysis among household contacts of new leprosy patients in French Polynesia, Zaire, Papua New Guinean, Venezuela, Brazil, India and Philippines shows that the risk of developing leprosy is about three times higher in those who are positive for anti-PGL-1 antibodies compared to the seronegative group, with the odds ratio varying from 2.72 to 3.53. However, the sensitivity of anti-PGL-1 tests as predictor of the development of clinical leprosy was found to be lower than 50% in all studies. Follow-up of the participants of COLEP study conducted in Bangladesh for assessment of efficacy of single dose rifampicin (SDR) also corroborated the results of this meta-analysis.[87] This study showed that anti-PGL-1 antibody levels at intake did not significantly differ between contacts who developed leprosy during the study and those who remained free of disease.

Summary: Although significant advances have been made in serological and molecular diagnosis of leprosy, the search for an ideal laboratory test with unambiguous utility over and above the clinical criteria, slit skin smears and histopathology for diagnosis of disease and its complications and for utility in curbing transmission of the disease is still ongoing. The recent WHO report notes that enzyme-linked immunosorbent assays (ELISA) and lateral flow assays are associated with low diagnostic accuracy for PB leprosy.[89] Further, although some polymerase chain reaction (PCR)-based assays are associated with higher diagnostic accuracy, they lack standardization, are not commercially available, and would be difficult to perform in most primary healthcare settings. Thus, no additional tests are yet recommended in addition to standard methods for diagnosis of leprosy. The guidelines also do not recommend any test for the diagnosis of leprosy in asymptomatic contacts citing poor positive predictive values of available tests.[89]

Thus, there is an urgent need for diagnostic methods which could assist clinical diagnosis of leprosy especially in field conditions and possibly help in detecting susceptible individuals who may benefit from an early pharmacological intervention. Detection of blood based cytokines is a promising approach in this regard. Their detection by POC lateral flow assays may offer diagnostic advantages if universally validated. Although rapid tests detecting cytokines/chemokines have been field-tested in certain endemic regions, larger scale studies are needed to provide proper sensitivity and specificity data.[90,91]

Cytology in Leprosy

Fine needle aspiration cytology (FNAC) has been explored for use in diagnosis of cutaneous lesions and neural leprosy. Cytology requires less infrastructure than a biopsy and thus has potential use in field conditions. Further, it may be an important tool for diagnosis of pure neural leprosy (PNL) where tissue for histopathology is difficult to obtain.

It has been long understood that the cellular exudates in slit-skin smears could generate more information than just the BI and MI and could place the leprosy lesions in their approximate position on the Ridley-Jopling classification.[92]

Singh et al have suggested cytology criteria for subclassification of leprosy which have been utilized by later studies[93] (Table 3.3). Broadly, cytology demonstrates cohesive epithelioid cell granulomas with lymphocytes, not infiltrating the granuloma, in tuberculoid leprosy.[93] As the disease progresses toward the lepromatous pole, cohesion between the cells of the granulomas diminishes, concurrent with increasing infiltration of lymphocytes within them.[93] Thus, the epithelioid cell granuloma of TT is gradually transformed into the macrophage granuloma of LL. *M. leprae* appears as

Table 3.3: Cytology criteria for sub-classification of leprosy[93]	
Spectrum	Cytology
Tuberculoid leprosy (including TT and BT)	• Cellular smears • Cohesive epithelioid cell granulomas • Numerous lymphocytes not infiltrating the granuloma • No stainable AFB (BI = 0)
Mid-borderline leprosy (BB)	• Fair cellular yield • Poorly cohesive granulomas composed of an admixture of epithelioid cells and macrophages • Few lymphocytes infiltrating the granulomas • BI = 1+ to 2+
Borderline lepromatous leprosy (BL)	• Moderate cellularity • Singly dispersed macrophages with 'negative images'; no epithelioid cells • Numerous lymphocytes diffusely admixed with macrophages BI = 3+ to 4+
Lepromatous leprosy (LL)	• Heavy cellularity • Numerous foamy macrophages in a fatty background with intracellular and extracellular 'negative images' • Few lymphocytes • BI = 5+ to 6+ (globi)
Reaction	• Numerous fragmented AFB (MI <1) and neutrophils suggest a type II reaction in LL (erythema nodosum leprosum)

"negative images" on the routine May-Grünwald-Giemsa stained cytology smears.[93] A cytohistological correlation of about 78% has been reported between the clinical, histological and cytomorphological features of skin aspirates in different studies.[94,95]

FNAC of affected nerves can be a valuable and less invasive procedure for the diagnosis of PNL. Singh et al reported the presence of the entire spectrum of leprosy in nerve aspirates, while the frequent presence of necrosis was a prominent finding setting nerve aspirates apart from skin lesions.[96] The authors performed FNA in sensory as well as mixed nerves including ulnar, common peroneal, radial and median nerves, and reported no worsening of nerve function following the procedure. Vijaikumar et al have proposed a set of criteria for interpreting the cytology of nerve aspirates.[97]

In a recent series involving 13 suspected PNL patients, an improved diagnosis was reported with use of multiplex PCR.[98] On cytological examination of the aspirates, 23% cases showed specific epithelioid cells, whereas 61.5% showed non-specific inflammation, and 15.3% cases had no inflammatory cells.[98] *M. leprae* could be elicited in the nerve tissue aspirates in 38.4% cases with the help of conventional Ziehl-Neelsen staining while with multiplex PCR, the positivity rose to 84.6%.[98]

Older Diagnostic Tests

Older tests not in routine use in the present times are listed in Table 3.4.

Diagnostic Tests and Histopathology

Table 3.4: Other diagnostic tests

Lepromin test (for details please refer to the 5th edition)	• A nonspecific test which is positive in the majority of healthy adults in nonendemic, and cannot be used as a diagnostic test • Previously used for classifying leprosy; a guide to the resistance of the patient • It is a delayed type hypersensitivity reaction to *M. leprae* or its antigens	• Late Mitsuda reaction: Read at 4 weeks • Early Fernandez reaction in some (best seen with Dharmendra's lepromin test)
Sweating test	• A method of testing the integrity of dermal nerves • Anhidrosis is characteristic of skin lesions in tuberculoid leprosy	• Inject 0.2 ml of a 1 in 1000 solution of pilocarpine nitrate intradermally into the lesion to be tested, the area is painted with tinctur of iodine and then to dusted with starch powder • Quinizarin powder can be used in place of starch, in which case there is no need to paint with iodine • Sweating causes a blue discoloration of the powder, whereas there is no blue color if sweating is absent due to damage to dermal nerves
Histamine test	Histamine can be used to test the integrity of dermal nerves, and the degree of damage to these nerves can be gauzed by the reduction in size and brightness of the histamine flare. This can be useful in deciding if a hypopigmented macule is due to leprosy *Caveat:* Depression of histamine flare occurs in all other types of peripheral neuropathy as well	• One drop of histamine acid phosphate (diphosphate) 1 in 1000 (1 mg in 1 ml) is placed on the area of skin to be tested and another on a control site. • A superficial prick is made through each drop, and a bright flare will appear if dermal nerves are intact. The flare will appear within a minute on face or trunk but takes a little longer on limbs • In a leprosy macule, the flare is delayed, feeble (indeterminate and borderline leprosy) or entirely absent (tuberculoid leprosy). • In Lucio leprosy there is depression or absence of flare all over the skin

Future Tests and their Implications

The field of diagnostics is rapidly advancing and multiple new aspects are being debated and investigated. These are listed in Box 3.2.

The need is of tools that can predict, among the risk population, individuals that have the highest chance of progressing to disease, which may then enable the use of single dose rifampicin (SDR) or other immune/chemoprophylactic means to prevent transmission. Genomics could be used to better understand phylogeography and perhaps depict novel virulence factors. Whole, large scale genomics could be used to help determine strains/SNP type/haplotype associations isolated from different clinical forms of the disease.

An overview of the potential techniques and modifications that can be used to translate diagnostics to various aspects of leprosy are listed in Table 3.5. In essence,

Box 3.2: Future advances in diagnosis[59]

- Artificial intelligence to screen skin biopsies or slit-skin smears slides for unrecognized patterns.
- Cutaneous thermography as a complementary diagnostic method, with or without ultraviolet photography.
- Panel of SNPs be used to estimate the risk of developing disease.
- Use of tick cell lines to grow *M. leprae*.[99]

Table 3.5: Translational implications and future advances in diagnostic tests[59]	
qPCR	• Need for independent confirmation, larger sample sizes, and external quality assessment • Better sampling methods available for direct/indirect detection of *M. leprae* or DNA/RNA for use in diagnostic confirmation • Use of loop-mediated isothermal amplification (LAMP) in leprosy molecular diagnosis which is simple, rugged, and low cost
Drug-resistance surveillance	• To map out the prevalence of *M. leprae* resistant strains in endemic countries • To decipher mechanisms for drug resistance, especially for clofazimine
Reactions and relapse	• Duplex or triplex qPCR to target the most frequent resistant SNPs in rpoB • Test for viability in fresh or fixed clinical samples to enable management of relapse cases (live mycobacteria) from reactional states (dead mycobacteria)
Diagnostic test based on host immunity	• Need for large scale multicentric studies to validate diagnostic potential for MB and PB leprosy of POC lateral flow assays for (simultaneous) detection of multiple cytokines/chemokines • Early detection of leprosy in high risk populations using a defined biomarker signature • Tests for monitoring treatment responses in patients using a defined biomarker signature
Screening population	• Panel of genetic polymorphisms or transcripts or metagenomic markers be defined to scrutinize high risk contacts • Next generation skin test (for example, based on recombinant proteins) to screen infected people • Low complexity lateral flow assays based on finger-stick blood provide a means for POC triage testing for infection by measuring both antibodies and cyto-/chemokines in capillary blood

the main focus that is envisaged is to achieve the goal of zero leprosy by using tests for early and specific diagnosis of leprosy and *M. leprae* infection and to block transmission using affordable, rapid POC tests in low-resourced settings.

REFERENCES

1. Sayer J, Gent R, Jesudasan K. Are bacterial counts on slit-skin smears in leprosy affected by preparing slides under field conditions? Lep Rev 1987;58:271–278.
2. Fisher CA, Barksdale L. Elimination of the acid-fastness but not the gram positivity of leprosy bacilli after extraction with pyridine. Journal of Bacteriology 1971;106:707–8.
3. Dutta AK, Katoch VM, Sharma VD, Katoch K (1984). Effect of pyridine extraction on the acid-fastness of *M. leprae*: It is possible mechanism. Abstract IV/219(A) in XII International Leprosy Congress Abstracts.
4. Hansen GA, Looft C. (1895). Leprosy: In its clinical and pathological aspects. Reprinted by John Wright, Bristol, 1973.
5. Waters MF, Rees RJ. Changes in the morphology of *Mycobacterium leprae* in patients under treatment. Int J Lepr 1962;30:266–77.
6. Rees RJW, Pearson JMH, Waters MFR. Experimental and Clinical Studies on Rifampicin in Treatment of Leprosy Br Med J 1970;1:89–92.
7. Browne SG. Some observations on the morphological index in lepromatous leprosy. Lepr Rev 1966;37:23–25.
8. Karat Aba, Samuel I, Albert R, Kumar ASJ. Experiments in cultivation of *M. leprae* in monkeys and in foot-pads of mice—an interim report of 6 years of study. Lepr India 45:138–42.
9. Desikan KV. Correlation of morphology with viability of *Mycobacterium leprae*. Lepr India 1976;48:391–97.
10. Odinsen O, Nilson T, Humber DP. Viability of *Mycobacterium leprae*: A comparison of morphological index and fluorescent staining techniques in slit-skin smears and *M. leprae* suspensions. Int J Lepr Other Mycobact Dis 1986;54:403–8.
11. Sathish M, Prasad HK, Mittal A, Nath I. Lack of correlation between morphological index and viability as assessed by the uptake of 3H-thymidine by macrophage resident *M. leprae*. Lepr India 1982;54:420–27.
12. Nakamura M, Tsuchiya T, Nagamatsu T, Aono Y, Ishida M. Staining conditions influencing morphological index of acid-fast bacilli. Kurume Med J 1968;15:39–41.
13. Ridley DS. The morphological index. Lepr Rev 1971;42:75–77.
14. Ridley DS. The SFG (solid, fragmented, granular) index for bacterial morphology. Lepr Rev. 1971;42:96–97.
15. Ridley M, Jopling WH, Ridley DS. Acid-fast bacilli in the fingers of long-treated lepromatous patients. Lep Rev 1976;47: 93–96.
16. Kumar B, Kaur S, Gupta SK, Rajwanshi A, Darshan H. Acid-fast bacilli in lymph node aspirate and smears from ear lobules and fingers in long treated patients. Indian J Lepr 1984;56:71–77.
17. Jopling WH, Rees RJ, Ridley DS, Ridley MJ, Samuel NM. The fingers as sites of leprosy bacilli in 20 prerelapse patients. Leprosy Review 1979;50:289–92.
18. Jopling WH, Ridley M, Bonnici E, Depasquale G. A follow-up investigation of the Malta-Project. Lep Rev 1984;55:247–53.
19. Macrery RT. Slit-skin smears from the fingers in leprosy. Lepr Rev 1988;59:360–1.
20. Chemotherapy of leprosy for control programmes: Report of a WHO Study Group. Geneva, World Health Organization, 1982 (WHO Technical Report Series, No. 675).
21. WHO Expert Committee on leprosy. Sixth report. Geneva, World Health Organization, 1988 (WHO Technical Report Series, No. 768).
22. Chemotherapy of leprosy: Report of a WHO study group. Geneva, World Health Organization, 1994 (WHO Technical Report Series, No. 847).

23. Croft RP, Smith WC, Nicholls P, Richardus JH. Sensitivity and specificity of methods of classification of leprosy without use of skin smear examination. Int J Lepr Other Mycobact Dis 1998;66:445–50.
24. Norman G, Joseph G, Richard J. Validity of the WHO operational classification and value of other clinical signs in the classification of leprosy. Int J Lepr Other Mycobact Dis 2004;72:278–83.
25. Mahajan VK. Slit-skin smear in leprosy: Lest we forget it! Indian J Lepr 2013;85:177–83.
26. WHO Expert Committee on leprosy (1980). A guide to leprosy control. World Health Organization, Geneva.
27. Rees RJW and Young DB. The microbiology of leprosy: Standard bacteriological assessment and investigations in clinical leprosy In: Hasting and RC. Leprosy, 2nd edition. Churchill Livingstone: Edinburgh (London); 1994:pp.71–74.
28. Kumar B, Kaur S. Selection of sites for slit skin smears in untreated and treated leprosy patients. Int J Lepr Other Mycobact Dis 1986;54:540–44.
29. Chacko CJ. Microbiology. A manual of leprosy, 4th edition. Thangaraj RH (Ed), New Delhi: The Leprosy Mission; 1985: pp 43–60.
30. Poricha D, Nayak S, Sahoo LB, et al. Can the skin smear examination in NLEP be reconsidered? Indian J Lepr 2011;83:45–52.
31. http://www.ilepfederation.org/wp-content/uploads/2016/11/How-to-do-a-smear-examination-for-leprosy-NEW-LOGO.pdf (last accessed 15/9/2019)
32. Banerjee S, Biswas N, Kanti Das N, Sil A, Ghosh P, Hasanoor Raja AH, et al. Diagnosing leprosy: Revisiting the role of the slit skin smear with critical analysis of the applicability of polymerase chain reaction in diagnosis. Int J Dermatol 2011;50:1522–7.
33. Shepard CC, McRae DH. A method for counting acid-fast bacteria. Int J Lepr Other Mycobact Dis 1968;36:78–82.
34. Scollard DM, Gillis TP, Williams DL. Polymerase chain reaction assay for the detection and identification of *Mycobacterium leprae* in patients in the United States. Am J Clin Pathol. 1998;109:642–46.
35. Santos AR, De Miranda AB, Sarno EN, Suffys PN, Degrave WM. Use of PCR-mediated amplification of *Mycobacterium leprae* DNA in different types of clinical samples for the diagnosis of leprosy. J Med Microbiol 1993;39:298–304.
36. Barbieri RR, Manta FSN, Moreira SJM, Sales AM, Nery JAC, Nascimento LPR, et al. Quantitative polymerase chain reaction in paucibacillary leprosy diagnosis: A follow-up study. PLoS Negl Trop Dis 2019;13:e0007147.
37. Martinez AN, Britto CF, Nery JA, Sampaio EP, Jardim MR, Sarno EN, et al. Evaluation of real-time and conventional PCR targeting complex 85 genes for detection of *Mycobacterium leprae* DNA in skin biopsy samples from patients diagnosed with leprosy. J Clin Microbiol 2006;44:3154–59.
38. Almeida EC, Martinez AN, Maniero VC, Sales AM, Duppre NC, Sarno EM, et al. Detection of *Mycobacterium leprae* DNA by polymerase chain reaction in the blood and nasal secretion of Brazilian household contacts. Mem Inst Oswaldo Cruz 2004;99:509–11.
39. Martinez AN, Talhari C, Moraes MO, Talhari S. PCR-based techniques for leprosy diagnosis: from the laboratory to the clinic. PLoS Negl Trop Dis 2014;8:e2655.
40. Yan W, Xing Y, Yuan LC, De Yang R, Tan FY, Zhang Y, et al. Application of RLEP real-time PCR for detection of *M. leprae* DNA in paraffin-embedded skin biopsy specimens for diagnosis of paucibacillary leprosy. Am J Trop Med Hyg 2014;90:524–29.
41. Davis GL, Ray NA, Lahiri R, Gillis TP, Krahenbuhl JL, Williams DL, et al. Molecular assays for determining *Mycobacterium leprae* viability in tissues of experimentally infected mice. PLoS Negl Trop Dis 2013;7:e2404.
42. Moher D, Liberati A, Tetzlaff J, Altman DG, Group P. Preferred reporting items for systematic reviews and meta-analyses: The PRISMA statement. BMJ 2009;339: b2535.
43. Martinez AN, Ribeiro-Alves M, Sarno EN, Moraes MO. Evaluation of qPCR-based assays for leprosy diagnosis directly in clinical specimens. PLoS Negl Trop Dis. 2011;5:e1354.

44. Yan W, Xing Y, Yuan LC, De Yang R, Tan FY, Zhang Y, et al. Application of RLEP real-time PCR for detection of *M. leprae* DNA in paraffin-embedded skin biopsy specimens for diagnosis of paucibacillary leprosy. Am J Trop Med Hyg 2014;90:524–29.
45. Davis GL, Ray NA, Lahiri R, Gillis TP, Krahenbuhl JL, Williams DL, et al. Molecular assays for determining *Mycobacterium leprae* viability in tissues of experimentally infected mice. PLoS Negl Trop Dis 2013;7:e2404.
46. Martinez AN, Britto CF, Nery JA, Sampaio EP, Jardim MR, Sarno EN, et al. Evaluation of real-time and conventional PCR targeting complex 85 genes for detection of *Mycobacterium leprae* DNA in skin biopsy samples from patients diagnosed with leprosy. J Clin Microbiol 2006;44: 3154–59.
47. Caleffi KR, Hirata RD, Hirata MH, Caleffi ER, Siqueira VL, Cardoso RF. Use of the polymerase chain reaction to detect *Mycobacterium leprae* in urine. Braz J Med Biol Res. 2012;45:153–57.
48. Arunagiri K, Sangeetha G, Sugashini PK, Balaraman S, Showkath Ali MK. Nasal PCR assay for the detection of *Mycobacterium leprae* PRA gene to study subclinical infection in a community. Microb Pathog. 2017;104:336–39.
49. Qinxue W, Xinyu L, Wei H, Tao L, Yaoping Y, Jinping Z, et al. A study on PCR for detecting infection with *M. leprae*. Chin Med Sci J 1999;14: 237–41.
50. Turankar RP, Pandey S, Lavania M, Singh I, Nigam A, Darlong J, et al. Comparative evaluation of PCR amplification of RLEP, 16S rRNA, rpoT and Sod A gene targets for detection of *M. leprae* DNA from clinical and environmental samples. Int J Mycobacteriol 2015;4: 54–59.
51. Chaitanya VS, Cuello L, Das M, Sudharsan A, Ganesan P, Kanmani K, et al. Analysis of a novel multiplex polymerase chain reaction assay as a sensitive tool for the diagnosis of indeterminate and tuberculoid forms of leprosy. Int J Mycobacteriol 2017;6:1–8.
52. da Silva Martinez T, Nahas AA, Figueira MM, Costa AV, Goncalves MA, Goulart LR, et al. Oral lesion in leprosy: Borderline tuberculoid diagnosis based on detection of *Mycobacterium leprae* DNA by qPCR. Acta Derm Venereol 2011;91:704–7.
53. Cruz AF, Furini RB, Roselino AM. Comparison between microsatellites and Ml MntH gene as targets to identify *Mycobacterium leprae* by PCR in leprosy. An Bras Dermatol 2011;86:651–56.
54. Young SK, Taylor GM, Jain S, Suneetha LM, Suneetha S, Lockwood DN, et al. Microsatellite mapping of *Mycobacterium leprae* populations in infected humans. J Clin Microbiol 2004;42: 4931–36.
55. Tatipally S, Srikantam A, Kasetty S. Polymerase Chain Reaction (PCR) as a Potential Point of Care Laboratory Test for Leprosy Diagnosis—A Systematic Review. Trop Med Infect Dis 2018;3: pii: E107.
56. Rudeeaneksin J, Srisungngam S, Sawanpanyalert P, Sittiwakin T, Likanon-sakul S, Pasadorn S, et al. LightCycler real-time PCR for rapid detection and quantitation of *Mycobacterium leprae* in skin specimens. FEMS Immunol Med Microbiol 2008; 54:263–70.
57. Martinez AN, Ribeiro-Alves M, Sarno EM, Moraes MO. Evaluation of qPCR-based Assays for Leprosy Diagnosis Directly in Clinical Specimens. PLOS Negl Trop Dis 2011; 5:e1354.
58. Kramme S, Bretzel G, Panning M, Kawuma J, Drosten C. Detection and quantification of *Mycobacterium leprae* in tissue samples by real-time PCR. Med Microbiol Immunol 2004; 193:189–93.
59. https://zeroleprosy.org/wp-content/uploads/2019/07/GPZL-RWG-Diag-nostics-FINAL-REV2.pdf (last accessed 1/10/2019)
60. Cambau E, Saunderson P, Matsuoka M, Cole ST, Kai M, Suffys P, et al. Antimicrobial resistance in leprosy: Results of the first prospective open survey conducted by a WHO surveillance network for the period 2009-2015. Clin Microbiol Infect 2018;24:1305–10.
61. Martinez AN, Lahiri R, Pittman TL, Scollard D, Truman R, Moraes O et al. Molecular determination of *Mycobacterium leprae* viability by use of real-time PCR. J Clin Microbiol 2009;47:2124–30.
62. Barbieri RR, Sales AM, Illarramendi X, Moraes MO, Nery JAC, Moreira SJM, et al. Diagnostic challenges of single plaque-like lesion paucibacillary leprosy. Mem Inst Oswaldo Cruz 2014; 109:944–47.
63. Lavania M, Jadhav RS, Chaitanya VS, Turankar R, Selvasekhar A, Das L, et al. Drug resistance patterns in *Mycobacterium leprae* isolates from relapsed leprosy patients attending The Leprosy Mission (TLM) Hospitals in India. Lepr Rev 2014; 85:177–85.

64. Cheng X, Sun L, Zhao Q, Mi Z, Yu G, Wang Z, et al. Development and evaluation of a droplet digital PCR assay for the diagnosis of paucibacillary leprosy in skin biopsy specimens. PLoS Negl Trop Dis 2019;13:e0007284.
65. Oskam L, Dockrell HM, Brennan PJ, Gillis T, Vissa V, Richardus JH. Molecular methods for distinguishing between relapse and reinfection in leprosy. Trop Med Int Health 2008;13:1325–26.
66. da Silva Rocha A, Cunha Dos Santos AA, Pignataro P, Nery JA, de Miranda AB, Soares DF, et al. Genotyping of *Mycobacterium leprae* from Brazilian leprosy patients suggests the occurrence of reinfection or of bacterial population shift during disease relapse. J Med Microbiol 2011; 60:1441–46.
67. Monot M, Honore N, Garnier T, Zidane N, Sherafi D, Paniz-Mondolfi A, et al. Comparative genomic and phylogeographic analysis of *Mycobacterium leprae*. Nat Genet 2009;41:1282–89.
68. Zhang L, Budiawan T, Matsuoka M. Diversity of potential short tandem repeats in *Mycobacterium leprae* and application for molecular typing. J Clin Microbiol 2005; 43:5221–29.
69. Kimura M, Sakamuri RM, Groathouse NA, Rivoire BL, Gingrich D, Krueger-Koplin S, et al. Rapid variable number tandem repeat genotyping for *Mycobacterium leprae* clinical specimens. J Clin Microbiol 2009; 47:1757–66.
70. Stefani MMA, Avanzi C, Bührer-Sékula S, Benjak A, Loiseau C, Singh P, et al. Whole genome sequencing distinguishes between relapse and reinfection in recurrent leprosy cases. PLoS Negl Trop Dis 2017;11:e0005598.
71. Brennan PJ, Barrow WW. Evidence for species-specific lipid antigens in *Mycobacterium leprae*. Int J Lepr Other Mycobact Dis 1980;48:382–87.
72. Buhrer-Sekula S, Smits HL, Gussenhoven GC, van Leeuwen J, Amador S, Fujiwara T, Klatser PR, Oskam L. Simple and fast lateral flow test for classification of leprosy patients and identification of contacts with high risk of developing leprosy. Jorunal of Clinical Microbiology 2003; 41:1991–95.
73. Silva EA, Iyer A, Ura S, Lauris JR, Naafs B, Das PK, Vilani-Moreno F. Utility of measuring serum levels of anti-PGL-I antibody, neopterin and C-reactive protein in monitoring leprosy patients during multi-drug treatment and reactions. Trop Med Int Health 2007;12:1450–58.
74. Chatterjee D, Cho SN, Brennan PJ, Aspinall GO. Chemical synthesis and seroreactivity of O-(3,6-di-O-methyl-beta-D-glucopyranosyl)-(1-4)-O-(2,3-di-O-methyl-alpha-L-rhamnopyranosyl)-(1-9)-oxynonanoyl-bovine serum albumin—the leprosy-specific, natural disaccharide-octyl-neoglycoprotein. Carbohydr Res. 1986;156:39–56.
75. Fujiwara T, Aspinall GO, Hunter SW, Brennan PJ. Chemical synthesis of the trisaccharide unit of the species-specific phenolic glycolipid from *Mycobacterium leprae*. Carbohydr Res 1987; 163: 41–52.
76. Gigg J, Gigg R, Payne S, Conant R. The allyl group for protection in carbohydrate chemistry. 17. Synthesis of propyl O-(3,6-di-O-methyl-beta-D-glucopyranosyl)-(1–4)-O-(2,3-di-O-methyl-alpha-L-rhamnopyranosyl)-(1-2)-3-O-methyl-alpha-L-rhamnopyranoside: The oligosaccharide portion of the major serologically active glycolipid from *Mycobacterium leprae*. Chem Phys Lipids 1985; 38:299–307.
77. Tsukamoto Y, Maeda Y, Makino M. Evaluation of major membrane protein I as a serodiagnostic tool of paucibacillary leprosy. Diagn Microbiol Infect Dis 2014;80:62–65.
78. Sengupta U. Recent Laboratory Advances in Diagnostics and Monitoring Response to Treatment in Leprosy.Indian Dermatol Online J 2019;10:106–14.
79. Mizoguti Dde F, Hungria EM, Freitas AA, Oliveira RM, Cardoso LP, Costa MB, et al. Multibacillary leprosy patients with high and persistent serum antibodies to leprosy IDRI diagnostic-1/LID-1: higher susceptibility to develop type 2 reactions. Mem Inst Oswaldo Cruz 2015; 110:914–20.
80. Devides AC, Rosa PS, de Faria Fernandes Belone A, Coelho NMB, Ura S, Silva EA. Can anti-PGL-1 and anti-NDO-LID-1 antibody titers be used to predict the risk of reactions in leprosy patients? Diagn Microbiol Infect Dis. 2018;91:260–65.

81. Hungria EM, Bührer-Sékula S, de Oliveira RM, Aderaldo LC, Pontes AA, Cruz R. Leprosy reactions: The predictive value of *Mycobacterium leprae*-specific serology evaluated in a Brazilian cohort of leprosy patients (U-MDT/CT-BR).PLoS Negl Trop Dis. 2017;11:e0005396.
82. Hungria EM, Oliveira RM, Penna GO, Aderaldo LC, Pontes MA, Cruz R, et al. Can baseline ML flow test results predict leprosy reactions? An investigation in a cohort of patients enrolled in the uniform multi-drug therapy clinical trial for leprosy patients in Brazil. Infect Dis Poverty 2016;5:110.
83. Douglas JT, Cellona RV, Fajardo TT (Jr), Abalos RM, Balagon MV, Klatser PR. Prospective study of serological conversion as a risk factor for development of leprosy among household contacts. Clin Diagn Lab Immunol 2004;11:897–900.
84. Duppre NC, Camacho LA, Sales AM, Illarramendi X, Nery JA, Sampaio EP, et al. Impact of PGL-I seropositivity on the protective effect of BCG vaccination among leprosy contacts: a cohort study. PLoS Negl Trop Dis 2012;6:e1711.
85. Carvalho AP, da Conceicao Oliveira Coelho Fabri A, Correa Oliveira R, Lana FC. Factors associated with anti-phenolic glycolipid-I seropositivity among the household contacts of leprosy cases. BMC infectious diseases 2015;15:219.
86. Penna ML, Penna GO, Iglesias PC, Natal S, Rodrigues LC. Anti-PGL-1 positivity as a risk marker for the development of leprosy among contacts of leprosy cases: Systematic review and meta-analysis. PLoS Negl Trop Dis 2016;10:e0004703.
87. Richardus RA, van der Zwet K, van Hooij A, Wilson L, Oskam L, Faber R, et al. Longitudinal assessment of anti-PGL serology in contacts of leprosy patients in Bangladesh. PLoS Negl Trop Dis 2017 Dec 11;11:e0006083.
88. Gurung P, Gomes CM, Vernal S, Leeflang MMG. Diagnostic accuracy of tests for leprosy: A systematic review and meta-analysis. Clin Microbiol Infect 2019 May 31. pii: S1198-743X(19)30283-6.
89. http://www.searo.who.int/entity/global_leprosy_programme/ap-proved-guidelines-leprosy-executives-summary.pdf?ua=1 (WHO, 2018; last accessed 18/9/2019).
90. van Hooij A, Tjon Kon Fat EM, Batista da Silva M, Carvalho Bouth R, Cunha Messias AC, Gobbo AR, et al. Evaluation of Immunodiagnostic Tests for Leprosy in Brazil, China and Ethiopia. Sci Rep 2018,8.17920.
91. Corstjens PLAM, van Hooij A, Tjon Kon Fat EM, Alam K, Vrolijk LB, Dlamini S, et al. Fingerstick van Hooij A, Tjon Kon Fat EM, Richardus R, et al. Quantitative lateral flow strip assays as userfriendly tools to detect biomarker profiles for leprosy. Sci Rep 2016;6:34260.
92. Ridley MJ. The cellular exudate—*Mycobacterium leprae* relationship and the critical reading of skin smears. Lepr Rev 1989;60:229–40.
93. Singh N, Bhatia A, Gupta K, Ramam M. Cytomorphology of leprosy across the Ridley-Jopling spectrum. Acta Cytol 1996;40:719–23.
94. Ray R, Mondal RK, Pathak S. Benefits and limitations of fine needle aspiration cytology in the diagnosis and classification of leprosy in primary and secondary healthcare settings. Cytopathology 2015;26:238–43.
95. Nigam PK, Kumar P, Pathak N, Mittal S. Fine needle aspiration cytology in reactional and non-reactional leprosy. Indian J Dermatol Venereol Leprol 2007;73:247–49.
96. Singh N, Malik A, Arora VK, Bhatia A. Fine needle aspiration cytology of leprous neuritis. Acta Cytol 2003;47:368–72.
97. Vijaikumar M, D'Souza M, Kumar S, Badhe B. Fine needle aspiration cytology (FNAC) of nerves in leprosy. Lepr Rev 2001;72:171–78.
98. De A, Hasanoor Reja AH, Aggarwal I, Sen S, Sil A, Bhattacharya B. Use of Fine Needle Aspirate from Peripheral Nerves of Pure-Neural Leprosy for Cytology and Polymerase Chain Reaction to Confirm the Diagnosis: A Follow-up Study of 4 Years. Indian J Dermatol 2017;62:635–43.
99. Ferreira JDS, Souza Oliveira DA, Santos JP, et al. Ticks as potential vectors of *Mycobacterium leprae*: Use of tick cell lines to culture the bacilli and generate transgenic strains. PLoS Negl Trop Dis 2018;12:e0007001.

3.2 HISTOPATHOLOGY OF LEPROSY

Sarita Sasidharanpillai, Aparna Govindan

INTRODUCTION

Majority of individuals exposed to *Mycobacterium leprae* are able to mount an effective immune response that protects them from the disease.[1] Thus, it is the immune response of the host to *M. leprae* or its antigens that defines the clinical and histopathology features in the affected patients.

In patients whose immunity is effective in containing the infection to limited sites, CD4+ T cells are able to activate the macrophages. After the activated macrophages eliminate the bacilli, they transform into epithelioid cells. Towards the lepromatous pole of the disease, the number of CD4+ T cells mounting the immune response is less than that observed towards the tuberculoid pole.[1]

The cytokine profile documented suggests a Th1 (type 1 helper T cell) response in tuberculoid cases and Th2 (type 2 helper T cell) response in lepromatous cases. Th1 response (with expression of cytokines IL-1, -2, -6, -10, -18, TNF-α and interferon γ) upregulates cell-mediated immunity, whereas Th2 response (with expression of cytokines IL-4, -5, -8 and -10) upregulates humoral immunity. Humoral immunity fails to evoke effective response against an intracellular pathogen like *M. leprae*. Unchecked multiplication of *M. leprae* within macrophages takes place in lepromatous cases and when these macrophages eventually die, hundreds of *M. leprae* are released which are taken up by fresh macrophages.[1]

Except in indeterminate leprosy, which is considered as the pre-granulomatous stage of the disease, the affected individual's body responds to *M. leprae* by formation of granulomas.

Disease morphology is studied by staining formalin fixed, paraffin-embedded tissue specimens with hematoxylin and eosin. Fite-Faraco stain is used to demonstrate the acid-fast bacilli in tissue specimen. Immunohistochemistry, *in situ* hybridization and polymerase chain reaction have helped to demonstrate mycobacterial antigens in tissue sections from leprosy lesions that do not show acid-fast bacilli; thereby improving the diagnostic accuracy.

Histopathological changes involve only less than one tenth of a tissue section taken from the skin lesion of early leprosy. Hence, a 1.5 cm long and 0.5 cm wide specimen including subcutaneous tissue is ideal for histopathology analysis in early leprosy. A 6 mm punch biopsy may serve the purpose for well established lesions. Preferred site for biopsy is the most active part of the lesion, which is usually at the periphery.[1]

HISTOLOGICAL CLASSIFICATION IN SKIN

Early Lesions

The histological features in an early skin lesion of leprosy can be of three types:
a. Histologically *normal* or almost normal, with no bacilli
b. Presence of *lymphocytic* infiltrate or *AFB*, or both, but without any granuloma
c. Presence of *granuloma* at one or more sites, with or without AFB.[2]

Demonstration of AFB requires examination of serial sections cut through the entire block and hence is often impractical. Normal or near normal biopsy is not uncommon in lesions less than 6 months duration.[2] The clues to diagnose leprosy in an early lesion are—solid infiltrate of lymphocytes that selectively encompasses one or more nerve bundles or lymphocytic infiltrate penetrating the perineurium or presence of epithelioid cells in the nerve. Proliferation of Schwann cells, along with disorganization of the neural structure, strongly supports the diagnosis of leprosy, whereas proliferation of Schwann cells without disorganization may be observed in repair of Wallerian degeneration following minor trauma or other causes. A small granuloma, localized to sweat glands or duct, or invading arrector pili muscle, may point to leprosy, whereas granuloma in a nerve bundle is a conclusive evidence for the same.[2]

Late Lesions

As already stated, in established lesions, granuloma formation characterizes tissue response to *M. leprae*. Granulomas are constituted by compact aggregate of macrophages or cells derived from them. Epithelioid cells, giant cells, macrophages and lymphocytes are the major constituents of granuloma. Epithelioid cells are special forms of activated macrophages. They are elongated cells with 'bean-shaped' vesicular nuclei and densely stained eosinophilic cytoplasm. Borders of cells are not distinct as they tend to interdigitate.[1,2]

Mature epithelioid cells are large polygonal cells with elongated nucleus, margination of chromatin and sometimes a prominent nucleolus. The abundant cytoplasm appears eosinophilic and finely granular or pale due to minute vesicles. Concentric organization of cells is the hall mark.[1,2]

Mature fully differentiated epithelioid cells are less common and most of the epithelioid cells that constitute the granuloma are immature. Immature epithelioid cells have smaller nucleus, less conspicuous and basophilic nucleolus, little margination of chromatin and less bulky cytoplasm. Immature epithelioid cells do not show concentric organization.[2]

As macrophages mature, they lose the ability to divide and fuse to form giant cells under suitable stimulus, which usually is the large amount of indigestible matter.[2] Two or more macrophages trying to ingest the same particle join together to form cells with two to three nuclei.[2]

Histological Criteria of Classification Based on Characteristics of Granuloma

Histological classification of leprosy relies on certain salient features of granuloma.[3]
1. **Cell type of the granuloma:**[3] The most mature and differentiated cell type present defines the character of the granuloma. On most occasions, predominant cell constituting the granuloma could be a less mature form, but the most mature cell type has to be considered while assessing the granuloma.
2. **Bacterial load:**[3] Bacterial density in the granuloma determined by bacterial index of granuloma is the best indicator of immunological competence of macrophages in untreated patients.[3,4] It is a more useful index than slit-skin smear.[4,5]

    Immunologically competent macrophages are able to kill the organism effectively. Bacterial load in the granuloma helps to distinguish noncompetent active macrophages from epithelioid cells. But in treated patients, density of bacilli is much less useful in evaluating the immunological competence of macrophages, since most of the organisms would be dead and cleared from the lesion.[3]

3. **Lymphocytic infiltrate:**[3] The number and distribution of lymphocytes in the granuloma are important features in classification. When considered in relation to the size of granuloma (not as an absolute number), the number of lymphocytes is *high* in primary tuberculoid (TTp) and BL and low in BB and LL, especially LLp. In BT, lymphocytes may or may not be numerous.
4. **Nerve involvement:**[3] Preferential involvement of dermal nerve bundles, in comparison to perivascular sites, indicates either a high immune response or an infection that is yet to establish. Granuloma formation within the nerve bundle favors an established, high resistant lesion. The maximum size attained by a swollen dermal nerve is limited for any group of the spectrum, the size being the greatest in TTs and lowest in LL.
5. **Perineurial involvement:**[3] The thickness of perineurium increases progressively down the spectrum. The maximum thickness is seen in BL and LLs and here the laminated perineurium resembles an "onion skin". The rapidity with which nerve damage occurs in TT and BT is proposed as the reason for the absence of lamination of perineurium (which is a repair mechanism of damaged nerve) in these groups.[6] The mechanisms proposed for the multilayering of perineurium in leprosy include an attempt for repair by endoneurium that becomes exposed following the breakdown of perineurium. Another simpler explanation suggested for multilayering in dermal nerve bundles is infiltration by inflammatory cells.[7]

    The appearance becomes more striking since the thin perineurium of TT surrounds a much larger nerve than the swollen perineurium of BL or LLs. Perineurial infiltration by lymphocytes is another distinguishing feature between different groups. The perineurium is infiltrated by lymphocytes in TT (slightly), BT (more so) and BL (significant). In BB, there are often epithelioid cells within the laminations of perineurium; in LLs the laminations are empty, since the lymphocytic infiltrate retreats during downgrading. In LLp, the perineurium, like the nerve, is not much affected.[3]
6. **Epidermal erosion:**[3] Erosion of a portion of epidermis extending into superficial layer is important owing to the probability of siting bacilli.
7. **Fibrinoid necrosis:**[3] Lepra reactions and post-reactional secondary tuberculoid (TTs) lesions manifest *necrosis*. Two forms of necrosis may occur—*caseation* necrosis and *fibrinoid* necrosis. Necrosis of epithelioid cells results in caseation necrosis and in leprosy, this takes place only in nerve centers. Necrosis of collagen leads to fibrinoid necrosis and this can occur in any part of the dermal lesion.

    Both types of necrosis are features of strong delayed hypersensitivity response. Caseation in a non-neural granuloma virtually rules out leprosy; hence it is important to distinguish between the two types of necrosis. Fibrinoid necrosis appears more coarse and deeply eosinophilic when compared to caseation which is paler. Fibrinoid stains deep orange red with martius scarlet blue (MSB) stain while caseation does not.[2]

CHARACTERISTIC HISTOLOGY FEATURES OF DIFFERENT GROUPS OF THE LEPROSY SPECTRUM (Table 3.6)[1,3,6,8]

Indeterminate Leprosy[1,3,8] (Fig. 3.4a and b)

This is histologically classified into early stage and late stage. Occasional acid-fast bacilli in normal nerve, arrector pilorum muscle, hair follicles, subepidermal zone and/or perivascular infiltrate may be seen in early stage, whereas lymphocyte infiltration

Table 3.6: Comparison of histopathology features of leprosy granulomas

Type of leprosy	Granuloma	T lymphocytes	Epithelioid cells	Giant cells	Macrophages	Subepidermal clear zone (Grenz zone)	Bacterial index	Perineural lamination
Tuberculoid leprosy (TT)	Compact organized epithelioid granuloma eroding epidermis	Plenty, form dense mantle around epithelioid cells	Plenty	Less than that in BT, mainly Langhans' giant cells	Nil	Obliterated by granuloma	0	Not seen
Borderline tuberculoid leprosy (BT)	Epithelioid granuloma, less compact than that of TT	Moderate in number	Moderate in number	Giant cells more than that in TT, mainly foreign body giant cells	Present	Present, though at focal points granuloma touches epidermis	1+	Not seen
Borderline borderline leprosy (BB)	Mixed cellular type (epithelioid cells and macrophages, epithelioid cells predominate)	Scanty	Less than that in TT and BT	Absent	More than that in BT	Clear Grenz zone	2+ – 3+	Present
Borderline lepromatous leprosy (BL)	Macrophage granuloma	Numerous	A few	Absent	More than that in BB	Clear Grenz zone	3+ – 4+	Concentric perineural cell proliferation gives a "cut onion" appearance to nerves
Lepromatous leprosy (LL)	Macrophage granuloma	Less than that in BL	Absent	Absent	Plenty	Clear Grenz zone	5+ – 6+	Concentric perineural cell proliferation gives "onion peel" appearance to nerves in subpolar LL

or Schwann cell proliferation characterize the late stage. Lymphocyte infiltration usually involves perineurial sheath with preservation of nerve parenchyma; but at times the nerve fiber is almost completely replaced by lymphocytes. Proliferation of Schwann cells results in loss of wavy pattern of nerves and loss of longitudinal orientation of individual Schwann cell nuclei which appear as "baton"-shaped in normal nerves.

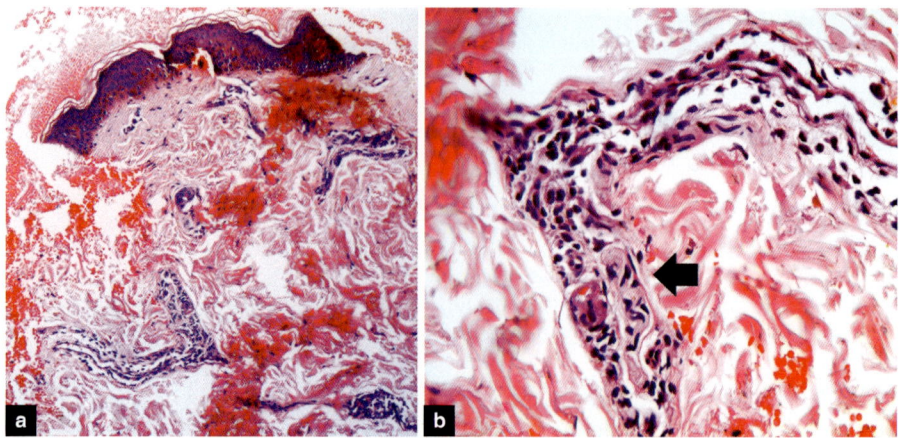

Fig. 3.4: (a) Skin biopsy showing inflammation along the neurovascular bundle, no evidence of granuloma indicating indeterminate leprosy (H & E, ×100); (b): Higher magnification showing lymphocytic infiltrate around nerve twig (H & E, ×400)

M. leprae being the only bacterium to parasitize a peripheral nerve, the described neural changes are diagnostic of leprosy while lymphocyte infiltration of other appendages is considered suspicious, but not diagnostic.

Primary Tuberculoid Leprosy (TTp)[1,3,8]

Epidermis shows areas of atrophy. Though clear subepidermal zone is not seen, erosion of epidermis is less marked than in TTs. Fibrinoid necrosis is not a feature of TTp.

Usual manifestation is one or two small clusters of granuloma among abundant lymphocytes (Fig. 3.5). Large lesions may be seen occasionally (Fig. 3.6). Lymphocytes are numerous relative to the granuloma and form a dense peripheral *mantle* around it, which is more obvious in deep dermis. The granuloma features immature epithelioid cells with a cluster of mature epithelioid cells. Identification of these mature epithelioid cells is essential for accurate classification. Langhans' giant cells are seldom seen. AFB are not found.

Nerves are small and relatively normal except for a dense cuff of lymphocytes and some Schwann cell proliferation.

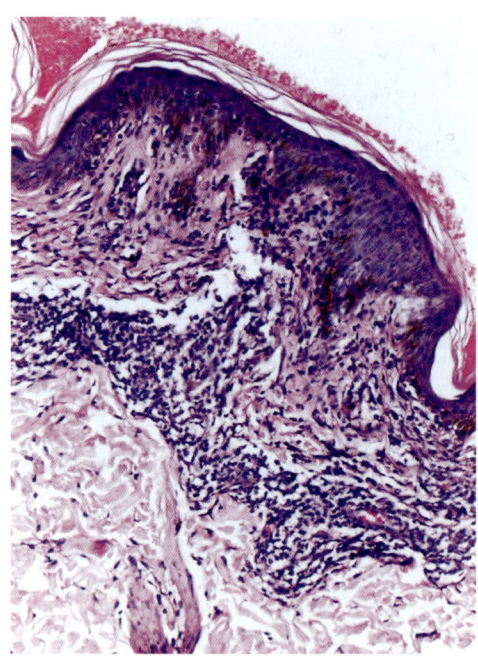

Fig. 3.5: Small epithelioid cell granuloma among abundant lymphocytes and absence of clear subepidermal zone indicating primary tuberculoid leprosy (H & E, ×200)

Secondary Tuberculoid Leprosy (TTs)[1,3,8]

TTs is a *post-reactional* lesion, has variable size and is often large. A hallmark feature is large erosion of the epidermis with a patch of fibrinoid or caseation necrosis. Similar

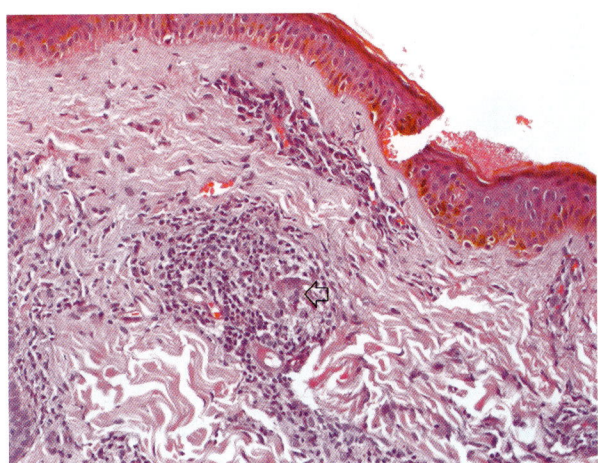

Fig. 3.6: Epithelioid cell granuloma of tuberculoid leprosy with lymphocytes and Langhans' giant cells (H & E, ×200)

to TTp, granuloma consists of immature epithelioid cells; but in place of the cluster of mature epithelioid cells seen in TTp, TTs manifests only a few mature epithelioid cells. Large Langhans' giant cells are often seen. Number of lymphocytes vary and at times, they are fairly scanty. Lymphocytes are more diffusely spread than in TTp.

Nerve bundles, greatly swollen with a granuloma and sharply circumscribed perineurium, differentiates TTs from TTp. Though usually not seen, AFB may occasionally be found in areas of caseation.

Borderline Tuberculoid (BT)[1,3,8]

Epidermal atrophy is variable and depends on the size and extent of granuloma. When the inflammation in dermis is small and focal, epidermal changes are minimal. Involvement of subepidermal zone is variable. Granuloma may encroach upon the basal layer.

Immature epithelioid cells constitute the granuloma. Mature epithelioid cells are conspicuously absent. Moderate number of lymphocytes with or without Langhans' giant cells may be present. More characteristic is the presence of foreign body giant cells (Fig. 3.7).[8] Lymphocytes may form mantles around, as well as clusters inside, the granuloma.

In late lesions, nerve bundles may be considerably swollen and destroyed by granuloma, but strands of nerve fiber often

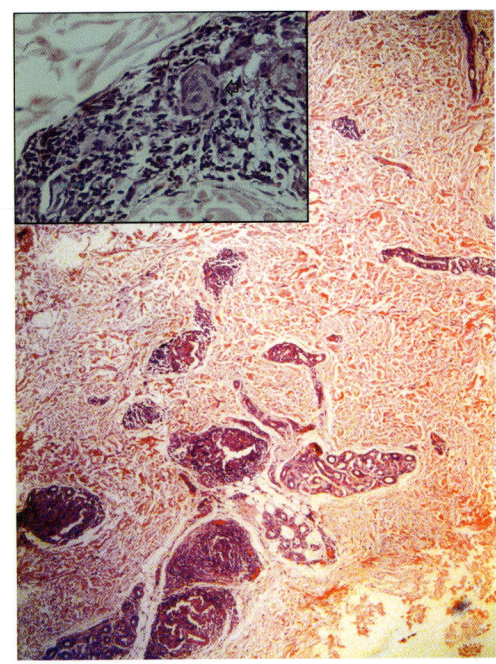

Fig. 3.7: Skin biopsy specimen showing multiple epithelioid granulomas of borderline tuberculoid leprosy (H & E, ×40); inset: higher magnification showing foreign body giant cells and lymphocytes in granuloma (H & E, ×200)

survive intact. Surviving strands of nerve, subepidermal zone or granuloma may show AFB. But outside the nerve, they are seldom seen more than one per field. All nerve fibers and AFB will be completely destroyed in advanced lesions. Necrosis is not a feature of BT.

Borderline Borderline (BB)[1,3,8]

Epidermis is atrophic. A clear subepidermal zone and presence of AFB (at times numerous) mark BB. The lesions are comprised of mixed granulomas composed of immature epithelioid cells and bacteria-laden activated macrophages.

The histology features are often obscured by *edema* that denotes the reactional instability.

Absence of giant cells, scanty inflammatory cells including lymphocytes and lack of lymphocyte cuffing around granuloma are the other features (Fig. 3.8). Laminated perineurium is swollen with epithelioid cells and surrounds nerve bundles that are not very large.

Borderline Lepromatous (BL)[1,3,8]

Epidermis is atrophic. A clear grenz zone separates epidermis from granuloma. BL features macrophage granuloma with slightly foamy cytoplasm (Fig. 3.9). A small focus of epithelioid cells may be there in a few cases. Giant cell is *not* a feature of BL. BL shows a dense infiltrate of lymphocytes extending over the whole of at least one segment of granuloma, reaching to its peripheral edge while other parts remain free of the same. Plasma cells may also be seen.

Nerves are not swollen greatly, but some of the lymphocytes that infiltrate their laminated perineurium may penetrate into the nerve bundle. A dense peripheral cuff of lymphocytes around a nerve bundle in a macrophage granuloma favors BL. AFB may be almost as much as in LL.

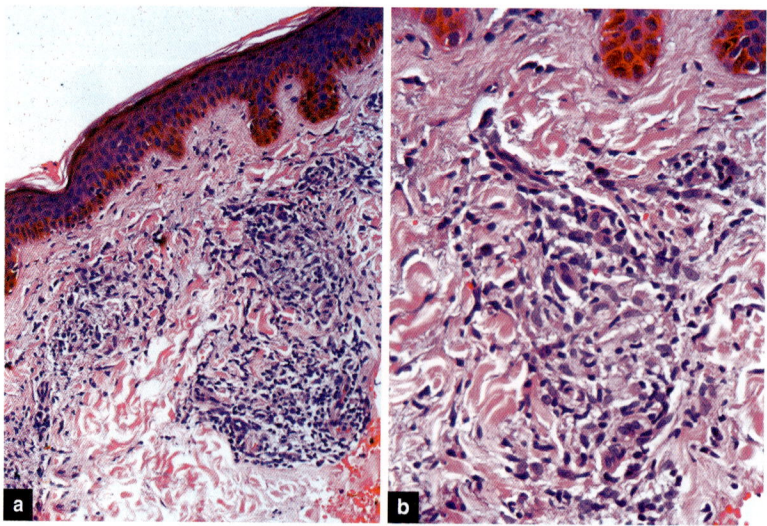

Fig. 3.8: (a) Diffuse epithelioid cell granuloma of borderline borderline leprosy without giant cells or lymphocyte mantle (H & E, ×100); (b) Higher magnification showing absence of giant cells and paucity of lymphocytes in granuloma (H & E, ×400)

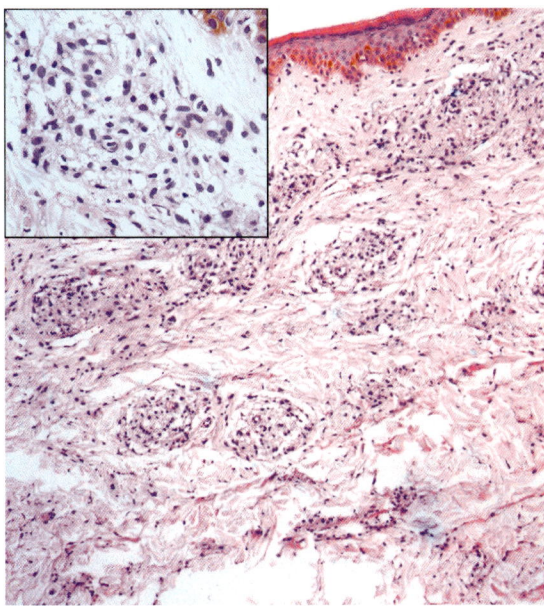

Fig. 3.9: Macrophage granuloma of borderline lepromatous leprosy (H & E, ×100); inset: Higher magnification showing scattered epithelioid cells along with foamy macrophages and sprinkling of lymphocytes (H & E, ×400)

Lepromatous Leprosy (LL)[1,3,8]

In well established LL, epidermis is thin and atrophied with complete flattening of rete ridges. Clear subepidermal grenz zone is visible between epidermis and the cellular infiltrate. Pink and granular cytoplasm of macrophages becomes foamy and vacuolated as lesions get older (Fig. 3.10a and b). A few lymphocytes are seen among macrophages.

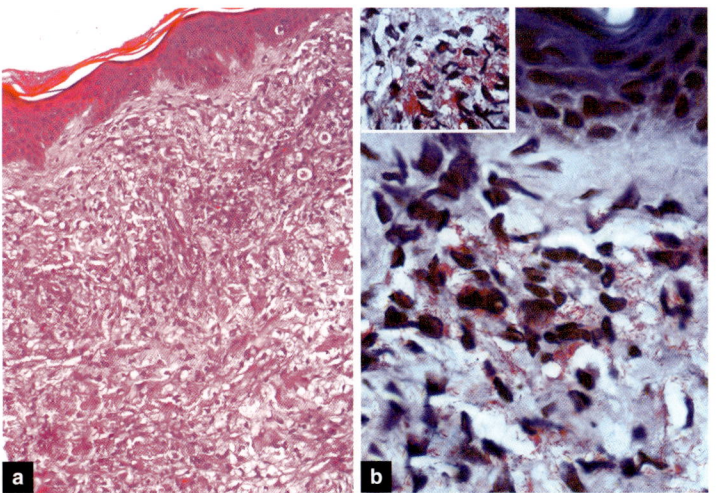

Fig. 3.10: (a) Macrophage granuloma of lepromatous leprosy showing subepidermal grenz zone and sheets of foamy macrophages (H & E, ×200); (b) Oil immersion view of the same specimen showing acid fast bacilli just below the grenz zone (Wade Fite, ×1000); inset: Another focus of same biopsy showing globi within the macrophages (Wade Fite, ×1000)

Plasma cells are present focally. Early lesions show small, focal clusters of cellular infiltrate in the dermis and as disease advances, these focal infiltrates join to form a band of macrophages infiltrating the dermis and extending into the subcutaneous fat. Hair follicles and sweat and sebaceous glands are surrounded by macrophages. These skin appendages show atrophy.

Larger, more rounded and more foamy macrophages are seen in polar LL (LLp) when compared to subpolar LL (LLs). Lymphocytes are sparse in LLp, whereas in LLs, lymphocytes and plasma cells may be adequately numerous to form clusters. But unlike in BL, they do not extend over segments of granuloma.

Significant swelling of nerves is not a feature of either LLs or LLp. In both, macrophage collections are seen perineurially; but intraneural infiltration by inflammatory cells is minimal. Reactive proliferation of perineurium is minimal in LLp, while in LLs, nerve bundles show multilaminated perineurium as the disease is downgraded from BL. The empty laminated perineurium produced by the retreatment of lymphocytes during downgrading is a characteristic feature of LLs.

Histoid Leprosy[1,3,8,9]

In this variant of LL, the characteristic histology observed is a hypercellular granuloma, predominantly composed of spindle-shaped cells (Fig. 3.10c to e). The centrifugal growth of these cells compresses the fibrous tissue into a clear pseudocapsule. Uniform arrangement of cells in whorls as in histiocytoma was the reason for using the term 'histoid' to describe this entity. Highly bacillated cells harboring solid staining forms are arranged in parallel stalks, which are referred to as histoid habitus. Some lesions of histoid leprosy may show islands of epithelioid cells without any organism inside, which are known as epithelioid contaminants.

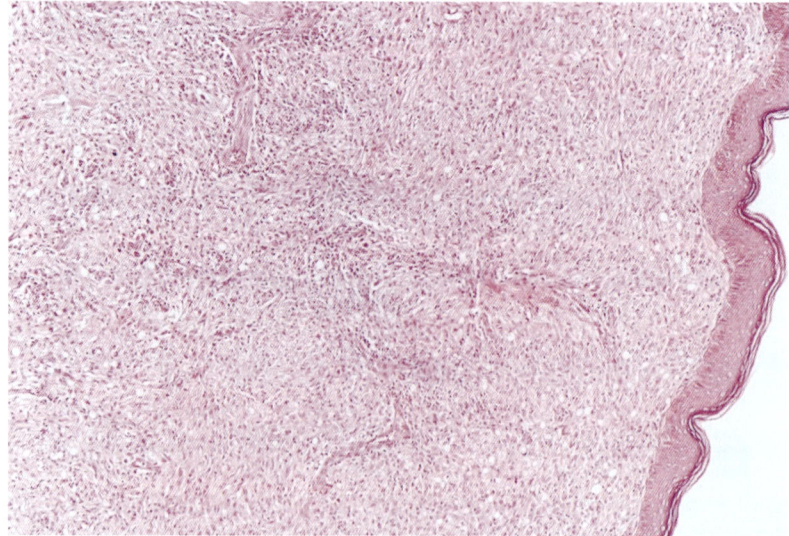

Fig. 3.10c: Interlacing histiocytic spindle shaped cells arranged in a centrifugal fashion efface the dermis (H & E, ×100) (*Courtesy:* Dr Purnima Paliwal)

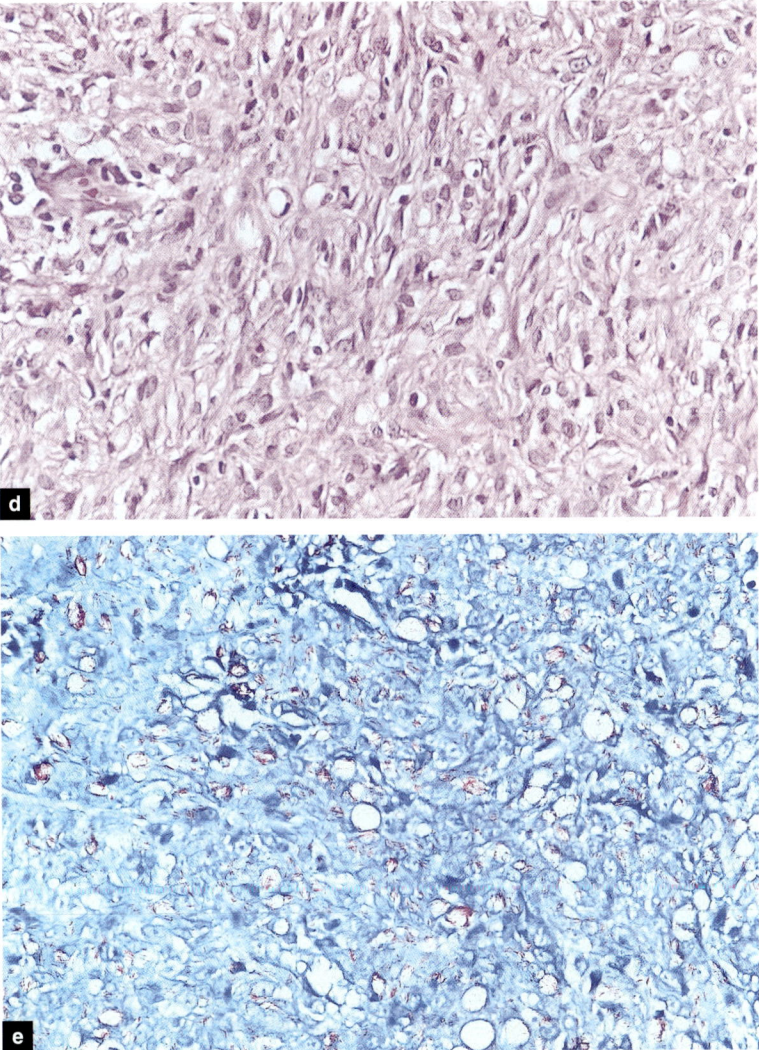

Fig. 3.10: (d) Higher magnification showing oval to spindle cells arranged in fascicles, a few cells showing foamy cytoplasm (H & E, ×400); (e) Fite stain showing many solid staining acid-fast bacilli all across the field (Fite, ×1000) (*Courtesy:* Dr Purnima Paliwal)

REACTIONS IN LEPROSY

A. Type 1 Reaction (T1R)

Lockwood et al have considered histological diagnosis of T1R in the setting of two of the following features—granulomas with extra and intracellular edema, dilated vascular channels, separation of dermal collagen, evidence of an intense delayed-type hypersensitivity response with acute damage to dermal nerves and granuloma (Fig. 3.11).[10] But it is pertinent to point out that there are discrepancies between clinical and histopathology features in patients manifesting leprosy reactions.[10–12] Dermal edema, considered as an important feature of reaction may be missed if there is a delay between the onset of reaction and time of biopsy.[12,13]

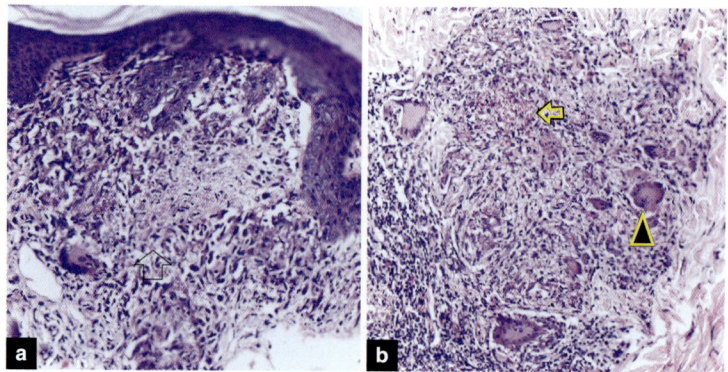

Fig. 3.11: (a) Arrow denoting focus of necrosis within epithelioid cell granuloma in borderline tuberculoid leprosy with type 1 lepra reaction (H & E, ×200); (b) Biopsy from skin lesion of borderline tuberculoid leprosy in type 1 lepra reaction showing epithelioid cell granuloma, intragranuloma oedema, Langhan's giant cells (indicated by black arrow head), foreign body giant cell and beginning of necrosis (indicated by yellow arrow) in a focus of granuloma (H & E, ×200)

T1R is classified into three types based on the immunological events. They are upgrading reaction (rapid increase in specific CMI against *M. leprae*), downgrading reaction (rapid decline in CMI) and static reaction (without any change in the immunity).

1. *Upgrading T1R*: An increase in defensive cells like lymphocytes, epithelioid cells and giant cells and decrease in bacillary load (Fig. 3.12).
2. *Downgrading T1R*: Fewer defensive cells like lymphocytes and epithelioid cells (Fig. 3.13), bacilli may increase, macrophages may replace defensive cells.
3. *Static reactions*: Features of underlying leprosy only; considered as ineffective attempts at upgrading.[12, 13]

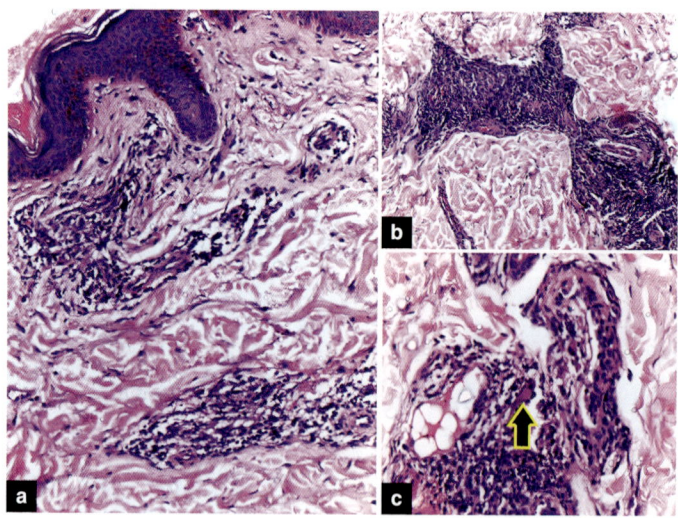

Fig. 3.12: (a) Epithelioid granuloma with intragranuloma oedema in borderline tuberculoid leprosy with type 1 lepra reaction (H & E, ×200); (b) Another focus in the granuloma showing abundance of lymphocytes (H & E, ×200); (c) Black arrow denoting Langhans' giant cell (H & E, ×400)—features suggestive of upgrading type 1 lepra reaction

Diagnostic Tests and Histopathology

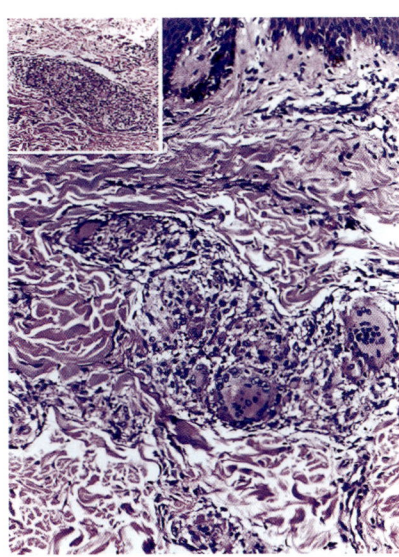

Fig. 3.13: Epithelioid granuloma with intragranuloma edema in borderline tuberculoid leprosy with type 1 lepra reaction showing Langhans' giant cell and foreign body giant cell, lymphocytes are scanty (H & E, ×200); inset: Close up view of granuloma showing scanty lymphocytes (H & E, ×200)—probably downgrading type 1 lepra reaction

These variations are better appreciated when pre-reaction biopsy specimen is available for comparison and is one reason why some experts do not seem to diagnose and recognize the downgrading reaction. Other types of T1R may be overlooked, if the term reversal reaction is used as synonym for T1R (Table 3.7).

Table 3.7: Histological classification of type 1 lepra reaction					
	Histological feature				
Type 1 lepra reaction	Edema	Lymphocytes	Macrophages	Giant cells	Acid-fast bacilli
Upgrading reaction	Intense Edema	Marked increase	Old foamy macrophages, if present in pre-reactional state, may persist	Many Langhans' giant cells	Considerably decrease or disappear in borderline lepromatous cases
Downgrading reaction	Present	Decrease	Increase	Pre-existing Langhans' giant cells may persist	May increase if downgraded to lepromatous disease
Static reaction (reaction with no evidence of upgrading or down-grading)	Conflicting reports	Remain at same level	Remain at same level	Remain at same level	Remain at same level

Ridley and Radia suggested dermal edema to be an infrequent manifestation of static reaction.[13] But we have observed dermal edema in T1R that did not show features of upgrading or downgrading (Fig. 3.14).[12] This was in accordance with the findings of Ramu and Desikan.[14]

T1R has been categorized into *four* stages histologically by Ridley:[15]

1. *The prodromal phase of the reaction*: This may precede the clinical onset. The features described are: Mild edema and proliferation of fibrocytes that is not confined to the zone around the granuloma. Dilated lymphatics and spaces around the granuloma and in the dermis, point to the extracellular nature of edema. Variable number of lymphocytes are seen.

   All patients with signs of prodromal phase need not necessarily develop full fledged T1R subsequently.

2. *Acute stage reaction*: More severe edema and dispersion of granuloma by swelling and disruption characterize this stage. Different types of giant cells may be seen. Langhans'-type cells need not always indicate upgrading since they may persist in downgrading reactions.[16]

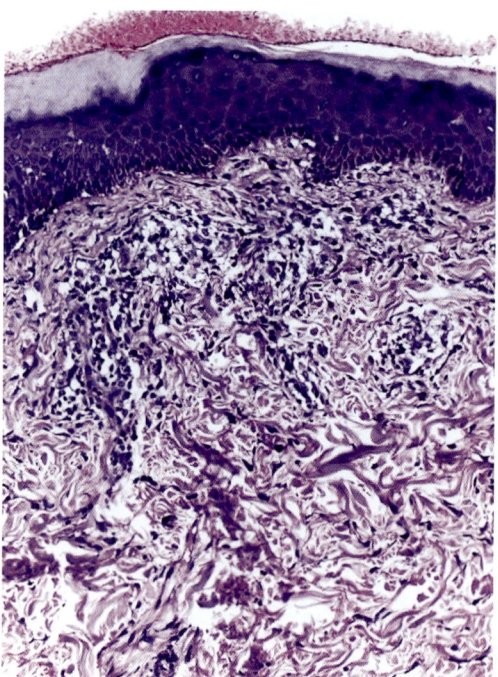

Fig. 3.14: Epithelioid granuloma with dermal and intragranuloma edema in borderline tuberculoid leprosy with type 1 lepra reaction, lymphocytes as expected in borderline tuberculoid spectrum favoring static reaction (H & E, ×200)

   Giant cells may contain small cytoplasmic vesicles, due to intracellular edema. Replacement of fibrocytes by fibroblasts in the dermis and variable degrees of damage to collagen and elastic fibers are the other features.

3. *Necrosis*: Severe upgrading reactions usually manifest necrosis. In granulomas with initial high bacterial load, profuse edema may occur along with liquefaction necrosis in the granuloma. In lesions in the tuberculoid spectrum with low bacterial load, small foci of necrosis involve the collagen than the granuloma, producing fibrinoid necrosis in case of high delayed hypersensitivity. This usually marks the late stage of reaction leading to TTs. Local infiltrate of neutrophils is a feature that accompanies any necrosis. Presence of epithelioid cells differentiates such reactions from ENL; though rarely ENL and T1R may coexist.

4. *Subsidence of the reaction*: Reformation of granuloma marks subsidence. There is a reduction in dermal edema. Fibrosis resulting from proliferation of fibroblasts resolves later.

B. Type 2 Reaction (T2R)[1,15]

The most common cutaneous lesions of T2R are painful, evanescent nodules known as ENL. The characteristic histopathology is dense infiltration, of superficial and/or

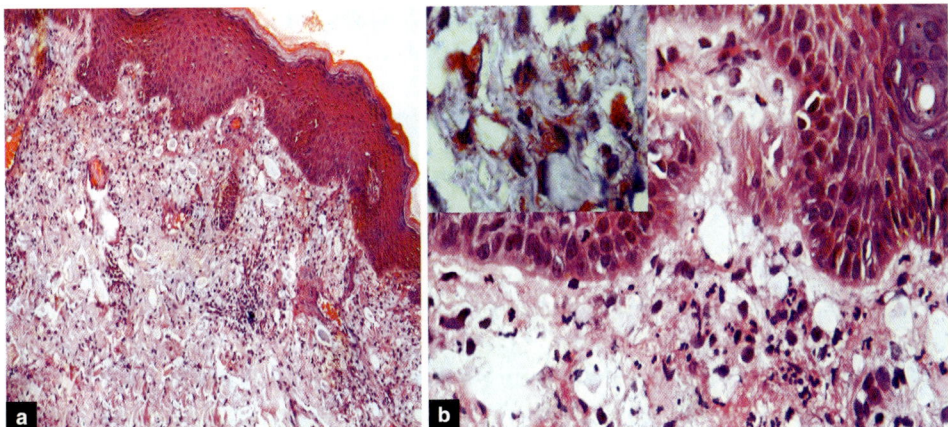

Fig. 3.15: (a) Macrophage granuloma in lepromatous leprosy with type 2 lepra reaction (H & E, ×100); (b) Higher magnification showing neutrophil infiltration in macrophage granuloma (H and E, ×400); inset: Wade Fite staining of same specimen showing acid-fast bacilli (Wade Fite, ×1000)

deep dermis and/or subcutaneous tissue by neutrophils that is superimposed on preexisting macrophage granuloma (Fig. 3.15). Polymorphs emerging from capillaries form clusters around degenerate macrophages, often producing microabscesses. Eosinophils and mast cells may also be seen. Vasculitis is a prominent feature in some cases. Damage to collagen and elastic fibers is a common finding. Considerable reduction occurs in bacterial load and most of the AFB present are fragmented and granular.

Classic ENL

In the classic ENL, the reaction center where neutrophil influx occurs is in subcutis. During resolution, neutrophils get replaced by lymphocytes and plasma cells. Hence, neutrophil infiltration may be missed in late lesions.[17]

Necrotizing ENL[1,15]

Severity of reaction is more when the granuloma involved is larger. In necrotizing ENL, numerous AFBs (including some solid forms) can be seen. Other differentiating features favoring necrotizing ENL over classic form are—intense edema, heavy and diffuse scattering of neutrophils over the superficial zone of the dermis (though they may also produce microabscesses centered on areas of lepromatous granuloma), karyorrhexis at the site of granuloma and necrosis within the granuloma (in severe forms). Though vasculitis is not a universal feature, the chance for the same is higher than in classic ENL. Lepromatous infiltration of large vessels in the subcutis or deep dermis, or a necrotizing capillaritis is not uncommon. Intense connective tissue damage may occur.

Dermal ENL[15]

Ridley documented that dermal ENL can be clinically mild or severe, similar to classic ENL, but with striking differences histologically.[15]

Acute stage shows dermal edema and infiltration by primitive fibroblasts and tissue macrophages. Severe elastosis featuring swollen, fractured and clumped elastic fibers is a major finding. Fibrinoid degeneration and necrosis are often seen. In some cases, a subacute vasculitis leads to enormous distension of dermal blood vessels. Electron microscopy has revealed abundance of membrane bound sacs loaded with mycobacterial debris, especially cell wall material. When these sacs rupture, the phagosomes deposit their loads onto the degenerate collagen fibrils. The changes described in classic ENL, are observed in other areas of the granuloma. Fibrosis almost equivalent to a keloid, accompanies the resolution; but lesions are repaired completely, except for the changes observed in elastic fibers.

C. Lucio Phenomenon[1,8,15]

Lucio phenomenon (*also see Chapters 2 and 5, Sections 2.1 and 5.3*) associated with Lucio leprosy. The diffuse spread of infection is associated with the formation of very small granulomas or isolated macrophages. Larger granulomas may also be present. Heavy colonization of *M. leprae* observed in the endothelium of small capillaries in the superficial dermis, is a peculiar feature of Lucio leprosy in both reactional and in nonreactional states. Involvement of these capillaries in reaction, manifests as haemorrhage and infarction of the overlying epidermis. If deep vessels also become involved, the reaction may resemble classic ENL; but with a marked component of vascular necrosis.

D. Acute Exacerbation[1,15] (*also see Chapter 5.3*)

Acute exacerbation of the disease is seen mainly in nodular and plaque lesions of advanced lepromatous leprosy. Histology reveals small, localized areas of necrosis in the middle of large sheet of macrophages that attracts localized infiltration by neutrophils. Vasculitis is a rare feature. Macrophages contain numerous AFB, among which many are solid staining. Presence of solid staining AFB, distinguishes acute exacerbation from ENL, where most of the bacilli are fragmented.

Only the most active part of the lesion may be affected in an acute exacerbation. When it occurs in a histoid nodule, it is known as Wade's reaction centers.[15] Localized cell necrosis and acute inflammation resulting from sudden localized burst of bacterial multiplication that outgrows the macrophage population is cited as the mechanism underlying acute exacerbation.[15]

Acute exacerbation is less significant than ENL clinically, since there occur only few systemic manifestations and as the exacerbations are localized to a few large lesions only. But the importance lies in the fact that the involved lesions may ulcerate and discharge viable bacilli.

Ridley opined that massive and persistent antigenic load is the cause of all reactions of lepromatous leprosy and the variations observed depend on the size of the antigenic mass that participates in a reaction.[15]

NERVE INVOLVEMENT IN LEPROSY[1]

The different mechanisms suggested for entry of *M. leprae* in cutaneous nerves are the following (*also see Chapter 4, Section 4.4*):
  i. *Epidermis*: Through naked axons
 ii. *Papillary dermis*: Through naked axons when epithelium is denuded.
iii. *Dermis*: Phagocytosed by the perineurial cells in dermis and from there by invading endoneurium and Schwann cells or through endoneurial blood vessels during bacteremia.

Biopsies from purely sensory nerves in pure neuritic leprosy have showed histology that could be assigned to all types including indeterminate leprosy.[1] Pathological causes for leprous neuropathy are classified into intra-fascicular (Schwann cell involvement), extra-fascicular (reactional episodes) and extra-neural (compression in osteofibrous corridors).[7]

Irrespective of the position in the spectrum, earliest stage of leprous neuropathy is the appearance of AFB in Schwann cells without any cellular response. This phase is followed by Schwann cell proliferation, segmental demyelination and axonal degeneration. Sensory fibers are the earliest to be affected and the most affected. It is proposed that the Schwann cells of myelinated fibers are the first to be affected; but larger number of organisms are seen in the Schwann cells of unmyelinated fibers. In some lepromatous cases, bacilli are seen in the myelinated and unmyelinated axons, more frequently in myelinated axons. Their number is scanty in comparison to the bacterial load in Schwann cells. Intra-axonal bacilli contribute to bacterial dissemination and neural destruction.[7]

When skin and nerve lesions coexist, the bacterial load is generally higher in nerve except at the lepromatous pole and in reactions, since peripheral nerve is an immunologically protected site. The histological classification of concurrent skin and nerve lesions into groups, often yields discordant results.[1,2]

Groups assigned on the basis of skin lesions, rather than the nerve lesions, indicate the overall immune responsiveness of the affected individual. Many AFB reside in Schwann cells instead of the granuloma cells and this is more obvious in LL. Moreover, neural architecture inhibits infiltration by lymphocytes. But mature epithelioid cells and caseation necrosis are more common in nerves than in skin lesions (Fig. 3.16). The histological changes in nerves vary depending on the type of leprosy.[1] They are broadly classified into tuberculoid neuritis, borderline neuritis, lepromatous neuritis and end stage neuritis (Table 3.8)[1] (*see Chapter 2.4, Section 2.4*).

In tuberculoid neuritis, the extent of the nerve affected differs. It varies from a portion of a fascicle in a nerve trunk to one or all fascicles to one or a few nerve trunks. In lepromatous leprosy, many cutaneous nerves may be affected. Borderline group, manifests features of both tuberculoid and lepromatous disease (destructive effect of

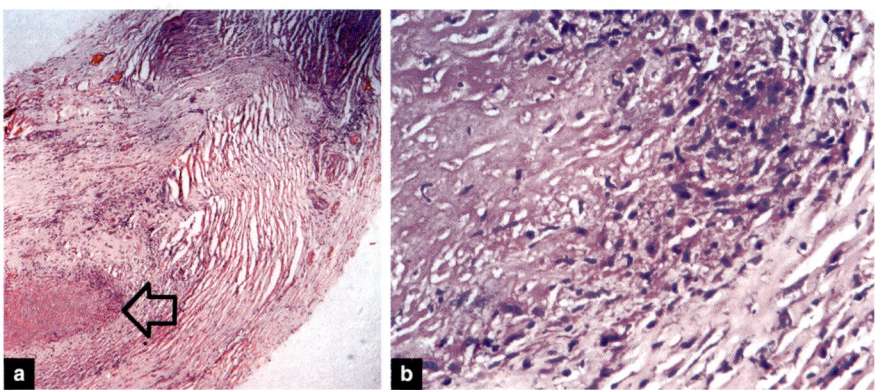

Fig. 3.16: (a) Nerve biopsy from radial cutaneous nerve showing epithelioid cell granuloma (black arrow) with caseation necrosis (H & E, ×40); (b) Higher magnification showing necrosis, epithelioid cells and lymphocytes (H & E, ×400)

Table 3.8: Histopathology features of leprosy neuropathy

Tuberculoid neuritis	Borderline neuritis	Lepromatous neuritis	End stage neuritis
1. Granuloma infiltrating the nerve composed of epithelioid cells, hymphocytes and Langhans' giant cells 2. Caseation necrosis may be seen 3. A few AFB seen in caseous material and Schwann cell 4. Thickening of perineurium by infiltration of lymphocytes epithelioid cells and fibroblasts and by proliferation of perineurial cells 5. Nerve abscess is a common feature (large acres of caseous necrosis surrounded by granuloma and fibrous tissue remnants of nerve tissue at the periphery of the granuloma)	1. Varying proportion of macrophages, epithelioid cells and lymphocytes infiltrate the nerve tissue depending on patient's immunity against *M. leprae* 2. Moderate number of AFB seen in Schwann cells and intraneural macrophages 3. Sudden increase in size of granuloma due to marked edema and influx of inflammatory cells (lymphocytes or macrophages depending on whether reaction is upgrading or downgrading) and ischemia induced by raised intraneural pressure in type 1 lepra reaction may cause rapid deterioration of nerve function	1. Early lesion. AFB in Schwann cells and endoneurial macrophages 2. Foamy degeneration of Schwann cells and macrophages 3. Infected Schwann cells lose function and ability to regenerate 4. Schwann cells and their axons die and disappear 5. Reactive proliferation of perineurium follows infection of perineural cells 6. Basement membrane of capillary endothelium thickens, reduplicates and causes luminal narrowing 7. Further damage to nerve parenchyma due to resultant ischemia 8. Infiltration of neutrophils that form focal micro-abscesses in macrophage granuloma which in turn produces rapid destruction of nerve tissue at sites of abscess formation in type 2 lepra reactions	1. Fibrosis and hyalinization—end stage of al types of neuritis in leprosy 2. Schwann cells, axons, myelin sheath and perineurium replaced by fibrous tissue 3. Nerve destroyed by leprous granuloma unable to regenerate since no Schwann tubes for re-growing nerve fibers to grow into nerves 4. No evidence of inflammation

tuberculoid granuloma coupled with generalized multiple nerve involvement seen in lepromatous disease), which makes it the high risk group for severe nerve paralysis. Another factor that contributes to nerve damage in borderline groups is their vulnerability to reversal reactions which accentuates the inflammation in nerves.[1]

SYSTEMIC INVOLVEMENT

Leprosy, though primarily affects skin and nerves, may involve various other tissues in the body though this is more common in lepromatous disease.

Histopathology changes are similar in various sites manifested as infiltration by AFB laden macrophages with a few plasma cells and lymphocytes in lepromatous cases, epithelioid cells, lymphocytes and giant cells in tuberculoid leprosy and varying combinations of epithelioid cells, macrophages and lymphocytes in borderline cases.[1]

T2R, when present shows neutrophil infiltration and edema in the background of macrophage granuloma, at times producing focal microabscess formation.[1,8,15]

Rapid accumulation of edema fluid and influx of inflammatory cells (macrophages or lymphocytes, depending on whether the reaction is upgrading or downgrading) results in increase in size and pressure effect exerted by the granuloma in borderline cases.[1,15]

Eyes, nose and testes are the sites other than skin and peripheral nerves, that are affected commonly in leprosy.[1]

Eyes[1]

Direct invasion of eye by *M. leprae* is limited to lepromatous group of patients and is mostly confined to the anterior aspect of eye.

Microgranulomas composed of AFB packed foamy macrophages lead to:
a. Increased tear secretion by obstruction of nasolacrimal duct
b. Subconjunctival nodules, frequently at limbus
c. Corneal opacity
d. Complete destruction of sclera
e. Iris pearls (miliary lepromas of 0.25 mm diameter around pupillary margin of eye)
f. Retinal miliary lepromas, rarely.

The changes documented in T2R are:
a. Formation of keratotic precipitates in the anterior chamber
b. Adhesion between anterior capsule of lens and iris (posterior synechiae)
c. Anchoring of pupils to lens by fibrosis
d. Blindness caused by covering of pupil by fibrinous exudate.

Nose[1]

The changes induced by granulomas of lepromatous disease are:
a. Submucosal lepromatous nodules
b. Atrophy of mucous glands
c. Thinning and ulceration of mucosal lining
d. Damage to septal cartilage and perforation
e. Destruction of bony and cartilaginous framework by granuloma and secondary pyogenic infection, leading to collapse of nose.
f. Flat nose deformity produced by contraction of fibrous tissue formed during resolution of inflammation that pulls nose further to face.

In addition, a direct extension from adjacent skin lesion to nasal mucosa may occur in tuberculoid disease.

Testes[1]

Testes are usually spared in tuberculoid disease. In borderline cases, seminiferous tubules may be infiltrated by granuloma.

In lepromatous disease, in early stage, focal, perivascular, macrophage granuloma formation occurs in testes. Thickening of basement membrane and loss of spermatogenesis take place in seminiferous tubules surrounding the areas of vasculitis. Other changes described are obliterative endarteritis and periarteritis of interstitial blood vessels, atrophy and hyalinization of seminiferous tubules in advanced disease (leaving behind Sertoli cells alone) hypertrophy, clumping and hyperplasia of Leydig cells and fibrous thickening of tunica vaginalis. The entire organ may be destroyed structurally and functionally.

Lymph Nodes[1]

Generalized lymphadenopathy is seen in lepromatous patients, whereas in tuberculoid and borderline cases, lymph nodes draining the skin lesions show granulomas. Granulomas are seen throughout the cortex and medulla of involved lymph nodes. Reactive hyperplasia of reticuloendothelial cells and prominent germinal centers are observed. In addition, thickening and fibrosis of the capsule of lymph node is described in lepromatous cases. Caseous necrosis is absent; but in T2R, microabscesses formed by focal collections of neutrophils may occasionally produce large abscesses that break open through the lymph node capsule and skin. In tuberculoid cases, epithelioid cell granuloma is seen.

Rarely other organs may also be affected and the histopathological characteristics are summarized in Table 3.9.[1]

HISTOLOGICAL DIFFERENTIAL DIAGNOSES OF LEPROSY[1-3]

The most common difficulty arises in accurately diagnosing indeterminate leprosy and some tuberculoid lesions. Job has commented that the responsibility of diagnosis in doubtful cases rests with the clinician.[1] The 'leprosy pattern' of granuloma is suggested as a clue to diagnosis in granulomatous stage of disease.[18] The pattern is described as *superficial* and *deep*, well-circumscribed, oval, oblong, or curvilinear infiltrates in a perivascular and periappendageal distribution with minimal extension into the interstitial dermis under low power (Fig. 3.17). The oblong presentation of infiltrates is attributed to the involvement along the neurovascular bundle. The common histological differential diagnoses for leprosy and differentiating features are charted in Table 3.10 (Figs 3.18 to 3.21).

REGRESSING LESIONS[1,2]

Regression of leprous granuloma usually follows treatment (Fig. 3.22a and b) and is complete within one to three years of treatment in tuberculoid disease and later in lepromatous disease (Flowchart 3.1).[1,19]

Increase in epidermal basement membrane pigmentation and morphea-like changes in the dermis (sclerotic dermis with paucity of adnexal structures and inflammatory infiltrate) have been reported in treated leprosy cases (Fig. 3.23).[20,21]

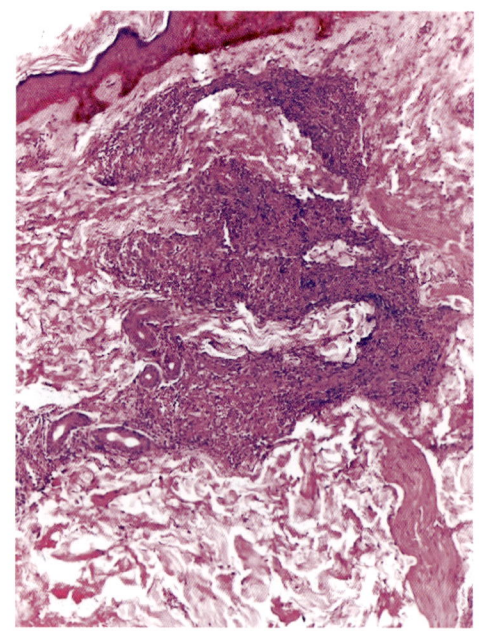

Fig. 3.17: Well-circumscribed, curvilinear infiltrates in a perivascular and periappendageal distribution—'leprosy pattern' of granuloma (H & E, ×100)

Table 3.9: Less common manifestations in leprosy: Tissues involved beyond skin and nerves

Site affected	Histopathology findings	Clinical manifestations	Group of patients affected
Mouth, hard and soft palate	Infiltration by macrophages containing *M. leprae*	Gingivitis, nodular lesions of hard and soft palate, perforation of hard palate, destruction of uvula, nodularity and fissuring of tongue	Lepromatous group
Larynx	• Infiltration of subepithelial tissue of laynx with bacillated macrophages • Acute edema and neutrophil infiltration in type 2 lepra reaction • Fibrosis of vocal cords during resolution of inflammation	• Lepromatous laryngitis presents as hoarseness of voice • Acute laryngeal obstruction • Permanent hoarseness	• Lepromatous leprosy
Liver	• Prominent Kupffer cells, numerous miliary lepromas, no liver cell necrosis, condensation of reticulum around the capsule forming a false capsule, slight increase in fibrous tissue around portal tracts • Infiltration of liver with neutrophils • Tuberculoid granulomas • Granulomas composed of variable mixture of epithelioid cells, lymphocytes and macrophages	• No gross abnormality described. Miliary lepromas, being expansile lesions push out the liver tissue without destroying parenchyma or architecture, elevated liver transaminases • Type 2 lepra reaction	• Lepromatous leprosy • Lepromatous disease • Tuberculoid disease • Borderline cases
Spleen	• Miliary lepromas throughout red and white pulp, cuffing of penicillar arteries and branching capillaries by collections of macrophages • Macrophages replacing lymphocytes in thymus dependent areas	• No gross abnormality reported • Nonspecific suppression of CMI	• Lepromatous disease • Advanced lepromatous disease
Bone marrow	Numerous miliary granulomas, AFB inside macrophages and lying freely in the interstitium of bone marrow	Refractory anemia	Lepromatous leprosy
Bone	• Macrophage granuloma invading bony trabeculae and periosteum,	• Lepromatous osteomyelitis (destructive lesions mainly affecting	• Advanced lepromatous leprosy

(Contd.)

Table 3.9: Less common manifestations in leprosy: Tissues involved beyond skin and nerves (Contd.)			
Site affected	Histopathology findings	Clinical manifestations	Group of patients affected
	proliferation of capillaries, reactive proliferation of osteoid tissue, no calcification or new bone formation, presence of AFB in osteoblasts and osteocytes as well • Proliferation of periosteum (many layers of osteoblasts laying down new bone at the anterior aspect of tibia), AFB within osteoblasts	small bones of hands, feet and bones forming framework of nose), atrophy, fragmentation and absorption of bone • Periostitis of tibia (acute pain along anterior aspect of leg)	 • Children and young adults with lepromatous leprosy
Muscle	• Infiltration and destruction of muscle tissue by foamy macrophages, occasional neutrophils and a few lymphocytes, loss of striation, swelling and thickening of endomysium and clumping of sarcolemmal nucleus in muscle cells surrounding inflammatory infiltrate, AFB within striated muscle cells as well as in macrophages • Fibrous replacement of muscle tissue	• Painful nodules in muscles, usually affecting superficial muscles of limbs • Resolution of painful nodules in muscles	• Lepromatous disease • Lepromatous disease
Breast	Proliferation of connective tissue and duct epithelium as in gynecomastia due to other causes, small focal collections of macrophages with AFB in connective tissue occasionally	Gynecomastia	Lepromatous leprosy
Adrenal glands	Miliary lepromas in adrenal cortex	Normal function of adrenals (lepromas push out the gland rather than infiltrating or destroying it) except in patients with chronic ENL in whom adrenal reserve is compromised	Lepromatous patients
Kidneys	Diffuse endocapillary, proliferative, crescenteric, membranous, mesangiocapillary, sclerosing or focal proliferative minimal change disease	Glomerulonephritis, renal failure, amyloidosis*	Lepromatous leprosy, borderline cases

*The organs commonly affected by amyloidosis in leprosy are liver, spleen, kidneys and adrenals. Amyloid deposition gives rosy violet color on a blue background when stained with metachromatic stain like methyl violet.

Table 3.10: Histological differential diagnoses in leprosy

Group of leprosy	Differential diagnosis	Distinguishing feature in against diagnosis of leprosy
Indeterminate leprosy	Nonspecific dermatitis	A strong perivascular infiltrate favors dermatitis, even if there is some involvement of perineurial or periappendageal sites. In the absence of reaction (which is unlikely in indeterminate cases), edema or an infiltrate of neutrophils or eosinophils suggests dermatitis.
Tuberculoid leprosy AFB, when found in nerve bundles or just below epidermis or arrector pili muscles, may help to diagnose leprosy. Another clue in favor of leprosy is infiltration and destruction of nerve bundles by granuloma (when nerves are totally destroyed by granuloma staining of S-100 protein may identify nerve fragments)	Cutaneous tuberculosis	• Tubercles infiltrate superficial dermis, hug the epidermis and ulcerate at times. • The granuloma produces a relatively large solid mass in the deep dermis or subcutis, which is unlike leprosy. Caseous necrosis may be present, extensive fibrosis in long-standing lesions. Caseation, if it is present outside nerve centers, is the best point of distinction from leprosy • In tuberculosis verrucosa cutis, presence of epidermal changes like hyperkeratosis, acanthosis and papillomatosis. Fibrosis surrounds granuloma
	Cutaneous leishmaniasis	• Tuberculoid granuloma in superficial dermis, Giemsa staining revealing numerous intracellular Leishman-Donovan bodies • The lesion as a whole, though not the granuloma in it, is much more compact than in leprosy. One of the most useful distinguishing features, often present, is epidermal involvement: Downgrowths of epidermis or pseudoepitheliomatous hyperplasia
	Tertiary syphilis	Granuloma surrounded by large number of plasma cells, endarteritis and periarteritis, gumma shows central necrosis
	Sarcoidosis	• Whorled nests of plump epithelioid cells in well circumscribed clusters. Naked tubercles with scanty lymphocytes • The nests are surrounded by strands of reticulin or a fine band of collagen
	Granuloma annulare	Palisaded granuloma surrounding collagen undergoing mucinous degeneration. Mucin stains metachromatically with Giemsa or toluidine blue.
	Granuloma multiforme	Clear subepidermal zone, large number of plasma cells in granuloma
Lepromatous leprosy	Skin nodules of post-Kala-azar dermal leishmaniasis	AFB negativity and Giemsa stain revealing numerous intracellular Leishman-Donovan bodies
Histoid leprosy	Dermatofibroma Neurofibroma	Negative staining for AFB Negative staining for AFB

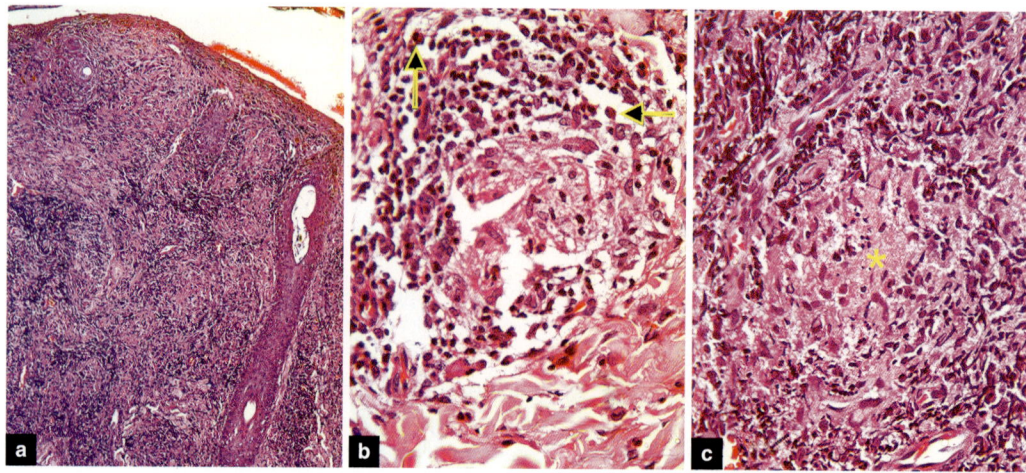

Fig. 3.18: (a) Skin biopsy from lupus vulgaris showing thinned out epidermis and dense dermal inflammatory infiltrate with granulomas (H & E, ×100); (b) Higher magnification showing epithelioid cells, lymphocytes and plasma cells (indicated by yellow arrows) (H & E, ×400); (c) Higher magnification of granuloma showing impending central necrosis (denoted by yellow starred area)

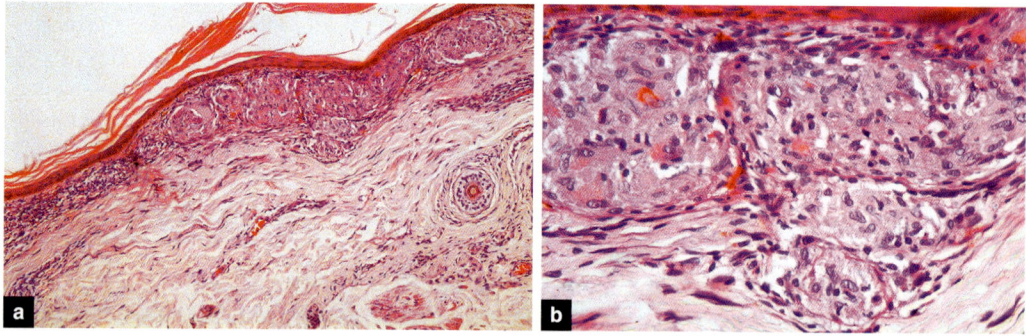

Fig. 3.19: (a) Skin biopsy from cutaneous lesion of sarcoidosis showing multiple, non-caseating naked granulomas without lymphocyte cuffing (H & E, ×100); (b) Higher magnificaton showing epithelioid histiocytes without lymphocyte cuffing (H & E, ×400)

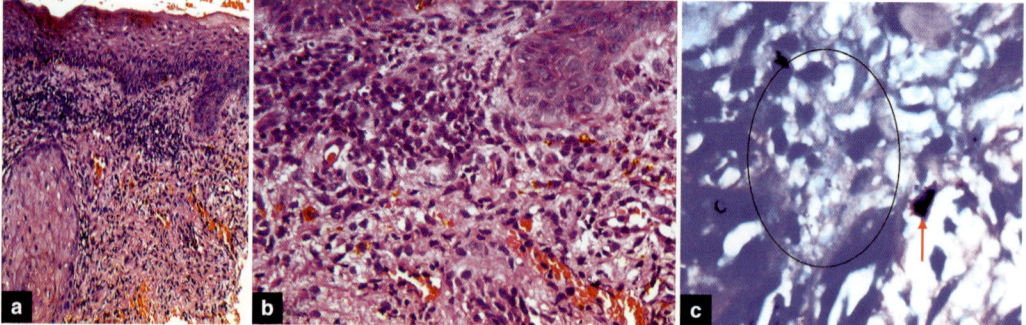

Fig. 3.20: (a) Skin biopsy from cutaneous Leishmaniasis showing dense inflammatory infiltrate in the dermis (H & E, ×200); (b) Higher magnification reveals the infiltrate to be composed of lymphocytes, plasma cells and histiocytes (H & E, ×400); (c) Giemsa stain showing scattered organisms within the macrophages (red arrow) (Giemsa, ×1000)

Diagnostic Tests and Histopathology

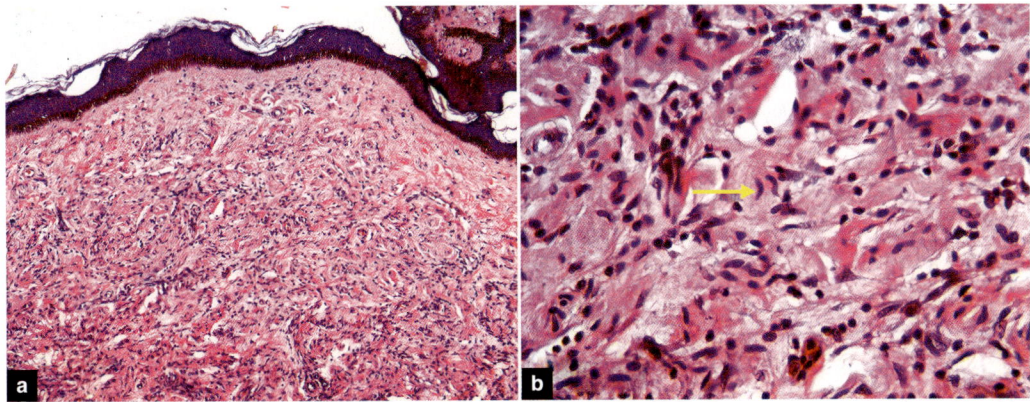

Fig. 3.21: (a) Skin biopsy from neurofibroma, showing thinned out epidermis with a subepidermal clear zone and a diffuse infiltrate of cells resembling macrophages admixed with a few lymphocytes (H & E, ×100); (b) At higher magnification the cells have wavy buckled nuclei (yellow arrow) suggesting nerve sheath origin (H & E, ×400)

Flowchart 3.1: Regression of leprosy lesions

TT, BT, BB	BL	LL
Epithelioid cells disappear leaving behind nonspecific inflammatory infiltrate composed of lymphocytes	Macrophages with small vesicles, no vacuoles and fairly numerous lymphocytes	Macrophages with much foam or larger vacuoles and a few lymphocytes
The classification reverts to indeterminate	Macrophages gradually disappear leaving behind a few scattered collections of lymphocytes and foam cells	Macrophages gradually disappear leaving behind a few scattered collections of lymphocytes and foam cells. Sometimes foam cells may persist lifelong

TT: Tuberculoid leprosy; BT: Borderline tuberculoid leprosy
BB: Midborderline leprosy
BL: Borderline lepromatous leprosy
LL: Lepromatous leprosy

RELAPSE

Reappearance of granulomas *on a regressed background* should raise the suspicion of a relapse (Fig. 3.22b and c).[6]

Appearance of active macrophages, in areas with remnants of foam cells, along with appearance of solid staining AFB, in places, where only granular forms were seen, indicates relapse in BL and LL. A 2 log rise in BI also favors a relapse.

But the differentiation becomes difficult at times, since LLp case may relapse with BL and BT and BL may relapse with BT lesions. Diagnosing relapse in BT and TT and

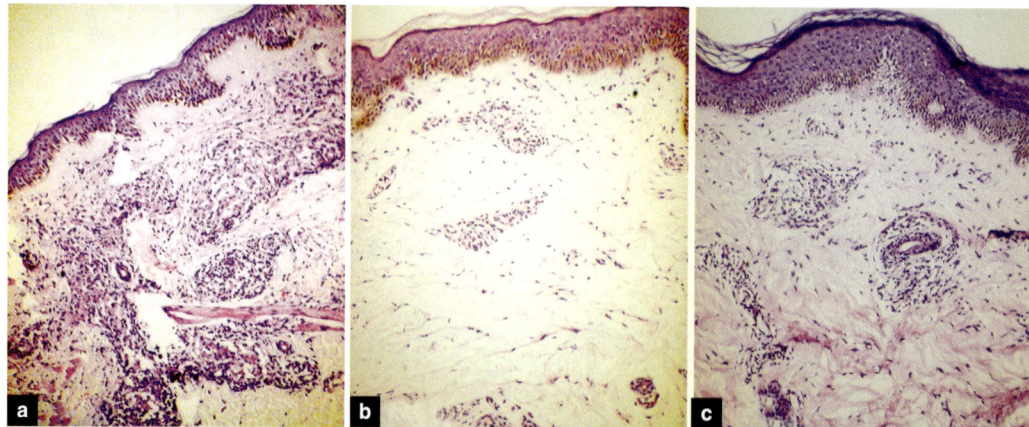

Fig. 3.22: (a) Pre-treatment biopsy from borderline tubeculoid leprosy revealing epithelioid granulomas (H & E, ×100); (b) Post-treatment biopsy showing complete clearance of granulomas leaving only minimal inflammatory infiltrate (H & E, ×100); (c) Biopsy from a lesion that appeared after completion of fixed duration treatment in the same patient showing epithelioid granulomas (H & E, ×100)

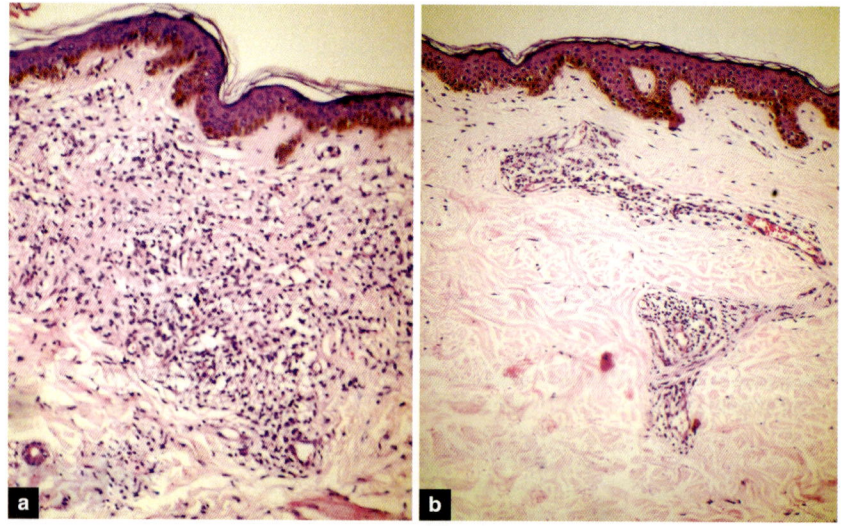

Fig. 3.23: (a) Pre-treatment biopsy of lepromatous leprosy patient revealing macrophage granulomas (H & E, ×200); (b) Post-treatment biopsy showing complete clearance of granulomas, minimal inflammatory infiltrate and dermal fibrosis (H & E, ×100)

distinguishing relapse from late reaction is very difficult and at times relapse may occur with reaction. The authors have noted formation of active granulomas in patients who manifest leprosy reactions at the time of completion of treatment.[21] Trindade et al suggested that distinguishing granulomatous reactivation due to lepra reaction from leprosy relapse is often difficult in AFB negative specimens since bacterioscopy alone is useful in such scenarios.[22]

Its often difficult to distinguish the CMI mediated granuloma formed in response to the continuous release of antigens of live *M. leprae* seen in relapse, from the hypersensitive, reactive inflammation seen against the antigens of dead bacilli in late reaction.[15]

Ridley, has detailed some subtle differences to differentiate relapse from late reaction which are often useful for a trained eye.[15]

1. Disrupted and dispersed granuloma, without any definite edge, is certainly in reaction. Concentric organization of epithelioid cells, or presence of many neutrophils or giant cells is a feature of reaction. But these features of severe reaction, may be unlikely in late reaction.
2. Compact granuloma with slightly irregular edge and small spurs extending out between the fascicles of the dermis, but not far beyond, indicates relapse.
3. Compact and well demarcated granuloma with a completely smooth edge suggests that the lesion is neither in reaction nor in relapse (histoid excluded). It is postulated that in lesions that were known to have resolved previously, this would indicate a relapse that had become quiescent or, in case of evidence of upgrading, a reaction that had subsided.

IMMUNOHISTOCHEMISTRY IN LEPROSY: A PRIMER[1,23,24]

The clinical picture and prognosis in leprosy is mainly dependent on the host's immune response to *M. leprae*. Immunohistochemistry studies have unravelled major differences between tuberculoid and lepromatous spectrum of cases (Table 3.11) (Figs 3.24 to 3.28).

Total lymphocyte content in tuberculoid leprosy is greater than that in lepromatous leprosy with higher percentage of CD4+ T cells in the former (Fig. 3.24). CD4+ to CD8+ ratio decreases towards the lepromatous end (Figs 3.24 and 3.25).[1] CD4+ to CD8+ ratio is 2:1 in tuberculoid lesions, whereas in lepromatous lesions, this has been found to be 0.6:1. This does not correlate with the blood and thus its more useful studying these cells at the sites of disease activity instead of in the peripheral blood. Moreover, the memory T cell to T naïve ratio documented in tuberculoid lesions is 14:1 and the similar ratio observed in lepromatous lesions is 1:1. Most of the CD8+ T cells in lepromatous lesions are of suppressor phenotype (CD28–) which is in contrast to the

Table 3.11: Immunohistochemistry features in leprosy					
Type of leprosy	CD4+ T cells	CD8+ T cells	CD68+ cells*	CD28+ T cells	CD1a+ cells
Tuberculoid lesions	• CD4+ T cells are the *predominant* cells • Associated with *macrophages* in the core of the granuloma	• CD8+ T cells restricted to the *mantle* surrounding the granuloma	Strong expression throughout granuloma	More number of CD28+, CD8+ cells which are of *cytotoxic* phenotype	More in number in *epidermis* of skin lesions and *periphery* of epithelioid cell granuloma
Lepromatous lesions	• CD4+ T cells *equal* in number to CD8+ cells • Scattered throughout granuloma	CD8+ T cells admixed with CD4+ T cells and macrophages throughout granuloma	Strong expression throughout granuloma	Mostly CD28–ve, CD8+ cells of *suppressor* phenotype	Less number of CD1a+ cells in epidermis of skin lesions and infrequent in macrophage granuloma

*CD68 positivity observed irrespective of the group in the spectrum since both epithelioid cells and macrophages take the stain.

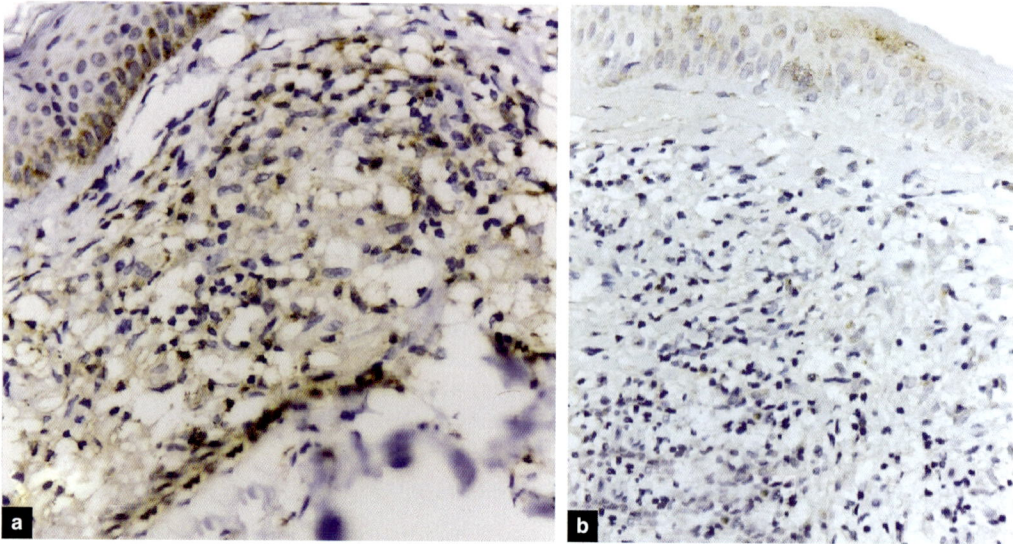

Fig. 3.24: (a) Moderate CD4 expression in tuberculoid granuloma (immunohistochemistry, ×200); (b) Weak CD4 expression in a few cells within lepromatous granuloma (immunohistochemistry, ×200)

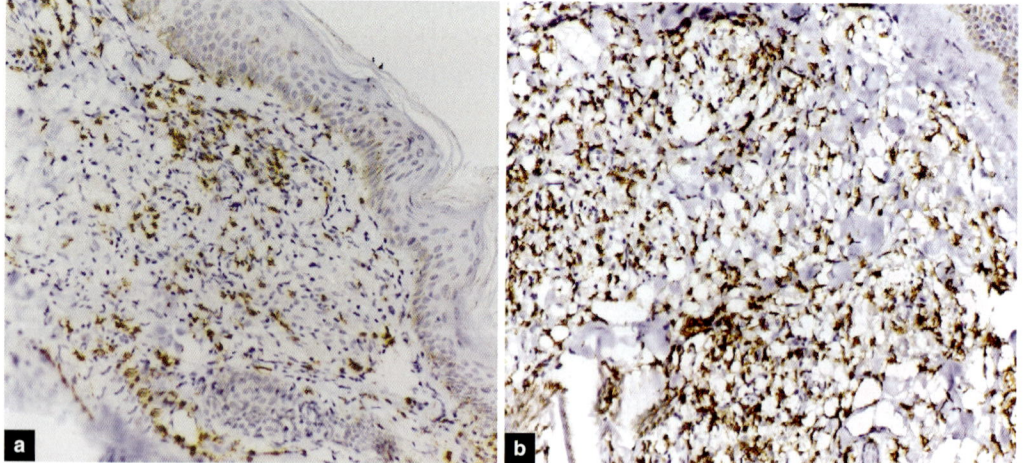

Fig. 3.25: (a) Moderate CD8 expression in the periphery of tuberculoid granuloma (immunohistochemistry, ×200); (b) Strong CD8 expression in many cells throughout the lepromatous granuloma (immunohistochemistry, ×200)

predominance of cytotoxic CD8+ T cells (CD28+) seen in tuberculoid lesions (Fig. 3.24). The distribution of cells in the granuloma also differs in tuberculoid and lepromatous cases. The immunological distribution of cells is shown in Table 3.11.[1,24]

The CD4+ cells seen in the center of the granuloma are of the T memory phenotype and as they adjoin the macrophages it is conceivable that they may play a role in mediating macrophage localization, activation and maturation leading to restriction or elimination of the pathogen. In contrast, in lepromatous granulomas, the CD8+ cells are of the T suppressor phenotype, thus they may act to suppress the cell-mediated immune response *(also see Chapter 4, Section 4.3)*.

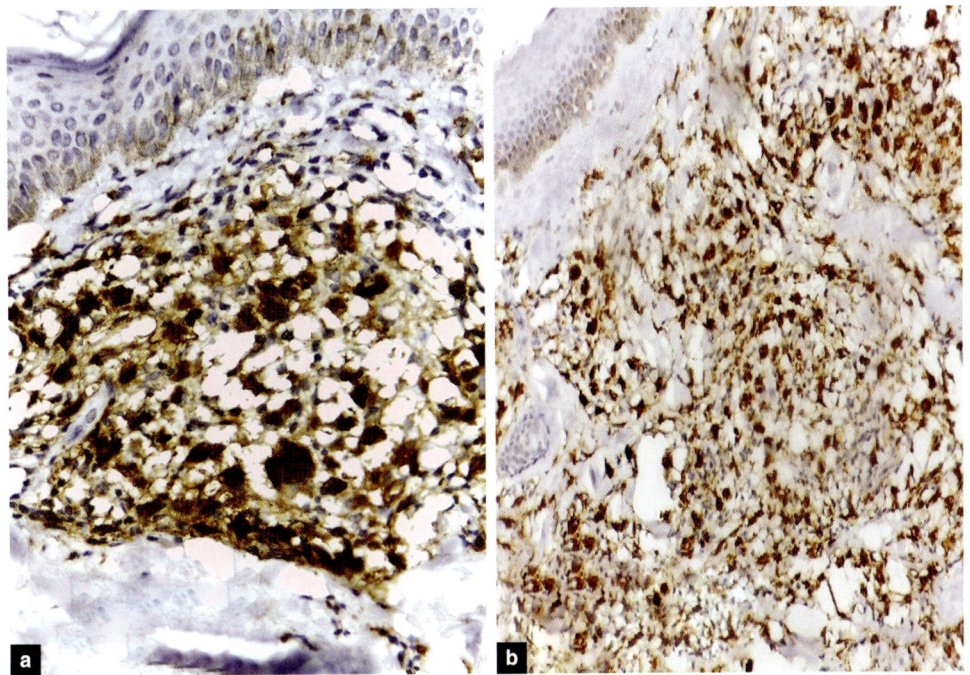

Fig. 3.26: (a) Strong CD68 expression in many cells throughout the tuberculoid granuloma (immunohistochemistry, ×200); (b) Strong CD68 expression in many cells throughout the lepromatous granuloma (immunohistochemistry, ×200)

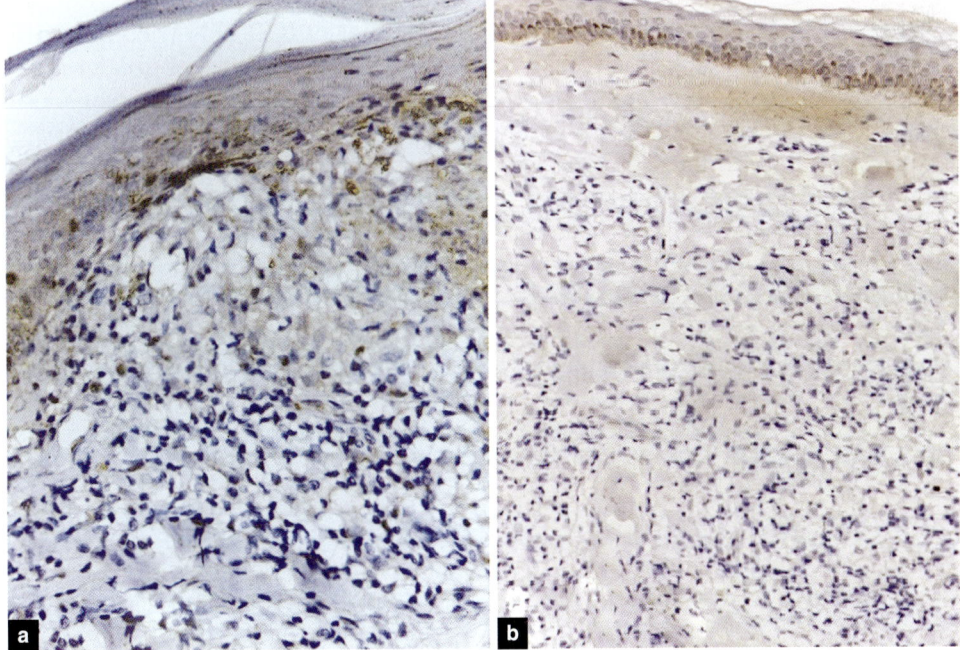

Fig. 3.27: (a) Weak CD28 expression in a few cells in tuberculoid granuloma (immunohistochemistry, ×200); (b) Negative staining for CD28 in macrophage granuloma (immunohistochemistry, ×200)

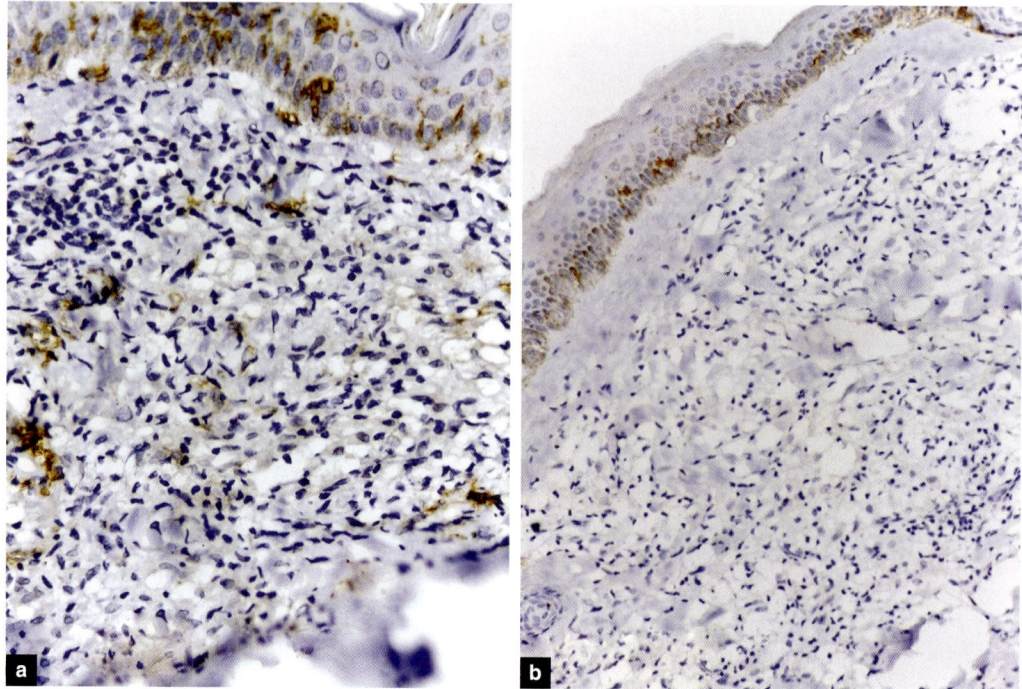

Fig. 3.28: (a) Moderate CD1a expression in epidermis and in a few cells in the periphery of tuberculoid granuloma (immunohistochemistry, ×200); (b) Mild CD1a expression in epidermis and lack of CD1a staining in lepromatous granuloma (immunohistochemistry, ×200)

Further studies have demonstrated greater number of IL-2, IFN-γ, IL-1β and TNF positive cells in tuberculoid than in lepromatous lesions. Presence of greater number of cells containing serine esterase mRNA in tuberculoid than in lepromatous lesions points to the role of cytotoxic T cells in defence against *M. leprae* infection.[1] Comparison of immunohistochemistry findings in upgrading T1R and T2R have showed predominant CD4+ T cells and similar T memory: T naïve ratios in both, which indicate an influx of T memory cells, irrespective of the type of reaction. But predominance of CD28+, CD8+ T cells (cytotoxic) is documented in reversal reaction which is not observed in T2R.[1,23,24] Increased number of cells positive for human serine esterase mRNA in reversal reaction (but not in lesions of T2R),[1,23,24] indicates the predominance of cytotoxic T cells in reversal reaction. This is consistent with the role of these cells in the destruction of bacilli. Also there is a increased number of γδ cells that is important for granuloma formation. A summary of the features in immunohistochemistry in different types of T1R and T2R is detailed in Table 3.12.[23]

CONCLUSION

The importance of histopathology analysis in conjunction with IHC helps in confirming the diagnosis in doubtful cases, for proper classification of disease into various groups as per the Ridley-Jopling classification, to assess activity of disease, to determine response to treatment, and to distinguish between lepra reactions and relapse. Thus, biopsy in conjunction with clinical diagnosis is useful in diagnosing and differentiating the common disorders that need to excluded in leprosy endemic countries.

Table 3.12: Immunohistochemistry features in leprosy and lepra reactions observed by authors

Type of leprosy	CD4+ T cells	CD8+ T cells	CD68+ T cells	CD28+ T cells	CDla positivity in epidermis	CDla positivity in granuloma
Tuberculoid lesions	Moderate to strong expression in many cells, mainly in the *periphery* of granuloma	Moderate to strong expression in many cells, mainly in the *periphery* of granuloma	Strong expression in many cells throughout the granuloma	Weak expression in a few cells scattered throughout the granuloma in most of the lesions	Moderate to strong CDla expressions in many cells in epidermis	Moderate to strong CDla expressions in a few cells in the periphery of granuloma
Lepromatous leions	Weak expression in a few cells scattered throughout the granuloma	Moderate to strong expression in many cells, distributed throughout the granuloma	Strong expression in many cells throughout the granuloma	Negative staining in most of the lesions	Moderate to strong CDla expression in many cells in epidermis in the majority	Negative staining in majority
Lesions manifesting lepra reaction	The intensity of expression and the number of cells taking the stain highest in *reversal reaction* compared to leprosy without reaction or other types of reaction	Moderate to strong expression in many cells in all lesions irrespective of presence of reaction or type of reaction	Moderate to strong expression in many cells in all lesions irrespective of presence of reaction or type of reaction	Higher percentage of upgrading and static reactions showing positive staining	Moderate to strong expression in epidermis in majority of type 1 reactions and weak expression in epidermis in type 2 reaction	Higher percentage of upgrading and static reactions manifesting positive staining compared to nonreacting lesions and lesions showing down-grading reaction. Negative staining in type 2 reaction

REFERENCES

1. Job CK. Pathology of leprosy. In: Leprosy. Hastings RC. editor. 2nd edn. Edinburgh: Churchill Livingstone 1994;12:193–224.
2. Ridley DS. Histological diagnosis. In: Pathogenesis of leprosy and related diseases. Ridley DS. Editor. UK: Butterworth and Co-publishers Ltd 1988;15:145–54.
3. Ridley DS. Classification. In: Pathogenesis of leprosy and related diseases. Ridley DS. Editor. UK: Butterworth and Co-publishers Ltd 1988;15:155–75.
4. Ridley DS. The bacteriological interpretation of skin smears and biopsies in leprosy. Trans R Soc Trop Med Hyg 1955;49:449–52.
5. Sardana KS, Koranne RV, Mahajan S, Bhushan P. Correlation of bacterial index (BI) and bacterial index of granuloma (BIG) in leprosy. Is there a therapeutic relevance? Indian J Lepr 2004; 76:363–9.
6. Porichha D, Natrajan M. Pathological aspects of leprosy. In: IAL Textbook of Leprosy. Kumar B, Kar HK. Editors. 2nd edn. New Delhi: Jaypee 2016:9:132–51.
7. Ridley DS. Neuropathy in leprosy. In: Pathogenesis of leprosy and related diseases. Ridley DS Editor. UK: Butterworth and Co-publishers Ltd 1988;9:71–83.
8. Jopling WH, McDougall AC. The Disease. In: Handbook of Leprosy. Jopling WH, McDougall AC. Editors. 5th edn. New Delhi: CBS Publishers and Distributors 1996: 10–53.

9. Wade HW. The histoid variety of lepromatous leprosy. Int J Lepr 1963;31:129–42.
10. Lockwood DN, Lucas SB, Desikan KV, Ebenezer G, Suneetha S, Nicholls P, et al. The histological diagnosis of leprosy type 1 reactions: Identification of key variables and an analysis of the process of histological diagnosis. J Clin Pathol 2008; 61:595–600.
11. Lockwood DNJ, Nicholls P, Smith WCS, Das L, Barkataki P, Van Brakel W, et al. Comparing the clinical and histological diagnosis of leprosy and leprosy reactions in the INFIR cohort of Indian Patients with multibacillary leprosy. PLoSNegl Trop Dis 2012; 6:e1702.
12. Sarita S, Muhammed K, Najeeba R, Rajan GN, Anza K, Binitha MP, et al. A study on histological features of lepra reactions in patients attending the Dermatology Department of the Government Medical College, Calicut, Kerala, India. Lepr Rev 2013;84:51–64.
13. Ridley DS, Radia KB. The histological course of reaction in borderline leprosy and their outcome. Int J Lepr 1981:49:383–92.
14. Ramu G, Desikan KV. Reactions in borderline leprosy. Indian J Lepr 2002;74:115–28.
15. Ridley DS. Reactions. In: Pathogenesis of leprosy and related diseases. Ridley DS. Editor.UK: Butterworth and Co-publishers Ltd 1988;15:118–34.
16. Lyons NF, Naafs B. Persistence of Langhans giant cells in rapidly downgrading leprosy lesions. Int J Lepr 1985;53:114–5.
17. Hussain R, Lucas SB, Kifayet A, Jamil S, Raynes J, Uquili Z, et al. Clinical and histological discrepancies in diagnosis of ENL reaction classified by assessment of acute phase protein SAA and CRP. Int J Lepr 1995;63:222–30.
18. Yadav D, Ramam M. Epithelioid cell granuloma. Indian J Dermatopathol Diagn Dermatol 2018;5: 7–18.
19. Desikan P, Desikan KV. Persistence of lepromatous granuloma in clinically cured cases of leprosy. Int J Lep 1995; 63:417–21.
20. Joshy R. Clues to histopathological diagnosis of treated leprosy. Indian J Dermatol Venereol Leprol, 2011;56:505–9.
21. Sasidharanpillai S, Govindan A, Riyaz N, Binitha MP, Parambath SP, Khader A, et al. Histopathology of skin lesions of leprosy before and after fixed duration treatment. Lepr Rev 2017;88:142–53.
22. Trindade MAB, Benard G, Ura S, Ghidella CC, Avelleira JCR, Vianna FR, et al. Granulomatous Reactivation during the Course of a Leprosy Infection: Reaction or Relapse. PLoS Negl Trop Dis 2010;4:e921.
23. Govindan A, Sasidharanpillai S, Ajithkumar K, Parambath SP, Abdul Latheef EN, Rahima S, et al. Immunohistochemistry of skin lesions in leprosy. Lepr Rev 2018;89:256–71.
24. Modlin RL, Rea TH. Immunopathology of leprosy granulomas. Springer Semin Immunopathol. 1988;10:359–74.

CHAPTER 4

Microbiology and Immunopathogenesis

4.1 BACTERIOLOGY OF LEPROSY

Ananta Khurana

Mycobacterium leprae is an acid-fast, gram-positive obligate intracellular micro-organism with a marked Schwann cell tropism and is the only human pathogen capable of invading the superficial peripheral nerves.[1] The bacillus was discovered by Armauer Hansen in 1873, in Bergen, Norway. Important aspects in microbiology of *M. leprae* are highlighted in Table 4.1. To date, four different *M. leprae* strains—TN (India), Tahi-53 (Thailand), NHDP63 (USA) and Br4923 (Brazil)—have been fully sequenced. Comparative genomics of four different strains revealed remarkable conservation of the genome (99.99% identity) with less than 0.005% differences, which comprise 289 polymorphic sites including single nucleotide polymorphisms (SNPs) and small insertion-deletion events (InDels).[2]

M. leprae was the only organism known to cause leprosy until 2008, when a new species, namely *Mycobacterium lepromatosis*, was found to be the cause of diffuse lepromatous leprosy (DLL) in two patients of Mexican origin who died of the disease.[3] Further analysis revealed a 9.1% difference between the two organisms to substantiate a species-level divergence that occurred approximately 10 million years ago.[4,5] Thus far, *M. lepromatosis* has been found in patients with leprosy from Mexico, Canada, Brazil, Singapore, and Myanmar and contrary to initial reports is likely to present with a similar clinical spectrum as *M. leprae*.[6–8]

M. leprae has undergone reductive evolution, whereby many genes and associated functions were lost through shrinkage of the genome and gene decay, possibly due to a drastic change in lifestyle from free-living, like most mycobacteria, to a host-associated bacillus.[9] Hence, with 50% of the genome seemingly devoid of function, *M. leprae* has the largest proportion of pseudogenes in comparison to other pathogenic and nonpathogenic bacteria.[10] The mechanism of formation of pseudogenes is not yet known but lack of the dna Q mediated proofreading activity of Dna polymerase III due to pseudogenization and the loss of sigma factors are the plausible explanations.[10–12] Following reductive evolution, *M. leprae* has only retained a minimum set of genes representing essential gene families, eliminating several metabolic pathways, and leaving it with markedly specific growth requirements.[13]

Table 4.1: Microbiology of *Mycobacterium leprae*

Ultrastructure
Rod-shaped bacilli, 1–8 μm long, 0.3 μm diameter.

Cell Wall and Capsule[14]
- *Cell wall core*: Complex of long-chain fatty acids (mycolic acids) linked to arabinogalactan, which is further attached to peptidoglycan.
- *Lipoglycans and glycolipids*: LAM, PDIM, PIM, cord factor/dimycolyl-trehalose and sulfolipids; noncovalently attached to the plasma membrane through their GPI anchors; extend to exterior of cell wall.
- *Phenolic glycolipid 1 (PGL-1)*: A unique glycolipid found only in *M. leprae*; important immunological functions.
- *Cell wall proteins*: Structural and nutrient uptake function.

Cell Membrane
- *Lipids*: Mainly phospholipids
- *Proteins*: MMP-I and MMP-II

Generation (Doubling) Time[15]
- Slow; 12–13 days in footpads of mice during the logarithmic phase
- For the entire period from inoculation to the early plateau phase, the average is 20–40 days
- Logarithmic phase is preceded by a lag phase of 60–90 days

Cultivation in Animal Models
- Uncultivable in microbiological culture media or in cell culture systems
- Nine banded armadillo (*Dasypus novemcinctus*): Ideal core body temperature of 32°–35°C; disseminated infection in susceptible animals
- Mouse foot pad (MFP) inoculation:[16] Most favorable inoculums size: 5000 bacilli; Minimal infectious dose: 50–500 bacilli (Shepherd, 1971)[17]/5 bacilli (Welch, 1980);[18] growth peaks at approximately 10^6 bacilli within 5–6 months and then enters a plateau phase. In immunodeficient strains such as thymectomized and irradiated mice, congenitally athymic nude mice and SCID mice, prolific *M. leprae* multiplication continues, reaching up to 10^{10} bacilli in each foot pad.[19–21]

Viability Assays
- Molecular: Reverse transcriptase (RT)—PCR of 16S rRNA[22]
- MFP inoculation
- Morphological index
- Fluorescent vital dyes: Fluorescein diacetate (FDA) and Ethidium Bromide (EB), rhodamine 123 (R-123)/EB, SYTO9 and propidium iodide
- Metabolic profiling: ^{3}H-purine/pyrimidine uptake, mass spectrometry to measure Na^+/K^+ ratio, ATP content, PGL-1 synthesis
- Radio respirometry: ^{14}C-labeled palmitic acid oxidation

LAM: Lipoarabinomannan, PDIM: Phthiocerol dimycocerosate, PIM: Phosphatidyl-myoinositol; MMP: Major membrane protein.

GENETIC SUSCEPTIBILITY TO LEPROSY

Twin studies, familial clustering and segregation analyses studies have suggested that host genetics play an important role in susceptibility to leprosy.[23–25] Further, following infection, the development of different clinical forms also is based on the genetic makeup of an individual which regulates the type of immune response.[26]

Genetic polymorphisms in components of the innate and adaptive immune response have been shown to be important susceptibility/protection factors in different populations. Important among these are summarized in Table 4.2. TLR and complement

Table 4.2: Summary of literature on association of leprosy with genes related to innate immune response and cytokines[26,29,30-58]

S. No.	Gene	Protective polymorphisms (population studied)	Polymorphisms associated with susceptibility to leprosy (population studied)
1.	TLR1	• I602S/rs5743618, 602S/SS/rs5743618 (Indian) • I602S/SS/rs5743618 (Turkish) • N248S/SS/rs4833095 (Bangladesh; ENL)	• N248S/SS/rs4833095 (Bangladesh) • N248S/SS/rs4833095 (Brazilian) • N199N/rs3804099 (Ethiopian, T1R)
2.	TLR2	–	**Susceptibility to T1R:** N199N/rs3804099 (Ethiopian)
3.	TLR4	A299G/rs4986790-T390I/rs4986791 Ethiopian	–
4.	NOD2	• Protection from disease *per se*: rs8057341, rs2111234, rs3135499, rs8057341-genotype AA, rs8057341-allele A (Brazilian) • **Protection from T1R:** rs2287195, rs8043770, rs7194886, rs1861759 (Nepalese)	• Susceptibility to leprosy *per se*: rs12448797, rs2287195, rs8044354, rs8043770, rs13339578, rs4785225, rs751271, rs1477176, rs1131716 (Nepalese) • rs9302752, rs7194886 (Chinese) • **Susceptibility to ENL:** rs8044354, rs17312836, rs1861759, rs1861758 (Nepalese) • **Susceptibility to reactions:** rs751271 at NOD2, rs2069845 (Brazilian)
5.	PARK2		• rs9347684, rs9346929, rs4709648, rs12215676, rs10806765, rs6936373, rs1333957, rs9365492, rs9355403 (Indian) • PARK2_e01 (-2599) allele T, rs1040079 (allele C) (Brazilian) • PARK2_e01 (-2599) allele T, rs1040079 (allele C) (Vietnamese)
6.	PARK2/PAR-CRG		• rs6915128, rs10945859, rs9347683, rs10806768 (Indian) • rs6915128, rs10806768, rs1333955, rs1333955 (Vietnamese) • rs1333955 (Brazilian)
7.	VDR	TaqI"Tt"rs731236 (Indian)	• TaqI"tt"rs731236 (Brazilian) • TaqI"TT"rs731236 (Mexican) • TaqI"tt"rs731236, TaqI"TT"rs731236, • Fok-I/rs2228570 (Nepalese; susceptibility to T1R) • TaqI"Tt"rs731236 (Indian) • Fok1"ff" and Taq1"tt" (Indian)
8.		–	• Genotype 22 and 23 (Brazilian) • INT4/469 + 14 (Indonesian; PB) • 3-UTR/1729 + 55del4 (Malian; MB) • 274 C/T (Brazilian; TT)

(Contd.)

Table 4.2: Summary of literature on association of leprosy with genes related to innate immune response and cytokines[26,29,30–58] *(Contd.)*

S. No.	Gene	Protective polymorphisms *(population studied)*	Polymorphisms associated with susceptibility to leprosy *(population studied)*
9.	MRC1	• G396S/rs1926736 (Vietnamese) • G396S/rs1926736 (Vietnamese) • L407Frs2437257 (Brazilian) • L407F rs2437257 (Brazilian)	• G396Srs1926736 (Brazilian) • G396Srs1926736 (Brazilian) • rs692527, rs34856358 (PB, Chinese)
10.	MICA	• MICA*A5 (Chinese; MB) • MICA*027, MICA*027, MICA*010 (Brazilian)	MICA*5A5.1 (Indian)
11.	MICA/MICB	MICB*CA21 (Indian)	• MICB*CA16 (Indian) • MICB*CA19 (Indian)
12.	KIR	KIR2DL1-C2, KIR2DL1-C2, KIR2DL3-C1, KIR2DL1, KIR2DL1 (Brazilian)	• KIR2DS3, KIR3DL2-A3/11, KIR2DS2-C1, KIR2DS2-C1 (TT), KIR2DL2-C1, KIR2DL2-C1 (TT), KIR2DL2-C1 (Brazilian)
13.	TNF	• TNF-G-308 (A) (Thailand) • TNF*2/LTA*2 (Brazilian)	• TNF-308 (G/A), TNF-308 (A) (Thailand) • TNF-308 (Brazilian)
14.	IFN-γ	IFNG + 874(T) rs2430561(Brazilian)	• (10CA) rs3138557, (13CA) rs3138557, (15CA) rs3138557, (17CA) rs3138557 (Chinese) • IFNG + 874 (AA), alleles 5, 6, and 7 (Brazilian)
15.	LTA	–	rs13192469 (Indian)
16.	CR1	–	rs3849266*T in intron 21 and rs3737002*T in exon 26 (Brazilian)
17.	IL-6	**Protection from ENL:** (GG) rs2069840, (GG + CG) rs2069840 (Brazilian)	**Susceptibility to ENL:** (CC) rs1800795, (CC + CG) rs1800795, (AA) rs2069832, (AA + AG) rs2069832, (GG) rs2069845, (GG + AG) rs2069845
18.	IL-10	• 3575A-2849G-2763C, 1082G-819C-592C (Brazilian) • 819 (CC vs CT + TT),-592 (CC vs CA + AA),-3575T-2849G-2763C-1082A-819C-592C (Indian)	• 819T, 819TT,-3575-2849-2763 (Brazilian) • (C/C and C/T) rs1800871, (C/C and C/A) rs1800872, haplotype (819C-519C), 1082A-819C-592C (Columbian) • 819 (TT vs CT + CC), –592 (AA vs CA + CC) (Indian)
19.	IL-12	3′UTR2.2 (Indian)	3′UTR 1188 A/C (CC) (Mexican)
20.	IL-17A	–	rs2275913 (T1R; Brazilian)
21.	IL-17F	–	rs763780 (Indian)
22.	IL-8	–	rs4073 (progression to MB; Brazilian)

TLR: Toll-like Receptor; *NOD2*: Nucleotide-binding oligomerization domain containing 2; *PARK2*: Parkin, *PACRG*: Parkin coregulated; KIR: Killer-immunoglobulin-like receptor; MICA: MHC class I polypeptide-related sequence A; MRC1: Mannose receptor, C type 1; Natural resistance-associated macrophage protein 1; CR1: Complement receptor 1; T1R: Type 1 reaction; ENL: Erythema nodosum leprosum; PB: Paucibacillary; MB: Multibacillary; TT: Tuberculoid leprosy.

receptors form initial points of contact of *M. leprae* with the immune system and thus are significant in clearance or establishment of initial infection. Vitamin D receptor (VDR) activation leads to production of protective antimicrobial peptides. *NRAMP1* gene is expressed in macrophage phagosome membranes where it acts as a transporter of iron and other divalent ions. Iron is essential for biological functions, both for host immune defense and mycobacterial growth. *NOD2* is another innate receptor which plays a role in differentiation of monocytes to dendritic cells and in release of pro-inflammatory cytokines. Major histocompatibility complex class I chain-related genes A (*MICA*) and B (*MICB*) are located on chromosome 6 near to the HLA-B and HLA-C loci. These genes are highly polymorphic producing different MICA and MICB proteins which are induced by cellular stress. Wong et al reported HLA-DRB1/DQA1 as major determinants of leprosy susceptibility in Indian patients.[27] KIR is a crucial receptor on natural killer (NK) cells.

Mutations in the *PARK2* gene have been shown to be the cause of autosomal recessive early onset Parkinson's disease.[28] *PARK2*, as a ubiquitin ligase, has been shown to provide resistance to intracellular pathogens through ubiquitin-mediated autophagy. The function of *PACRG* is unknown but also has been linked to the ubiquitin-proteasome system. *PARK2* is expressed by primary Schwann cell explants and by monocyte-derived macrophages, whereas *PACRG* is strongly expressed in primary Schwann cells and very weakly by monocyte derived macrophages.[29] Possession of as few as two of the 17 risk alleles has been shown to be highly predictive of leprosy.[29]

Recent genome wide association studies (GWAS) have brought into highlight many more leprosy associated genes including—caspase recruitment domain family member (CARD9), fillagrin, hypoxia-inducible factor 1 alpha subunit (HIF1A), HLA-C and HLA-DR-DQ, IL-10, IL-12B, IL-18 accessory protein and receptor, IL-23 receptor, IL-27, laccase domain containing—coiled-coil domain containing 122 (LACC1-CCDC122), leucine rich repeat kinase 2/Dardarin (LRRK2), lymphotoxin-α, NCK interacting protein with SH3 domain, tyrosine kinase 2, solute carrier family 29 member 3 (SLC29A3) and tumor necrosis factor (Ligand) superfamily-Member 8/Member 15.[59]

REFERENCES

1. Chavarro-Portillo B, Soto CY, Guerrero MI. *Mycobacterium leprae's* evolution and environmental adaptation. Acta Trop 2019;197:105041.
2. Singh P, Cole ST. *Mycobacterium leprae*: Genes, pseudogenes and genetic diversity. Future Microbiol 2011;6:57–71.
3. Han XY, Seo Y-H, Sizer KC, Taylor S, May GS, Spencer JS, Li W, Nair RG. A new *Mycobacterium* species causing diffuse lepromatous leprosy. Am J Clin Pathol. 2008;130:856–64.
4. Han XY, Sizer KC, Thompson EJ, Kabanja J, Li J, Hu P, Gómez-Valero L, Silva FJ. Comparative sequence analysis of *Mycobacterium leprae* and the new leprosy-causing *Mycobacterium lepromatosis*. J Bacteriol 2009;191:6067–74.
5. Singh P, Benjak A, Schuenemann VJ, Herbig A, Avanzi C, Busso P, et al. Insight into the evolution and origin of leprosy bacilli from the genome sequence of *Mycobacterium lepromatosis*. Proc Natl Acad Sci USA 2015;112:4459–64.
6. Jessamine PG, Desjardins M, Gillis T, et al. Leprosy-like illness in a patient with *Mycobacterium lepromatosis* from Ontario, Canada. J Drugs in Dermatol 2012;11:229–33.
7. Han XY, Aung FM, Choon SE, Werner B. Analysis of the leprosy agents *M. leprae* and *M. lepromatosis* in four countries. Am J Clin Pathol 2014;142:524–32.

8. Han XY, Sizer KC, Tan HH. Identification of the leprosy agent *Mycobacterium lepromatosis* in Singapore. J Drugs Dermatol 2012;11:168–72.
9. Cole ST, Eiglmeier K, Parkhill J, et al. Massive gene decay in the leprosy bacillus. Nature 2001; 409:1007–11.
10. Liu Y, Harrison PM, Kunin V, Gerstein M. Comprehensive analysis of pseudogenes in prokaryotes: widespread gene decay and failure of putative horizontally transferred genes. Genome Biol 2004;5:R64.
11. Babu MM. Did the loss of sigma factors initiate pseudogene accumulation in *Mycobacterium leprae*? Trends Microbiol 2003;11:59–61.
12. Tyagi JS, Saini DK. Did the loss of two-component systems initiate pseudogene accumulation in *Mycobacterium leprae*? Microbiology 2004;150(1):4–7.
13. Marri PR, Bannantine JP, Golding GB. Comparative genomics of metabolic pathways in *Mycobacterium* species: Gene duplication, gene decay and lateral gene transfer. FEMS Microbiol. Rev 2006;30:906–25.
14. Kaur G, Kaur J. Multifaceted role of lipids in *Mycobacterium leprae*. Future Microbiol 2017;12:315–35.
15. Shepard CC, McRae DH. *Mycobacterium leprae* in mice: Minimal infectious dose, relationship between staining quality and infectivity, and effect of cortisone. J Bacteriol 1965;89:365–72.
16. Shepard CC. The experimental disease that follows the injection of human leprosy bacilli into footpads of mice. J Exp Med 1960;112:445–54.
17. Shepard CC. The first decade in experimental leprosy. Bull Wld Hlth Org 1971;44:821–7.
18. Welch TM, Gelber RH, Murray LP, Ng H, O'Neill SM, Levy L. Viability of *Mycobacterium leprae* after multiplication in mice. Infect Immun 1980;30:325–8.
19. Rees RJ. Enhanced susceptibility of thymectomized and irradiated mice to infection with *Mycobacterium leprae*. Nature 1996;211:657–8.
20. Colston MJ, Hilson GR. Growth of *Mycobacterium leprae* and *M. marinum* in congenitally athymic (nude) mice. Nature 1976;262:399–401.
21. Yogi Y, Nakamura K, Inoue T, Kawatsu K, Kashiwabara Y, Sakamoto Y, Izumi S, Saito M, Hioki K, Nomura T. Susceptibility of severe combined immunodeficient (SCID) mice to *Mycobacterium leprae*: Multiplication of the bacillus and dissemination of the infection at early stage. Nihon Rai Gakkai Zasshi 1991;60:139–45.
22. Sharma R, Lavania M, Katoch K, Chauhan DS, Gupta AK, Gupta UD, Yadav VS, Katoch VM. Development and evaluation of real-time RT-PCR assay for quantitative estimation of viable *Mycobacterium leprae* in clinical samples. Ind J Lepr 2008;80:315–21.
23. Chakravartti M, Vogel F. A twin study on leprosy. Stuttgart: 1973 Georg Thieme. pp 1–123.
24. Shields ED, Russell DA, Pericak-Vance MA. Genetic epidemiology of the susceptibility to leprosy. J Clin Invest 1987;79:1139–43.
25. Abel L, Vu DL, Oberti J, Nguyen VT, Van VC, et al. Complex segregation analysis of leprosy in Southern Vietnam. Genet Epidemiol 1995;12:63–82.
26. Mazini PS, Alves HV, Reis PG, Lopes AP, Sell AM, Santos-Rosa M, Visentainer JE, Rodrigues-Santos P. Gene Association with Leprosy: A Review of Published Data. Front Immunol 2016; 12;6:658.
27. Wong SH, Gochhait S, Malhotra D, Pettersson FH, Teo YY, Khor CC, et al. Leprosy and the adaptation of human toll-like receptor 1. PLoS Pathog 2010;6:e1000979.
28. Kitada T, et al. Mutations in the parkin gene cause autosomal recessive juvenile parkinsonism. Nature 1998;392:605–8.
29. Mira MT, Alcais A, Nguyen VT, Moraes MO, Di Flumeri C, Vu HT, et al. Susceptibility to leprosy is associated with *PARK2* and *PACRG*. Nature 2004;427:636–40.
30. Schuring RP1, Hamann L, Faber WR, Pahan D, Richardus JH, Schumann RR, et al. Polymorphism N248S in the human toll-like receptor 1 gene is related to leprosy and leprosy reactions. J Infect Dis 2009;199:1816–9.

31. Marques Cde S, Brito-de-Souza VN, Guerreiro LT, Martins JH, Amaral EP, Cardoso CC, et al. Toll-like receptor 1 N248S single-nucleotide polymorphism is associated with leprosy risk and regulates immune activation during mycobacterial infection. J Infect Dis 2013;208:120–9.
32. Bochud PY, Hawn TR, Siddiqui MR, Saunderson P, Britton S, Abraham I, et al. Toll-like receptor 2 (TLR2) polymorphisms are associated with reversal reaction in leprosy. J Infect Dis 2008; 197:253–61.
33. Bochud PY, Sinsimer D, Aderem A, Siddiqui MR, Saunderson P, Britton S, et al. Polymorphisms in toll-like receptor 4 (TLR4) are associated with protection against leprosy. Eur J Clin Microbiol Infect Dis 2009;28:1055–65.
34. Zhang FR, Huang W, Chen SM, Sun LD, Liu H, Li Y, et al. Genomewide association study of leprosy. N Engl J Med 2009;361:2609–18.
35. Grant AV, Alter A, Huong NT, et al. Crohn's disease susceptibility genes are associated with leprosy in the Vietnamese population. J Infect Dis 2012;206:1763–7.
36. Sales-Marques C, Salomão H, Fava VM, Alvarado-Arnez LE, Amaral EP, Cardoso CC, et al. NOD2 and CCDC122-LACC1 genes are associated with leprosy susceptibility in Brazilians. Hum Genet 2014;133:1525–32.
37. Berrington WR, Macdonald M, Khadge S, Sapkota BR, Janer M, Hagge DA, et al. Common polymorphisms in the NOD2 gene region are associated with leprosy and its reactive states. J Infect Dis 2010;201:1422–35.
38. Mira MT, Alcais A, Nguyen VT, et al. Susceptibility to leprosy is associated with PARK2 and PACRG. Nature 2004; 427(6975):636–40.
39. Alter A, Fava VM, Huong NT, Singh M, Orlova M, Van Thuc N, et al. Linkage disequilibrium pattern and age-at-diagnosis are critical for replicating genetic associations across ethnic groups in leprosy. Hum Genet 2013;132:107–16.
40. Chopra R, Ali S, Srivastava AK, Aggarwal S, Kumar B, Manvati S, et al. Mapping of PARK2 and PACRG overlapping regulatory region reveals LD structure and functional variants in association with leprosy in unrelated Indian population groups. PLoS Genet 2013; 9:e1003578.
41. Sapkota BR, Macdonald M, Berrington WR, Misch EA, Ranjit C, Siddiqui MR, et al. Association of TNF, MBL, and VDR polymorphisms with leprosy phenotypes. Hum Immunol 2010;71:992–8.
42. Zhang DF, Huang XQ, Wang D, Li YY, Yao YG. Genetic variants of complement genes ficolin-2, mannose-binding lectin and complement factor H are associated with leprosy in Han Chinese from Southwest China. Hum Genet 2013;132:629–40.
43. de Messias-Reason IJ, Boldt AB, Moraes Braga AC, Stahlke EVRS, Dornelles L, Pereira-Ferrari L, et al. The association between mannan-binding lectin gene polymorphism and clinical leprosy: New insight into an old paradigm. J Infect Dis 2007;196:1379–85.
44. Goulart LR, Ferreira FR, Goulart IM. Interaction of TaqI polymorphism at exon 9 of the vitamin D receptor gene with the negative lepromin response may favor the occurrence of leprosy. FEMS Immunol Med Microbiol 2006;48:91–8.
45. Roy S, Frodsham A, Saha B, Hazra SK, Mascie-Taylor CG, Hill AV. Association of vitamin D receptor genotype with leprosy type. J Infect Dis 1999;179:187–91.
46. Sapkota BR, Macdonald M, Berrington WR, Misch EA, Ranjit C, Siddiqui MR, et al. Association of TNF, MBL, and VDR polymorphisms with leprosy phenotypes. Hum Immunol 2010;71:992–8.
47. Fitness J, Floyd S, Warndorff DK, Sichali L, Mwaungulu L, Crampin AC, et al. Large-scale candidate gene study of leprosy susceptibility in the Karonga district of Northern Malawi. Am J Trop Med Hyg 2004;71:330–40.
48. Ferreira FR, Goulart LR, Silva HD, Goulart IM. Susceptibility to leprosy may be conditioned by an interaction between the NRAMP1 promoter polymorphisms and the lepromin response. Int J Lepr Other Mycobact Dis 2004;72:457–567.
49. Alcais A, Sanchez FO, Thuc NV, Lap VD, Oberti J, Lagrnge PH, et al. Granulomatous reaction to intradermal injection of lepromin (Mitsuda reaction) is linked to the human NRAMP1 gene in Vietnamese leprosy sibships. J Infect Dis 2000;181:302–8.

50. Hatta M, Ratnawati, Tanaka M, Ito J, Shirakawa T, Kawabata M. NRAMP1/SLC11A1 gene polymorphisms and host susceptibility to *Mycobacterium tuberculosis* and *M. leprae* in South Sulawesi, Indonesia. Southeast Asian J Trop Med Public Health 2010;41:386–94.
51. Teixeira MA, Silva NL, Ramos Ade L, Hatagima A, Magalhães V. NRAMP1 gene polymorphisms in individuals with leprosy reactions attended at two reference centers in Recife, Northeastern Brazil. Rev Soc Bras Med Trop 2010;43:281–6.
52. Alter A, de Léséleuc L, Van Thuc N, Thai VH, Huong NT, Ba NN, et al. Genetic and functional analysis of common MRC1 exon 7 polymorphisms in leprosy susceptibility. Hum Genet 2010; 127:337–48.
53. Wang D, Feng JQ, Li YY, Zhang DF, Li XA, Li QW, et al. Genetic variants of the MRC1 gene and the IFNG gene are associated with leprosy in Han Chinese from Southwest China. Hum Genet 2012;131:1251–60.
54. Sales-Marques C, Cardoso CC, Alvarado-Arnez LE, Illaramendi X, Sales AM, Hacker MA, et al. Genetic polymorphisms of the IL-6 and NOD2 genes are risk factors for inflammatory reactions in leprosy. PLoS Negl Trop Dis. 2017;11:e0005754.
55. Singh I, Lavania M, Pathak VK, Ahuja M, Turankar RP, Singh V, et al. VDR polymorphism, gene expression and vitamin D levels in leprosy patients from North Indian population. PLoS Negl Trop Dis 2018;12:e0006823.
56. Aquino JS, Ambrosio-Albuquerque EP, Alves HV, Macedo LC, Visentainer L, Sell AM, et al. IL8 and IL-17A polymorphisms associated with multibacillary leprosy and reaction type 1 in a mixed population from Southern Brazil. Ann Hum Genet 2019;83:110–14.
57. Chaitanya VS, Jadhav RS, Lavania M, Singh M, Valluri V, Sengupta U. Interleukin-17F single-nucleotide polymorphism (7488T>C) and its association with susceptibility to leprosy. Int J Immunogenet 2014;41:131–7.
58. Sales-Marques C, Cardoso CC, Alvarado-Arnez LE, Illaramendi X, Sales AM, Hacker MA, et al. Genetic polymorphisms of the IL-6 and NOD2 genes are risk factors for inflammatory reactions in leprosy. PLoS Negl Trop Dis 2017;11:e0005754.
59. Cambri G, Mira MT. Genetic susceptibility to leprosy-from classic immune-related candidate genes to hypothesis-free, whole genome approaches. Front Immunol. 2018;9:1674.

4.2 TRANSMISSION OF LEPROSY

Ananta Khurana

Multi-drug therapy has effectively reduced the prevalence of leprosy but has not been effective in stopping transmission, as reflected by the almost static incidence rates globally.[1] Interruption of transmission is the final push needed to further the cause of a leprosy-free world.

However, owing to its long incubation period, even after interruption of transmission, new cases would continue to be detected for many years and leprosy may continue to be a public health problem, with the prevalent issue of post-cure morbidity.

Some progress has been made in understanding the transmission of leprosy and establishment of infection and is detailed in the sections below. However, definitive links are still lacking.

Nasal Entry and Mucosal Immunity

The importance of nasal secretions in leprosy has been known for long. *M. leprae* discharged during coughing or sneezing may get airborne as droplets and cause infection.[2,3] This is supported by findings of large number of bacilli in nasal discharge of lepromatous cases with a high proportion being morphologically intact and viable.[4-6] Pedley et al[2] demonstrated that a large number of *M. leprae*, including some of normal morphology, were projected during sneezing, up to a distance of 30 cm from the face and smaller numbers to a distance of 50 cm. None could however be recovered during 20 min of normal speech. Viable bacilli have been demonstrated for up to two days in discharged nasal secretions.[7] An experimental evidence of airborne infection and nasal route of entry was later provided by Rees and McDougall (1977) when they demonstrated that immunologically suppressed mice can be infected with *M. leprae* by airborne infection.[8] In another experiment, introduction of *M. leprae* into the lung of mice by tracheostomy did not result in disease, whereas delivery of *M. leprae* into the nostril in a saline suspension was associated with invasion of the nasal mucosa producing a localized nodule and disseminated disease 15 months later.[9]

However, the lepromatous cases have been declining over time and the severe nasal disease with nodules and ulcers is not commonly encountered. The importance of this route however remains with findings of nasal carriage of *M. leprae* in general population in endemic regions.[10-15] Pattyn et al found a nonsignificant difference between nasal swab PCR positivity among contacts of PB and MB patients indicating that most infections are community acquired.[14]

The nasal PCR positivity has been studied in healthy residents of endemic regions. While only 1.2% of 2552 nasal swabs were PCR positive in MILEP-2 study involving 3 villages in South Maharashtra, India (Smith et al, 2004) and 2.9% and 7.8% from endemic regions in Indonesia.[10,13,15,16] Lavania et al reported about 30% PCR positivity amongst residents of a highly endemic district from West Bengal, India.[17] Interestingly, a higher positivity in the wet monsoon season was observed by both Smith et al and Lavania et al.[10,17] A high PCR positivity (19%) has also been reported from nasal swabs of hospital workers working with leprosy patients on a daily basis.[18]

An important observation however from community based studies is the transitory nature of PCR positivity. Smith et al reported that of all who were PCR positive initially, none remained positive in the first follow-up survey and only one was positive in the second follow-up survey.[10] Similar findings were reported from Indonesia by Hatta et al.[13] The authors reported that PCR positivity can occur in clusters in the community. And the clustering seems to be a time-dependent phenomenon, not necessarily related to the presence of patients.[13]

Predictive value of nasal PCR positivity in development of disease at a later date cannot be confidently commented on at this point of time. New patients have been diagnosed in follow-up surveys who were PCR negative in the initial ones.[13] Further, if these carriers actually disseminate bacilli too also remains to be established. The carriers may possibly have some role in the environmental presence of M. leprae which shall be discussed later. Thus, with evidence so far available, it seems that asymptomatic nasal carriers may be important for continued transmission of leprosy in endemic communities but the many missing links demand more work on the topic.

The nasal mucosa however is likely the main port of entry of M. leprae. Histological changes of leprosy have been demonstrated in about half of pure neuritic Hansen patients.[19] Further, the nasal mucosal biopsies even from patients with indeterminate, tuberculoid and borderline tuberculoid patients have revealed leprosy suggestive histopathology.[20] Thus, it seems that contact with M. leprae leads first to a primary nasal infection. The entry into epithelial cells involves a surface protein (Mce1A) encoded by Mce1A gene.[21,22] Some adhesins present on M. leprae surface, like heparin-binding hemagglutinin and histone-like protein may also be involved.[23] The entry and replication of M. leprae in nasal epithelial cells has been demonstrated in in vitro models.[23] From the primary focus in nose, the organism may spread via the bloodstream and/or lymphatics to lodge in nerves, skin and other sites, where the secondary lesions occur. The histological findings of nasal lesions showing bacilli in endothelial cells and presence of a perivascular infiltrate is consistent with hematogenous dissemination of infection from nose.[19]

Since the nasal mucosa is probably the main port of entry, nasal immunity is likely to be an important defense against further dissemination of bacilli and mucosal IgA responses (serum M. leprae IgA/sMLIgA) may be important markers of early exposure and infection.[24] Although a direct correlation of serial measurements of PCR positivity and serological tests has not been demonstrated, the studies which have simultaneously measured both parameters provide a framework for understanding early infection and immunity.[3,10,13,15] First infection with M. leprae is likely to be followed by immunity in most individuals. Thus, those not yet infected (PCR/sMLIgA–) will become transiently PCR +/sMLIgA– during primary infection and then develop immunity while infection resolves (PCR+/sMLIgA+).[3] Retesting those patients are expected to show a putative protection with PCR–/sMLIgA+ status, although this has not been satisfactorily demonstrated.[3] Van Beers et al suggested that the lack of correlation between PCR positivity and serology may be because of several reasons.[15] Firstly, it is possible that only a transient state of carriership occurs without actual colonization or infection. Secondly, there may be a time lag between the carriage of M. leprae in the nose and the onset of a serological response. And finally, not every infection would necessarily lead to a serological response.

To conclude, the evidence so far indicates that a primary nasal infection occurs at the point of first contact with *M. leprae* and a protective mucosal immunity ensues, which possibly overcomes infection in most cases and is likely long lasting. Hematogenous spread from the initial bacilliferous lesion in the nasal mucosa occurs in those unable to mount a protective response and the subsequent disease manifest depending on the kind of immune response mounted by the host.[25]

The Role of Skin

For long, it was widely held that direct person-to-person skin contact is important in transmission of leprosy. However, in a widely referenced paper, Pedley (1970) reported their findings of lack of a significant number of acid-fast bacilli on the skin of lepromatous patients, using composite skin contact smear (CSCS) technique, and concluded that the bacilli do not pass through intact skin.[26] This view came to be widely accepted although contradictory findings were demonstrated later using the same technique.[27] Later, Job et al reported clumps of AFB in one or more focal areas of the keratin layer in 5 of the 13 biopsies of leprosy patients with BI >4.[28]

M. leprae has also been detected in the epidermis, sweat and sebaceous glands and hair follicles of leprosy patients suggesting a possible excretion of bacilli from these sites.[29,30] Using PCR, about 80% of multibacillary patients were shown to have *M. leprae* DNA in skin washings. *M. leprae* DNA was also present in a 17% of samples taken from skin of contacts of untreated MB leprosy cases. A transepidermal elimination of *M. leprae* from intact nodules of histoid leprosy and of lepromatous granulomas has also been reported.[31,32]

M. leprae may be engulfed by the epidermal cells and have been demonstrated to lie within them in electron microscopic studies.[33] This epidermal cell invasion was further detailed by Lyrio et al who reported that HaCaT, a human keratinocyte cell line, phagocytoses *M. leprae* and the *M. leprae*-phagocytosed keratinocytes produce cathelicidin, an antimicrobial peptide, as well as tumor necrosis factor α (TNF-α).[34] It has been suggested that *M. leprae* binds to keratinocytes via interaction of LN-5 in the basal lamina of the epidermis and a surface receptor of keratinocytes, such as α-dystroglycan, integrin-β1, or -β4 similar to its interaction with the Schwann cells.[35]

The inoculation into skin as a mode of entry of bacilli is supported by case reports[40-42] and series describing disease following injuries and tattooing.[36-39] The lag period described in these reports is variable, between 2 and 40 years. Another point in support of skin as an entry site is predilection of initial lesions on exposed or trauma prone areas.

To conclude, the evidence for skin as site of exit and entry of *M. leprae* is still not defined. But, there is now some clarity on the presence of bacilli in superficial skin structures which may act as exit points for *M. leprae*. And further, with increasing evidence of environmental sources of *M. leprae* as discussed below, the role of skin in transmission of leprosy may need to be revisited.

Oral Cavity

Oral lesions are generally seen in advanced stages of MB leprosy and form a source of infection for others then. There is recent evidence pointing to possibility of a primary oral mucosal infection, akin to a primary nasal infection and presence of oral carriers of *M. leprae*.[43,44]

Martinenz et al (2011) reported a buccal swab *M. leprae* DNA positivity of 18.3% among patients and 6.8% among contacts.[44] The positivity rates of *M. leprae* DNA in the oral cavity were not significantly different between PB and MB patients, indicating that PB patients may also be oral *M. leprae* carriers and that the mouth might function as a route of initial and transitory infection for this clinical form. A much higher positivity was observed by Morgado de Abreu et al (2014) using oral biopsies. But similar to Martinenz et al, they also dint find any significant difference in positivity among PB and MB patients.[45] Similarly, Carvalho et al (2018) reported hard palate mucosa PCR positivity of 35% and 31% among patients and contacts, reinforcing role of oral mucosa as the primary site of infection as well as in transmission.[46]

The role of saliva and especially salivary IgA would be of relevance in the development of protective immunity towards *M. leprae* within the oral cavity, preventing dissemination.

Contacts and Clustering

There is significant literature confirming clustering of leprosy cases. There is an elevated risk of leprosy among contacts of index cases, both within the household and social contacts. Molecular evidence showed that cases within households were often due to the same strain of *M. leprae* and that a variety of strains existed in the same area.[47] A clear stratification of the risk of disease has emerged, with household contacts of MB cases being at higher risk than household contacts of PB cases, and individuals with more intensive social contact or living closer to leprosy cases being at higher risk.[48-56] But it must be remembered that genetic relationship is also a relevant risk factor for household contacts, independent of physical distance. Moet et al showed that closely related contacts of the index patient had a higher risk than the non-relative household contacts.[57] Importantly, most secondary cases are of the paucibacillary/tuberculoid type.[58]

However, a large proportion of newly diagnosed cases cannot be attributed to any known index case especially in high transmission areas. Only 15% of all incidence cases arise among recognized household contacts.[58] This may be explained with presence of subclinical infection in the community, presence of environmental sources or possibly undiagnosed cases. The role of nasal and oral carriers as discussed before may be important in this regard. Lastly, it must be pointed out that although residential contact with a MB case is a strong determinant of leprosy risk, the vast majority of such contacts never manifest disease, which indicates a crucial role for genetic and/or environmental factors in the transmission of *M. leprae* infection and/or the pathogenesis of clinical leprosy.[58]

Environmental Presence of *M. leprae*/Extra Human Reservoirs

Apart from human carriers and undiagnosed cases, environmental reservoirs may also play a role in continued transmission of leprosy as evidenced by past and recent literature. An existence of zoonotic *M. leprae* reservoirs among 9 banded armadillos is well established but is unlikely to have much epidemiological relevance especially in parts of the world most affected by the disease.[59] Interestingly, *M. lepromatosis* has been reported in red squirrels in Scotland, but again epidemiological relevance is unclear.[60]

Lahiri et al (2008) demonstrated for the first time that free-living pathogenic amoebae are capable of ingesting and supporting the viability of *M. leprae* expelled into the environment.[61] Wheat et al induced cyst formation in *M. leprae* infected *Acanthamoeba castellani* and *A. polyphaga* and, after 35 days of encystation, recovered bacilli that showed normal growth in the footpads of athymic mice.[62] They also showed that *M. leprae* resides in an acid-rich compartment within the trophozoite cytoplasm, similar to how they reside in macrophages, and that viable *M. leprae* could be recovered for at least eight months in the cysts of *A. castellani*, *A. polyphaga*, *A. lenticulata*, and 2 different strains of *Hartmannella vermiformis*, thus suggesting a protective mechanism to sustain adverse environmental conditions while outside the human hosts. The role of insects in transmission has never been proven and there are no recent publications demonstrating the same.[56]

Presence of viable *M. leprae* in soil and water of endemic regions has been demonstrated using PCR in studies from India and Indonesia.[62–66] Poor sanitation and hygiene are long known factors promoting the persistence of leprosy in a community and the demonstration of the bacillus in soil and water may be a plausible scientific reasoning for it. Viable *M. leprae* can be found in moist soil for up to 46 days.[67] It is suggested that the soil and water may get contaminated with *M. leprae* from high BI MB patients via nasal and oral secretions (spitting, sneezing, blowing nose) or during bathing and washing.[68] Infact, moist places like bathing place, areas near the drain water and washing places showed numerically higher PCR positivity when compared to that of the dry areas like entrance of the house and sitting places in a study done in a few endemic villages from India.[68] Turankar et al (2019) further demonstrated an association of viability (with presence of 16S rRNA) of *M. leprae* in soil and water with presence of Acanthamoeba which may provide a protective niche for the bacilli as mentioned above.[68] The route of transmission of infection from contaminated soil and water to susceptible persons is not clear yet, although contact with exposed skin is a likely mechanism.

REFERENCES

1. WHO weekly epidemiological record 2019;94:389–412 (https://apps.who.int/iris/bitstream/handle/10665/326775/WER9435-36-en-fr.pdf).
2. Pedley JC, Geater JG. Does droplet infection play a role in the transmission of leprosy? Lepr Rev 1976;47:97–102.
3. Ramprasad P, Fernando A, Madhale S, et al. Transmission and protection in leprosy: Indications of the role of mucosal immunity. Lepr Rev 1997;68:301–15.
4. Dharmendra N, Sen N. Frequency of the presence of the leprosy bacillus in nasal smears of leprosy patients. Int J Lepr 1948;16:286.
5. Shepard CC. The nasal excretion of *Mycobacterium leprae* in leprosy. Int J Lepr 1962;30:10–8.
6. Shepard CC. Acid-fast bacilli in nasal excretions in leprosy, and results of inoculation of mice. Am J Hyg 1960;71:147–57.
7. Davey TF, Rees RJ. The nasal dicharge in leprosy: Clinical and bacteriological aspects. Lepr Rev 1974;45:121–34.
8. Rees RJ, McDougall AC. Airborne infection with *Mycobacterium leprae* in mice. J Med Microbiol 1977;10:63–8.
9. Chehl S, Job CK, Hastings RC. Transmission of leprosy in nude mice. Am J Trop Med Hyg, 1985;34:1161–6.

10. Smith WC, Smith S, Cree IA et al, An approach to understanding the transmission of *Mycobacterium leprae* using molecular and immunological methods: Results from the MILEP2 Study. Int J Lepr Other Mycobact Dis 2004;72:269–77.
11. de Wit MY, Douglas JT, McFadden J, et al. Polymerase chain reaction for detection of *Mycobacterium leprae* in nasal swab specimens. J Clin Microbiol 1993;31:502–6.
12. Klatser PR, van Beers S, Madjid B, et al. Detection of *Mycobacterium leprae* nasal carriers in populations for which leprosy is endemic. J Clin Microbiol 1993;31:2947–51.
13. Hatta M, van Beers SM, Madjid B, et al. Distribution and persistence of *Mycobacterium leprae* nasal carriage among the population in which leprosy is endemic in Indonesia. Trans R Soc Trop Med Hyg 1995;89:381–5.
14. Pattyn SR, Ursi D, Ieven M, Grillone S, Raes V. Detection of *Mycobacterium leprae* by the polymerase chain reaction in nasal swabs of leprosy patients and their contacts. Int J Lepr Other Mycobact Dis 1993;61:389–93.
15. van Beers SM, Izumi S, Madjid B, Maeda Y, Day R, Klatser PR. An epidemiological study of leprosy infection by serology and polymerase chain reaction. Int J Lepr Other Mycobact Dis 1994;62:1–9.
16. Klatser PR, van Beers S, Madjid B, Day R, de Wit MY. Detection of *Mycobacterium leprae* nasal carriers in populations for which leprosy is endemic. J Clin Microbiol 1993;31:2947–51.
17. Lavania M, Turankar RP, Karri S, Chaitanya VS, Sengupta U, Jadhav RS. Cohort study of the seasonal effect on nasal carriage and the presence of *Mycobacterium leprae* in an endemic area in the general population. Clin Microbiol Infect 2013;19:970–4.
18. de Wit MY, Douglas JT, McFadden J, Klatser PR. Polymerase chain reaction for detection of *Mycobacterium leprae* in nasal swab specimens. J Clin Microbiol 1993;31:502–6.
19. Suneetha S, Arunthathi S, Job A, Date A, Kurian N, Chacko CJ. Histological studies in primary neuritic leprosy: Changes in nasal mucosa. Lepr Rev 1998;69:358–66.
20. Chacko CJG, Bhanu T, Victor V, Alexander R, Taylor PM, Job CK. The significance of changes in the nasal mucosa in indeterminate, tuberculoid and borderline leprosy. Lepr Ind 1979;51: 8–22.
21. Fadlitha VB, Yamamoto F, Idris I, Dahlan H, Sato N, Aftitah VB, et al. The unique tropism of *Mycobacterium leprae* to the nasal epithelial cells can be explained by the mammalian cell entry protein 1A. PLoS Negl Trop Dis 2019;13:e0006704.
22. Sato N, Fujimura T, Masuzawa M, Yogi Y, Matsuoka M, Kanoh M, et al. Recombinant *Mycobacterium leprae* protein associated with entry into mammalian cells of respiratory and skin components. J Dermatol Sci 2007;46:101–10.
23. Silva CA1, Danelishvili L, McNamara M, Berredo-Pinho M, Bildfell R, Biet F, et al. Interaction of *Mycobacterium leprae* with human airway epithelial cells: Adherence, entry, survival, and identification of potential adhesins by surface proteome analysis. Infect Immun 2013;81: 2645–59.
24. Barton RP. Importance of nasal lesions in early lepromatous leprosy. Annals of the Royal College of Surgeons of England 1975;57:309–12.
25. Cree IA, Smith WC. Leprosy transmission and mucosal immunity: Towards eradication? Lepr Rev. 1998;69:112–21.
26. Pedley JC. Composite skin contact smears: A method of demonstrating non-emergence of *Mycobacterium leprae* from intact lepromatous skin. Lepr Rev 1970;41;31–43.
27. Hameedullah A, Lal S, Garg BR. Composite skin contact smears in multibacillary leprosy patients. Lepr India 1982;54:605–12.
28. Job CK, Jayakumar J, Aschhoff M. "Large numbers" of *Mycobacterium leprae* are discharged from the intact skin of lepromatous patients; a preliminary report. Int J Lepr Other Mycobact Dis 1999;67:164–7.
29. Hosokawa A. A clinical and bacteriological examination of *Mycobacterium leprae* in the epidermis and cutaneous appendages of patients with multibacillary leprosy. The Journal of dermatology 1999;26:479–88.

30. Kotteeswaran G, Chacko CJ, Job CK. Skin adnexa in leprosy and their role in the dissemination of *M. leprae*. Lepr India 1980;52:475–81.
31. Namisato M, Kakuta M, Kawatsu K, Obara A, Izumi S, Ogawa H. Transepidermal elimination of lepromatous granuloma: A mechanism for mass transport of viable bacilli. Lep Rev 1997;68:167–72.
32. Ghorpade AK. Transepidermal elimination of *Mycobacterium leprae* in histoid leprosy: A case report suggesting possible participation of skin in leprosy transmission. Indian J Dermatol Venereol Leprol 2011;77:59–61.
33. Okada S, Komura J, Nishiura M. *Mycobacterium leprae* found in epidermal cells by electron microscopy. Int J Lepr Other Mycobact Dis 1978;46:30–4.
34. Lyrio EC, Campos-Souza IC, Correa LC, Lechuga GC, Vericimo M, Castro HC, et al. Interaction of *Mycobacterium leprae* with the HaCaT human keratinocyte cell line: New frontiers in the cellular immunology of leprosy. Experimental dermatology, 2015;24:536–42.
35. Jin SH, Kim SK, Lee SB. *M. leprae* interacts with the human epidermal keratinocytes, neonatal (HEKn) via the binding of laminin-5 with α-dystroglycan, integrin-β1, or -β4.PLoS Negl Trop Dis 2019;13:e0007339.
36. Ghorpade A. Inoculation (tattoo) leprosy: A report of 31 cases. J Eur Acad Dermatol Venereol 2002; 16:494–499.
37. Ghorpade A. Post-traumatic inoculation tuberculoid leprosy after injury with a glass bangle. Lepr Rev 2009;80:215–8.
38. Ghorpade A. Post-traumatic borderline tuberculoid leprosy over knee in an Indian male. Lepr Rev 2013;84:248–51.
39. Singh RK. Tattoos and paucibacillary leprosy. Travel Med Infect Dis 2009;7:325–6.
40. Horton RJ, Povey S. The distribution of first lesions in leprosy. Lepr Rev 1966;37:113–4.
41. Bechelli LM, Garbajosa PG, Gyi MM, Dorniguez VM, Quagliato R. Site of early skin lesions in children with leprosy. Bull WHO 1973;48:107–11.
42. Abraham S, Mozhi NM, Joshep GA, Kurian N, Rao PS, Job CK. Epidemiological significance of first lesion in leprosy. Int J Lepr 1998;66:131–9.
43. Carvalho RS, Foschiani IM, Costa MRSN, Marta SN, da Cunha Lopes Virmond M. Early detection of *M. leprae* by qPCR in untreated patients and their contacts: Results for nasal swab and palate mucosa scraping. Eur J Clin Microbiol Infect Dis 2018;37:1863–7.
44. Martinez TS, Figueira M, Costa A, Gonçalves M, Goulart L, Goulart I. Oral mucosa as a source of *Mycobacterium leprae* infection and transmission, and implications of bacterial DNA detection and the immunological status. Clin Microbiol Infect 2011; 17:1653–8.
45. Morgado de Abreu MA, Roselino AM, Enokihara M, Nonogaki S, Prestes-Carneiro LE, Weckx LL, et al. *Mycobacterium leprae* is identified in the oral mucosa from paucibacillary and multibacillary leprosy patients.Clin Microbiol Infect 2014;20:59–64.
46. Carvalho RS, Foschiani IM, Costa MRSN, Marta SN, da Cunha Lopes Virmond M. Early detection of *M. leprae* by qPCR in untreated patients and their contacts: results for nasal swab and palate mucosa scraping. Eur J Clin Microbiol Infect Dis 2018;37:1863–7.
47. Bratschi MW, Steinmann P, Wickenden A, Gillis TP. Current knowledge on *Mycobacterium leprae* transmission: A systematic literature review. Lepr Rev 2015;86:142–55.
48. Vijayakumaran P, Jesudasan K, Mozhi NM, Samuel JD. Does MDT arrest transmission of leprosy to household contacts? Int J Lepr Other Mycobact Dis 1998;66:125–30.
49. Moet FJ, Meima A, Oskam L, Richardus JH. Risk factors for the development of clinical leprosy among contacts, and their relevance for targeted interventions. Lepr Rev 2004;75:310–26.
50. Rao PS, Karat AB, Kaliaperumal VG, Karat S. Transmission of leprosy within households. Int J Lepr Other Mycobact Dis 1975;43:45–54.
51. Ali PM, Prasad KVN. Contact surveys in leprosy. Lepr Rev 1966;37:173–82.
52. Ranade MG, Joshi GY. Long-term follow-up of families in an endemic area. Indian J Lepr 1995; 67:411–25.

53. Jesudasan K, Bradley D, Smith PG, Christian M. Incidence rates of leprosy among household contacts of "primary cases". Indian J Lepr 1984;56:600–14.
54. van Beers SM, Hatta M, Klatser PR. Patient contact is the major determinant in incident leprosy: Implications for future control. Int J Lepr Other Mycobact Dis 1999;67:119–28.
55. de Matos HJ, Duppre N, Alvim MF, MachadoVieira LM, Sarno EN, Struchiner CJ. Leprosy epidemiology in a cohort of household contacts in Rio de Janeiro (1987-1991) [authors' transl]. Cad Saude Publica 1999;15:533–42.
56. Bratschi MW, Steinmann P, Wickenden A, Gillis TP. Current knowledge on *Mycobacterium leprae* transmission: A systematic literature review. Lepr Rev 2015;8:142–55.
57. Moet FJ, Pahan D, Schuring RP, Oskam L, Richardus JH. Physical distance, genetic relationship, age, and leprosy classification are independent risk factors for leprosy in contacts of patients with leprosy.J Infect Dis 2006;193:346–53.
58. Fine PE, Sterne JA, Pönnighaus JM, Bliss L, Saui J, Chihana A, Munthali M, Warndorff DK. Household and dwelling contact as risk factors for leprosy in Northern Malawi. Am J Epidemiol 1997;146:91–102.
59. Truman RW, Singh P, Sharma R, et al. Probable zoonotic leprosy in the southern United States. N Engl J Med 2011;364:1626–33.
60. Meredith A, Del Pozo J, Smith S, Milne E, Stevenson K, McLuckie J. Leprosy in red squirrels in Scotland.Vet Rec 2014;175:285–6.
61. Lahiri R, Krahenbuhl JL. The role of free-living pathogenic amoeba in the transmission of leprosy: A proof of principle. Lepr Rev 2008;79:401–9.
62. Wheat WH, Casali AL, Thomas V, Spencer JS, Lahiri R, Williams DL, et al. Long-term survival and virulence of *Mycobacterium leprae* in amoebal cysts. PLoS Negl Trop Dis 2014;18;8:e3405.
63. Lavania M, Katoch K, Sachan P, Dubey A, Kapoor S, Kashyap M, et al. Detection of *Mycobacterium leprae* DNA from soil samples by PCR targeting RLEP sequences. J Commun Dis 2006; 38:269–73.
64. Lavania M, Katoch K, Katoch VM, Gupta AK, Chauhan, DS, Sharma R, et al. Detection of viable *Mycobacterium leprae* in soil samples: Insights into possible sources of transmission of leprosy. Infect Genet Evol 2008;8:627–31.
65. Turankar RP, Lavania M, Singh M, Sengupta U, Siva Sai K, Jadhav RS. Presence of viable *Mycobacterium leprae* in environmental specimens around houses of leprosy patients. Indian J. Med Microbiol 2016;34:315–21.
66. Matsuoka M, Izumi S, Budiawan T, et al. *Mycobacterium leprae* DNA in daily using water as a possible source of leprosy infection. Indian J Lepr 1999;71:61–7.
67. Desikan KV, Sreevatsa. Extended studies on the viability of *Mycobacterium leprae* outside the human body. Lepr Rev 1995;66:287–95.
68. Turankar RP, Lavania M, Darlong J, Siva Sai KSR, Sengupta U, Jadhav RS. Survival of *Mycobacterium leprae* and association with Acanthamoeba from environmental samples in the inhabitant areas of active leprosy cases: A cross sectional study from endemic pockets of Purulia, West Bengal. Infect Genet Evol 2019;72:199–204.

4.3 IMMUNOLOGY OF DISEASE

Ananta Khurana

M. leprae genome has been fully sequenced and shown to be remarkably conserved (99.99% identity) between different strains.[1,2] This suggests that the diverse clinical manifestations of infection result from the variable host responses. Leprosy is thus a unique infection showing spectral evolution of the host immune response. The tuberculoid form (TT) represents the pole of resistance and is characterized by intense cellular immunity, with few bacilli and a limited number of lesions. The lepromatous form (LL) represents the pole of susceptibility with extensive lesions and intense growth of the bacillus in macrophages (an infection specific immunological anergy; "split anergy").[3] The intermediate borderline forms are immunologically dynamic with characteristics between the two polar forms and progressive reduction of the cell-mediated response from the borderline tuberculoid (BT) to the borderline borderline (BB) and borderline lepromatous (BL) forms.

INNATE IMMUNITY

Although the diversity in adaptive immune response contributing to the spectral manifestations of leprosy has been extensively studied, the role of innate immunity to *M. leprae* is a focus of active research. The innate immunity cells and their secreted mediators contribute to microbial clearance as well as in shaping the adaptive immune response (Table 4.3).

Of the various pattern recognition receptors (PRR) which recognize *M. leprae*, role of toll-like receptors (TLR) is prominent. *M. leprae* predominantly activates the TLR2/1 heterodimer expressed mainly on macrophages and dendritic cells.[4] TLR-1 and TLR-2 are more strongly expressed in lesions of TT than LL.[5] Interestingly, the local cytokine milieu influences the expression and activation of TLRs. Type 1 cytokines upregulate expression and enhance activation of TLR1 in response to *M. leprae*, while type 2 cytokines downregulate TLR2 expression.[6] This suggests an influence of adaptive immune response on innate immunity. A genome-wide scan of *M. leprae* detected 31 lipoproteins that could serve as pathogen-associated molecular patterns (PAMP) recognized by TLR2-TLR1 heterodimers.[5] Synthetic lipopeptides representing the 19-kD and 33-kD lipoproteins also activate the TLR2 receptors on both monocytes and dendritic cells.[5] The presence and role of TLR2 on Schwann cells has been discussed in the subsequent section on nerve damage. The activation of the TLR 2/1 heterodimer activates downstream transcription factors, mainly NF-κB and vitamin D receptor (VDR). This triggers production of proinflammatory cytokines and antimicrobial peptides from the macrophages (Fig. 4.1).

The cytokine milieu thus created modulates the development of Th1/Th17 effector pathways.[5] The role of other TLRs is mentioned in Table 4.4.

Macrophages (MΦ) form the key cell population preferentially infected by *M. leprae* and perform antimicrobial and phagocytic functions (Fig. 4.1). Similar to T-helper cell profiles, distinct MΦ profiles have now been detailed. Under resting conditions, the monocytes are modulated by endothelial cells to differentiate into **M2 MΦ** (CD209+, CD163+) which are highly phagocytic, and are involved in clearing various

Table 4.3: Important innate immune cells	
Cell	Role in immune response to M. leprae
Macrophages	• Phagocytic and antimicrobial function • M1 MΦ ↑ in TT spectrum: Antimicrobial • M2 MΦ ↑ in LL spectrum: Phagocytic • Cytokine release modulates the adaptive Th response
Dendritic cells (DC)	• Professional antigen presenting cells; release proinflammatory cytokines • Marked deficit in LL[14] • Activation and maturation of DCs inhibited by *M. leprae*[15] • PGL-I impairs DC maturation and activation[16]
Schwann cells	See *Section 4.4* on nerve damage
Keratinocytes	• ↑ICAM expression in TT[17] • Upregulation of human beta-defensins 2 and 3 on stimulation with *M. leprae*[18] • Major producer of CXCL-10 in TT[19] • Present *M. leprae* to CD4+ T cells[20]

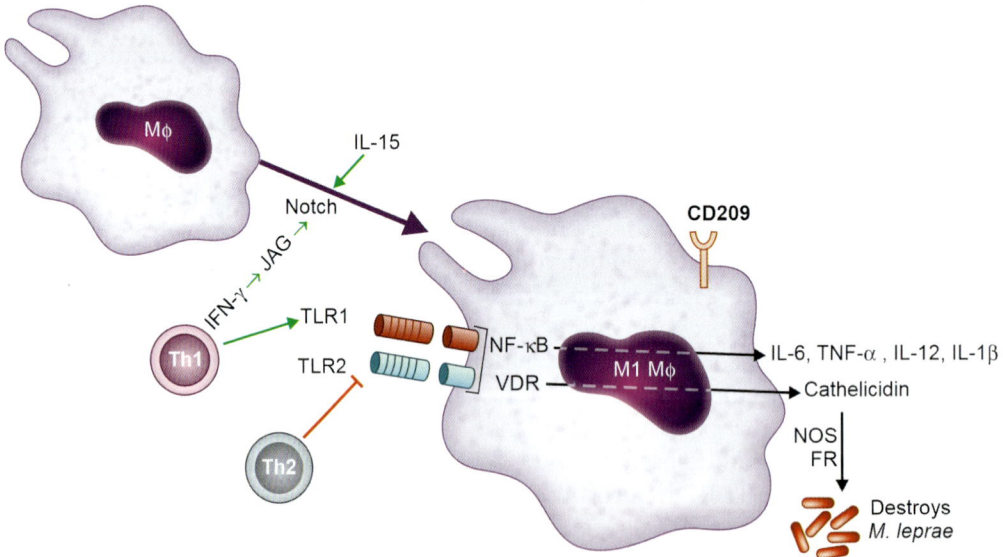

Fig. 4.1: The induction of M1 macrophages (M1 MΦ) and the subsequent downstream steps leading to *M. leprae* killing in the high immunity pole. NOS: Nitric Oxide Synthase; FR: Free Radicals

biomolecules relevant for tissue repair, removal of excess metabolic products as well as clearance of debris.[7] However, in the context of *M. leprae* infection, M2 MΦ can phagocytose the bacteria, but are unable to mount an antimicrobial response. Furthermore, M2 MΦ take up host-derived lipids, providing necessary nutrients for sustaining mycobacterial growth[8] (Fig. 4.2). These cells also produce anti-inflammatory cytokines (IL-4, IL-10, and IL-13), growth factors [TGF-β and basic fibroblast growth factor (bFGF)], and enzymes such as arginase 1 and IDO that contribute to the development of immunosuppressive mechanisms as well as tissue repair.[9] Therefore, the induction of **M1 MΦ** (CD209+, CD163–), which are weakly phagocytic but exhibit

Table 4.4: Innate immune receptors

Receptor	Role in immune response to M. leprae
Toll-like receptors (TLR) TLR1/2	• Most important for recognition of *M. leprae* by innate immune cells (*see* text) • Schwann cell apoptosis
TLR4[21]	• Role and ligands not precisely defined yet • Neutralizing antibodies to TLR4 → ↓ TNF, IL-6, CXCL-10 production by macrophages stimulated with *M. leprae*
TLR6[22]	• Biogenesis of lipid droplets in *M. leprae* infected Schawann cells (mainly) and macrophages (partial dependence); improved survival of intracellular bacilli • Expression upregulated in LL[12]
TLR9[23]	Increased expression during ENL
C type lectin receptors (CD209/DC-SIGN, CD-206)[4]	• Phagocytic receptors on macrophages • Phagocytosis induced by IL-10[4, 12]
Scavenger receptors (CD163, SR-A, CD-36, MARCO)	• Uptake of *M. leprae*, apoptotic cells and nutrient sources for bacilli (hemoglobin-haptoglobin for iron, ApoB, lipids, lipoproteins) • Pathways upregulated in LL • Lipid uptake → ↓ TLR induced antimicrobial activity, ↑ IL-10, ↓ IL-12, nitric oxide production
Vitamin D receptors	• Activated via TLR1/2 pathway and IL-15 (secreted by macrophages; present mainly in TT lesions) • Release of antimicrobial peptide cathelicidin
NOD-like receptors (NLR)[24]	• Activation of monocytes via NOD2 causes their preferential differentiation into DCs, mediated by IL-32 • Higher expression of NOD2 and IL-32 in TT
Leukocyte immunoglobulin-like receptor subfamily A member 2 (LILRA2)[12]	• Ligand not defined • Expression more in monocytes from LL lesions • Activation on monocytes impaired GM-CSF induced differentiation into immature DC[25] • Activation inhibits TLR2/1-induced IL-12 release but maintains IL-10 release

a strong antimicrobial response is required for host defense. The antimicrobial response of M1 MΦ is by means of generation of free radicals via inducible nitric oxide synthase pathway (Fig. 4.1). Kibbie et al demonstrated that INF-γ induces expression of Jagged-1 (JAG-1) on endothelial cells, which via mediation of Notch-1 signaling, induces M1 MΦ differentiation.[10] JAG-1 protein is preferentially expressed in the lesions from the self-limited form of leprosy, and localized to the vascular endothelium. IFN-γ also augments TLR-induced regulation of JAG-1 expression in differentiated MΦ.[11]

Apart from this, the innate response cytokine IL-15 (a monocyte released cytokine with high expression in TT lesions) directly triggers M1 MΦ differentiation.[10] IL-15 also activates vitamin D-dependent antimicrobial pathways in M1 MΦ.[6] On the other hand, IL-10-stimulation enhances phagocytosis of both oxidized low-density lipoprotein (LDL) and mycobacteria, but without triggering the vitamin D-dependent antimicrobial pathway.[12,13]

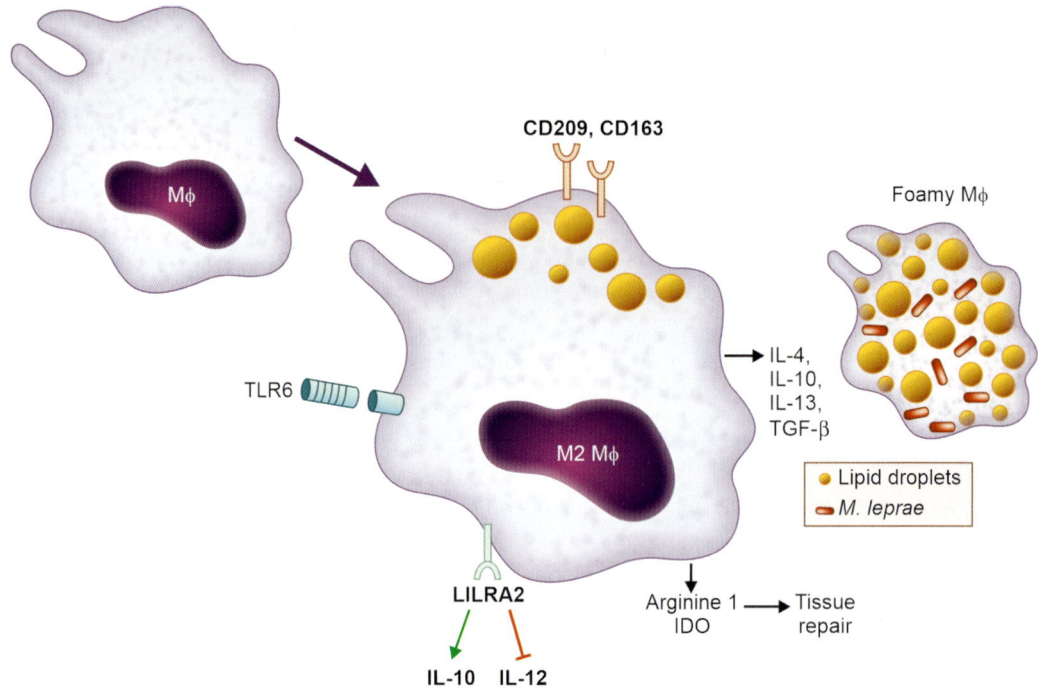

Fig. 4.2: The M2 macrophages (M2 MΦ) present in the lepromatous pole promote intracellular bacterial growth by providing the essential nutrients and lipids and subsequent conversion into the classical foamy macrophages (LILAR 2: Leukocyte immunoglobulin-like receptor subfamily A member 2; CD209: A C type lectin receptor; CD163: A scavenger receptor)

While DC-SIGN+ macrophages carry out the phagocytic and presumably micro-bicidal activity, CD1b+ immature DCs are more potent proinflammatory cytokine-producing and antigen presenting cells. Interestingly, it has been shown that TLR2/1-activation of peripheral monocytes from LL patients triggered differentiation into DC-SIGN+ macrophages but not to CD1b+ DCs, whereas activation of monocytes from TT patients triggered differentiation into both effector populations.[26] Correspondingly, DC-SIGN+ macrophages but not CD1b+ DCs were detected in skin lesions from LL patients, whereas both cell types were detected in TT lesions.[26]

Of the molecules expressed by *M. leprae*, PGL-1 deserves a special mention. It has not only been used for serological diagnosis of disease (*see Chapter 3, Section 3.1*), but also plays an important role in pathogenesis of leprosy. PGL-I has been shown to play an important role in downregulating the inflammatory immune response, inhibits DC maturation and activation, facilitates entry of bacilli into macrophages and SCs and scavenges potentially cytocidal oxygen metabolites *in vitro*, all of which enhance the survival of intracellular bacilli.[27–31] The role of PGL-1 is likely crucial to the ability of *M. leprae* to invade, survive and proliferate in the hostile intracellular environment.

Apart from the major pathways of innate immunity discussed above, there are some *minor/less defined* components described below:

a. **Complement system:** The complement cascade activated by mannose capped lipoarabinomannan (LAM) mediates nerve damage in infected nerves and plays an important role in ENL. These aspects are further discussed in the section on immunopathogenesis of reactions.

b. **Autophagy:** This is an evolutionarily conserved mechanism through which organelles and proteins are degraded and recycled by the lysosomal system to promote cellular and organismal homeostasis.[37] Xenophagy is the term specifically used for the process applied by the immune system to microbes. Autophagy is differentially expressed in leprosy spectrum with increased expression of autophagy initiator Beclin 1 in tuberculoid form contributing to control of bacterial growth and of inhibitor BCL-2 in lepromatous forms.[38,39] Other regulators of autophagy (*NOD2, IRGM, PARK2, LRRK2,* and *RIPK2*) determine susceptibility to leprosy.[32,40,41]

c. **Apoptosis:** Apoptotic cells are more frequently expressed in TT and reversal reaction (RR). de Oliveira Fulco et al demonstrated that M1 MΦ stimulated by *M. leprae*, in the presence of apoptotic cells, changed their phenotype to M2 MΦ and secreted anti-inflammatory mediators such as IL-10, TGF-β, and arginase, thus contributing to sustenance of infection.[42]

ADAPTIVE IMMUNITY

The Th1/Th2 paradigm: The two distinctive T cell subsets, differing in cytokine secretion pattern and other functions, were identified in animal models in the late 80s. Each of these two effector T cell subsets produces cytokines that serve as their own growth factors, thus forming a feed forward loop which promotes further differentiation of that subset.[43] The Th1/Th2 balance hypothesis was subsequently applied to various human diseases including leprosy, the spectral manifestations of which typify the paradigm. An increased expression of type 1 cytokines (INF-γ, IL-2) has been demonstrated in the tuberculoid spectrum and a higher expression of type 2 cytokines (IL-4, IL-5, IL-10) in the lepromatous spectrum (Fig. 4.3).[44]

A Th1 response pattern, seen in the tuberculoid spectrum, via production of IFN-γ and TNF α activates macrophages and induces the production of inducible nitric oxide synthase (iNOS) that destroys the bacillus by means of free radical release. IFN-γ is a very crucial cytokine for protection against mycobacterial infections including leprosy. The Th2 predominance in the lepromatous pole leads to production of IL-4, IL-10 and TGF-β that facilitates survival of the bacillus.[45] IL-4 may also contribute to the elevated anti-*M. leprae* antibodies seen in lepromatous patients via its role in differentiation and immunoglobulin class switching of B cells, while IL-10 is a prominent anti-inflammatory cytokine (Fig. 4.3).[44] Role of transcription factors in modulating a Th1/Th2 differentiation has been investigated in recent times. STAT4 has been shown to contribute towards a Th1 differentiation, while STAT6 modulates Th2 differentiation.[46]

For a long time, the interpretation of host response in leprosy was based on the Th1/Th2 paradigm. However, the Th1/Th2 paradigm alone cannot explain the polarization of immune response and varied clinical presentations of leprosy. Also, many patients have a mixed Th1/Th2 pattern (IFN-γ/IL-4) of cytokines (a nonpolarized Th0 phenotype). A study from India demonstrated that about 43% of leprosy patients produce both classes of cytokines but there were no clinically detectable differences between patients having polarized T helper subsets from those having nonpolarized Th0 functional phenotype.[47]

The advances in immunology with identification of newer immunological pathways have furthered our understanding of the varied host response in leprosy (Fig. 4.3). These are discussed below.

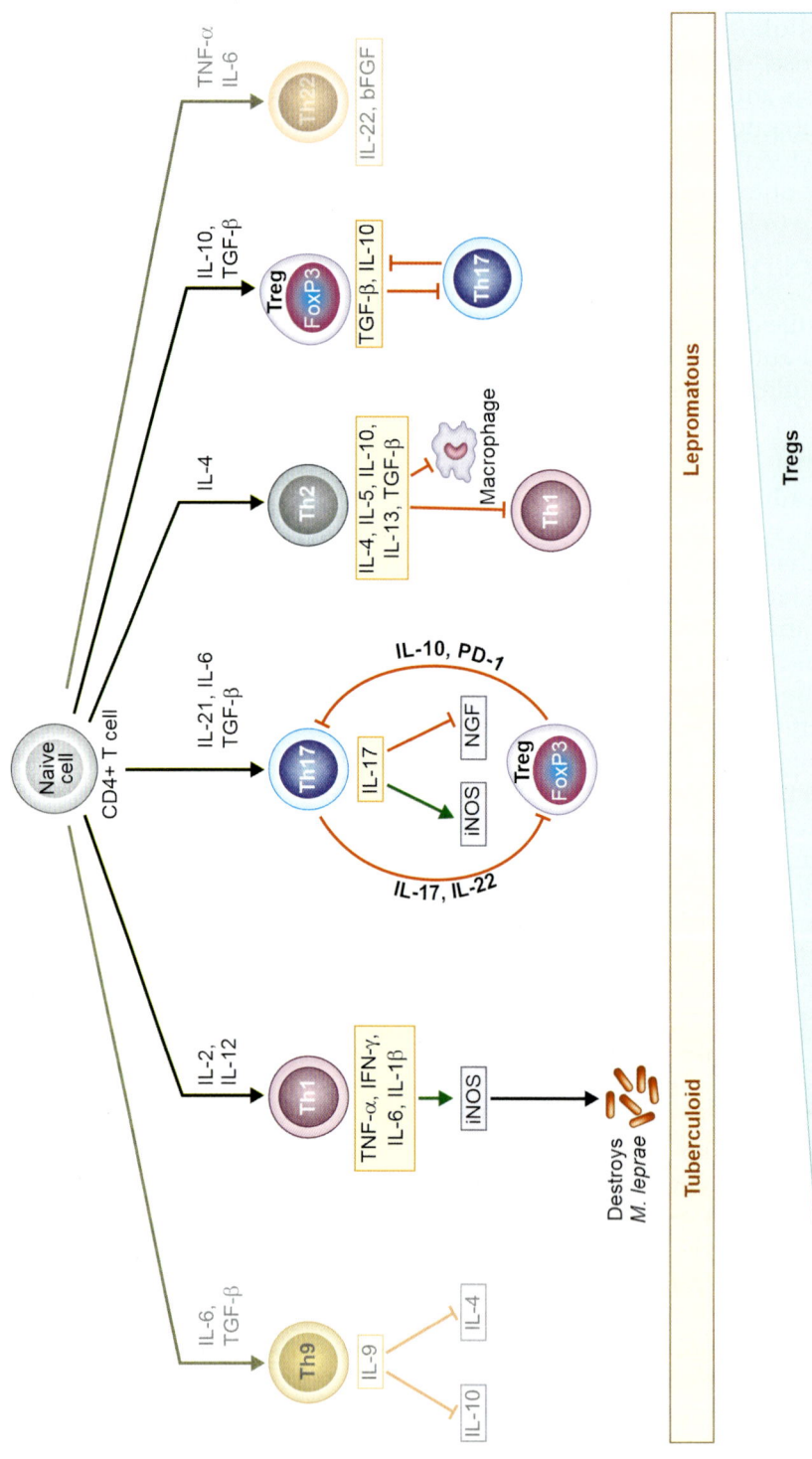

Fig. 4.3: The T helper profiles across the spectrum of leprosy. Note the reciprocal relationship between Th17 and FoxP3+ Treg cells. The role of Th9 and Th22 is not well delineated in leprosy (Treg: T regulatory; NGF: Nerve growth factor; iNOS: inducible nitric oxide synthase; bFGF: basic fibroblast growth factor)

Th17 cells: Th17 cells possibly form the third effector T helper cell subset in leprosy, in addition to the Th1 and Th2 subsets. The differentiation factors (TGF-β plus IL-6 or IL-21), the growth and stabilization factor (IL-23), and the transcription factors (STAT3, ROR-γt, and ROR-α) involved in the development of Th17 cells have now been established (Fig. 4.3).[48]

IL-17 is the signature cytokine associated with this subtype and has proinflammatory functions. Interestingly, IL-17 is also an important component of the innate immune response, its production being induced by interaction of pathogens with the pathogen recognition receptors (PRR) present on certain innate immune cells.[49] Subsequent neutrophil recruitment via IL-6, granulocyte colony stimulating factor (G-CSF) and CXCL8, triggers a rapid nonspecific immunity to infectious agents.[49] Thus, IL-17 also forms a part of a very early event in the inflammatory response to pathogens. In a study from India, leprosy patients showed lower IL-17A expression compared with healthy contacts of patients.[50] Similar findings have been demonstrated in Brazilian and Egyptian patients as well.[51, 52] It has been proposed that a constitutively *low* IL-17A profile could be a marker of susceptibility to *M. leprae*, or that *M. leprae* suppresses IL-17A as an escape mechanism.[51, 52]

Comparison of expression of IL-17 between different subtypes of leprosy has shown significantly higher levels in both skin lesions and antigen stimulated peripheral blood mononuclear cells (PBMC) in BT leprosy compared to LL leprosy, suggesting its differential role in the leprosy spectrum.[50] Interestingly, Th17 cells have been shown to be strongly associated with the nonpolarized Th0 phenotype (showing concomitant IFN-γ and IL4/IL-5 production) and the Th17 distinction between the paucibacillary BT and multibacillary LL was less obvious in polarized Th1 and Th2 states.[50, 53] Hence, based on existing data, it is yet unclear whether Th17 lineage is an alternate pathway for bacillary clearance, when the patient is unable to mount a Th1 response or when Th polarization has not set in OR a stable alternate immune mechanism by itself.[50, 53]

T regulatory cells: In the early 90s, it was discovered that the cells responsible for inhibition of organ specific autoimmunity were CD4+ T cells which expressed CD25 on surface.[54] While CD25 (the IL-2 receptor α chain) is also a marker for activation of effector T cells, only the subset with high levels of CD25 (CD25^{high}) exhibit regulatory functions. They were later shown to also express transcription factor fork-headbox P3 (FoxP3) (CD4+, CD25^{high} and FoxP3+ cells or Tregs).[55, 56] FoxP3 drives various mechanisms that are essential for suppressive potential of Treg cells.[57] Treg was understood to be a class of T cells essential in maintaining peripheral tolerance and preventing autoimmune diseases.[54] Later, FoxP3+ Tregs were demonstrated to be the most potent cell type suppressing effector T cell response in intracellular infections like tuberculosis and leishmaniasis.[59–61] Similarly, a higher absolute number and a higher frequency of Tregs have now been reported in leprosy patients as compared to controls.[62, 63]

TGF-β and IL-10 are the main cytokines involved in differentiation of FoxP3+ Tregs as also in mediating the suppression induced by these cells.[45, 64] Expression of both these cytokines has been shown to be higher in lepromatous pole of leprosy.[65] Higher expression of FoxP3+ Tregs has been demonstrated in both sera and skin lesions of lepromatous forms of leprosy in comparison with the tuberculoid pole.[65–67] The chemokine receptor (CCR4) may play a role in recruiting FoxP3+ Tregs to the lesional sites.

The participation of TGF-β in the differentiation of Th17 cells places the Th17 lineage in close relationship with CD4+, CD25+ and FoxP3+ Tregs, as TGF-β also induces differentiation of naïve T cells into FoxP3+ Tregs. However, in the presence of TGF-β plus IL-6 or IL-21, the Treg developmental pathway is abrogated, and instead T cells develop into Th17 cells.[48] A reciprocal relationship between FoxP3+ Treg cells and the effector Th17 cell function in leprosy is supported by the reported negative correlation between the Treg produced IL-10 production and the presence of Th17 cells in BL/LL leprosy spectrum.[66] The Programmed Death 1/PD-1+ Treg cells and its ligand PDL-1 are found in a higher frequency in BL/LL spectrum and this pathway is likely another factor involved in Treg mediated immune suppression via a contact dependent mechanism as the inhibition of the PD-1/PD-1 ligand pathway rescues the IFN-γ producing Th1 cells and IL-17 producing Th17 cells. Further, the presence of Th17 related cytokines, including Th17 inducing (TGF-β, IL-6, and IL-23) and Th17 secreted cytokines (IL-17, Il-22), decreases the number of FoxP3+ Treg cells concomitantly increasing IL-17 producing CD4+ cells in lepromatous leprosy.[65]

Thus, FoxP3+ Treg cells may be the long searched for contributor towards immunological unresponsiveness or anergy in the lepromatous pole. The counterbalance between the effector T cell types Th1 and Th17 and the suppressor FoxP3+ Treg cells may be an important factor in polarization of the host immunity towards a protective or suppressive response. However, it must be pointed out here that the role of Tregs needs further elucidation as some contradictory views exist at present. In contrast to the above studies (from India and Brazil), some authors have demonstrated either no difference (Parente et al, 2015; Brazil)[68] in Treg expression among different clinical forms or a higher expression in TT spectrum and a marked reduction towards lepromatous pole (Attia et al, 2010 and 2014; Egypt).[63, 70] The authors of the latter studies suggested that Tregs provide a protective counter mechanism trying to regulate effective anti-pathogen immune response and to attenuate the *M. leprae*-induced chronic immune activation.[63]

Th9: The precise place of Th9 cells and IL-9 in the leprosy spectrum is not well delineated. However, existing data suggests that IL-9 may have an atypical Th2 behavior and play a role in the modulation of the immune response to the infection by participating in an interplay of cytokines that control the powerful effect or mechanism of cytotoxicity.[70] IL-9 was demonstrated to counteract the negative effect of IL-4, IL-10 and IL-13 on the specific cytotoxic activity elicited by *M. leprae* in cells from normal controls and leprosy patients. And it further enhanced the stimulatory effect of IL-2 or IL-6 on this lytic activity. These effects likely occur via mediation of IFN-γ.[70]

Th22: Th22 cells have been identified as a cell line producing the prototype cytokine IL-22 and is differentiated from Th1 and Th17 cell lines by lack of production of IFN-γ and IL-17. Smaller amounts of IL-22 are also produced by the Th17 cells. IL-22 levels are higher in LL lesions than in TT, with intense staining in vacuoles and globules of infected macrophages.[71, 72] Here, IL-22 may induce mechanisms that lead to tissue reparative mechanisms, since it regulates the response of growth factors such as basic fibroblast growth factor (bFGF), which is important for the proliferation of keratinocytes, production of extracellular matrix and induction of angiogenesis. Small amounts of bFGF are also likely released from Th22 cells.[73] However, increased IL-22 levels have not been seen by other authors[69] and in the absence of a definitive phenotypic marker however, the role of this putative Th cell line remains unclear.[74]

CONCLUSION

The understanding of immunopathogeneis of leprosy is evolving. From a simplistic Th1/Th2 dichotomy, our understanding has expanded regarding the role of other Th phenotypes as well as the important effects of innate immunity *per se* and in modulating the development of the adaptive immune response (Fig. 4.3). However, there are complexities yet to be resolved. It seems plausible that specific cytokine profiles seen in individuals or population groups may modify the expression of various Th profiles and broad generalizations may not always be possible. Thus, there may be an increasing focus on the role of genetic variations on immune profiles in the future.

REFERENCES

1. Cole ST, Eiglmeier K, Parkhill J, James KD, Thomson NR, Wheeler PR, et al. Massive gene decay in the leprosy bacillus. Nature 2001;409(6823):1007–11.
2. Singh P, Cole ST. *Mycobacterium leprae*: Genes, pseudogenes and genetic diversity. Future Microbiol 2011;6:57–71.
3. de Sousa JR, Sotto MN, Simões Quaresma JA. Leprosy as a Complex Infection: Breakdown of the Th1 and Th2 Immune Paradigm in the Immunopathogenesis of the Disease. Front Immunol 2017;8:1635.
4. Fonseca AB, Simon MD, Cazzaniga RA, de Moura TR, de Almeida RP, Duthie MS, et al. The influence of innate and adaptive immune responses on the differential clinical outcomes of leprosy. Infect Dis Poverty 2017;6:5.
5. Krutzik SR, Ochoa MT, Sieling PA, Uematsu S, Ng YW, Legaspi A, et al. Activation and regulation of toll-like receptors 2 and 1 in human leprosy. Nat Med 2003;9:525–32.
6. Modlin RL. The innate immune response in leprosy. Curr Opin Immunol 2010;22:48–54.
7. He H, Xu J, Warren CM, Duan D, Li X, Wu L, et al. Endothelial cells provide an instructive niche for the differentiation and functional polarization of M2-like macrophages. Blood 2012;120: 3152–62.
8. McKinney JD, Hönerzu Bentrup K, Munoz-Elias EJ, Miczak A, Chen B, Chan WT, et al. Persistence of *Mycobacterium tuberculosis* in macrophages and mice requires the glyoxylate shunt enzyme isocitrate lyase. Nature 2000;406:735–8.
9. de Sousa JR1, Sotto MN2, Simões Quaresma JA. Leprosy as a Complex Infection: Breakdown of the Th1 and Th2 Immune Paradigm in the Immunopathogenesis of the Disease. Front Immunol. 2017;8:1635.
10. Kibbie J, Teles RM, Wang Z, Hong P, Montoya D, Krutzik S. Jagged1 Instructs Macrophage Differentiation in Leprosy. PLoS Pathog 2016;12:e1005808.
11. Foldi J, Chung AY, Xu H, Zhu J, Outtz HH, Kitajewski J, et al. Autoamplification of Notch signaling in macrophages by TLR-induced and RBP-J-dependent induction of Jagged1. J Immunol 2010;185:5023–31.
12. Bleharski JR, Li H, Meinken C, Graeber TG, Ochoa MT, Yamamura M, Burdick A, Sarno EN, Wagner M, Rollinghoff M, et al. Use of genetic profiling in leprosy to discriminate clinical forms of the disease. Science 2003;301:1527–30.
13. Mosser DM, Edwards JP. Exploring the full spectrum of macrophage activation. Nat Rev Immunol 2008;8:958–69.
14. Simões Quaresma JA, de Oliveira MF, Ribeiro Guimarães AC, de Brito EB, de Brito RB, Pagliari C, et al. CD1a and factor XIIIa immunohistochemistry in leprosy: A possible role of dendritic cells in the pathogenesis of *Mycobacterium leprae* infection. Am J Dermatopathol 2009;31: 527–31.
15. Murray RA, Siddiqui MR, Mendillo M, Krahenbuhl J, Kaplan G. *Mycobacterium leprae* inhibits dendritic cell activation and maturation. J Immunol 2007;178:338–44.

16. Kumar S, Naqvi RA, Bhat AA, Rani R, Ali R, Agnihotri A, et al. IL-10 production from dendritic cells is associated with DC SIGN in human leprosy. Immunobiology 2013;218:1488–96.
17. Sullivan L, Sano S, Pirmez C, Salgame P, Mueller C, Hofman F, et al. Expression of adhesion molecules in leprosy lesions. Infect Immun 1991;59:4154–6.
18. Cogen AL, Walker SL, Roberts CH, Hagge DA, Neupane KD, Khadge S, et al. Human beta-defensin 3 is up regulated in cutaneous leprosy type 1 reactions. PLoS Negl Trop Dis 2012;6:e1869.
19. Kaplan G, Luster AD, Hancock G, Cohn ZA. The expression of a gamma interferon-induced protein (IP-10) in delayed immune responses in human skin. J Exp Med 1987;166:1098–108.
20. Mutis T, De Bueger M, Bakker A, Ottenhoff TH. HLA class II+ human keratinocytes present *Mycobacterium leprae* antigens to CD4+ Th1-like cells. Scand J Immunol 1993;37:43–51.
21. Polycarpou A, Holland MJ, Karageorgiou I, Eddaoudi A, Walker SL, Willcocks S, et al. *Mycobacterium leprae* Activates Toll-like Receptor 4 Signaling and Expression on Macrophages Depending on Previous Bacillus Calmette-Guerin Vaccination. Front Cell Infect Microbiol 2016;6:72.
22. Mattos KA, Oliveira VGC, D'Avila H, Rodrigues LS, Pinheiro RO, Sarno EN, et al. TLR6-driven lipid droplets in *Mycobacterium leprae*-infected Schwann cells: Immunoinflammatory platforms associated with bacterial persistence. J Immunol 2011;187:2548–58.
23. Dias AA, Silva CO, Santos JPS, Batista-Silva LR, Acosta CCD, Fontes ANB, et al. DNA sensing via TLR-9 constitutes a major innate immunity pathway activated during erythema nodosum leprosum. J Immunol 2016;197:1905–13.
24. Schenk M, Krutzik SR, Sieling PA, Lee DJ, Teles RM, Ochoa MT, et al. NOD2 triggers an interleukin-32-dependent human dendritic cell program in leprosy. Nat Med 2012;18:555–63.
25. Lee DJ, Sieling PA, Ochoa MT, Krutzik SR, Guo B, Hernandez M, et al. LILRA2 activation inhibits dendritic cell differentiation and antigen presentation to T cells. J Immunol 2007;179:8128–36.
26. Krutzik SR, Tan B, Li H, Ochoa MT, Liu PT, Sharfstein SE, et al. TLR activation triggers the rapid differentiation of monocytes into macrophages and dendritic cells. Nat Med 2005;11:653–60.
27. Schlesinger LS, Horwitz MA. Phenolic glycolipid I of *Mycobacterium leprae* binds complement component C3 in serum and mediates phagocytosis by human monocytes. J Exp Med 1991;174:1031–8.
28. Murray RA, Siddiqui MR, Mendillo M, et al. *Mycobacterium leprae* inhibits dendritic cell activation and maturation. J Immunol 2007;178:338–44.
29. Sinsimer D, Fallows D, Peixoto B, et al. *Mycobacterium leprae* actively modulates the cytokine response in native human monocytes. Infect Immun 2010;78:293–300.
30. Tabouret G, Astarie-Dequeker C, Demangel C, et al. *Mycobacterium leprae* phenolglycolipid 1 expressed by engineered M. bovis BCG modulates early interaction with human phagocytes. PLoS Pathog 2010;6:e1001159.
31. Chan J, Fujiwara T, Brennan PJ, et al. Microbial glycolipids: Possible virulence factors that scavenge oxygen radicals. Proc Natl Acad Sci 1989;86:2453–7.
32. Pinheiro RO, Schmitz V, Silva BJA, Dias AA, de Souza BJ, de Mattos Barbosa MG, et al. Innate Immune Responses in Leprosy. Front Immunol 2018;9:518.
33. Silva BJ, Barbosa MG, Andrade PR, Ferreira H, Nery JA, Côrte-Real S, et al. Autophagy is an innate mechanism associated with leprosy polarization. PLoS Pathog 2017;13:e1006103.
34. Pattingre S, Tassa A, Qu X, Garuti R, Liang XH, Mizushima N, et al. Bcl-2 antiapoptotic proteins inhibit Beclin 1-dependent autophagy. Cell 2005;122:927–39.
35. Mira MT, Alcais A, Nguyen VT, Moraes MO, Di Flumeri C, Vu HT, et al. Susceptibility to leprosy is associated with PARK2 and PACRG. Nature 2004;427:636–40.
36. Yang D, Chen J, Zhang L, Cha Z, Han S, Shi W, et al. *Mycobacterium leprae* upregulates IRGM expression in monocytes and monocyte derived macrophages. Inflammation 2014;37:1028–34.
37. Pinheiro RO, Schmitz V, Silva BJA, Dias AA, de Souza BJ, de Mattos Barbosa MG, et al. Innate Immune Responses in Leprosy. Front Immunol 2018;9:518.

38. Silva BJ, Barbosa MG, Andrade PR, Ferreira H, Nery JA, Côrte-Real S, et al. Autophagy is an innate mechanism associated with leprosy polarization. PLoS Pathog 2017;13:e1006103.
39. Pattingre S, Tassa A, Qu X, Garuti R, Liang XH, Mizushima N, et al. Bcl-2 antiapoptotic proteins inhibit Beclin 1-dependent autophagy. Cell 2005;122:927–39.
40. Mira MT, Alcais A, Nguyen VT, Moraes MO, Di Flumeri C, Vu HT, et al. Susceptibility to leprosy is associated with PARK2 and PACRG. Nature 2004; 427:636–40.
41. Yang D, Chen J, Zhang L, Cha Z, Han S, Shi W, et al. *Mycobacterium leprae* upregulates IRGM expression in monocytes and monocyte-derived macrophages. Inflammation 2014; 37:1028–34.
42. de Oliveira Fulco T, Andrade PR, de Mattos Barbosa MG, Pinto TG, Ferreira PF, Ferreira H, et al. Effect of apoptotic cell recognition on macrophage polarization and mycobacterial persistence. Infect Immun 2014;82:3968–78.
43. Kidd P. Th1/Th2 balance: The hypothesis, its limitations, and implications for health and disease. Altern Med Rev 2003;8:223–46.
44. Modlin RL. Th1-Th2 paradigm: Insights from leprosy. J Invest Dermatol 1994;102:828–32.
45. de Sousa JR, Sotto MN, Simões Quaresma JA Leprosy as a Complex Infection: Breakdown of the Th1 and Th2 Immune Paradigm in the Immunopathogenesis of the Disease Front Immunol. 2017;8:1635.
46. Upadhyay R, Dua B, Sharma B, Natrajan M, Jain AK, Kithiganahalli Narayanaswamy, et al. Transcription factors STAT-4, STAT-6 and CREB regulate Th1/Th2 response in leprosy patients: effect of *M. leprae* antigens. BMC Infect Dis 2019;19:52.
47. Misra N, Murtaza A, Walker B, Narayan NP, Misra RS, Ramesh V, et al. Cytokine profile of circulating T cells of leprosy patients reflects both indiscriminate and polarized T-helper subsets: T-helper phenotype is stable and uninfluenced by related antigens of *Mycobacterium leprae*. Immunology 1995;86:97–103.
48. Korn T, Bettelli E, Oukka M, Kuchroo VK. IL-17 and Th17 Cells. Annu Rev Immunol 2009;27: 485–517.
49. Cua DJ, Tato CM. Innate IL-17-producing cells: The sentinels of the immune system. Nat Rev Immunol 2010;10:479–89.
50. Saini C, Ramesh V, Nath I. CD4+ Th17 cells discriminate clinical types and constitute a third subset of non-Th1, non-Th2 T cells in human leprosy. PLoS Negl Trop Dis 2013;7:e2338.
51. da Motta-Passos I, Malheiro A, Gomes Naveca F, de Souza Passos LF, Ribeiro De Barros Cardoso C, da Graça Souza Cunha M, et al. Decreased RNA expression of interleukin 17A in skin of leprosy. Eur J Dermatol 2012;22:488–94.
52. Abdallah M, Emam H, Attia E, Hussein J, Mohamed N. Estimation of serum level of interleukin-17 and interleukin-4 in leprosy, towards more understanding of leprosy immunopathogenesis. Indian J Dermatol Venereol Leprol 2013;79:772–6.
53. Saini C, Tarique M, Rai R, Siddiqui A, Khanna N, Sharma A. T helper cells in leprosy: An update. Immunol Lett 2017;184:61–6.
54. Sakaguchi S, Sakaguchi N, Asano M, Itoh M, Toda M. Immunologic self-tolerance maintained by activated T cells expressing IL-2 receptor alpha-chains (CD25). Breakdown of a single mechanism of self-tolerance causes various autoimmune diseases. J Immunol 1995;155:1151–64.
55. Hori S, Nomura T, Sakaguchi S. Control of regulatory T cell development by the transcription factor FoxP3. Science 2003;299:1057–61.
56. Yagi H, Nomura T, Nakamura K, Yamazaki S, Kitawaki T, et al. Crucial role of FoxP3 in the development and function of human CD25+ CD4+ regulatory T cells. Int Immunol 2004;16:1643–56.
57. Kumar S, Naqvi RA, Ali R, Rani R, Khanna N, Rao DN. FoxP3 provides competitive fitness to CD4+ and CD25+ T cells in leprosy patients via transcriptional regulation. Eur J Immunol 2014;44:431–9.
58. Baecher-Allan C, Brown JA, Freeman GJ, Hafler DA. CD4+ and CD25+ high regulatory cells in human peripheral blood. J Immunol 2001;167:1245–53.

59. Sharma PK, Saha PK, Singh A, Sharma SK, Ghosh B, et al. FoxP3+ regulatory T cells suppress effector T cell function at pathologic site in miliary tuberculosis. Am J Respir Crit Care Med 2009;179:1061–70.
60. Mendez S, Reckling SK, Piccirillo CA, Sacks D, Belkaid Y. Role for CD4+ and CD25+ regulatory T cells in reactivation of persistent leishmaniasis and control of concomitant immunity. J Exp Med 2004;200:201–10.
61. Rai AK, Thakur CP, Singh A, Seth T, Srivastava SK, et al. Regulatory T Cells Suppress T Cell Activation at the Pathologic Site of Human Visceral Leishmaniasis. PLoS One 2012;7: e44728.
62. Palermo ML, Pagliari C, Trindade MA, Yamashitafuji TM, Duarte AJ, Cacere CR, et al. Increased expression of regulatory T cells and downregulatory molecules in lepromatous leprosy. Am J Trop Med Hyg 2012;86:878–83.
63. Attia EA, Abdallah M, Saad AA, Afifi A, El Tabbakh A, El-Shennawy D, et al. Circulating CD4+, $CD25+^{high}$ and FoxP3+ T cells vary in different clinical forms of leprosy. Int J Dermatol 2010; 49:1152–8.
64. Treganergy lepromatous Saini A, Ramesh V, Nath I. Increase in TGF-β Secreting CD4+, CD25+ and FoxP3+ T Regulatory Cells in Anergic Lepromatous Leprosy Patients. PLoS Negl Trop Dis 2014; 8: e2639.
65. Treg ref 88 Quaresma JA, Esteves PC, de Sousa Aarão TL, de Sousa JR, da Silva Pinto D, Fuzii HT. Apoptotic activity and Treg cells in tissue lesions of patients with leprosy. Microb Pathog 2014;76:84–8.
66. Ref 89 Sadhu S, Khaitan BK, Joshi B, Sengupta U, Nautiyal AK, Mitra DK. Reciprocity between Regulatory T Cells and Th17 Cells: Relevance to Polarized Immunity in Leprosy. PLoS Negl Trop Dis 2016;10:e0004338.
67. Bobosha K, Wilson L, van Meijgaarden KE, Bekele Y, Zewdie M, van der Ploegvan Schip JJ, et al. T cell regulation in lepromatous leprosy. PLoS Negl Trop Dis 2014;8:e2773.
68. Parente JN, Talhari C, Schettini AP, Massone C. T regulatory cells (Treg) (TCD4+, CD25+ and FoxP3+) distribution in the different clinical forms of leprosy and reactional states. An Bras Dermatol 2015;90:41–7.
69. Attia EA, Abdallah M, El-Khateeb E, Saad AA, Lotfi RA, Abdallah M, et al. Serum Th17 cytokines in leprosy: Correlation with circulating CD4+, $CD2^{high}$ and FoxP3+ Tregs cells, as well as down-regulatory cytokines. Arch Dermatol Res 2014;306:793–801.
70. Finiasz MR1, Franco MC, de la Barrera S, Rutitzky L, Pizzariello G, del Carmen Sasiain M, et al. IL-9 promotes anti-*Mycobacterium leprae* cytotoxicity: Involvement of IFNgamma.Clin Exp Immunol 2007;147:139–47.
71. de Sousa JR, de Sousa RPM, de Souza Aarão TL, Dias LB Jr, Oliveira Car-neiro FR, Simões Quaresma JA. Response of iNOS and its relationship with IL-22 and STAT3 in macrophage activity in the polar forms of leprosy. Acta Trop 2017;171:74–9.
72. de Lima Silveira E, de Sousa JR, de Sousa Aarão TL, Fuzii HT, Dias Junior LB, Carneiro FR, et al. New immunologic pathways in the pathogenesis of leprosy: Role for Th22 cytokines in the polar forms of the disease. J Am Acad Dermatol 2015;72:729–30.
73. Eyerich K. Eyerich's Th22 cells in allergic disease. Allergo J Int 2015; 24:1–7.
74. Azevedo MCS, Marques H, Binelli LS, Malange MSV, Devides AC, Silva EA, et al. Simultaneous analysis of multiple T helper subsets in leprosy reveals distinct patterns of Th1, Th2, Th17 and Tregs markers expression in clinical forms and reactional events. Med Microbiol Immunol 2017;206:429–39.

4.4 M. LEPRAE AND NERVE INJURY

Kabir Sardana, David Scollard

M. leprae is the only bacterium that infects nerves and Schwann cells (SC) and produces a range of clinical manifestations—from a silent neuropathy to rapidly damaging acute neuritis. Multiple factors can predict nerve damage in both the normal disease process and in reactions and an understanding of this is crucial as leprosy is largely a neural disease. M. leprae interacts specifically with the mature glia of the human peripheral nervous system (PNS), i.e. Schwann cells, and *not* the glia of the CNS (oligodendrocytes or astrocytes), and thus the clinical presentation mainly involves the peripheral nerves.[1,2]

The effect of the bacilli can be broadly divided into a *direct* effect and *an indirect* effect which is largely mediated by the immune response. While the direct mechanism of nerve damage in leprosy is attributed to the ability of M. leprae to bind and infect SC and is predominantly found in multibacillary (MB) forms, the indirect mechanism of nerve involvement is commonly observed in paucibacillary (PB) forms, where the immune response of the host plays the predominant role.[3,4]

The route of entry is believed to be via the respiratory mucosa *(see Chapter 4, Section 4.2)* and from there the bacilli may cross the basement membrane and the underlying connective tissue in order to reach the blood vessels.[5] M. leprae can then spread hematogenously and reach skin and peripheral nerve trunks in an asymmetrical fashion.

1. DIRECT DAMAGE

Scollard et al[6] described the invasion of nerves by M. leprae occurs via the colonization of the endothelial cells of the blood and lymphatic vessels in the epineurium. This vascular and lymphatic colonization increases the risk of nerve ischemia and facilitates the invasion of M. leprae into macrophages residing in the epineural layer.[7] This vascular route of invasion enables M. leprae to cross the impermeable perineural sheath and reach the endoneurium, thus leading to the invasion and proliferation of mycobacteria within SCs, which form the primary target of M. leprae in peripheral nerves (Fig. 4.4). SCs provide a safe niche for survival of the bacillus, protected from the host immunity due to blood nerve barrier. Differentiated SCs have a high bacterial retention capacity promoting replication and colonization. The bacillus thus initially inhabits the SC without causing much damage, thus facilitating its own survival. It later takes advantage of the plasticity of SCs (ability to dedifferentiate into an immature phenotype) for furthering bacterial colonization and spread.[8]

The direct action of M. leprae on the SCs can cause nerve damage. The nonmyelinated Schwann cells (SCs) are highly susceptible to M. leprae colonization, whereas myelinated SCs are naturally resistant to the mycobacterial invasion (Fig. 4.5).[8] The clinical translation of this explains the earlier loss of thermal sensation which is mediated by unmyelinated C type fibers.[10] In the endoneurium, M. leprae can bind to SC basement membrane, specifically to its basal lamina[11] (Fig. 4.5). While the basal lamina is composed of various elements, the most important is the laminin 2 isoform, which is formed by assembly of three subunits of laminin chains—the β_1, γ_1, and α_2 chains. Of these components, a specific subcomponent-G domain of the laminin α_2 chain (**α_2LG**) determines the neural affinity of M. leprae (Fig. 4.6).[12] Surface molecules of M. leprae,

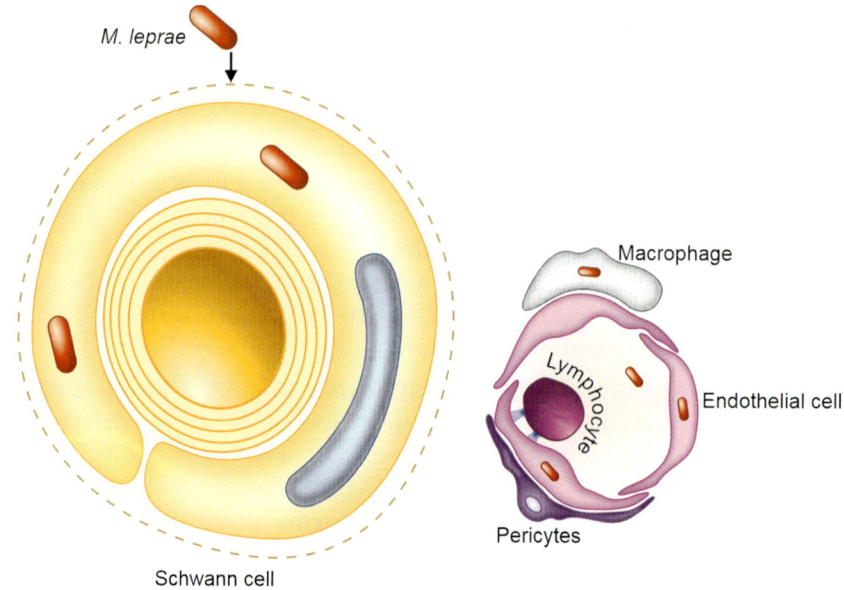

Fig. 4.4: The vascular route of invasion of *M. leprae* into the Schwann cells

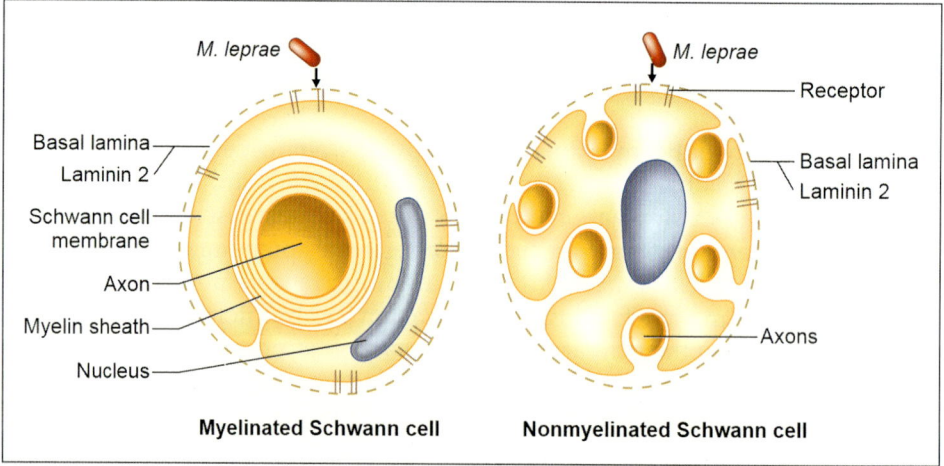

Fig. 4.5: A depiction of interaction of *M. leprae* with myelinated and nonmyelinated Schwann cells

mainly PGL-1 and H1p, bind to basal lamina of SC activating the phosphoinositol 3 kinase signaling leading to reorganization of the actin cytoskeleton of SC and subsequently the internalization of *M. leprae* (Fig. 4.7).[13] Teles et al suggested that CD209 on SCs may also be involved in uptake of bacilli.[14]

Apart from the interaction with the basal lamina, the SC dystrophin-related complex leads to a sequence of steps that culminate in direct damage to the SC (Box 4.1).[15] The initial interaction of *M. leprae* with the basal lamina of SC-axon units appears to deregulate the delicate SC-axon communication system, leading to breakdown of the myelin sheath.[16] Although such early demyelination *in vivo* may not initially lead to clinical manifestation, as peripheral nerves possess a remarkable capacity to regenerate

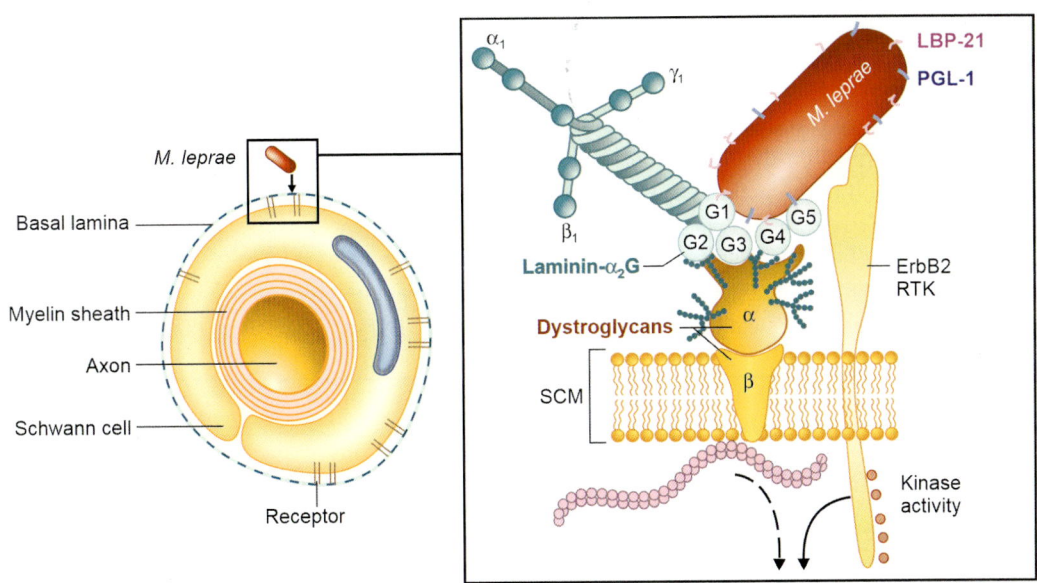

Fig. 4.6: Schwann cell receptors α/β-dystroglycan and receptor tyrosine kinase ErbB2 serve as receptors for *M. leprae* on the Schwann cell membrane (SCM) in an $α_2$LG domain dependent and independent manner (LBP-21: Laminin-binding protein 21; ErbB2 RTK: ErbB2 receptor tyrosine kinase; PGL-1: Phenolic glycolipid 1)

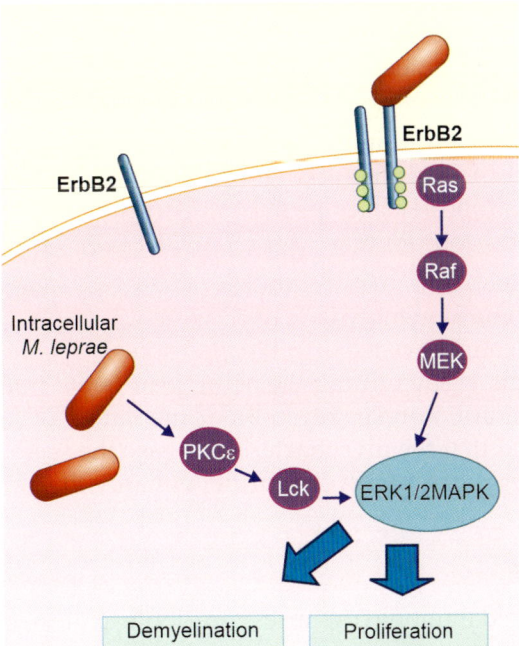

Fig. 4.7: Schematic showing the activation of ERK1/2 MAPK signaling pathways by *M. leprae*. The bacilli bind to ErbB2 receptor which via the Ras-Raf-MEK-ERK pathway induces Schwann cell demyelination and proliferation. Intracellular *M. leprae* induces proliferation of nonmyelinated Schwann cells through a different route to ERK that involves PKCε and Lck (ERK: Extracellular signal-regulated kinase)

Box 4.1: Consequences of *M. leprae* interaction with Schwann cell (Figs 4.6 and 4.7)

- **Neurotropism** of *M. leprae* due to affinity for **laminin α_2** chain
  a. **PGL-1** interacts with α_2**LG** in the basal lamina and **ErbB2** on the Schwann cell membrane
  b. Interaction with α-dystroglycan receptors (DG)
- Reorganization of the actin cytoskeleton in SCs, allowing phagocytosis and internalization of *M. leprae*.
- Activation of phosphoinositol 3 kinase (PI3K) signaling pathway[23]*
- Activation of ERK1/2 mitogen activated protein kinase signaling*
- Increase expression of metalloproteinases (MMP2, MMP9), TNF-α*—activation of Notch signaling pathway[24]

*Can cause nerve fiber atrophy and irreversible damage (PGL-1: Phenolic glycolipid 1; α_2LG: Laminin α_2 chain)

following injury, it may lead to activation of additional signaling from SCs similar to nerve injury.[8] Functional consequences like demyelination provide a survival advantage for *M. leprae*, as it induces dedifferentiation and proliferation and generates myelin-free SCs which are also highly susceptible to *M. leprae* invasion.[17] Also, the de-differentiated SCs more effectively transfer *M. leprae* to macrophages and neural fibroblasts aiding in bacterial dissemination.[18] Thus, *M. leprae* is capable of reprogramming adult SC by downregulation of lineage/differentiation-associated genes and the upregulation of genes related to mesoderm development, rendering these cells highly plastic, migratory and with properties of bacterial transfer.[19, 20] Notably immune cells are not involved in the early stage of this infection. An alternate view is that the early demyelination is initiated by infected macrophages that patrol axons rather than by *M. leprae* itself.[21]

M. leprae has been shown to induce the production of matrix metalloproteinases (MMP-2 and MMP-9) in SCs, irrespective of the inflammatory process, in synergy with TNF.[22] The metalloproteinases promote demyelination and breakdown of the blood-nerve barrier and contribute to fibrous replacement of nerve tissue.[22]

Nerve fibrosis, which is the reason for chronic nerve damage in leprosy, has also been shown to be a consequence of TGF-β, which is known to reprogramme SC phenotype as well as connective tissue cell expansion. This is consequent to the effect of the bacilli, which via α-smooth muscle actin, lead to SC trans-differentiation into myofibroblasts, which are, in turn, key cellular mediators of fibrosis. In addition, it has been demonstrated that the mycobacteria increase the secretion of type I collagen and fibronectin by these cells, which can further enhance the nerve fibrogenic process in vivo.[25]

2. INDIRECT DAMAGE

Both innate and acquired immune responses contribute to the nerve damage of leprosy. *M. leprae* antigens can induce SC apoptosis by pathways involving TLR2 and TNF.[26, 27] There is also some evidence of a role of the complement pathway in inducing nerve damage. Deposits of the membrane attack complex (MAC) or the soluble terminal complement complex (TCC) has been demonstrated in association with damaged nerves in leprosy patients.[28] *M. leprae* component lipoarabinomannan (LAM) is likely the key pathogen associated molecule that activates the complement.[28]

Intraneural macrophages, especially, are capable of secreting a wide array of damaging cytokines and chemokines. These prominently include TNF, which has been discussed above. The major toxic effector molecule known to kill *M. leprae* is nitric oxide (NO), produced by activated macrophages expressing the inducible NO synthase (iNOS). Nitrotyrosine, an end product of the metabolism of NO known to cause lipid peroxidation of myelin, has been observed in nerves in BL lesions suggesting its role in leprosy associated nerve damage as well.[29] CCL-2 is an essential chemokine for recruitment of macrophages to nerves and has been shown to have high immunoreactivity in infected nerves.[30]

Human SCs express MHC class I and II molecules in addition to ICAM and CD80 after infection with *M. leprae* and thus bring in the MHC class II-restricted CD4+ T cells into play at the site of infection causing further damage to the SCs.[31] CXCL10 also has an important role in the activation of Th1 response by recruitment of T cells, and can be a biological marker for imminent leprosy reversal reactional episodes.[32] The immune response without a reactional state is described in tuberculoid leprosy where there is an increased expression of a cellular immune response mediated by CD4+ T cells with Th1 and Th17 effector phenotypes; and CD8+ T cells with a Tc1 cytotoxic phenotype.[3] In leprosy reactions, the type 1 reactions (T1Rs) are related to an increase in cell-mediated immune activity due to an increased expression of CD4+ T cells and the Th1 and Th17 phenotypes against antigens of *M. leprae*, inducing inflammation in skin and peripheral nerves.[33,34] On the other hand, type 2 reactions (T2Rs) are systemic inflammatory responses that induce the deposition of immune complexes in peripheral nerves thus inducing migration of inflammatory cells and nerve damage which have been shown to be complement mediated.

Apart from these, other novel pathways have been described, including affliction of neurofilaments (NF), neurotrophins and Ninjurin polymorphism, but these are yet to validated comprehensively.[35-37]

CONCLUSION

While the interaction of *M. leprae* and the nerve is more complex than depicted, it is important to understand that neural damage forms the primary cause of most of the deformities and reactional consequences in leprosy. While research has been directed at killing the bacilli and suppressing the host response, we still do not have a drug that can effectively inhibit the bacilli-SC interaction. Though ErbB2 inhibitors such as herceptin, PKI166, and U0126 block activation of this pathway in response to *M. leprae*, they are still not tested *in vivo*. Also, the exact stage where immunologically preserved SCs becomes a target of immune damage is uncertain and which explains the paradox of adequate treatment by MDT and the lack of translatable clinical outcome of consistently preserved neural function.

REFERENCES

1. Rambukkana A. Molecular basis for the peripheral nerve predilection of *Mycobacterium leprae*. Curr Opin Microbiol 2001;4:21–27.
2. Ooi WW, Srinivasan J. Leprosy and the peripheral nervous system: Basic and clinical aspects. Muscle Nerve 2004;30:393–409.

3. Fonseca AB, Simon MD, Cazzaniga RA, de Moura TR, de Almeida RP, Duthie MS, et al. The influence of innate and adaptative immune responses on the differential clinical outcomes of leprosy. Infect Dis Poverty 2017;6:5.
4. Khanolkar-Young S, Young DB, Colston MJ, Stanley JN, Lockwood DN. Nerve and skin damage in leprosy is associated with increased intralesional heat shock protein. Clin Exp Immunol 1994;96:208–13.
5. Silva CAM, Danelishvili L, McNamara M, Berredo-Pinho M, Bildfell R, Biet F, et al. Interaction of *Mycobacterium leprae* with Human Airway Epithelial Cells: Adherence, Entry, Survival, and Identification of Potential Adhesins by Surface Proteome Analysis. Infect Immun. 2013; 81:2645–59.
6. Scollard DM, McCormick G, Allen JL. Localization of *Mycobacterium leprae* to endothelial cells of epineurial and perineurial blood vessels and lymphatics. Am J Pathol 1999;154:1611–20.
7. Scollard DM. The biology of nerve injury in leprosy. Lepr Rev 2008;79:242–5.
8. Rambukkana A. Usage of signaling in neurodegeneration and regeneration of peripheral nerves by leprosy bacteria. Prog Neurobiol 2010;91:102–7.
9. Rambukkana A, Zanazzi G, Tapinos N, Salzer JL. Contact-dependent demyelination by *Mycobacterium leprae* in the absence of immune cells. Science 2002;296(5569):927–31.
10. Scollard DM, Truman RW, Ebenezer GJ. Mechanisms of nerve injury in leprosy. Clin Dermatol 2015;33:46–54.
11. Chacha JJ, Sotto MN, Peters L, Lourenço S, Rivitti EA, Melnikov P. [Peripheral nervous system and grounds for the neural insult in leprosy]. An Bras Dermatol. 2009;84:495–500.
12. Rambukkana A, Salzer JL, Yurchenco PD, Tuomanen EI. Neural targeting of *Mycobacterium leprae* mediated by the G domain of the laminin-α_2 chain. Cell 1997;88:811–21.
13. Alves L, de Mendonça Lima L, da Silva Maeda E, Carvalho L, Holy J, Sarno EN, et al. *Mycobacterium leprae* infection of human Schwann cells depends on selective host kinases and pathogen-modulated endocytic pathways. FEMS Microbiol Lett. 2004;238:429–37.
14. Teles RM, Krutzik SR, Ochoa MT, Oliveira RB, Sarno EN, Modlin RL. Interleukin-4 regulates the expression of CD209 and subsequent uptake of *Mycobacterium leprae* by Schwann cells in human leprosy. Infect Immun 2010;78:4634–43.
15. Sherman DL, Fabrizi C, Gillespie CS, Brophy PJ. Specific disruption of a Schwann cell dystrophin-related protein complex in a demyelinating neuropathy. Neuron 2001;30:677–87.
16. Rambukkana A. 2004. *Mycobacterium leprae*-induced demyelination: A model for early nerve degeneration. CurrOpin Immunol 16:511–8.
17. Hess S, Rambukkana A. Bacterial-induced cell reprogramming to stem cell-like cells: New premise in host-pathogen interactions. CurrOpin Microbiol 2015;23:179–88.
18. Masaki T, McGlinchey A, Tomlinson SR, Qu J, Rambukkana A. Reprogramming diminishes retention of *Mycobacterium leprae* in Schwann cells and elevates bacterial transfer property to fibroblasts. F1000Res 2013;2:198.
19. Masaki T, Qu J, Cholewa-Waclaw J, Burr K, Raaum R, Rambukkana A. Re-programming adult Schwann cells to stem cell-like cells by leprosy bacilli promotes dissemination of infection. Cell 2013;152:51–67.
20. Masaki T, McGlinchey A, Cholewa-Waclaw J, et al. Innate immune response precedes *Mycobacterium leprae*-induced reprogramming of adult Schwann cells. Cell Reprogram 2014;16:9–17.
21. Madigan CA, Cambier CJ, Kelly-Scumpia KM, Scumpia PO, Cheng TY, Zailaa J, et al. A Macrophage Response to *Mycobacterium leprae* Phenolic Glycolipid Initiates Nerve Damage in Leprosy. Cell 2017;170:973–85.e10.
22. Oliveira AL, Antunes SL, Teles RM, Costa da Silva AC, Silva TP, BrandãoTeles R, et al. Schwann cells producing matrix metalloproteinases under *Mycobacterium leprae* stimulation may play a role in the outcome of leprous neuropathy. J Neuropathol Exp Neurol 2010;69:27–39.

23. Tapinos N, Ohnishi M, Rambukkana A. ErbB2 receptor tyrosine kinase signaling mediates early demyelination induced by leprosy bacilli. Nat Med 2006;12:961–6.
24. Lindsay J, Jiao X, Sakamaki T, Casimiro MC, Shirley LA, Tran TH, et al. ErbB2 induces Notch1 activity and function in breast cancer cells. Clin Transl Sci 2008;1:107–15.
25. Petito RB, Amadeu TP, Pascarelli BM, Jardim MR, Vital RT, Antunes SL,et al. Transforming growth factor-$β_1$ may be a key mediator of the fibrogenic properties of neural cells in leprosy. J Neuropathol Exp Neurol 2013;72:351–66.
26. Oliveira RB, Ochoa MT, Sieling PA, Rea TH, Rambukkana A, Sarno EN, et al. Expression of Toll-like receptor 2 on human Schwann cells: A mechanism of nerve damage in leprosy. Infect Immun 2003;71:1427–33.
27. Oliveira RB, Sampaio EP, Aarestrup F, Teles RM, Silva TP, Oliveira AL, et al. Cytokines and *Mycobacterium leprae* induce apoptosis in human Schwann cells. J Neuropathol Exp Neurol. 2005;64:882–90.
28. Bahia El Idrissi N, Das PK, Fluiter K, Rosa PS, Vreijling J, Troost D, et al. *M. leprae* components induce nerve damage by complement activation: Identification of lipoarabinomannan as the dominant complement activator. Acta Neuropathol 2015;129:653–67.
29. Schön T, Hernández-Pando R, Baquera-Heredia J, Negesse Y, Becerril-Vil-lanueva LE, Eon-Contreras JC, et al. Nitrotyrosine localization to dermal nerves in borderline leprosy. Br J Dermatol 2004;150:570–4.
30. Medeiros MF, Rodrigues MM, Vital RT, da Costa Nery JA, Sales AM, de Andrea Hacker M, et al. CXCL10, MCP-1, and other immunologic markers involved in neural leprosy. Appl Immunohistochem Mol Morphol 2015;23:220–9.
31. Spierings E, de Boer T, Wieles B, Adams LB, Marani E, Ottenhoff TH. *Mycobacterium leprae*-specific, HLA class II-restricted killing of human Schwann cells by CD4+ Th1 cells: A novel immunopathogenic mechanism of nerve damage in leprosy. J Immunol 2001;166:5883–8.
32. Stefani MM, Guerra JG, Sousa ALM, et al. Potential plasma markers of type 1 and type 2 leprosy reactions: A preliminary report. BMC Infect Dis 2009;9:75.
33. Nery JA da C, Bernardes Filho F, Quintanilha J, Machado AM, Oliveira S de SC, Sales AM. Understanding the type 1 reactional state for early diagnosis and treatment: A way to avoid disability in leprosy. An Bras Dermatol 2013;88:787–92.
34. Pandhi D, Chhabra N. New insights in the pathogenesis of type 1 and type 2 lepra reactions. Indian J Dermatol Venereol Leprol 2013;79:739–49.
35. Save MP, Shetty VP, Shetty KT, Antia NH. Alterations in neurofilament protein(s) in human leprous nerves: Morphology, immunohistochemistry and Western immunoblot correlative study. Neuropathol Appl Neurobiol 2004;30:635–50.
36. Michellin LB, Barreto JA, Marciano LHSC, Lara FA, Nogueira MES, Souza VNB de, et al. Leprosy patients: Neurotrophic factors and axonal markers in skin lesions. Arq Neuropsiquiatr. 2012;70:281–6.
37. Cardoso CC, Martinez AN, Guimarães PEM, Mendes CT, Pacheco AG, de Oliveira RB, et al. Ninjurin 1 asp110ala single nucleotide polymorphism is associated with protection in leprosy nerve damage. J Neuroimmunol 2007;190:13113–8.

4.5 IMMUNOPATHOGENESIS OF REACTIONS

Ananta Khurana, Kabir Sardana

The reactional episodes mark periods of acute intense tissue damage in an otherwise chronic course of the disease. A brief summary of the immunopathogenesis of reactions covering the salient aspects are given below and depicted in Figs 4.8 and 4.9.

TRIGGERS

Factors which trigger the development of reactions are still not completely known. Most reactional episodes occur while the patients are on multi-drug therapy (MDT), although *de novo* presentation with reactions is also common.[1] It is hypothesized that the antigen that becomes available to the immune system by killing of the bacteria during antibiotic treatment gives rise to overactivation of the immune system, which attempts to clear these bacterial antigens, leading to an inflammatory state, especially in those with high bacillary load at initiation of MDT.

Type 2 reaction (T2R) mostly develops in patients with lepromtous leprosy (LL) and a BI of ≥4.[2] Pregnancy, lactation, puberty, intercurrent infection, vaccination, surgery and psychological stress are the proposed risk factors for T2R, but these have not been confirmed in prospective studies. Coinfections are more frequently associated

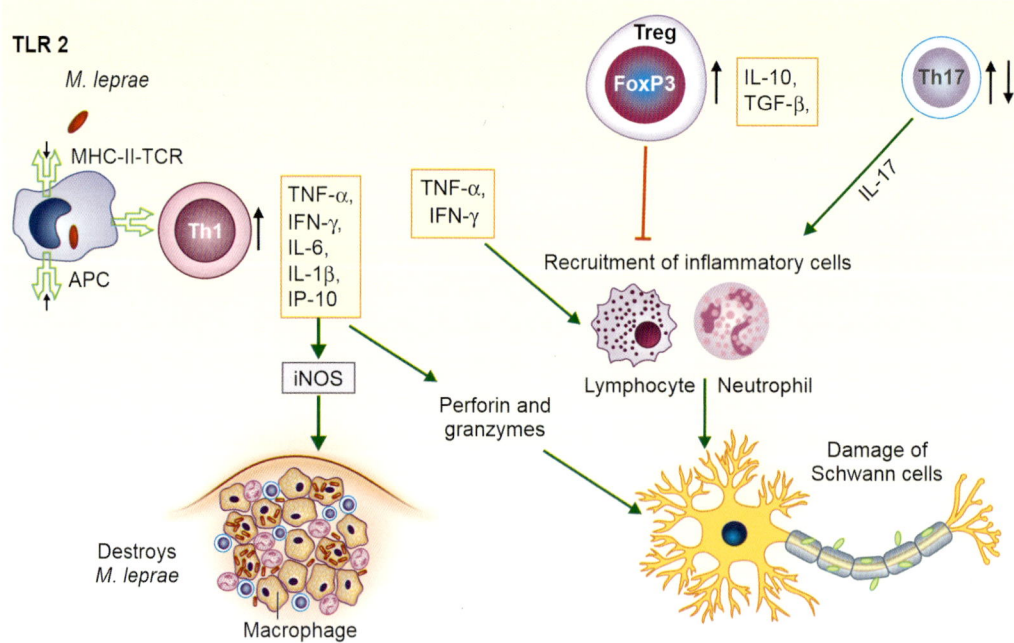

Fig. 4.8: Type 1 reaction occurs in a setting of a prominent Th1–Th17 immunity at baseline, with a shift towards Th1-Treg predominance during the reactional state. The role of Tregs here is to control the excessive immune damage mediated by the proinflammatory cytokines released into the tissues. There is a resultant destruction of bacilli, tissue inflammation and nerve damage (*see* text and Box 4.2 for details)

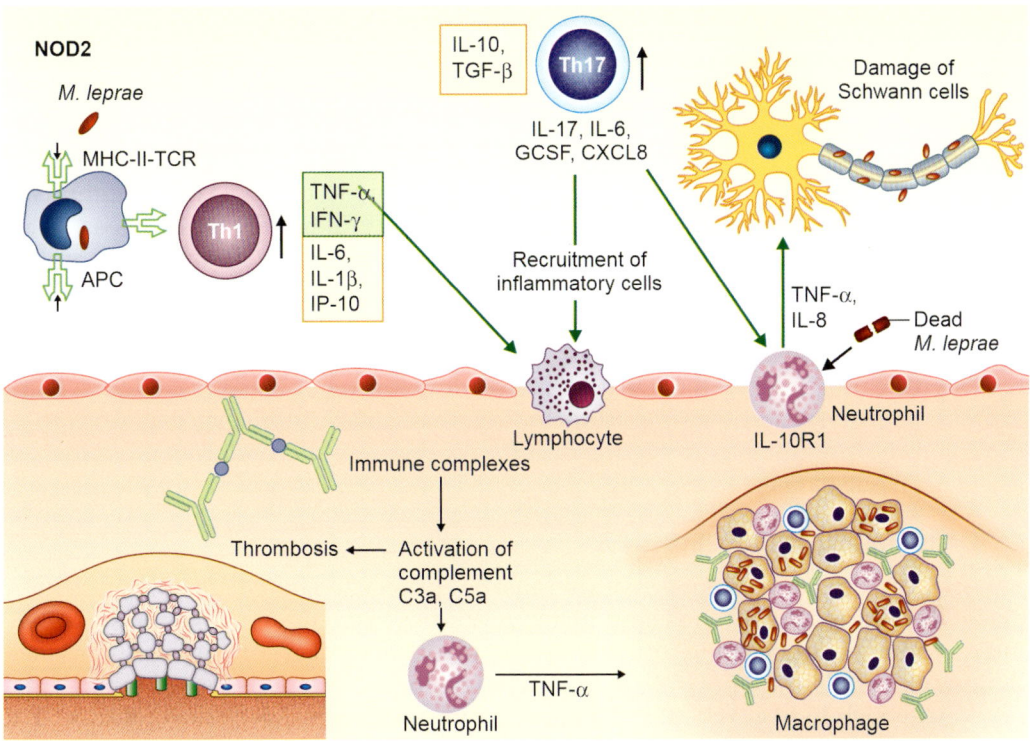

Fig. 4.9: An increased Th1–Th17 action characterizes type 2 reaction. There is prominent neutrophil recruitment and immune complex deposition leading to vascular and neural damage (*see* text and Box 4.3 for details)

with T2Rs than type 1 reactions (T1Rs), with oral coinfections being most frequently reported followed by urinary tract infections, sinusopathy, hepatitis C and hepatitis B.[1] A case series found coinfections to be present in 39.1% of reaction patients while 60.9% were free of them.[3] Chronic oral infections may also be involved in the maintenance of leprosy reactional episodes.[2–4] Leprosy patients with oral infections have higher C-reactive protein (CRP), IP-10, IL-1 and IL-6 levels than the leprosy patients without oral infections, suggesting that oral infections can maintain the proinflammatory state.[3] Another trigger is the immune reconstitution inflammatory syndrome (IRIS) seen in both T1R and T2R within 6 months after initiation of HAART.[5] Machado et al found that leprosy patients with a viral co-infection (HBV, HCV, HIV, HTLV) are at higher risk to develop nerve inflammation and damage, as well as relapse, compared to subjects without viral coinfection.[6] In some countries, helminthic infection has been implicated in triggering T2R.[7] Pneumonia, oropharyngeal infections, syphilis, leishmaniasis, tuberculosis, and staphylococcus infections are less commonly associated.[3]

While there is enthusiasm in certain quarters about the beneficial immunoprophylactic outcomes of vaccination, it is pertinent to emphasize that in a recent trial, of the 0.4% of healthy contacts of patients who received prophylactic BCG and developed leprosy, about 43% had signs of nerve function impairment and/or T1R.[8] Incomplete clearance of bacilli by MDT may become another cause of repeated reactions and this may be amenable to amelioration with modification of the drug regimen used.[9,10]

GENETIC SUSCEPTIBILITY TO LEPROSY REACTIONS

Certain possible genetic associations have been studied and include certain polymorphisms in TLR 1 and 2 genes associated with protection from ENL and higher risk of T1R respectively and polymorphisms in the nucleotide-binding oligomerization domain containing 2 gene (NOD2), associated either with protection from T1R or increased susceptibility to T2R.[11-13] Consistent with the role of TLR, a significant reduction in gene expression and protein levels of TLR2 and TLR4 has been noted during corticosteroid therapy in T1R patients.[14] Six different polymorphisms in IL-6 gene are associated with increased susceptibility to T2R, while 2 protective polymorphisms are described.[15] Polymorphisms in TNF and mannose binding lectin failed to show strong associations in a Nepalese population while VDR FokI-T allele was significantly associated with a risk of developing reversal reaction.[16] Gene expression analysis studies support the notion that transcriptomic biomarkers reflect the collapse of regulation in favour of inflammation, as the underlying etiology of reactional tissue damage as correlates of both ENL and T1R (*also see Chapter 4.1; Table 4.2*).

CYTOKINE MILIEU AND T CELL LINES

Before addressing the cytokine mileu, it must be appreciated that there is heterogeneity in results reported by different studies and in studies from different locations. Further, many studies are done using serum levels as surrogate markers of the levels in tissues. But, serum levels may not corroborate with the actual tissue levels of a particular cytokine, which in turn is better validated by mRNA expression of the molecule. The best evidence favoring the role of a particular cytokine emanates from tissue level measurements using paired samples taken before and during the reactional episode. We have attempted to present the best evidence available regarding each cytokine in the following section (also *see* Boxes 4.2 and 4.3 *for a summary of the immunological profile in T1R and T2R*).

T1Rs is considered to be a **delayed hypersensitivity reaction** with characteristic infiltrations of skin and nerve lesions by CD4+ T cells producing IFN-γ and TNF-α.[17-19]

Box 4.2: Mediators of type 1 reaction

Gene expression (genetic polymorphisms)	*Protection*: NOD2 *Susceptibility*: TLR 2
Cell type	*Background cytokine profile*: Th1/Th17 *During reaction*: ↑Treg
Cytokines	↑ **TNFα, IFN-γ,** IL-1β, IL-2, IL-2R, IL-6, IL-12 p40, IL-17 ↓ **IL-10** (↑ on treatment) ↓ TGF-β
Chemokines	↑ CXCL10/IP-10 (↓ on treatment) ↑ CXCL9[38]
Others	↑ VEGF,[38] iNOS ↓ G-CSF,[38] neopterin[63] ↑ C4[64] ↑ CRP, cortisol

Those in bold are the predominant cytokines.

Box 4.3: Mediators of type 2 reaction

Gene expression (genetic polymorphisms)	*Protection*: TLR 1, some IL-6 *Susceptibility*: NOD2, some IL-6
Cell type	*Background cytokine profile*: Th2/Treg *During reaction*: ↑Th17 cells; ↓ Treg Neutrophil (IL-10R1)
Cytokines	↑ **IFN-γ, TNF-α,** IL-1β, IL-6, IL-8, IL-2R ↑ **IL-17A,** TGF-β, IL-10 ↑ sIL-6R (levels ↓ on treatment)
Acute phase reactants	↑ PTX3[65] ↑ C3, ↑ C4[2,64] ↑ CRP, serum amyloid A protein, α_1 antitrypsin
Others	↑ E selectin,[66] neopterin[67]

Those in bold are the predominant cytokines.

It most commonly occurs in the immunologically unstable borderline forms of leprosy (borderline tuberculoid—BT, borderline borderline—BB and borderline lepromatous—BL).[20] **T2R** affects patients with BB, BL, and LL forms and has been classically believed to be an **immune complex** (IC) mediated disease. However, there is a lack of evidence to support the causative role of ICs in erythema nodosum leprosum (ENL) and it is yet unclear whether ICs are involved in the pathogenesis of ENL or are simply an epiphenomenon.[21, 22] There is also little direct evidence of the actual effector role of **neutrophils** in ENL, despite the cell being the histological hallmark of ENL.[21] It remains unclear whether the neutrophils initiate ENL or are recruited to the site of reaction under the action of chemokines, such as IL-8, secreted by other cell types. Supporting an effector function is the study by Oliviera et al wherein it was demonstrated that neutrophils isolated from leprosy patients (ENL and BL/LL) released TNF-α and IL-8 after stimulation with lipopolysaccharide (LPS) or *M. leprae*.[23] Further, a recent study showed that IL-10R1 expression in neutrophils leads to release of proinflammatory cytokines and dead *M. leprae* were more potent than live *M. leprae* in the regard.[22a] Interestingly, *in vitro* TNF-α production by neutrophils was inhibited by thalidomide at 3 and 6 hours after-stimulation with LPS.[23]

Recent evidence has detailed the role of the various **T helper cell lines** in the pathogenesis of both reactions.[24, 26–29] Most, barring few, authors have reported an increase in **Tregs** during T1R.[24–27] This suggests that Tregs perform the role of controlling the exacerbated cell-mediated immunity seen in T1R with beneficial consequences for the host. On the other hand, majority of published literature till date reports Tregs to be depleted in T2R. The unregulated inflammation thus produced may be the reason behind the extensive clinical manifestations associated with T2R associated with widespread tissue damage. Regarding **Th17**, an increase in T2R is consistently reported, but the expression in T1R has been variably reported to be increased/decreased or unchanged.[24, 26, 27] There is suggestion of a possible plasticity of Treg-Th17 populations in leprosy reactions, with the existing cytokine milieu driving the Th cells towards either Treg or Th17 phenotype.[26]

IFN-γ is the hallmark cytokine for T2R. Repeated intradermal injection of recombinant IFN-γ induced ENL in 60% of BL/LL patients within 6–7 months compared to an incidence of 15% per year in patients who received MDT alone.[30] The cytokine is also an important and essential cytokine mediating T1R and raised levels have been consistently reported from studies involving sera, peripheral blood mononuclear cells (PBMCs) as well as skin biopsies from patients with both T1R and T2R.[31–40] Much higher levels have been reported in T1R skin lesions than T2R lesions, suggesting that while T1R is a hyperimmune response characterized by a selective increase of CD4+ IFN-γ producing cells resulting in the clearing of bacilli and concomitant tissue damage, T2R may be a partial and transient augmentation in cell-mediated immunity, perhaps sufficient to result in antibody and immune complex formation, but insufficient to clear bacilli from lesions.[37]

IL-1β and TNF-α, which mediate both local and systemic effects accompanying many diseases, are produced rapidly by monocytes and macrophages in response to a number of stimuli and are able to induce wide-ranging changes in a variety of cells.[41] Both these proinflammatory cytokines are increased in sera in both T1R and T2R.[41–44] TNF-α has been shown to be upregulated in reactional skin lesions as well.[45] The levels of IL-1β and TNF-α do not correlate with severity of ENL but TNF-α decreases with treatment of reaction with steroids or thalidomide.[41] A high initial IL-1β may indicate a higher susceptibility of reactions after treatment initiation.[46] **IL-6**, another important cytokine released from monocytes and granulocytes, is also raised in both T1R and T2R.[24, 45, 47] The upregulation has been demonstrated in both sera and skin biopsies.

Serum **IL-6 receptor** is also significantly increased in T2R.[48] IL-6 and serum IL-6 receptor have been considered appropriate to be labeled as biomarkers for ENL, with levels declining significantly with treatment.[47,48]

An increase in Th17 related cytokines, mainly **IL-17** has been reported in T2R, which is in agreement with the decrease in Treg populations. In T1R on the other hand, although IL-17 levels are higher than paired nonreactional samples, the magnitude of rise is less than that in T2R.[24, 26, 27] Here it must be noted that some Indian studies have shown IL-17F to be increased in T1R while IL-17A has been linked with ENL in most available literature.[38, 49]

TGF-β is also expressed more in skin lesions of ENL versus nonreactional paired biopsies.[26] The expression in T1R lesions however was less than in paired nonreactional biopsies.[26] Another suppressor cytokine **IL-10** is decreased during T1R but increases with treatment, while the levels in T2R are higher.[39, 50, 51] The **IL-2 receptor** increases in both T1R and T2R.[50,51] And lastly, the chemokine **CXCL10 (IP-10)** is characteristically raised in T1R lesions and serum from patients in T1R and may have a potential role in laboratory diagnosis and monitoring of the condition.[53]

High serum TNF-α levels correlated with disease activity in ENL and decreased significantly during thalidomide treatment.[54] For T1R, IP-10 could function as a correlate of risk as it is substantially increased during this reaction. Moreover, longitudinal studies showed that increased IP-10 levels correlate with T1R onset and it decreases upon successful treatment.[39]

In *summary*, it can be said that **T1R** mostly occurs in patients with a prominent Th1–Th17 immunity at baseline, with a shift towards **Th1-Treg** predominance during the reactional episode, while **T2R** occurs in patients with predominant Th2-Treg immunity, with a shift perhaps towards **Th1–Th17** profile (Figs 4.8 and 4.9).[26]

ACUTE PHASE REACTANTS

Besides cytokines, acute phase proteins belonging to the Pentraxin family such as CRP as well as the stress hormone cortisol can be detected in elevated levels in T1R patients.[55] Another Pentraxin family member, PTX3, also known as TNF-inducible gene 14 protein, is specifically increased in ENL patients and reduced on treatment with thalidomide.[56] This protein binds with high affinity to the complement component C1q, possibly explaining why C1q levels in the circulation are inversely correlated with ENL.

OTHER BIOMARKERS

Studies have shown that there are high levels of polyunsaturated fatty acids and phospholipids in lepromatous patients with high numbers of bacteria.[57] More extended serum metabolic studies on reactional patients showed that numerous metabolic pathways were deranged largely due to lipid metabolism.[58] This coincided with an increase in the abundance of the proinflammatory leukotriene LT B4, prostaglandin D2 and lipoxin A4 but a decrease in proresolving resolvin D1 and prostaglandin E_2. The shifts in levels from proresolving lipid mediators to proinflammatory clearly links metabolic and cellular immune responses that result in Th1-mediated pathology of T1R.

IMPLICATIONS OF CYTOKINES AND BIOMARKERS

It may seem that the different markers may hold promise for diagnosis of reactions. But reactions have a multifactorial etiology which makes it highly unlikely that only one serum marker will suffice to identify onset or predict development of reactions before these have already caused loss of sensation or motor function.[59,60] Thus, probably ratios of proinflammatory cytokines (e.g. IFN-γ, IP-10 or IL-17) versus IL-10 rather than the absolute cytokine levels may provide early indication of impending clinical reactions and help in evaluating treatment.[61] Negera et al observed that TNF-α, IL-6, and IL-7A were more powerful than other cytokines to discriminate ENL from LL; although the discriminating power for these cytokines was found to be less than 80%.[62]

A more relevant implication is the effect of treatment on the cytokine levels; but importantly not all cytokines revert to the normal state equitably after treatment which possibly accounts for the variability of clinical response. The *in vitro* production of IFN-γ, IL-17A, TNF-α, and IL-1β were found to be higher before prednisolone treatment and shows a significant reduction after treatment indicating the possible association of these proinflammatory cytokines and ENL reaction.[62] But while examining the biomarkers and cytokines (Boxes 4.2 and 4.3), it must be appreciated that the effect of various drugs used in reactions have not been rigorously tested in relation to these markers and can explain the differential response to therapy.

REFERENCES

1. Motta AC, Pereira KJ, Tarquínio DC, Vieira MB, Miyake K, Foss NT. Leprosy reactions: Coinfections as a possible risk factor. Clinics (Sao Paulo) 2012;67:1145–1148.
2. Kahawita IP, Lockwood DN. Towards understanding the pathology of erythema nodosum leprosum. Trans R Soc Trop Med Hyg 2008;102:329–37.
3. Motta ACF, Furini RB, Simão JCL, Vieira MB, Ferreira MAN, et al. Could leprosy reactional episodes be exacerbated by oral infections? Rev Soc Bras Med Trop 2011;44:633–35.

4. Pfaltzgraff RE, Ramu G. Clinical leprosy, in: Hastings, RC(Ed), Leprosy. Churchill Livingstone, Edinburgh, 1994; pp. 237–290.
5. Lockwood DN, Lambert SM. Leprosy and HIV, where are we at? Lepr Rev 2010; 81:169–75.
6. Machado PR, Machado LM, Shibuya M, Rego J, Johnson WD, Glesby MJ. Viral Coinfection and Leprosy Outcomes: A Cohort Study. PLoS Negl Trop Dis 2015;9:e0003865.
7. Oktaria S, Effendi EH, Indriatmi W, van Hees CL, Thio HB, Sjamsoe-Daili ES. Soil-transmitted helminth infections and leprosy: A cross-sectional study of the association between two major neglected tropical diseases in Indonesia. BMC Infect Dis 2016;16:258.
8. Richardus RA, Butlin CR, Alam K, Kundu K, Geluk A, Richardus JH. Clinical manifestations of leprosy after BCG vaccination: An observational study in Bangladesh.Vaccine 2015;33: 1562–67.
9. Sinha S, Sardana K, Agrawal D, Malhotra P, Lavania M, Ahuja M. Multi-drug resistance as a cause of steroid-nonresponsive downgrading type I reaction in Hansen's disease. Int J of Mycobacteriology 2019;8:305–8.
10. Arora P, Sardana K, Agarwal A, Lavania M. Resistance as a cause of chronic steroid dependent ENL: A novel paradigm with potential implications in management. Lepr Rev 2019;90:201–5.
11. Schuring RP, Hamann L, Faber WR, Pahan D, Richardus JH, Schumann RR, et al. Polymorphism N248S in the human Toll-like receptor 1 gene is related to leprosy and leprosy reactions. J Infect Dis 2009;199:1816–19.
12. Pierre-Yves Bochud, Thomas R. Hawn, M. Ruby Siddiqui, Paul Saunderson, Sven Britton, et al.Toll-like Receptor 2 (TLR2) Polymorphisms are Associated with Reversal Reaction in Leprosy. J Infect Dis 2008 Jan 15; 197:253–61.
13. Berrington WR, Macdonald M, Khadge S, Sapkota BR, Janer M, Hagge DA, et al. Common polymorphisms in the NOD2 gene region are associated with leprosy and its reactive states. J Infect Dis 2010;201:1422–35.
14. Walker SL, Roberts CH, Atkinson SE, Khadge S, Macdonald M, Neupane KD, et al. The effect of systemic corticosteroid therapy on the expression of toll-like receptor 2 and toll-like receptor 4 in the cutaneous lesions of leprosy type 1 reactions. Br J Dermatol 2012;167:29–35.
15. Sousa AL, Fava VM, Sampaio LH, Martelli CM, Costa MB, Mira MT, et al. Genetic and immunological evidence implicates interleukin-6 as a susceptibility gene for leprosy type 2 reaction. J Infect Dis 2012;205:1417–24.
16. Sapkota BR, Macdonald M, Berrington WR, Misch EA, Ranjit C, Siddiqui MR, et al. Association of TNF, MBL, and VDR polymorphisms with leprosy phenotypes. Hum Immunol 2011;10:992–98.
17. Polycarpou A, Walker SL, Lockwood DN. New findings in the pathogenesis of leprosy and implications for the management of leprosy. Curr Opin Infect Dis 2013;26:413–19.
18. Yamamura M, Uyemura K, Deans RJ, Weinberg K, Rea TH, Bloom BR, et al. Defining protective responses to pathogens: Cytokine profiles in leprosy lesions. Science 1991;254:277–79.
19. Yamamura M, Wang XH, Ohmen JD, Uyemura K, Rea TH, Bloom BR, et al. Cytokine patterns of immunologically mediated tissue damage. J Immunol 1992;149:1470–75.
20. Raffe SF, Thapa M, Khadge S, Tamang K, Hagge D, Lockwood DN. Diagnosis and treatment of leprosy reactions in integrated services—the patients' perspective in Nepal. PLoS Negl Trop Dis 2013;7:e2089.
21. Polycarpou A, Walker SL, Lockwood DN. A Systematic Review of Immunological Studies of Erythema Nodosum Leprosum. Front Immunol. 2017;8:233.
22. Hoiby N, Doring G, Schiotz PO. The role of immune complexes in the pathogenesis of bacterial infections. Annu Rev Microbiol 1986;40:29–53.
22a. Pacheo FS. ENL neutrophil subset expressing IL-10R1 transmigrates into skin lesions and responds to IL-10 Immunoflorizons. 2020;4:47–56.

23. Oliveira RB, Moraes MO, Oliveira EB, Sarno EN, Nery JA, Sampaio EP. Neutrophils isolated from leprosy patients release TNF-α and exhibit accelerated apoptosis *in vitro*. J Leukoc Biol 1999; 65:364–71.

24. Saini C, Siddiqui A, Ramesh V, Nath I. Leprosy Reactions Show Increased Th17 Cell Activity and Reduced FoxP3+ Tregs with Concomitant Decrease in TGF-β and Increase in IL-6. PLoS Negl Trop Dis 2016;10:e0004592.

25. Azevedo MCS, Marques H, Binelli LS, Malange MSV, Devides AC, Silva EA, et al. Simultaneous analysis of multiple T helper subsets in leprosy reveals distinct patterns of Th1, Th2, Th17 and Tregs markers expression in clinical forms and reactional events. Med Microbiol Immunol 2017; 206:429–39.

26. Costa MB, Hungria EM, Freitas AA, Sousa ALOM, Jampietro J, Soares FA, et al. In situ T regulatory cells and Th17 cytokines in paired samples of leprosy type 1 and type 2 reactions. PLoS One 2018;13:e0196853.

27. Vieira AP, Trindade MA, Pagliari C, Avancini J, Sakai-Valente NY, Duarte AJ, et al. Development of type 2, but not type 1, Leprosy Reactions is Associated with a Severe Reduction of Circulating and *in situ* Regulatory T cells. Am J Trop Med Hyg 2016;94:721–27.

28. Attia EA, Abdallah M, Saad AA, Afifi A, El Tabbakh A, El-Shennawy D, et al. Circulating CD4+, CD25+[high] and FoxP3+ T cells vary in different clinical forms of leprosy. Int J Dermatol 2010;49:1152–58.

29. Attia EA, Abdallah M, El-Khateeb E, Saad AA, Lotfi RA, Abdallah M, et al. Serum Th17 cytokines in leprosy: Correlation with circulating CD4+, CD25+[high] and FoxP3+ Tregs cells, as well as downregulatory cytokines. Arch Dermatol Res 2014;306:793–801.

30. Sampaio EP, Moreira AL, Sarno EN, Malta AM, Kaplan G. Prolonged treatment with recombinant interferon gamma induces erythema nodosum leprosum in lepromatous leprosy patients. J Exp Med 1992;175:1729–37.

31. Iyer A, Hatta M, Usman R, Luiten S, Oskam L, Faber W, et al. Serum levels of interferon-gamma, tumour necrosis factor-alpha, soluble interleukin-6R and soluble cell activation markers for monitoring response to treatment of leprosy reactions. Clin Exp Immunol 2007;150:210–16.

32. Madan NK, Agarwal K, Chander R. Serum cytokine profile in leprosy and its correlation with clinicohistopathological profile. Lepr Rev 2011;82:371–82.

33. Moraes MO, Sarno EN, Almeida AS, Saraiva BC, Nery JA, Martins RC, et al. Cytokine mRNA expression in leprosy: A possible role for interferon-gamma and interleukin-12 in reactions (RR and ENL). Scand J Immunol 1999;50:541–49.

34. Nath I, Vemuri N, Reddi AL, Bharadwaj M, Brooks P, Colston MJ, et al. Dysregulation of IL-4 expression in lepromatous leprosy patients with and without erythema nodosum leprosum. Lepr Rev 2000; 71(Suppl):S130–37.

35. Nath I, Vemuri N, Reddi AL, Jain S, Brooks P, Colston MJ, et al. The effect of antigen presenting cells on the cytokine profiles of stable and reactional lepromatous leprosy patients. Immunol Lett 2000;75:69–76.

36. Moraes MO, Sarno EN, Teles RM, Almeida AS, Saraiva BC, Nery JA, et al. Anti-inflammatory drugs block cytokine mRNA accumulation in the skin and improve the clinical condition of reactional leprosy patients. J Invest Dermatol 2000;115:935–41.

37. Cooper CL, Mueller C, Sinchaisri TA, Pirmez C, Chan J, Kaplan G, et al. Analysis of naturally occurring delayed-type hypersensitivity reactions in leprosy by *in situ* hybridization. J Exp Med 1989;169:1565–81.

38. Geluk A, van Meijgaarden KE, Wilson L, Bobosha K, van der Ploegvan Schip JJ, van den Eeden SJ, et al. Longitudinal immune responses and gene expression profiles in type 1 leprosy reactions. J Clin Immunol 2014;34:245–55.

39. Khadge S, Banu S, Bobosha K, van der Ploegvan Schip JJ, Goulart IM, Thapa P, et al. Longitudinal immune profiles in type 1 leprosy reactions in Bangladesh, Brazil, Ethiopia and Nepal. BMC Infect Dis 2015;15:477.
40. Moraes MO, Sarno EN, Teles RM, Almeida AS, Saraiva BC, Nery JA, et al. Anti-inflammatory drugs block cytokine mRNA accumulation in the skin and improve the clinical condition of reactional leprosy patients. J Invest Dermatol 2000;115:935–41.
41. Sarno EN, Grau GE, Vieira LM, Nery JA. Serum levels of tumour necrosis factor-alpha and interleukin-1 beta during leprosy reactional states. Clin Exp Immunol 1991;84:103–8.
42. Moubasher AD, Kamel NA, Zedan H, Raheem DD. Cytokines in leprosy, I. Serum cytokine profile in leprosy. Int J Dermatol 1998;37:733–40.
43. Moraes MO, Sarno EN, Almeida AS, Saraiva BC, Nery JA, Martins RC, et al. Cytokine mRNA expression in leprosy: A possible role for interferon-gamma and interleukin-12 in reactions (RR and ENL). Scand J Immunol 1999;50:541–49.
44. Haslett PA, Roche P, Butlin CR, Macdonald M, Shrestha N, Manandhar R, et al. Effective treatment of erythema nodosum leprosum with thalidomide is associated with immune stimulation. J Infect Dis 2005;192:2045–53.
45. Moraes MO, Sarno EN, Almeida AS, Saraiva BC, Nery JA, Martins RC, et al. Cytokine mRNA expression in leprosy: A possible role for interferon-gamma and interleukin-12 in reactions (RR and ENL). Scand J Immunol 1999;50:541–49.
46. Moubasher AD, Kamel NA, Zedan H, Raheem DD. Cytokines in leprosy, II. Effect of treatment on serum cytokines in leprosy. Int J Dermatol 1998;37:741–46.
47. Sampaio EP, Moraes MO, Nery JA, Santos AR, Matos HC, Sarno EN. Pentoxifylline decreases *in vivo* and *in vitro* tumour necrosis factor-alpha (TNF-alpha) production in lepromatous leprosy patients with erythema nodosum leprosum (ENL). Clin Exp Immunol 1998;111:300–8.
48. Iyer A, Hatta M, Usman R, Luiten S, Oskam L, Faber W, et al. Serum levels of interferon-gamma, tumour necrosis factor-alpha, soluble interleukin-6R and soluble cell activation markers for monitoring response to treatment of leprosy reactions. Clin Exp Immunol 2007;150:210–16.
49. Chaitanya S, Lavania M, Turankar RP, Karri SR,. Sengupta U. Increased serum circulatory levels of interleukin-17F in type 1 reactions of leprosy, J Clin Immunol 2012;32:1415–20.
50. Moubasher AD, Kamel NA, Zedan H, Raheem DD. Cytokines in leprosy, II. Effect of treatment on serum cytokines in leprosy. Int J Dermatol 1998;37:741–46.
51. Moubasher AD, Kamel NA, Zedan H, Raheem DD. Cytokines in leprosy, I. Serum cytokine profile in leprosy. Int J Dermatol 1998;37:733–40.
52. Saini C, Ramesh V, Nath I. CD4+ Th17 cells discriminate clinical types and constitute a third subset of non-Th1, Non-Th2 T cells in human leprosy, PLoS Negl Trop Dis 2013;7: e2338.
53. Scollard DM, Chaduvula MV, Martinez A, Fowlkes N, Nath I, Stryjewska BM, et al. Increased CXC ligand 10 levels and gene expression in type 1 leprosy reactions. Clin Vaccine Immunol. 2011;18:947–53.
54. Sampaio EP, Kaplan G, Miranda A, Nery JA, Miguel CP, Viana SM, Sarno EN. The influence of thalidomide on the clinical and immunologic manifestation of erythema nodosum leprosum. J Infect Dis 1993;18: 408–14.
55. Chaitanya VS, Lavania M, Nigam A, Turankar RP, Singh I, Horo I, et al. Cortisol and proinflammatory cytokine profiles in type 1 (reversal) reactions of leprosy Immunol Lett. 2013;156:159–67.
56. Mendes MA, de Carvalho DS, Amadeu TP, Silva BJA, Prata RBDS, da Silva CO, et al. Elevated Pentraxin 3 Concentrations in Patients with Leprosy: Potential Biomarker of Erythema Nodosum Leprosum. J Infect Dis 2017;216:1635–43.

57. Al-Mubarak R, Vander Heiden J, Broeckling CD, Balagon M, Brennan PJ, Vissa VD. Serum metabolomics reveals higher levels of polyunsaturated fatty acids in lepromatous leprosy: Potential markers for susceptibility and pathogenesis. PLoS Negl Trop Dis 2011;5:e1303.

58. Silva CA, Webb K, Andre BG, Marques MA, Carvalho FM, de Macedo CS, et al. Type 1 Reaction in Patients with Leprosy Corresponds to a Decrease in Proresolving Lipid Mediators and an Increase in Proinflammatory Lipid Mediators. J Infect Dis 2017;215:431–39.

59. van Brakel WH, Nicholls PG, Wilder-Smith EP, Das L, Barkataki P, Lockwood DN, et al. Early diagnosis of neuropathy in leprosy-comparing diagnostic tests in a large prospective study (the IN-FIR cohort study). PLoS Negl Trop Dis 2008;2:e212.

60. Wagenaar I, Brandsma W, Post E, van Brakel W, Lockwood D, Nicholls P, et al. Two randomized controlled clinical trials to study the effectiveness of prednisolone treatment in preventing and restoring clinical nerve function loss in leprosy: The TENLEP study protocols. BMC Neurol 2012;12:159.

61. Corstjens PLAM, van Hooij A, Tjon Kon Fat EM, van den Eeden SJF, Wilson L, Geluk A. Field-Friendly Test for Monitoring Multiple Immune Response Markers during Onset and Treatment of Exacerbated Immunity in Leprosy. Clin Vaccine Immunol 2016;23:515–19.

62. Negera E, Walker SL, Bobosha K, Bekele Y, Endale B, Tarekegn A, et al. The Effects of Prednisolone Treatment on Cytokine Expression in Patients with Erythema Nodosum Leprosum Reactions.Front Immunol 2018;9:189.

63. Hamerlinck FF, Klatser PR, Walsh DS, Bos JD, Walsh GP, Faber WR. Serum neopterin as a marker for reactional states in leprosy. FEMS Immunol Med Microbiol 1999;24:405–9.

64. Amorim FM, Nobre ML, Nascimento LS, Miranda AM, Monteiro GRG, Freire-Neto FP, et al. Differential immunoglobulin and complement levels in leprosy prior to development of reversal reaction and erythema nodosum leprosum. PLoS Negl Trop Dis 2019;13:e0007089.

65. Mendes MA, de Carvalho DS, Amadeu TP, Silva BJ, de A, Prata RB, et al. Elevated Pentraxin 3 concentrations in patients with leprosy: Potential biomarker of erythema nodosum leprosum. J Infect Dis 2017; 216:1635–43.

66. Lee DJ, Li H, Ochoa MT, Tanaka M, Carbone RJ, Damoiseaux R, et al. Integrated pathways for neutrophil recruitment and inflammation in leprosy. J Infect Dis 2010;201:558–69.

67. Villahermosa LG, Fajardo TT Jr, Abalos RM, Balagon MV, Tan EV, Cellona RV, et al. A randomized, double-blind, double-dummy, controlled dose comparison of thalidomide for treatment of erythema nodosum leprosum. Am J Trop Med Hyg 2005;72:518–26.

CHAPTER 5

Reactions in Leprosy

5.1 OVERVIEW AND TYPE 1 REACTIONS

Kabir Sardana, Surabhi Sinha, Premanshu Bhushan

OVERVIEW

Reactions are acute inflammatory episodes superimposed on the relatively uneventful usual course of leprosy. They are generally acute hypersensitivity reactions to bacillary antigens and while immune mediators have been investigated and a genomic predisposition has been suggested, the exact reason for the variable immune response is yet to be determined.[1,2] Type 1 reactions (T1Rs) mainly occur in the borderline spectrum (although a few with polar forms may also experience T1R); and about 30% individuals with borderline disease experience a T1R at some point during their disease course.[3,4] T1R may be upgrading (reversal) or downgrading. In the lepromatous group (LLs/BL), there may occur erythema nodosum leprosum (ENL) or type 2 reactions (T2Rs), Lucio phenomenon and acute exacerbation of the existing disease.[5]

TYPE 1 LEPROSY REACTION

T1R may be the presenting feature of the disease, may occur during the course of treatment or even after treatment has been completed. The reactions are frequently recurrent leading to further nerve damage.[6] T1R is a delayed hypersensitivity reaction which is an example of Coombs and Gell type IV hypersensitivity reaction, although its immunology has now been researched in much more detail (*see Chapter 4, Section 4.5*). Antigens from degenerating leprosy bacilli interact with T lymphocytes and this is associated with a rapid change in cell-mediated immunity (CMI).

T1Rs are typically seen in borderline patients because of their immunological instability, and if the reaction is associated with a rapid increase in specific CMI, as it is in patients under treatment, we speak of *upgrading* or reversal reaction (RR). This is because the natural tendency for borderline leprosy to downgrade slowly towards the lepromatous pole, in the absence of treatment, is reversed. On the other hand, if the reaction is associated with a reduction in immunity, we speak of *downgrading reaction*. During the normal course of leprosy, downgrading is more frequent than upgrading, but it is commonly *silent*, without reaction. However, the number of downgrading reactions is not insignificant. Such reactions do not attain the maximum severity, but they may be sufficiently severe to cause clinical confusion as to the nature of the event.[7,8]

Occasionally though there may not be any detectable change at all in immune status following the reactive phase (static T1R).[7,8]

Here it must be emphasized that the recent trend of discarding downgrading reaction and labelling all TIRs as RR is *not* representative of the actual situation and should be discouraged. Downgrading reaction is a distinct reaction that occurs without treatment.[8] Significantly, downgrading reactions can occasionally be associated with resistance making it a diagnosis with important implications.[9] Also, the required steroid dose and duration in downgrading reactions is either less than RR or steroids may not be required at all in cases of downgrading TIR.[8] This is because suppressing a heightened immune response (upgrading T1R) is more difficult than suppressing a downgrading reaction. Undoubtedly upgrading reactions are better documented than downgrading ones; one reason for this could be that patients under treatment are more likely to have their progress observed. The various shifts across the leprosy spectrum in an upgrading T1R are, LLs → BL → BB → BT → TTs. LLp and TTp, the polar forms are immunologically stable. The reverse holds good in downgrading reactions: BT → BB → BL → LLs. Herein, it is pertinent to note that T1R encompasses affliction of both the skin and nerve; although the involvement of the latter may be overt or silent.[10,11]

Prevalence

The epidemiology of T1R has been reviewed and, overall, the cumulative prevalence varies from 8 to 33% for all leprosy patients. In BT and BB patients, the most likely time for upgrading reaction to occur is between 2 weeks to 6 months of treatment, but longer intervals have been recorded in BL.[8] About 50% of BL patients will get T1R, usually between 2 and 12 months after starting chemotherapy, but sometimes later if they had previously downgraded almost to lepromatous.[12] Reactions may occur even without treatment in BT patients and are often the inciting factor for presenting to the clinic.[7,8] Untreated BT patients may suffer episodes of TIR in association with downgrading, presumably because the immunological balance is responding to an increasing antigenic stimulus. In this case, the reactions cease as the patient reaches BL but is likely to recur during chemotherapy. Upgrading reaction may also occur in subpolar LL (LLs) under treatment; these patients rapidly regain lost immunity and new skin lesions have the features of BL. Borderline patients may upgrade to the tuberculoid type (TT) but form a subgroup—secondary tuberculoid or TTs—which, in contrast to its counterpart at the other end of the spectrum (subpolar LL or LLs) appears to be immunologically stable.[13] T1R can be seen even after treatment and recurrence is common, with up to a third of T1R patients having recurrences.[14]

Factors that upset the immunological balance and precipitate reactions include pregnancy, intercurrent infections especially tuberculosis, vaccinations, psychological stress, HIV (immune reconstitution inflammatory syndrome) and immunosuppressive therapy.[10] Recently resistance has been described as a trigger.[9]

Etiopathogenesis and Risk Factors (*also see Chapter 4, Section 4.5*)

While it is still not completely known which antigens or antigenic determinants are responsible for a T1R, it is accepted that the reactions appear to arise as a result of an absolute increase in the level of delayed type hypersensitivity (DTH) in the early stages of clinical disease, or a relative increase in the level of hypersensitivity in relation to the bacterial load as a result of a decline in the latter following treatment. Thus, T1Rs may occur in patients even with a *low* bacterial burden and occur frequently before therapy, without necessitating the rapid bacterial death associated with effective antimicrobial therapy. In the series by Lockwood *et al* (1992), reactional symptoms developed in 45.4% patients before they sought treatment for leprosy, in 38.6% while they were on treatment, and in 9% after completion of treatment.[15]

A disequilibrium between local and general levels of antigen in hypersensitive patients may determine the onset of reaction (as in nerves), the disequilibrium being consequential to either local bacterial multiplication or, perhaps more commonly, by the exposure of antigen in previously protected sites. The sudden unmasking of a pocket of bacterial antigen in a nerve trunk or a dermal bundle in a patient with at least some residual DTH may elicit a local DTH response; as a result of this response, the general level of DTH of the patient will be modified, depending on the quantum of antigen in the system. The increased sensitization or desensitization that follows will determine the response to the next exposure of antigen.[7a] In untreated active infections, normally a progressive fall in DTH occurs in parallel with the increase in the bacterial load so that no delayed hypersensitivity reaction is precipitated. But a delay in this "desensitization" process would lead to a temporary imbalance between hypersensitivity and bacterial load leading to a downgrading T1R. On the other hand, upgrading T1R can be explained on the basis of "sensitization" of the DTH where, on treatment, the antigens reduce and the DTH relatively increases to the point where pre-existing antigen becomes "noticed" and a reaction is mounted.[7b]

Another premise is that in both upgrading and downgrading reactions, the same antigenic components may be involved.[8] Thus, possibly an enhanced cell-mediated immunity (CMI) stimulated by bacterial or human host antigenic determinants competes with a suppressive effect induced by others.[8] In fact, a transcriptional study showed that both T1R and ENL may have disordered recognition responses to *M. leprae* antigen with increased production of antibodies or heightened responsiveness to antibodies, mediated by complement and other components of innate immunity.[16] A hypothesis of "antigenic heterogeneity" between skin predominant and nerve predominant T1R has also been suggested.[17] Another study has further opined that it is the quality of "viable bacilli" that plays a role in the precipitation of T1R.[18] The orchestration of the cytokines and other mediators which result from these immunologic events, is likely to be responsible for the final effect, upgrading or downgrading.

Though there is a wealth of data on cytokines, the levels assessed are not consistently in the tissue and blood levels may not be truly representative of the cytokine milieu.[9] *(also see Chapter 4, Section 4.5)*. The relevance is that treatment of the reaction may cause clinical improvement but changes in the inflammatory cytokines *lag* behind the clinical improvement and in some cases may remain unchanged.[19]

While multiple risk factors have been described in T1R (Box 5.1),[21–30] the ultimate focus is on the incidence rates of nerve function impairment (NFI), and silent NFI which is considerably higher amongst MB patients compared with PB patients.[20]

It is pertinent to note that some studies have shown that humoral immunity may also play a role in T1R, which is mainly believed to be a disorder with increased CMI, reiterating the fact that there exists a "downgrading" reaction wherein the decrease in the CMI can elicit a humoral response.[31]

Box 5.1: Risk factors for type 1 reaction[21-30]

- During MDT and the subsequent 6 months
- Positive BI (MB cases)
- Extensive disease, indicated by the number of body areas involved
- Borderline classification
- Nerve function impairment/WHO disability grades 1 and 2 present at diagnosis
- Having a facial patch (as a risk factor for lagophthalmos) (Fig. 5.6a)
- Pregnancy
- Bactericidal drug regimens
- Enlarged ulnar nerve at diagnosis
- Attending as a self-reporting case
- Presence of anti-PGL-I antibodies and a positive lepromin test
- BCG vaccination

Nerve function is impaired by the local ischemia secondary to the compression of perineural blood vessels by the inflammatory edema and by direct destruction of Schwann cells and axons by the CD4+ T cell-mediated granulomatous process.[8,32] (Box 5.2; *also see Chapter 4, Section 4.5*) (Fig. 5.1). Though edema regularly accompanies cutaneous leprosy lesions, and it has been invoked as a potential mechanism of injury to peripheral nerves, no formal measurements of endoneurial pressure have been done in leprosy to document increased pressure or edema, although surgeons who operate on patients with acute lepromatous neuritis describe the procedures as "decompression".[33] The inevitable post-inflammatory fibrosis ultimately leads to irreversible nerve damage.

Here it must be noted that the histological sequence suggests that the ultimate outcome, up- or downgrading, may only be determined when the reaction has passed its peak, and a new immunological equilibrium has been struck.[34] This might be a reason why the spectral change is not identified in clinical practice, possibly as the biopsy is done only during the reactional phase. Histological studies have shown that while upgrading is commoner than downgrading, in some, "static" findings are seen.[35] It has been noted that even experienced pathologists may underdiagnose reaction in skin sections from patients with clinically apparent reactions.[36] Important diagnostic features appear to be edema within the epithelioid cell granuloma, dermal edema, the presence of plasma cells and granuloma fraction (*see Chapter 3, Section 3.2*).

Box 5.2: Cutaneous and neural damage in type 1 reaction

Tissue	Mechanism of damage
Skin	• Granuloma damaging the skin stucture
	• Reactional edema
Nerve trunks	• Immunological and mechanical factors ↓
	1. Edema → perineurium (rigid layer) → axonal compression → interruption of intra-axonal flow
	2. Edema → perineurium (rigid layer) → pressure on venules → engorgement of capillaries by back pressure → venostatic edema
	3. Diffuse subacute and chronic segmental demyelination

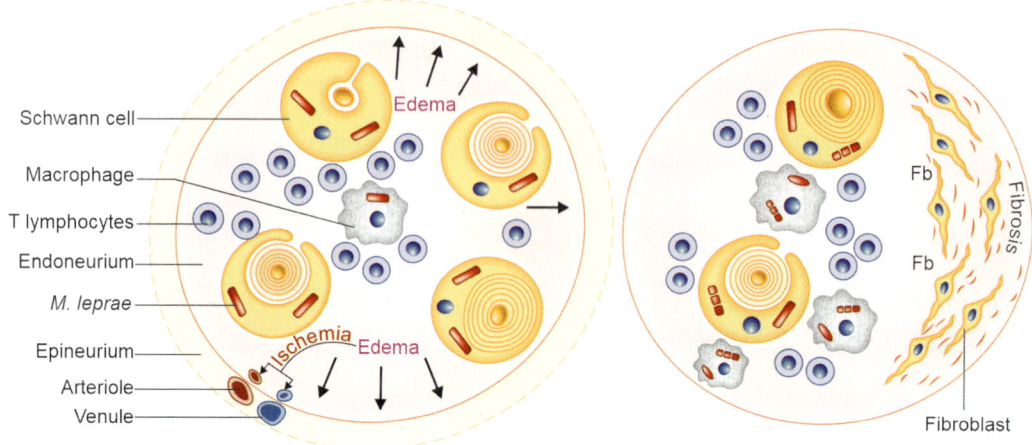

Fig. 5.1: Mechanisms of nerve damage due to local edema and granuloma in type 1 reaction and consequential fibrosis

Clinical Features

Clinically, the most prominent sign is a rapidly developing change in the appearance of some or all the skin lesions; which become erythematous, edematous, more prominent, shiny, warm to touch, and may resemble erysipelas (Fig. 5.2a). Sometimes, necrosis supervenes with breakdown and ulceration and the term "Lazarine leprosy" has been, possibly *incorrectly*, ascribed to this in the past. As the reaction starts to subside, the skin becomes dry and scaly and ultimately flattens leaving a wrinkled hypopigmented surface (Fig. 5.2b and c). Appearance of new lesions may also be seen—more commonly in downgrading reactions. Usually the new lesions resemble the pre-existing ones, but sometimes they are very numerous and small and clinically confusing (Figs 5.3 to 5.5). In the previous edition of this book it was highlighted that

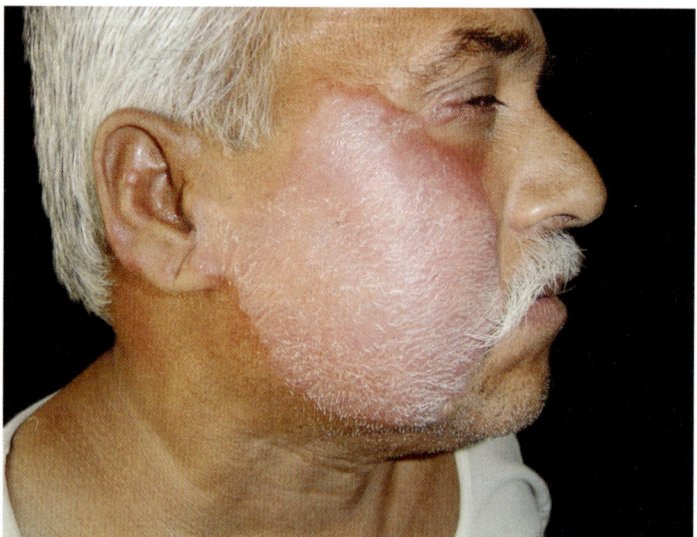

Fig. 5.2a: BT Hansen with type 1 reaction; showing marked edema in a facial plaque

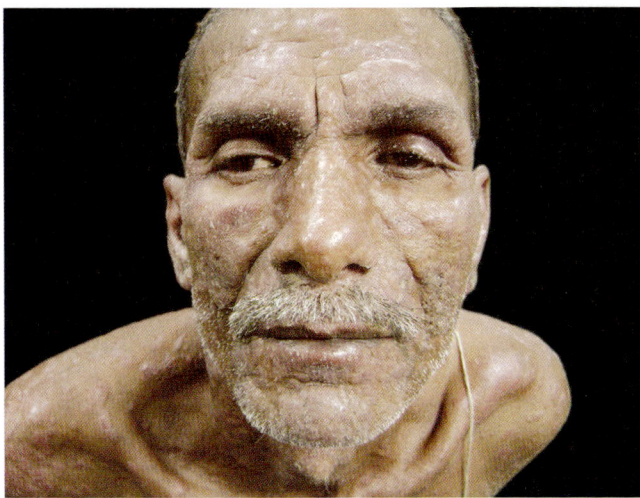

Fig. 5.2b: BL Hansen with subsiding type 1 upgrading reaction showing scaly erythematous edematous plaques. The patient also had neuritis of the left ulnar nerve

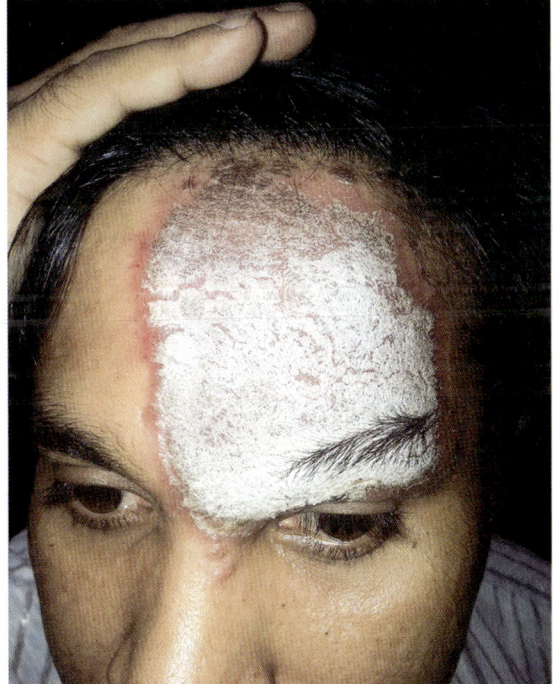

Fig. 5.2c: "Psoriasiform" type 1 reaction with intense scaling over an edematous plaque

sometimes even upgrading reaction may present with new lesions. Downgrading reactions may lead to atypical clinical presentations as well, since skin lesions suggestive of different portions of the classification spectrum may be present simultaneously in the same patient. If the reaction is accompanying an episode of downgrading, the new lesions are more lepromatous in appearance.[37] Table 5.1 elucidates the salient differences between the two types of T1R.[38,39]

Table 5.1: Type 1 upgrading and downgrading reaction		
	Upgrading (reversal) reaction	*Downgrading reaction*
Onset	Reversal reaction usually occurs during the first 6 months of therapy in BT and BB patients, but longer intervals have been observed in BL patients	It is seen either in patients on *no* treatment or who have *interrupted* treatment
Cause	Alteration in CMI (↑)	Alteration in CMI (↓)
Features	• Some or all of the existing leprosy lesions show signs of acute inflammation (pain, tenderness, erythema and edema) • Necrosis and ulceration occur in severe cases • Lesions desquamate as they subside • New lesions *might* appear occasionally	Lesions worsen and the morphology of the existing lesions and new lesions becomes more lepromatous New lesions appear more frequently
Nerve	Neuritis is often *marked*	Neuritis is *less* marked
Histology	In reversal reaction, there is edema, reduced bacilli and increased defensive cells such as lymphocytes, epithelioid cells and giant cells	There is increase in bacilli and defensive cells are replaced by macrophages
Treatment	Steroids are needed in most patients	Usually just continuing the MDT suffices; if steroids needed, response occurs with *lower* doses than upgrading reaction

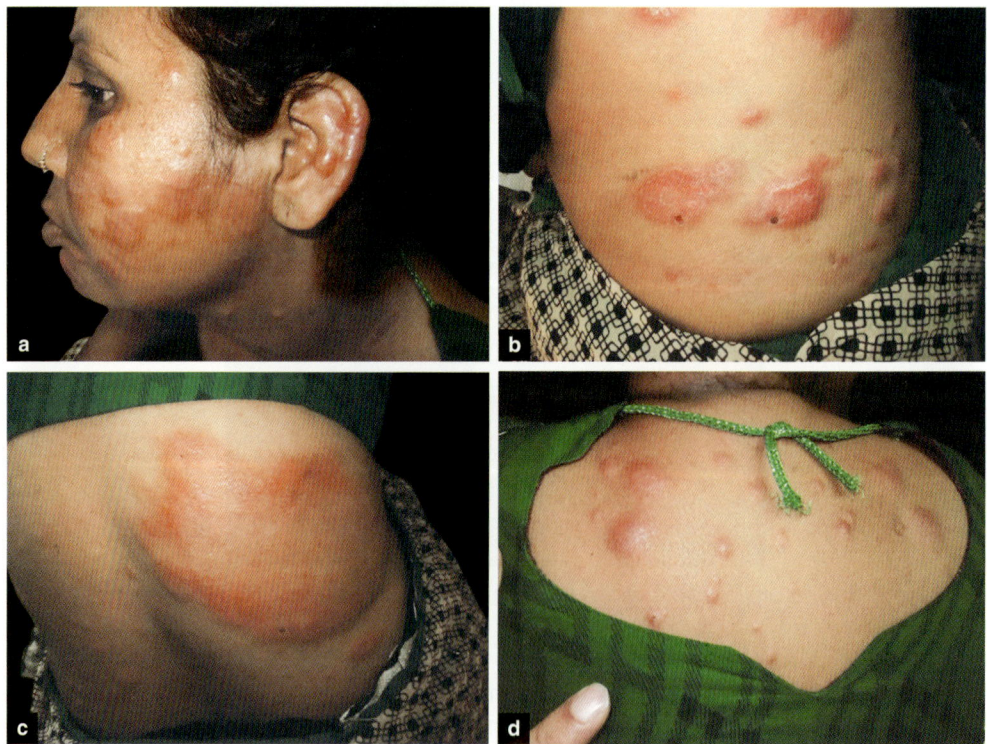

Fig. 5.3a to d: This patient presented with sudden erythema and edema of a pre-existing large plaque alongwith eruption of multiple smaller papules and nodules, with no neuritis. The new lesions were lepromatous in appearance. She was diagnosed as BT downgrading to BL with T1R

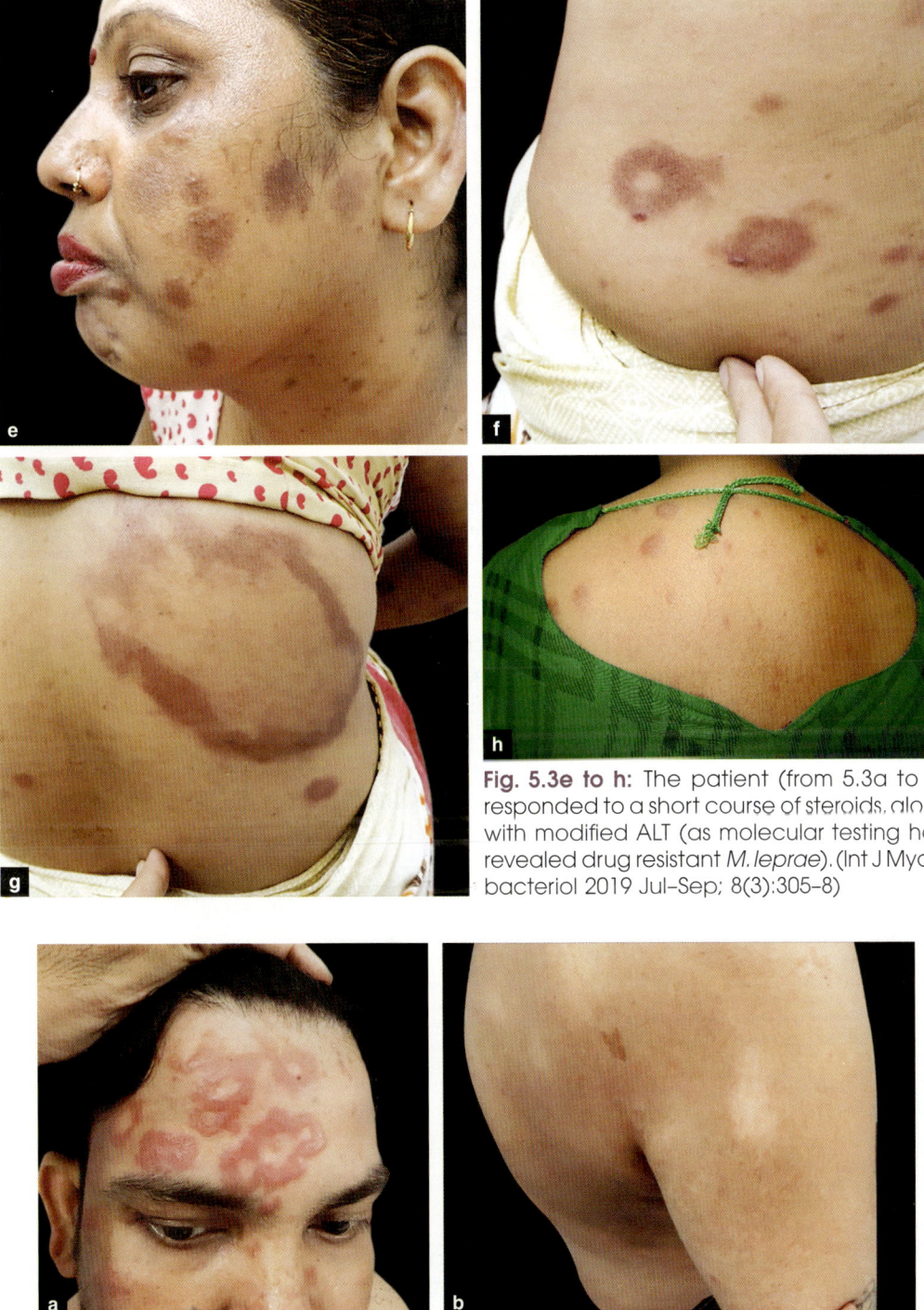

Fig. 5.3e to h: The patient (from 5.3a to d) responded to a short course of steroids, along with modified ALT (as molecular testing had revealed drug resistant *M. leprae*). (Int J Mycobacteriol 2019 Jul–Sep; 8(3):305–8)

Fig. 5.4a and b: This patient presented with edema and mildly tender annular lesions on the face with macules and papules on the back. There was no neuritis or nerve function impairment. He was diagnosed as a case of BT downgrading to BL (type 1 downgrading reaction) and responded adequately to low dose steroids (20 mg prednisolone)

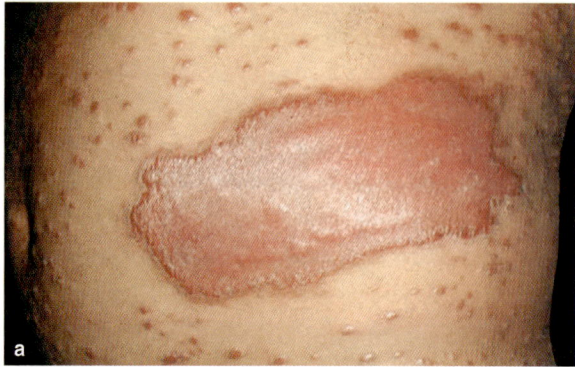
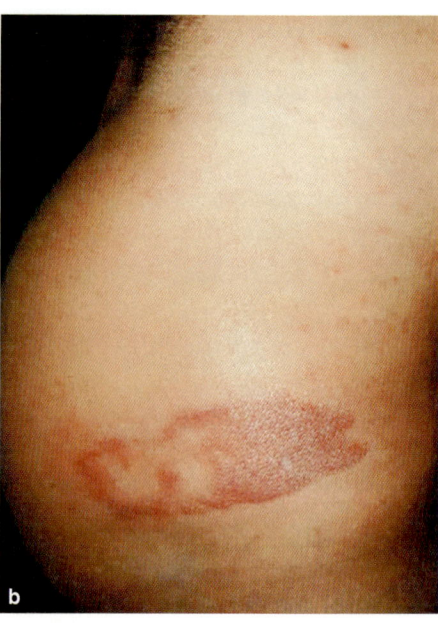

Fig. 5.5: (a) The patient has a visible annular edematous plaque with multiple barely visible papules which showed a BI of 5 with globi. A diagnosis of BB downgrading to LLs was made. The downgrading reaction was apparent at a later date (b) when the papules were histologically confirmed as LLs establishing the downgrading reaction (*Courtesy:* Dr Jaison A Barreto, Sao Paulo, Brazil)

Severe reactions may be accompanied by systemic illness, characterized by low grade fever, malaise and anorexia. Another associated manifestation is edema of hands, feet, or face (Fig. 5.6); sometimes all three sites are involved, or, rarely, one foot or one hand. Tenderness of palms and soles is often present, and may sometimes herald an upgrading reaction.

Neuritis is the most important part of a T1R and may be seen concomitantly with skin involvement or even independently; possibly reflecting hypersensitivity to different antigens of *M. leprae* as mentioned before.[41,42] This takes the form of rapid

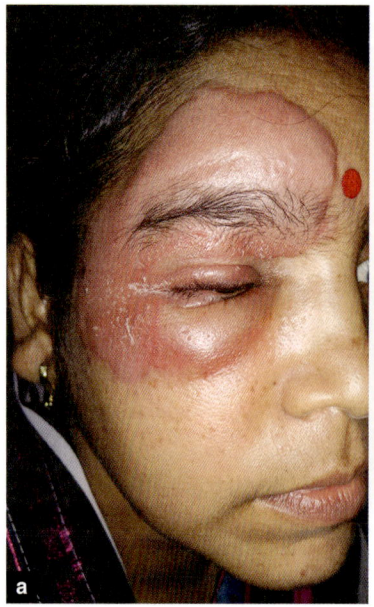
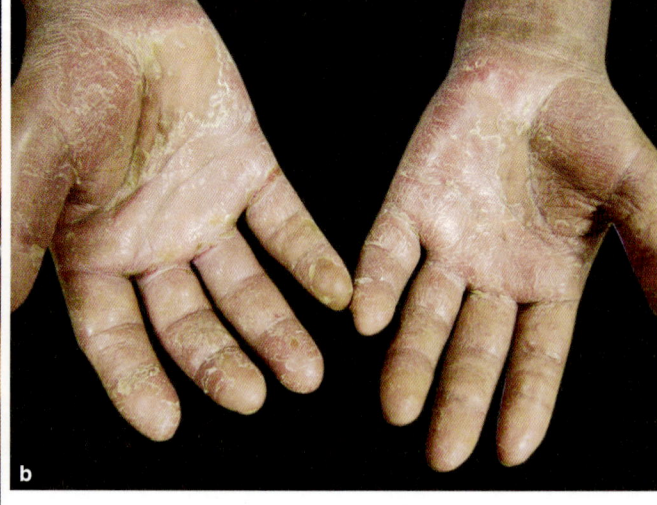

Fig. 5.6: (a) A type 1 reaction with intense signs involving the facial plaque—a candidate fit for oral steroids; (b) BT Hansen plaque on the palms with type 1 reaction

swelling of one or more nerves with pain and tenderness at the site of nerve swelling, usually where the nerve is most superficial. Sometimes, pain is referred to the region of the skin supplied by a sensory or mixed nerve such as pain at the medial border of the wrist and/or in the little finger in ulnar nerve involvement. In such a case, the ulnar nerve will be tender on palpation just above the elbow. More serious is motor disturbance, and the nerves most at risk are the ulnar (causing claw hand), the lateral popliteal (causing foot drop), and the facial (causing facial palsy). Facial palsy is most likely to occur if there is a lesion on one cheek. These paralyses are likely to be permanent if neglected or incorrectly treated, but will recover with correct and prompt treatment. The cause of nerve pain is increased intraneural pressure from edema and cellular reaction (granuloma formation), aggravated at sites where swollen nerve trunks are entrapped in bony or fascial tunnels, e.g. cubital tunnel and carpal tunnel. Rarely, a nerve abscess may form, producing a fluctuant swelling attached to the affected nerve. It is usually the ulnar nerve which is affected in this way, but the great auricular or the common peroneal (lateral popliteal) nerves have also been known to be involved in isolation.

A final clinical issue is distinguishing between late RR and relapse in patients who have completed MDT, particularly in skin smear negative PB patients. This is discussed in *Chapter 2, Section 2.2*.

Type 1 Reaction *versus* Type 2 Reaction

Sometimes, especially in BL patients, it is difficult to discern a T1R from a T2R. The reactions may even occur together or one after the other. Some clues to differentiating the two are given below.[8]

T2R is seen in lepromatous patients (LLs) and in some cases of BL. It is a generalized disease, affecting skin and nerves and other organs such as joints, lymph nodes, and liver. T1R is seen in borderline spectrum and co-existent systemic involvement is uncommon. During a T2R, the patient may be ill-looking (during a T1R, the patient usually is not) and may have a raised temperature and erythrocyte sedimentation rate, and even proteinuria. The skin lesions in T2R are evanescent while those in T1R are comparatively persistent. The lesions in T1R may have sensory loss compared with the surrounding skin; while in T2R this is usually not the case. When palpated, a T2R plaque consists of confluent papules and nodules, whereas a T1R lesion feels more homogeneous. Both T2R and T1R lesions may ulcerate, but a smear from a T2R lesion shows predominantly polymorphs, while that from a T1R lesion shows predominantly lymphocytes.

Two older tests—Ryrie and Ellis (detailed in *Chapter 5, Section 5.2*) may be of help as can be the findings on motor nerve conduction velocity testing; on which T1R shows only temporal dispersion, while T2R may also show a conduction block.

Therapy

The principles of management for T1Rs are two folds—one is initiation of anti-mycobacterial drugs and second is administering an effective and prolonged anti-inflammatory therapy with physical support during the phase of active neuritis (if present). It is imperative that MDT is maintained during and after a RR, as reduction in the antigenic load in skin and nerves removes the target for the T cell-driven inflammation and lessens the propensity to recurrence. This is especially relevant as viable or persistent *M. leprae* have been noted in T1R and moreover, resistant strains have been detected in downgrading T1R.[9]

Medical Therapy

1. Corticosteroids (*also see drug formulary, page 257*)

Steroids are indicated in the presence of neuritis or in severe T1R not controlled with anti-inflammatory drugs alone. The skin lesions rapidly respond to steroids while recovery of NFI is generally prolonged. In the presence of a recent NFI (<6 months), the use of steroids is imperative as it predicts recovery of nerve function (*for more detailed discussion on neuritis and NFI management, see Chapter 8, Section 8.1*).

The response of NFI to corticosteroids is highly variable with 33–73% of nerves recovering post-therapy.[41,42] The dose and duration is variable and needs to be individualized but as a general principle, immunosuppressive doses of corticosteroids are required for prolonged periods as the reaction will persist whilst the bacillary load gradually falls possibly due to antigenic stimulation. Thus, no single recommendation will suffice for all cases and only generic guidelines can be given. The ability to accurately predict the appropriate dose of prednisone for a given case of reaction and the rapidity with which it may be tapered improves with experience, but even with considerable experience such estimates are not always correct (Box 5.3).

Cytokines and steroid therapy and its implications

The notable recalcitrance in case of upgrading T1R can be explained by the fact that the levels of cytokines may rebound or may not decrease sufficiently on steroids.[43] A study found that prednisone therapy reduced the TNF-α after 30 days but the IL-10 and TGF-β did not rise on therapy.[19] It is the suppressive effect of TGF-$β_1$ that is crucial as it inhibits IFN-γ, TNF-α, and iNOS production and causes upregulation of IL-10 production. The level of TGF-β, and in recalcitrant cases IL-10, takes 6 months to rise on prednisolone. Thus, in all probability the rapid effects associated with prednisolone might be because it diminishes the formation of prostaglandins and leukotrienes, which are produced within the tissues and the cytokines may take longer to respond.[44]

Initial dose of prednisolone: May vary from 40 to 60 mg of prednisolone (or 1 mg/kg).[45]

Field studies with fixed regimens indicate that a dose of 40 mg prednisolone is sufficient to control 85% of T1Rs and this has been confirmed in a comparison of four corticosteroid regimens in Nepal.[46,47] But we reiterate that in most cases, a flexible approach is more practical (Box 5.3).[45,47]

Tapering of steroid:[47,48] Once there is evidence of improvement, the dose of prednisolone can be reduced at about 5 mg every 1–2 weeks until 20 mg is reached. This dose is usually continued for some months (*see below*) as gradual improvement in nerve function continues to occur. After this, the drug is withdrawn at 5 mg per fortnight. The maximum improvement occurs in the first 3 months but may continue for up to 6 months. Six months of treatment with prednisolone improves nerve function in about 50 to 80% of the patients.[19]

Box 5.3: Steroid dosimetry protocols in type 1 reaction[+]

1st protocol[+]	40–60 mg (till control) ↓ Reduce by 5 mg every 1–2 weeks till a dose of 20 mg (continued till optimal nerve function recovery) ↓ Reduce by 5 mg every 2 weeks ↓ Total duration: 12–20 weeks
2nd protocol[+]	30 mg/day for 2 weeks ↓ 25 mg/day for 2 weeks ↓ 20 mg/day for 8 weeks ↓ 10 mg/day for 4 weeks ↓ 5 mg/day for 4 weeks
3rd protocol[+]	**Initial phase** 80 mg daily (should improve in 1–2 days) • Deterioration after 12 hours → the dose may be divided and given BD • Continue till skin changes have completely resolved, neuritic pain has cleared and neural function lost in the course of the reactive episode has begun to return **Reduction of dose** • Attempt to reduce to a single morning dose if used BD initially (either ↓ evening dose by 5 mg every 2–3 days *or* the evening dose may be directly transferred and added to the morning dose) • Tapering daily dose by 5 mg every 1–2 weeks* **If prolonged duration:** Change to alternate day (80 mg daily to 80:75, 80:70, 80:65 ----> 80:0) (reductions of 5 mg, depending on response, every 2 weeks or more *or* even twice weekly if adequate response maintained)

BD: Twice daily
*If at any point, the reaction begins to recur, the dose may have to be temporarily increased once again and then tapered more slowly. Taper faster, if reaction is mild; slower, if it is severe. [+]Administer single dose albendazole to anyone being started on steroids.

Monitoring: The length and dose of therapy should be individualized based on careful assessment of motor function by voluntary muscle testing (VMT) and sensitive tests of sensory function such as the nylon monofilament test.[49]

Duration: BT patients require prednisolone for about 4–9 months, BB patients for 6–9 months and BL patients for 6–18 months, and at times even 24 months.[50] It is pertinent to reiterate that in real life practice, the WHO regimen of 12 weeks of prednisolone therapy for RRs in BB/BL patients is inadequate with one-third of patients relapsing with this fixed duration therapy. However, extension of therapy to 20 weeks resulted in a low recurrence rate.[51] Paradoxically, another trial, known as "TENLEP", showed that prolonging the course to 32 weeks provided little additional benefit over a 20-week course.[52] In essence, around 15% of patients in the trial (i.e. with 20 and

32 weeks treatment) required extra prednisolone because of a lack of improvement or worsening once the standard course ended. A randomized study of three different prednisolone regimes also suggested that *duration* of treatment, rather than the starting dose of prednisolone, may be more important in controlling T1Rs.[53] Thus, the *duration* of the therapy is more important than the dose as only 60% of individuals will show improvement in nerve function with 12 weeks of oral prednisolone.[49,53] The ALERT study observed that 15–20 mg prednisolone (±0.30–0.35 mg/kg) was the "critical dose" to control a RR after the initial period.[52,54]

Response: Patients with recent NFl of less than 6 months, BL spectrum and medial nerve damage are predictive of a favorable response.[50]

Follow-up
Record
- All episodes of reactions, including clinical features (skin lesions and nerve involvement), severity and duration
- Details of any nerve function assessments
- Details of treatment given, in particular the dosage and duration of steroid treatment.

Anyone on treatment with steroids should be seen at least every two weeks. Once steroids have been stopped, the patient should be seen every month initially, then every three months to monitor nerve function.

Prophylactic steroids to prevent T1R and neuritis:[55,56] The TRIPOD 1 trial concluded that the use of low dose prophylactic prednisolone during the first four months of multi-drug treatment for leprosy reduces the incidence of new reactions and nerve function impairment in the short term, but the effect is not sustained at one year. Thus, this does not seem to be a feasible option.

Adverse effects of steroid treatment of T1R: In view of the prolonged courses of steroids required in certain cases, careful monitoring for development of steroid related adverse effects is essential. A meta-analysis noted occurrence of dermatological side effects, diabetes, hypertension and psychosis in a statistically greater number of patients in the steroid than the placebo group. Sepsis, osteoporosis and tuberculosis also occurred more frequently in the steroid group, but the differences were not statistically significant.[57] The TRIPOD study also largely corroborates the same findings.[58] Further, it has been demonstrated that men with leprosy are at increased risk of osteoporosis which is related to the associated hypogonadism.[59] Prolonged steroids may worsen the condition or possibly is an additional factor leading to it. In endemic regions, the risk of tuberculosis must also be borne in mind as a high cumulative dose of steroids is an important risk factor for its reactivation.[58] Additional stresses of intercurrent illness or surgery would need additional steroid to prevent adrenal shock. Adrenocortical function recovers after stopping steroid but full recovery takes many months, but this has not been formally studied.

2. Alternative drugs

Some authors recommend a staged approach to therapy with a trial of aspirin and/or hydroxychloroquine for 'mild reactions' involving the skin alone without nerve impairment. While aspirin is a safe anti-inflammatory drug and can be used to treat

T1R while the patient is waiting for an expert assessment; a steroid course is recommended in order to manage any neuritis that often accompanies the reaction, except possibly in downgrading reactions.[45]

Azathioprine in combination with an 8-week course of prednisolone was as effective as a 12-week course of prednisolone in the management of T1Rs in a pilot study in Nepal.[60] But as azathioprine acts slowly and has no effect on intraneural edema, it is best used as an adjunct after initial treatment with corticosteroids.

Ciclosporin has been used in pilot studies in Nepal and Ethiopia with some success but is not universally effective.[61]

Methotrexate has been successfully used in T1Rs in an isolated case report.[62]

The use of clofazimine to manage T1R remains controversial. Its use in high doses (300 mg) may be attempted in occasional patients who require prolonged daily high dose prednisolone treatment.[62] While not commonly used for a localized reaction, topical corticosteroids may be a useful option in localized cases or even in pregnancy with a reaction.[63]

3. Immunobiological drugs

One novel option could revolve around targeting the cytokines involved in T1R. Recent studies have shown that type 1 interferons (IFNs) may counteract the antimicrobial effects of IFN-γ in leprosy and tuberculosis and also inhibit inflammasome activation pathways.[64] Betaferon/Betaseron and Rebif are recombinant IFN-β and -α, respectively and may be potentially useful as they have a immunosuppressive effect on type 1 IFNs.

Drugs that target IL-1β could be tested for the management of T1R since high levels of this cytokine have been reported in T1R patients' sera. The various drugs that can be potentially useful include anakinra, rilonacept and canakinumab.

Tacrolimus could prove promising for T1R management due to its effect on T lymphocytes. Indeed, a case report described an 11-year-old boy who developed a severe T1R after 4 months of MDT and was successfully treated with twice daily application of topical tacrolimus 0.1% along with oral steroids.[65]

The uncontrolled production of IL-6 has been associated with the onset of T1R.[66] Tocilizumab, a humanized anti-IL-6 receptor antibody, has proven efficacy and safety in rheumatoid arthritis and may have a potential use in T1R.

Surgical Options (also see Chapter 8, Section 8.3.2)

Surgery with decompression of swollen nerves has been advocated for patients with persistent nerve pain despite corticosteroid therapy. Although this may improve nerve conduction and function in individual cases, enhanced benefit has not been confirmed in clinical trials. A recent randomized comparative trial of corticosteroids and surgical intervention in patients with early neuritis showed that decompression of the ulnar nerve and medial epicondylectomy with medical therapy had no additional benefit over corticosteroids alone at follow-up after 1 or years.[67] Therefore, surgery should be reserved for the rare situations of nerve abscess in BT and TT patients, absence of nerve function improvement with steroids alone or intractable pain despite vigorous immunosuppressive therapy.

Downgrading Reactions

Since downgrading reactions occur in patients who are either not on effective therapy or have just begun treatment, initiation or continuation of appropriate anti-leprosy therapy should quickly control this reaction. If there is an accompanying neuritis or marked erythema and edema of skin lesions, a brief course of corticosteroids may be beneficial but this is usually not useful or necessary unless neuritis is present.[45]

LATE REACTIONS

While late reaction is a connotation ascribed to both T1R and T2R, most cases seen are usually of T1R.[68,69] Late T1R occurs at any time subsequent to MDT release and, especially in PB spectrum, there may be a difficulty in distinguishing it from relapse.

There is little published information on reactional states in MB patients following the completion of MDT. Saunderson found that after a fixed duration of 2 years WHO MDT, 43 of 300 patients (14%) developed reversal reactions while 24 patients (5%) developed T2R, the latter being associated with a high BI and LL classification.[70] But a study by Kumar found that after 2 years MDT, reactional states were distinctly infrequent.[71] A study examining late reactions after 1 year of MDT reported reversal reactions in 38% and T2R in 10%, 2 years after stopping therapy; which probably indicates that shortening the duration may cause more reactions.[72] One uniform trend noted is that T1R is commoner than T2R which is possibly because T2R generally occurs during the rapid killing of bacilli from effective chemotherapy, and like other antigen–antibody complex diseases, occurs particularly in a state of antigen excess which is seen during therapy.[73] On the other hand, T1R occur in patients even with a lower bacterial burden and occur frequently before therapy (downgrading T1R), without necessitating rapid bacterial death associated with effective antimicrobial therapy. A notable fact is that longer the duration of follow-up after release from treatment (RFT), lesser the incidence of T1R as possibly T1R is precipitated by *M. leprae* degradation products induced by the death of bacilli which have not yet been removed from the tissues; these moieties being found in tissues in higher concentrations in the early phase post-RFT.

Although, late T1R are presumed to be due to dead *M. leprae* and their antigens, some studies have shown that viable bacilli may also be important.[74] In fact, one author has opined that late reactions may be consequent to the re-multiplication of *M. leprae*, which increases the antigenic load and consequently causes reversal reaction.[75] With the use of PCR, viable bacilli as a cause can be assessed and recently, resistant *M. leprae* have been implicated in a case of late T1R which has important therapeutic implications.[9]

While the clinical presentation of late reaction and relapse may overlap, most relapses occur after the second year from RFT. In a recent paper there was no mouse footpad inoculation confirmed relapse in the first year after stopping treatment within 100 relapsed cases.[68] A more generalized conclusion is that while T1R and T2R occur most often during treatment with a decreasing rate thereafter; they can still be frequent in the first 2 years after treatment; after the fifth year of RFT though, reactions are rarely reported.[51]

While the therapy of late reaction is administering steroids, the logic being that this would suppress a reversal reaction and prevent or ameliorate any associated nerve damage, this treatment would only partially and temporarily suppress a reaction due to viable bacteria (and the latter would continue to multiply during this period of steroid immunosuppression, so that acid-fast bacteria might be more easily detected in smears). Thus, if the lesions subside and remain subsided after stopping steroid, it was most probably a case of late reaction. On the other hand, if the lesions do not subside, or, if they reappear during the period of observation, it is most probably a case of relapse needing anti-leprosy treatment.[76] Here we may point out that while WHO recommends initiation of clofazimine only if the steroid therapy is extended beyond 4 months, most clinicians administer concomitant MDT,[77] which may not be necessarily better or advisable in all such cases.

REFERENCES

1. Cambri G, Mira MT. Genetic Susceptibility to Leprosy-From Classic Immune-related Candidate Genes to Hypothesis-free, Whole Genome Approaches. Front Immunol 2018;9:1674.
2. E.A. Misch, W.R. Berrington, J.C. Vary Jr, T.R. Hawn, Leprosy and the human genome, Microbiol. Mol Biol Rev 2010;74:589–620.
3. Kumar B, Dogra S, Kaur I. Epidemiological characteristics of leprosy reactions: 15 years experience from north India. Int J Lepr Other Mycobact Dis 2004;72:125–33.
4. Walker SL, Lockwood DN. Leprosy type 1 (reversal) reactions and their management. Lepr Rev 2008;79:372–86.
5. Job CK. Pathology of leprosy In: Hastings RC, editor. Leprosy. New York: Churchill Livingstone; 1994. p. 205–206.
6. Van Brakel WH, Khawas IB, Lucas SB. Reactions in leprosy: An epidemiological study of 386 patients in west Nepal. Lepr Rev 1994;65:190–203.
7a. Ridley DS. Reactions. In: Pathogenesis of leprosy and related diseases. Butterworth & Co. (Publishers) Ltd. 1988.
7b. Ridley DS. Hypersensitivity and immunity reactions and classification. editorial. Lepr Rev 1976 Sep;47(3):171–4.
8. Naafs B, van Hees CL. Leprosy type 1 reaction (formerly reversal reaction). Clin Dermatol 2016;34:37–50.
9. Sinha S, Sardana K, Agrawal D, Malhotra P, Lavania M, Ahuja M. Multi-drug resistance as a cause of steroid—nonresponsive downgrading type I reaction in Hansen's disease. Int J Mycobacteriol 2019;8:305–8.
10. Roche PW, Theuvenet WJ, Britton WJ. Risk factors for type 1 reactions in borderline leprosy patients. Lancet 1991;338:654–57.
11. Katoch K, Ramu G, Ramanathan U, et al. Results of a modified WHO regimen in highly bacilliferous BL/LL patients. Int J Lepr Other Mycobact Dis 1989;57:451–7.
12. Mahapatra SB, Ramu G. Transformation from lepromatous to borderline leprosy under clofazimine therapy. Leprosy in India 1976;48: 172–76.
13. Ridley DS. The pathogenesis and classification of polar tuberculoid leprosy. Lepr Rev 1982;53: 19–26.
14. Britton WJ. The management of leprosy reversal reactions. Lepr Rev 1998;69:225–34.
15. Lockwood DN, Vinayakumar S, Stanley JN, McAdam KP, Colston MJ. Clinical features and outcome of reversal (type 1) reactions in Hyderabad, India. Int J Lepr Other Mycobact Dis 1993;61:8–15.
16. Dupnik KM, Bair TB, Maia AO, Amorim FM, Costa MR, Keesen TS, Valverde JG, QueirozMdo C, Medeiros LL, de Lucena NL, Wilson ME, Nobre ML, Johnson WD Jr, Jeronimo SM. Transcriptional changes that characterize the immune reactions of leprosy. J Infect Dis 2015;211:1658–76.
17. Barnetson RS, Bjune G, Pearson JM, Kronvall G Antigenic heterogeneity in patients with reactions in borderline leprosy. Br Med J 1975;4:435–7.

18. Save MP, Dighe AR, Natrajan M, Shetty VP. Association of viable *M. leprae* with Type 1 reaction in leprosy. Lepr Rev 2016;87:78–92.
19. Andersson AK, Chaduvula M, Atkinson SE et al. Effects of prednisolone treatment on cytokine expression in patients with leprosy type 1 reactions. Infect Immun 2005;73:3725–33.
20. Croft RP, Nicholls PG, Richardus JH, Smith WC. Incidence rates of acute nerve function impairment in leprosy: a prospective cohort analysis after 24 months (The Bangladesh Acute Nerve Damage Study). Lepr Rev 2000;71:18–33.
21. Groenen G, Janssens L, Kayembe T, Nollet E, Coussens L, Pattyn SR. Prospective study on the relationship between intensive bactericidal therapy and leprosy reactions. Int J Lepr 1986;54:236–44.
22. Boerrigter G, Ponnighaus M, Fine PEM. Preliminary appraisal of a WHO recommended multiple drug regimen in paucibacillary leprosy patients in Malawi. Int J Lepr 1988;56:406–17.
23. Hogeweg M, Kiran KU, Suneetha S. The significance of facial patches and type I reaction for the development of facial nerve damage in leprosy. A retrospective study among 1 226 paucibacillary leprosy patients. Lepr Rev 1991;62:143–49.
24. Roche PW, Le Master J, Butlin CR. Risk factors for type 1 reactions in leprosy. Int J Lepr 1997;65:450–55.
25. Roche PW, Theuvenet WJ, Britton WJ. Risk factors for type 1 reactions in borderline leprosy patients. Lancet 1991;338:654–57.
26. Becx-Bleumink M, Berhe D. Occurrence of reactions, their diagnosis and management in leprosy patients treated with multidrug therapy; experience in the leprosy control program of the All Africa Leprosy and Rehabilitation Training center (ALERT) in Ethiopia. Int J Lepr 1992;60:173–84.
27. Van Brakel WH, Khawas IB, Lucas SB. Reactions in leprosy: An epidemiological study of 386 patients in west Nepal. Lepr Rev 1994;65:190–203.
28. Lienhardt C, Fine PEM. Type 1 reaction, neuritis and disability in leprosy. What is the current epidemiological situation? Lepr Rev 1994;65:9–33.
29. Lockwood DNJ, Sinha HH. Pregnancy and leprosy: a comprehensive literature review. Int J Lepr 1999;67:6–12.
30. Reed NK, van Brakel WH, Reed DS. Progress of impairment scores following commencement of chemotherapy in multibacillary leprosy patients. Int J Lepr 1997;65:328–36.
31. Amorim FM, Nobre ML, Nascimento LS, Miranda AM, Monteiro GRG, Freire-NetoF, et al. Differential immunoglobulin and complement levels in leprosy prior to development of reversal reaction and erythema nodosum leprosum. PLoS Negl Trop Dis 2019;13:e0007089.
32. Job CK. Nerve damage in reversal reaction. Ind J Lepr 1996;68:43–47.
33. Scollard DM, Truman RW, Ebenezer GJ. Mechanisms of nerve injury in leprosy. Clin Dermatol 2015;33:46–54.
34. Ridley DS, Radia KB. The histological course of reactions in borderline leprosy and their outcome. Int. J. Lepr. 1981;49: 383–92.
35. Ramu G, Desikan KV. Reactions in borderline leprosy. Indian J Lepr. 2002;74:115–28.
36. Lockwood DN, Lucas SB, Desikan K, et al. The histological diagnosis of leprosy type 1 reactions: identifiication of key variables and an analysis of the process of histological diagnosis. J Clin Pathol 2008;61:595–600.
37. Pfaltzgraff RE, Ramu G. Clinical leprosy. In: Hastings RC, editor. Leprosy. New York: Churchill Livingstone;1994. p. 237–87.
38. Yawalkar SJ.Leprosy for medical practitioners and paramedical workers. Basle 5th edn p 84.
39. Sehgal VN, Bhattacharya SN, Jain S. Relapse or late reversal reaction? Int J Lepr Other Mycobact Dis 1990;58:118–21.
40. Barnetson RS, Bjune G, Pearson JM, Kronvall G. Antigenic heterogeneity in patients with reactions in borderline leprosy. Br Med J 1975;4:435–37.

41. Saunderson P, Gebre S, Desta K, Byass P, Lockwood DN. The pattern of leprosy-related neuropathy in the AMFES patients in Ethiopia: definitions, incidence, risk factors and outcome. Lepr Rev 2000;71:285–308.
42. Croft RP, Nicholls PG, Richardus JH, Smith WC. The treatment of acute nerve function impairment in leprosy: results from a prospective cohort study in Bangladesh. Lepr Rev 2000;71:154–68.
43. Manandhar R, Shrestha N, Butlin CR, Roche PW. High levels of inflammatory cytokines are associated with poor clinical response to steroid treatment and recurrent episodes of type 1 reactions in leprosy. Clin Exp Immunol 2002;128:333–38.
44. Guyton AC, Hall JE. The adrenocortical hormonesIn. Guyton AC Ed. Textbook of Medical Physiology, 9th ed. W. B. Saunders Company, 1996. Philadelphia, Pa.: p. 957–70.
45. Jacobson RR. Treatment of leprosy. In: Hastings RC, ed. Leprosy, 2nd edn. Churchill Livingstone, Edinburgh 1994; p 317–49.
46. Becx-Bleumink M, Berhe D. Occurrence of reactions, their diagnosis and management in leprosy patients treated with multi drug therapy; experience in the leprosy control program of the All Africa Leprosy and Rehabilitation Training Center (ALERT) in Ethiopia. Int J Lepr 1 992;173–84.
47. van Brakel WH, Khawasl B. Nerve function impairment: An epidemiological and clinical study. Part 2: result of various treatment regimens. Lepr Rev 1995;66:104–18.
48. Naafs B, Pearson JMH, Baar AJM. A follow-up study of nerve lesions in leprosy during and after reaction using motor nerve conduction. Int JLepr 1976;44:188–97.
49. van Brakel WH, Khawas IB, Gurung KS et al. Intra- and inter-tester reliability of sensibility testing in leprosy. Int JLepr 1996;64:287–98.
50. Rose P, Waters MFR. Reversal reactions in leprosy and their management. Lepr Rev 1991;62:113–21.
51. Becx-Bleumink M, Berhe D. Occurrence of reactions, their diagnosis and management in leprosy patients treated with multi drug therapy; experience in the leprosy control program of the All Africa Leprosy and Rehabilitation Training Center (ALERT) in Ethiopia. Int JLepr 1992;60:1 73–84.
52. Wagenaar I, Post E, Brandsma W, Bowers B, Alam K, Shetty B, et al. Effectiveness of 32 versus 20 weeks of prednisolone in leprosy patients with recent nerve function impairment: A randomized controlled trial. PLoSNeglTrop Dis 2017;11:e0005952.
53. Rao PS, Sugamaran DS, Richard J, Smith WC. Multicentre, double blind, randomized trial of three steroid regimens in the treatment of type 1 reactions in leprosy. Lepr Rev 2006;77:25–33.
54. Naafs B, Pearson JM, Wheate HW. Reversal reaction: the prevention of permanent nerve damage. Comparison of short and long-term steroid treatment. Int J Lepr Other Mycobact Dis 1979;47:7–12.
55. Croft RP, Nicholls P, Anderson AM, van Brakel WH, Smith WC, Richardus JH. Effect of prophylactic corticosteroids on the incidence of reactions in newly diagnosed multibacillary leprosy patients. Int J Lepr Other Mycobact Dis 1999;67:75–7.
56. Smith WC, Anderson AM, Withington SG, van Brakel WH, Croft RP, Nicholls PG, et al. Steroid prophylaxis for prevention of nerve function impairment in leprosy: Randomised placebo controlled trial (TRIPOD 1) BMJ 2004;328:1459.
57. Conn HO, Poynard T. Corticosteroids and peptic ulcer: meta-analysis of adverse events during steroid therapy. J Intern Med 1994;236:619–32.
58. Richardus JH, Withington SG, Anderson AM, Croft RP, Nicholls PG, Van Brakel WH, Smith WC. Adverse events of standardized regimens of corticosteroids for prophylaxis and treatment of nerve function impairment in leprosy: Results from the 'TRIPOD' trials. Lepr Rev 2003 Dec;74(4):319–27.
59. Ishikawa S, Tanaka H, Mizushima M, Hashizume H, Ishida Y, Inoue H. Osteoporosis due to testicular atrophy in male leprosy patients.Acta Med Okayama 1997;51:279–83.
60. Marlowe SN, Hawksworth RA, Butlin CR,Nicholls PG, Lockwood DN. Clinical outcomes in a randomized controlled study comparing azathioprine and prednisolone versus prednisolone alone in the treatment of severe leprosy type 1 reactions in Nepal. Trans R Soc Trop Med Hyg 2004;98:602–09.

61. Marlowe SN, Leekassa R, Bizuneh E, Knuutilla J, Ale P, Bhattarai B, et al. Response to cyclosporine treatment in Ethiopian and Nepali patients with severe leprosy Type 1 reactions. Trans R Soc Trop Med Hyg 2007;101:1004–12.
62. Guillermo Biosca, Sonia Casallo, Rogelio López-Vélez, Methotrexate Treatment for Type 1 (Reversal) Leprosy Reactions. Clinical Infectious Diseases 2007;45:e7–e9.
63. Srinivas CR, Padhee A, Menon SK, Naik RP, Ramnarayan K. Reversal reaction management with topical corticosteroids. Int J Lepr Other Mycobact Dis 1987;55:355–57.
64. Teles RM, Graeber TG, Krutzik SR, Montoya D, Schenk M, Lee D, et al. Type 1 interferon suppresses type 2 interferon-triggered human anti-mycobacterial responses. Science 2013;339:1448–53.
65. Safa G, Darrieux L, Coic A, Tisseau L. Type 1 leprosy reversal reaction treated with topical tacrolimus along with systemic corticosteroids. Indian J Med Sci 2009;63:359–62.
66. Stefani MM, Guerra JG, Sousa AL, Costa MB, Oliveira ML, Martelli CT, et al. Potential plasma markers of Type 1 and Type 2 leprosy reactions: A preliminary report. BMC Infect Dis 2009;9:75.
67. Ebenezer M, Andrews P, Solomon S. Comparative trial of steroids and surgical intervention in the management of ulnar neuritis. Int J Lepr 1996;62: 282–86.
68. Linder K, Zia M, Kern WV, Pfau RK, Wagner D. Relapses vs. reactions in multibacillary leprosy: Proposal of new relapse criteria. Tropical Medicine & International Health 2008;3:295–09.
69. Balagon MV, Gelber RH, Abalos RM, Cellona RV. Reactions following completion of 1 and 2 years multi-drug therapy (MDT). Am J Trop Med Hyg 2010;83:637–44.
70. Saunderson P, Gebre S, Byass P. Reversal reactions in the skin lesions of AMFES patients: Incidence and risk factors. Lepr Rev 2000;71:309–17.
71. Kumar B, Dogra S & Kaur I. Epidemiological characteristics of leprosy reactions: 15 years experience from North India. International Journal of Leprosy and other Mycobacterial Diseases 2004;72:125–133.
72. Balagon MV, Gelber RH, Abalos RM, Cellona RV. Reactions following completion of 1 and 2 years multi-drug therapy (MDT). Am J Trop Med Hyg 2010;83:637–44.
73. TaverneJ, Reichlin M, Turk JL, Rees RJW, Detection of immune complexes in mice infected with Mycobacterium lepraemurium. Clin Exp Immunol 1976;24:157–67.
74. Save MP, Dighe AR, Natrajan M, Shetty VP. Association of viable *Mycobacterium leprae* with Type 1 reaction in leprosy. Lepr Rev 2016;87:78–92.
75. Vijayakumaran P, Manimozhi N, Jesudasan K. Incidence of late lepra reaction among multibacillary leprosy patients after MDT. Int J Lepr Other Mycobact Dis 1995;63:18–22.
76. Reddy PK, Cherian A. Relapse in leprosy after multidrug therapy and its differential diagnosis with reversal reaction. Indian J Lepr 1991;63:61–9.
77. Shetty VP, Khambati FA, Ghate SD, et al. The effect of corticosteroids usage on bacterial killing, clearance and nerve damage in leprosy; Part 3—study of two comparable groups of 100 multibacillary (MB) patients each, treated with MDT+ steroids *vs* MDT alone, assessed at 6 months. Lepr Rev 2010;81:41–58.

5.2a TYPE 2 LEPRA REACTION

Tarun Narang, Divya Kamat

Reactions are the major cause of morbidity related to leprosy. Type 2 lepra reactions are seen exclusively in patients of multibacillary leprosy (mainly LL and BL).[1]

Epidemiology

While in the pre-sulfone era, the incidence of type 2 lepra reactions was reported to be about 50% in LL and up to 25% in BL cases, the incidence is lower with MDT, probably as a result of inclusion of clofazimine in the regimen.[2] A systematic review estimated the average incidence of erythema nodosum leprosum (ENL) in LL cases to be 15.4% (range 11.1–26%) and in BL cases to be 4.1% (range 2.7–5.1%) in field studies, while it was higher in hospital-based settings.[3] Type 2 reactions most commonly occur around 6 months after starting MDT, but may appear before (as a presenting feature in up to 1/3 of patients) or even after MDT (up to 7–8 years) due to persistence of bacterial antigens (granular bacilli). In a series of 414 patients, 34.7% individuals presented with ENL at the time of their leprosy diagnosis, 39.8% developed ENL during treatment with MDT and 25.5% after having successfully completed a 12-month course of MDT.[4] The first clinical and histological description of these cutaneous lesions was given by a Japanese leprologist, Murata, in a German journal of pathology in 1912.[6] He proposed the name ENL for these lesions, not for the symptom-complex. But the preferred term is type 2 lepra reaction as there are various systemic manifestations which accompany ENL.[5]

Risk or Precipitating Factors

Risk factors for type 2 reaction include: Lepromatous leprosy spectrum with a bacteriological index (BI) ≥4, <40 years of age, coinfections (like HIV, tuberculosis, hepatitis B and C, typhoid, etc.), pregnancy and lactation (30–40% of pregnant and lactating women are at risk to develop ENL), intercurrent infections (like streptococcal, viral, intestinal parasites, filariasis, malaria), vaccination, psychological stress, trauma/surgical interventions, decreased C4 and elevated anti-*M. leprae* antibodies in newly diagnosed leprosy,[7] a strongly positive Mantoux test, or ingestion of potassium iodide and antileprosy drugs. The immunopathogenesis is detailed in *Chapter 4, Section 4.5*.

Clinical Features

Type 2 reaction can cause inflammatory reaction in any organ invaded by the lepra bacilli. Cutaneous lesions known as ENL present as crops of erythematous, partially blanchable, warm, tender papules or nodules. These may be superficial or deep seated and have a bilaterally symmetrical predilection (Fig. 5.7). They are usually seen to involve the face, arms, thighs, palms and sole and may appear on any area *except* the hairy scalp, axillae, groins and perineum as these are the warmer regions of skin which are spared by leprosy as well as by ENL. The nodules characteristically blanch with light finger pressure (the red color reappearing immediately after pressure is released). In contrast to erythema nodosum, ENL lesions are evanescent (lasting 2–3 days), multiple in number and have a more widespread distribution beyond just the lower legs. The clinician sees *no* change whatsoever in the appearance of the old-standing leprosy

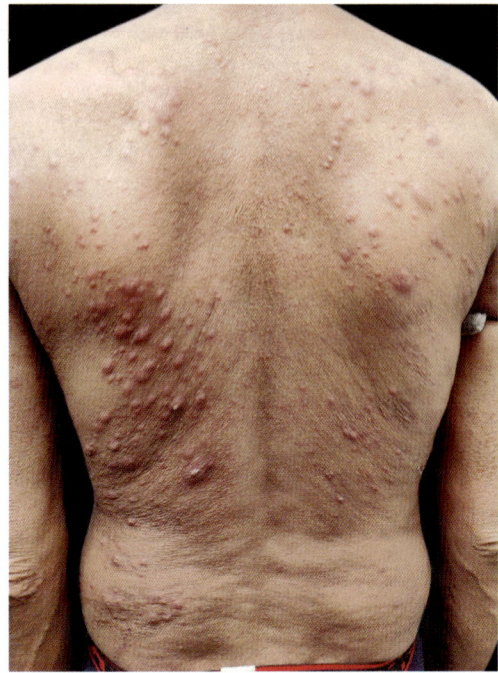

Fig. 5.7: Erythema nodosum leprosum: Extensive papules and nodules with bilateral involvement

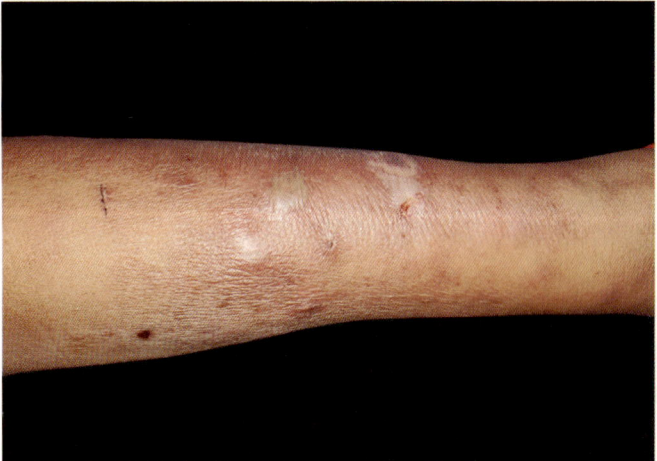

Fig. 5.8: Pustular ENL

lesions (even though the histologist may see some evidence of change), and ENL superimposed on them is unusual. Another close clinical differential diagnosis is Sweet's syndrome.

ENL lesions fade in 3–4 days with post-inflammatory hyperpigmentation (bruise or contusion-like) and desquamation. The onset of crops of ENL and intermittent fever is usually seen in the evenings (between 1700 and 1800 hours) when the endogenous cortisol is at its nadir. In severe reactions, skin lesions may become pustular (Fig. 5.8),

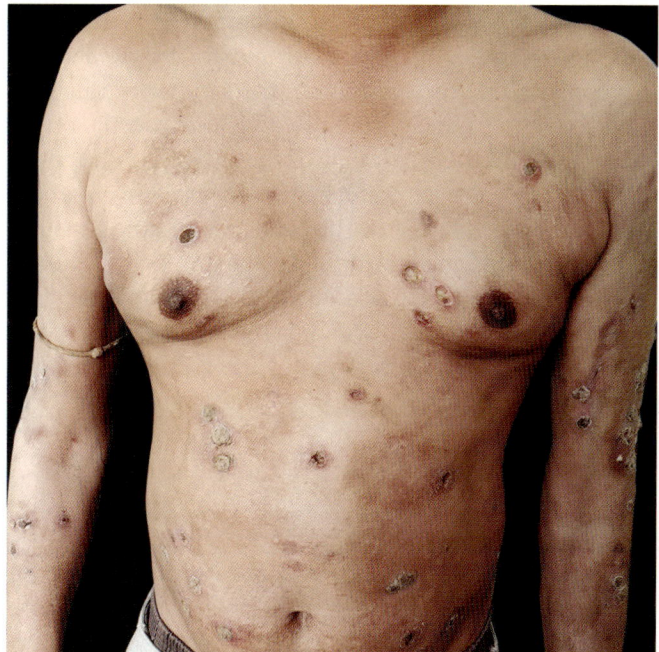 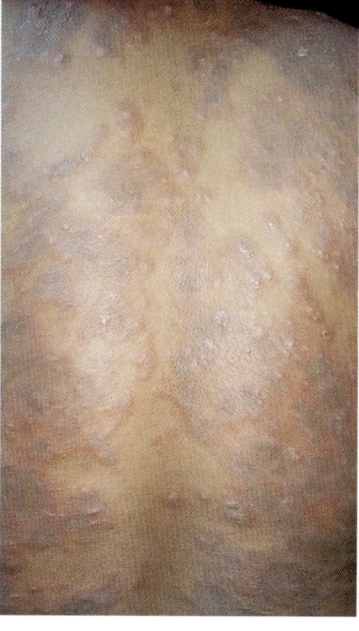

Fig. 5.9: Pustular "necrotic" lesions of ENL

Fig. 5.10: "Erythema multiforme" type of ENL

ulcerated, hemorrhagic, necrotic (Fig. 5.9), vesicular, bullous,[9] Sweet syndrome-like[10] and erythema multiforme-like (Fig. 5.10).[11] If there are recurrent lesions and they do not resolve completely, a chronic panniculitis may develop and this may lead to fibrosis and immobilization of the hand (reaction hand), foot or even face. This tissue is poorly vascularized and may ulcerate with slightest trauma; and for the same reason the wounds formed over these are poor to heal.

In contrast to type 1 reaction, wherein systemic features are unusual, type 2 reaction usually produces a generalized systemic illness with fever, myalgia, edema of the face, hands and feet and loss of protein in urine. Although fever is considered a hallmark sign of ENL, the Erythema Nodosum Leprosum International Study (ENLIST) group found that only 19.8% of patients had a documented fever on examination whilst 74.3% "complained of fever".[8] The authors reasoned that a large proportion of patients experience fever or feel feverish due to the systemic inflammatory nature of ENL but that this does not necessarily result in actual pyrexia or the pyrexia may have subsided by the time they present.[8] Further, although individuals classified as having severe ENL were more likely to be febrile than those with milder forms of ENL, the degree of fever was not found to be significantly different. Pain is the most common symptom reported by patients with ENL (96–98% patients).[4,8] About 80% report skin pain and more than 70% have nerve and joint pain. Other sites of pain reported include bone, digits, eyes, muscles, lymph nodes and testes.[4,8]

The ENLIST group reported cutaneous nodules, edema and nerve function impairment as the three most common clinical signs of type 2 reaction.[8]

Other extracutaneous manifestations include episcleritis, iritis, arthralgia or arthritis, dactylitis, lymphadenopathy, organomegaly and epididymo-orchitis. Neuritis is the most common extracutaneous manifestation but is often milder than seen in type 1 reaction. Bone pain is due to periosteitis and is usually confined to the tibiae, and there is exquisite tenderness (and a boggy feel) when palpated. Iritis may be unilateral or bilateral and can be mistaken for conjunctivitis, especially as it may occur, on its own (without any other signs of reaction). As the treatment of these two conditions is radically different, and as delay in treating acute iritis can have serious consequences for the patient, it is important for leprosy workers to know how to differentiate them. In iritis the redness is most marked at the corneoscleral margin, i.e. where the central colored part of the eye, covered by transparent cornea, joins the sclera (the white part of the eye). Further out, the redness is paler or may be absent. Also, the redness is less intense than in conjunctivitis and tends to have a dusky or even a violet hue. The redness in conjunctivitis is most evident further out, and a useful aid to remembering this is to think of the letter 'i' for inland and the letter 'c' for coast; in iritis the redness is mostly 'inland' and in conjunctivitis it is mostly 'coastal'. Epididymo-orchitis may be unilateral or bilateral, the testis being swollen and acutely tender. Alternatively, it may be low grade with little pain and swelling and gradual loss of function. Epistaxis may be aggravated and an affected palate may perforate. Protein and red blood cells in the urine are likely to be manifestations of acute glomerulonephritis, as immune complexes have been demonstrated in renal glomeruli during type 2 reaction[12] and subepithelial humps, typical of immune glomerulonephritis, have been seen on electron microscopy.[13]

Two simple tests have been described in type 2 reactions.[14] In the Ellis' test, the patient's arm is squeezed just above the wrist using the hands of the examiner resulting in excruciating pain. In the Ryrie's test, patient experiences a burning pain when the sole is stroked with a blunt object with light pressure. This may also be noticed when the patient walks and it appears as if he is walking on hot coal.[14] These tests are useful in screening patients with type 2 reaction and can also be used as a guide to determine the dose and duration of anti-reactional therapy. An overview of the systemic involvement is listed in Table 5.2.

Table 5.2: Systemic involvement in type 2 reaction	
Organs involved	Signs and symptoms
Joints	Polyarthritis or polyarthralgia
Lymph nodes	Tender generalized lymphadenopathy (especially femoral)
Eyes	Uveitis (iritis and iridocyclitis), glaucoma and blindness
Organomegaly	Hepatosplenomegaly—may be tender
Genitalia	Orchitis and epididymitis
Kidneys	Glomerulonephritis, acute tubulointerstitial nephritis and amyloidosis which can progress to chronic kidney disease
Bone	Dactylitis, periosteitis
Muscles	Myalgia, myositis
Nerves	Neuritis

Case Definitions[15]

New ENL is defined as 'the occurrence of ENL for the first time in a patient with LL'.

Acute ENL—'a single episode lasting less than 24 weeks while on corticosteroids treatment and in which treatment was slowly withdrawn with no recurrence of ENL whilst on treatment'.

Recurrent ENL—'if a patient experiences second or subsequent episode of ENL occurring 28 days or more after stopping treatment for ENL'.

Chronic ENL—'if occurring for 24 weeks or more during which a patient requires treatment for ENL either continuously or where any treatment-free period had been 27 days or less'.

Most of the patients with ENL experience multiple such acute episodes. They may also progress to chronic ENL which lasts for more than 6 months. It can even have a protracted course which lasts for several years. Walker et al observed ENL to be "chronic" in a majority of patients (70.7%); presenting as an "acute" event in 19.2% individuals and with a "recurrent" course in 10.1%.[8]

Severity Scale for Type 2 Lepra Reaction

The ENLIST group developed a 10-item scale known as the ENLIST ENL Severity Scale (EESS), for measuring the severity of ENL. It is the first published validated score to assess the severity of ENL. The original ENLIST ENL Severity Scale incorporated 16 items including assessments of pain and general well being using visual analogue scales (VAS), skin involvement (number, inflammation and extent of inflammation), peripheral edema, fever, epididymo-orchitis, ocular involvement, joint and bone involvement (bone pain, inflammation of joints and/or digits due to ENL), assessment of number of nerves with new sensory and new motor nerve function impairment (NFI) and assessment of nerve tenderness.[16] A later validation study on EESS shortened the list of items to 10 removing the well being point (to maintain a strictly clinical focus), orchitis (to produce a gender neutral scale) and points related to eye inflammation, urinalysis and sensory and motor nerve function (showing lowest levels of correlation).[15] The scores for each component are added together to obtain a final score. Mild ENL is categorized as an ENLIST ENL severity scale score of 8 or less while scores of >8 are associated with severe ENL.[15]

Laboratory Investigations

Slit smears of ENL lesions show mainly fragmented and granular AFB which are generally not as numerous as in the leprosy lesions. The histopathology is discussed in *Chapter 3, Section 3.2*.

The common hematological findings include normocytic normochromic anemia, polymorphonuclear leukocytosis and raised erythrocyte sedimentation rate (ESR). However, routine tests like blood sugar, serum chemistries and blood counts are mainly needed to monitor therapy. Occasionally, trigger factors can be infections and have been assessed by tests for malaria, typhoid, stool examination for parasites, HIV test and TB screening. At the referral level ESR, renal function, hepatic function, eye examination and bone density monitoring should be done.

REFERENCES

1. Pandhi D, Chhabra N. New insights in the pathogenesis of type 1 and type 2 lepra reaction. Indian J Dermatol Venereol Leprol 2013;79:739–49.
2. Lockwood DN. The management of erythema nodosum leprosum: Current and future options. Lepr Rev 1996;67:253–59.
3. Voorend CG, Post EB. A systematic review on the epidemiological data of erythema nodosum leprosum, a type 2 leprosy reaction. PLoS Negl Trop Dis 2013;7:e2440.
4. Walker SL, Lebas E, Doni SN, Lockwood DN, Lambert SM. The mortality associated with erythema nodosum leprosum in ethiopia: A retrospective hospital-based study. PLoS Negl Trop Dis 2014; 13;8:e2690.
5. Kahawita IP WS, Lockwood DN. Leprosy type 1 reactions and erythema nodosum leprosum. An Bras Dermatol 2008;83:75–82.
6. Jopling WH. Summary of Murata's paper on erythema nosodum leprosum. Leprosy Review 1958;29:116–18.
7. Amorim FM, Nobre ML, Nascimento LS, Miranda AM, Monteiro GRG, Freire-Neto FP, et al. Differential immunoglobulin and complement levels in leprosy prior to development of reversal reaction and erythema nodosum leprosum. PLoS Negl Trop Dis 2019;13:e0007089.
8. Walker SL, Balagon M, Darlong J, Doni SN, Hagge DA, Halwai V, et al. ENLIST 1: An International Multicentre Cross-sectional Study of the Clinical Features of Erythema Nodosum Leprosum. PLoS Negl Trop Dis 2015;9:e0004065.
9. Bakshi N, Rao S, Batra R. Bullous Erythema Nodosum Leprosum as the First Manifestation of Multibacillary Leprosy: A Rare Phenomenon. Am J Dermatopathol 2017;39:857–9.
10. Suryawati N, Saputra H. Erythema nodosum leprosum presenting as Sweet's syndrome-like reaction in a borderline lepromatous leprosy patient. Int J Mycobacteriol 2018;7:191–4.
11. Gunawan H, Yogya Y, Hafinah R, Marsella R, Ermawaty D, Suwarsa O. Reactive perforating leprosy, erythema multiforme-like reactions, Sweet's syndrome-like reactions as atypical clinical manifestations of Type 2 leprosy reaction. Int J Mycobacteriol 2018;7:97–100.
12. Drutz DJ, Gurman RA. Renal manifestations of leprosy: Glomerulonephritis, a complication of erythema nodosum leprosum. Am J Trop Med and Hyg 1973;22:496–502.
13. Date A, Johny KV. Glomerular subepithelial deposits in lepromatous leprosy. Am J Trop Med and Hyg 1975;24:853–6.
14. Naafs B, Lyons NF, Matamera BO, Madom B. The 'Ellis' and 'Ryrie' tests. Lepr Rev 1987; 58:53–60.
15. Walker SL, Sales AM, Butlin CR, et al. A leprosy clinical severity scale for erythema nodosum leprosum: An international, multicentre validation study of the ENLIST ENL Severity Scale. PLoS Negl Trop Dis 2017;11: e0005716.
16. Walker SL, Knight KL, Pai VV, Nicholls PG, Alinda M, Butlin CR, et al.The development of a severity scale for Erythema Nodosum Leprosum—the ENLIST ENL Severity Scale. Lepr Rev 2016; 87:332–46.

5.2b MANAGEMENT OF TYPE 2 LEPRA REACTION

Tarun Narang, Divya Kamat

The main aim of management of type 2 lepra reaction (T2LR) is to control acute systemic inflammation and neuritis with prompt diagnosis allowing early and adequate treatment to prevent further damage and disability.

General Measures
All patients with T2LR should be counseled regarding the nature of disease and advised to rest. All attempts should be made to find out and address the triggering factors including alcohol or drug withdrawal. MDT should be continued (if patient is still under treatment). When T2LR occurs or persists even after a 12-month course of MDT, repeat slit-smears with bacteriological index (BI) and morphological index (MI) estimation is required, as high bacterial load even after completion of treatment is an important risk factor and may be predictive of resistance.[1]

Specific Measures
Steroids (prednisolone) are the mainstay of treatment while thalidomide is another effective option in moderate to severe T2LR.

A convenient method of deciding the intervention is by broadly classifying the reactions as mild, moderate and severe. The natural course of T2LR is between one and two weeks, but many patients experience multiple recurrences for months[3] which necessitates flexible and individualized dosing.

Mild T2LR: This is largely managed with analgesics (aspirin, indomethacin, ibuprofen, diclofenac, acetaminophen, tramadol). If there is worsening and increase in the ENLIST score to >8, ENL should be reclassified as "severe" and managed accordingly. Monitoring should be done every two weeks.

Moderate T2LR: Steroid treatment is used starting with moderate doses of 30–40 mg prednisolone per day. Steroids have a rapid and defined therapeutic action.

Recurrent T2LR: This requires increased or prolonged doses of steroids to control the inflammation and symptoms.

Patients with chronic ENL may become dependent on steroids. In view of the potential serious side effects of prolonged steroid treatment, every effort must be made to reduce the overall dose of steroids. Here it must be remembered that the clinician must administer second line drugs in certain scenarios including:
  a. *Steroid nonresponders*: Those requiring higher doses of steroids with each episode of ENL.
  b. *Steroid dependent*: Those for whom tapering the steroid results in flares.
  c. *Patients with a serious comorbidity*

Retreatment with another 12 months of MDT was seen to control the reactional episodes and thus prevent further nerve damage in patients with chronic recurrent ENL. In cases, where rifampicin resistance is suspected, alternate leprosy treatment using minocycline, ofloxacin and clofazimine can also be considered to reduce the incidence of recurrent ENL.[1] Many patients with recurrent ENL have features of nerve function impairment, which if left unchecked might lead to permanent disability. Therefore, all attempts for early detection of nerve function impairment (NFI) must be done.² In all cases, anti-inflammatory medication like nonsteroidal anti-inflammatory drugs (NSAIDs) should be started. The painful nature of T2LR has been stressed upon previously and thus pain management forms an integral and important part of treatment of T2LRs.

The various drugs in T2LR are listed in Box 5.4. The dosimetry of salient drugs is given in Table 5.3; while important drugs are discussed in detail afterwards *(also see Drug Formulary, page 258–277)*. An algorithm of management is presented in Flowchart 5.1.

 Box 5.4: Overview of drugs used in T2LR

1. Systemic corticosteroids
    - Oral: Prednisolone
    - Intravenous therapies: Dexamethasone or methylprednisolone pulse
2. Systemic steroid sparing agents
    - Immunosuppressive therapies: Thalidomide, cyclosporine A, pentoxifylline, methotrexate, azathioprine
    - Antibacterial therapies with anti-inflammatory action: Clofazimine, minocycline
    - Anti-inflammatory therapies: Aspirin, chloroquine, colchicine, indomethacin
3. Other therapies
    - Oral zinc
    - *Mycobacterium indicus pranii* vaccine

Table 5.3: Dosimetry of drugs used for type 2 reaction

Drug	Dose	Most frequent adverse effects
Prednisone	• 1 to 1.5 mg/kg/day for 2–4 weeks • Thereafter, tapering by 10 mg every 2 weeks till 20 mg per day • Then slow tapering of 5 mg every 2 weeks	Exogenous Cushing's syndrome, acne, diabetes, hypertension, osteoporosis, gastritis, cataract, increased risk of opportunistic infections
Thalidomide	• 100–400 mg/day tapering by 50 mg every 2–4 weeks • Maintenance at 50 mg daily or alternate days	Sedation, constipation, teratogenicity, phocomelia, irreversible peripheral neuropathy, increased risk of thrombosis especially when combined with steroids
Pentoxifylline	• Conventional regimen: – 400 mg 3–4/day—control 2 days – Tapered by 50 mg 2–4 weeks – Chronic—maintenance 100 mg alternate day to 100 mg BD – Discontinue after 6 months • Short course schedule (3 months) – 100 mg thrice daily. Reduction of 100 mg every month	Dry mouth, constipation, anorexia, cholecystitis
Clofazimine	• 12-month long-term schedule: – Starting dose 100 mg thrice daily for 3 months – Tapering 100 mg over a period from 1 to 6 months	Skin pigmentation—reddish brown, icthyosis, gastrointestinal effects: Pain abdomen, nausea, vomiting, diarrhea, rarely bowel perforation

Flowchart 5.1: Treatment algorithm for management of type 2 reaction*

```
                          Type 2 reaction
                          /            \
                  Mild/moderate        Severe
                    /      \            /    \
                   /        \          /      \
              Add         General    Start prednisolone 1 mg/kg
         Aspirin, NSAIDs  measures   (with gradual tapering)
          /        \      1. Rest, splinting of   Add clofazimine 50 mg/minocycline 100 mg
         /          \        limb if neuritis    (if MDT is completed)
   No response    Adequate   present                    /         \
   add            response   2. Continue MDT           /           \
   prednisolone   Continue   3. Identify and      No response    Adequate
   1 mg/kg        the same      address the       Add            respone
                                triggering        clofazimine 100 mg TDS/   continue
                                factors           pentoxifylline 400 mg TDS  with gradual
                                                        |                    tapering
                                                        |
                                         ┌──────────────┴──────────────┐
                                         |                             |
                                   No response                   Adequate response
                                   • Thalidomide                continue with tapering of
                                   • Azathioprine/methotrexate/ clofazimine/ pentoxifylline as
                                     Cyclosporine               recommended over 12 months
                                   • Apremilast
```

*Restart MDT in case of treatment completion in late reaction, WHO recommends only clofazimine in such scenarios

Corticosteroids

Steroid therapy is a well-established method of controlling severe lepra reaction. It is useful in neuritis when muscle paralysis is threatened or real, iritis is not responding to steroid eye drops, in presence of epididymo-orchitis and in erythema necroticans (vesicular or bullous ENL).

Prednisolone is started at dose of 1 mg/kg/day, which should be given in single morning dose to coincide with the endogenous cortisol peak, and reductions can be made according to response *(also see Box 5.3, Chapter 5.1)*.[5] While a fixed duration regimen is recommended by some (Box 5.5), in patients with high bacterial counts, therapy will be required regularly or intermittently for years leading to complications. ENL is often recurrent or chronic in nature and frequently severe. Patients often require prolonged treatment with high doses of oral corticosteroids. Mortality in patients of ENL is often caused by steroid- related complications like sepsis which occur mostly in young people.[6]

Thalidomide *(also see page 270, Drug Formulary)*

Thalidomide was introduced by Sheskin in 1965 and has been regularly used in a number of leprosy centres. This drug is not generally available on prescription in most countries, and is banned in some parts of the world. Thalidomide is effective in improving symptoms of ENL. The proposed mechanisms of thalidomide include inhibition of TNF-α and neutrophil recruitment. Other proposed mechanisms include polarization of immune response towards Th2 with enhanced production of IL-2, IL-4 and 5; suppression of formation of IgM antibodies; decreased helper T cells and increased suppressor T cells production.[7-9]

The dosimetry in the management of T2LR is with a dosage of 3–4 tablets of 100 mg daily in divided dosage, tailing off as the reaction subsides and continuing on one tablet daily, or every alternate day, to prevent further outbreaks. It has no value in type 1 reaction. Other analogues that can be used include lenalidomide which has shown promising results and reduced side effects.

As with clofazimine, thalidomide can be used to wean a patient from a long period of steroid therapy. For patients with severe neuritis, epididymo-orchitis and uveitis, prednisone should be added with thalidomide.

The common reasons of *failure* of thalidomide include wrong selection of patient (patient may not have T2LR or patient may have both T1LR and T2LR in a case of BL), noncompliance (patient not taking the medicine) and borderline cases (often respond

Box 5.5: Fixed duration therapy for ENL effective for episodic ENL

Drug	Dosage	Duration
Prednisolone	40 mg/day	2 weeks
	30 mg/day	2 weeks
	20 mg/day	4 weeks
	15 mg/day	4 weeks
	10 mg/day	4 weeks
	5 mg/day	4 weeks
Total duration		**20 weeks**

poorly). Even in nonresponding cases, response to thalidomide can be seen if reaction is initially controlled with steroids and then thalidomide added at 100–200 mg daily, followed by slow tapering of steroids. In cases, where prednisone has been stopped and replaced by thalidomide, there has been a surprising lack of effect until small doses of prednisone have been added to treatment. Thus, it seems that thalidomide requires, for effectiveness in T2LR, a functioning adrenal cortex or concurrent small doses of steroid when the adrenal cortex is not functioning.

Although a number of side-effects, in addition to its teratogenic effect, were known prior to its introduction in leprosy therapy, these have not proved troublesome in leprosy. Commonly encountered side effects include constipation, drowsiness, dryness of oral and nasal mucosa, peripheral edema, dizziness, erythema of face and chest, skin rashes, and irreversible peripheral sensory neuritis. Thus, as long as it is not taken by women of childbearing age, the side-effects are definitely less than those of prednisone, especially in long-term use.[10] Because of its teratogenicity, thalidomide is contraindicated in women of childbearing group. In the United States FDA, the THALOMID Risk Evaluation and Mitigation Strategy (REMS) has been very effective at reducing thalidomide associated fetal exposure.

However, care must be taken to prevent deep vein thrombosis as coadministration of thalidomide with prednisone increases its risk.[11] The incidence of deep vein thrombosis (DVT) in ENL patients receiving thalidomide has been found to be as high as 6.6%. Prophylaxis with 75–150 mg/day of aspirin can help to reduce the incidence of DVT.[11] The neuropathy caused by thalidomide usually occurs after high doses are given for long periods. It is less commonly reported in leprosy as compared to conditions like multiple myeloma. The neuropathy caused by thalidomide is pure sensory with longest nerve fibers being affected the earliest. The deep tendon reflexes are often absent. The above findings usually helps to differentiate from leprosy associated neuropathy which is often sensory motor and is not length dependent and may be associated with thickened and tender nerve trunks with preserved deep tendon reflexes.[12]

Clofazimine (also see page 258, Drug Formulary)

High dose clofazimine has potent anti-inflammatory properties. As per WHO guidelines, it is advised to add clofazimine 100 mg thrice a day along with standard course of prednisolone and to continue for a maximum of 12 weeks. Further, the dose is tapered to clofazimine 100 mg twice daily for 12 weeks and then 100 mg once a day for 12–24 weeks. The total duration of treatment of high dose of clofazimine should not ideally exceed 12 months. It takes about 4–6 weeks for clofazimine to exert its anti-inflammatory action and to control ENL. A recent study, however, noted that when patients were randomized to receive clofazimine 100 mg per day or placebo, the drug showed no benefit in reducing ENL frequency or severity.[13] The main disadvantage with high dose clofazimine is the development of reddish brown pigmentation which further increases the stigma associated with leprosy. Management with clofazimine alone is indicated in patients with severe ENL when use of corticosteroids is contraindicated.[13]

Other Options

Other steroid sparing agents used are azathioprine *(also see page 273, Drug Formulary)*, methotrexate *(also see page 274, Drug Formulary)*, cyclosporine, hydroxychloroquine, high dose zinc and anti-TNF-α inhibitors for the treatment of recalcitrant ENL.

Azathioprine interferes with production of purines thus ultimately inhibiting synthesis of DNA and RNA. It also has anti-TNF-α action. Few studies have demonstrated that azathioprine may be a good steroid sparing agent for recurrent or chronic ENL.[14,15] The main reason for discontinuation of the drug is bone marrow suppression. Regular monitoring of blood counts and liver function tests further adds to the cost of treatment.

Methotrexate has also been used for treatment of T2LR and may offer a steroid sparing regimen for treatment. Methotrexate has been shown to be successful in patients with chronic steroid resistant ENL[16] and recent studies show that it is useful in recalcitrant cases.[17] It can be combined with steroids or thalidomide.

In a pilot study from Ethiopia, cyclosporine showed encouraging results in the treatment of acute ENL, but did not have a significant effect on reduction in cumulative steroid dose in case of chronic ENL. More studies are required to assess the efficacy and long-term effects of cyclosporine.[18]

Older drugs like colchicine and antimonials are now seldom used, as they are not very effective and have more adverse effects.

TNF-α inhibitors like infliximab[19] and etanercept,[20] have been successfully used in cases of treatment resistant recurrent ENL cases which have failed to respond to prednisolone, thalidomide and pentoxifylline. Infliximab in a dose of 5 mg/kg was used in a single case with repeated doses given on weeks 2 and 6. Response to treatment was seen within hours after starting treatment. No further episodes of ENL were seen in the one year of follow-up.[19] Etanercept has been used in a dose of 50 mg/week given subcutaneously. In all cases response was seen within a few weeks and the cumulative dose of prednisolone and thalidomide was significantly reduced. Biological agents can be used in difficult to treat cases of ENL which has failed the standard therapy. However, they must be used with caution especially in tuberculosis endemic countries which can lead to reactivation of latent infections. These drugs also increase the financial burden on the patient and thus must be used after considering all factors.

Minocycline (also see page 266, Drug Formulary)

In a prospective pilot study where the efficacy and safety of minocycline in patients with recurrent and/or chronic ENL was evaluated, the authors observed that minocycline is effective in controlling recurrent and/or chronic ENL.[21] Minocycline is used as a second line anti-leprosy drug and helps to reduce bacterial antigen load. Other than its antimicrobial activity, it also possesses anti-inflammatory, anti-apoptotic properties and inhibits proteolysis, angiogenesis, and production of collagenase.[22]

The main concern with long-term administration of steroids and other steroid sparing immune suppressants is the risk of blunting the host immune response. This increases the chances of multiplication of persisting *M. leprae* bacilli. The main advantages of using antibacterial drugs like clofazimine and minocycline are the combined immunomodulatory, anti-inflammatory and neuroprotective effect in addition to the antibacterial effect. Both have a relatively good safety profile which makes them a promising option in the management of refractory, recurrent and/or chronic ENL. The common side effect seen with both is the dyspigmentation which occurs with long-term administration. It has also been demonstrated that alternate day treatment with second line anti-leprosy drugs (clofazimine, ofloxacin, minocycline) led to a significant reduction in number of reactional episodes and mean dose of prednisolone required in patients who had persistent lesions in spite of completing standard WHO therapy.[23]

Apremilast

It is an oral phosphodiesterase-4 inhibitor which has immunomodulatory and anti-inflammatory actions. It inhibits the proinflammatory cytokines which play a key role in the pathogenesis of T2LR. In a report of two cases with recalcitrant ENL, apremilast showed promising effects with subsidence of skin lesions within 4 weeks. Extracutaneous symptoms like neuritis and arthralgia also improved. It can be considered as a good option in treatment resistant ENL or in cases where steroids or immunosuppressants are contraindicated.[24]

Leprosy Vaccines (also see Chapter 7, Section 7.2)

Immunotherapy with vaccination with *Mycobacterium indicus pranii* (MIP) or BCG was found to be useful in patients with a high BI as it upregulates host immune response thus enhancing bacterial clearance. Few studies showed that immunotherapy with MIP vaccine led to a quicker reduction in bacillary load. It also led to reduction in frequency and severity of ENL.[25,26]

REFERENCES

1. Arora P, Sardana K, Agarwal A, Lavania M. Resistance as a cause of chronic steroid dependent ENL: a novel paradigm with potential implications in management. Lepr Rev 2019;90:201–5.
2. Negera E, Walker SL, Girma S, Doni SN, Tsegaye D, Lambert SM, et al. Clinicopathological features of erythema nodosum leprosum: A case control study at ALERT hospital, Ethiopia. PLoS Negl Trop Dis 2017;11(10):e0006011.
3. Scollard DM, Marterlli CM, Stefani MM, Maroja Mde F, Villahermosa L, Pardillo F, Tamang KB. Risk factors for leprosy reactions in three endemic countries. Am J Trop Med Hyg 2015;92: 108–14.
4. Van Veen NHJ, Lockwood DNJ, Van Brakel WH, Ramirez J, Richardus JH. Interventions for erythema nodosum leprosum. A Cochrane review. Lepr Rev 2009;80:355–72.
5. Kamath S, Vaccaro SA, Rea TH, Ochoa MT. Recognizing and managing the immunologic reactions in leprosy. J Am Acad Dermatol 2014;71:795–803.
6. Walker SL, Lebas E, Doni SN, Lockwood DNJ, Lambert SM. The Mortality Associated with Erythema Nodosum Leprosum in Ethiopia: A Retrospective Hospital-based Study. PLoS Negl Trop Dis 2014;8(3):e2690.
7. Radomsky CL, Levine N. Thalidomide. Dermtol Clin 2001; 19:87–103.
8. Shanbhag PS, Viswanath V, Torsekar RG. Thalidomide: Current status. Indian J Dermatol Venerol Leprol 2006;72:75–80.
9. Walker SL, Waters MFR, Lockwood DNJ. The role of thalidomide in the management of erythema nodosum leprosum. Lepr Rev 2007;78:197–215.
10. Chaudhry NS, Rath SR, Visvanath V, Torsekar RG. Our experience of the use of thalidomide in the steroid-dependent severe erythema nodosum leprosum. Indian J Dermatol Venereol Leprol 2009;75:189.
11. Pôrto LAB, Grossi MA de F, Alecrim ES de, Xavier MH de SB, Paiva e Silva F, Pires AS, et al. Deep Venous Thrombosis in Patients with Erythema Nodosum Leprosum in the use of Thalidomide and Systemic Corticosteroid in Reference Service in Belo Horizonte, Minas Gerais. Case Rep Dermatol Med 2019;1–7.

12. Sabin T. Thalidomide Neuropathy and Leprous Neuritis. The Lancet 1974;303(7849):165–6.
13. Maghanoy A BM, Saunderson P, Scheelbeek P. A prospective randomised, double-blind, placebo controlled trial on the effect of extended clofazimine on Erythema Nodosum Leprosum in multibacillary leprosy. Lepr Rev 2017;88:208–16.
14. Jitendra SSV, Bachaspatimayum R, Devi AS, Rita S. Azathioprine in Chronic Recalcitrant Erythema Nodosum Leprosum: A Case Report. J Clin Diagn Res JCDR 2017;11:FD01-FD02.
15. Duraes SM, Salles Sde A, Leite VR, Gazzeta MO. Azathioprine as a steroid sparing agent in leprosy type 2 reactions: Report of nine cases. Lep Rev 2011;82:304–9.
16. Kar BR, Babu R. Methotrexate in resistant ENL. Int J Lepr Mycobact Dis Off Organ Int Lepr Assoc 2004;72:480–2.
17. Hossain D. Using methotrexate to treat patients with ENL unresponsive to steroids and clofazimine: a report on 9 patients. Lep Rev 2013;84:105–12.
18. Lambert SM, Nigusse SD, Alembo DT, Walker SL, Nicholls PG, Idriss MH, et al. Comparison of Efficacy and Safety of Cyclosporine to Prednisolone in the Treatment of Erythema Nodosum Leprosum: Two Randomised, Double Blind, Controlled Pilot Studies in Ethiopia. PLoS Negl Trop Dis 2016;10:e0004149.
19. Santos JRS, Vendramini DL, Nery J, Avelleira JCR. Etanercept in erythema nodosum leprosum. An Bras Dermatol 2017;92:575–7.
20. Faber WR, Jensema AJ, Goldschmidt WFM. Treatment of recurrent erythema nodosum leprosum with infliximab. N Engl J Med 2006;355:739.
21. Narang T, Sawatkar GU, Kumaran MS, Dogra S. Minocycline for Recurrent and/or Chronic Erythema Nodosum Leprosum. JAMA Dermatol 2015;151:1026–8.
22. Perret LJ, Tait CP. Nonantibiotic properties of tetracyclines and their clinical application in dermatology. Australas J Dermatol 2014;55:111–18.
23. Narang T, Bishnoi A, Dogra S, Saikia UN, Kavita. Alternate Anti-leprosy Regimen for Multi-drug Therapy Refractory Leprosy: A Retrospective Study from a Tertiary Care Center in North India. Am J Trop Med Hyg 2019;100:24–30.
24. Narang T, Kaushik A, Dogra S. Apremilast in chronic recalcitrant erythema nodosum leprosum: A report of two cases. Br J Dermatol 2019. doi:10.1111/bjd.18233.
25. Katoch K, Katoch VM, Natrajan M, Bhatia AS, Sreevatsa null, Gupta UD, et al. Treatment of bacilliferous BL/LL cases with combined chemotherapy and immunotherapy. Int J Lepr Mycobact Dis Off Organ Int Lepr Assoc 1995;63:202–12.
26. Narang T, Kaur I, Kumar B, Radotra BD, Dogra S. Comparative evaluation of immunotherapeutic efficacy of BCG and mw vaccines in patients of borderline lepromatous and lepromatous leprosy. Int J Lepr Mycobact Dis Off Organ Int Lepr Assoc 2005;73:105–14.

5.3 ACUTE EXACERBATIONS AND LUCIO REACTION

Kabir Sardana, Premanshu Bhushan

LUCIO LEPROSY

As discussed previously, the term Lucio leprosy, lazarine leprosy and Lucio-Latapi leprosy allude to the same spectrum of leprosy, wherein the morphology is characterized by diffuse infiltration, without visible nodulation, which subsequently gives a myxedematous appearance, and years later it becomes atrophic and ichthyosiform.[1]

Lucio phenomenon occurs 3–4 years after onset of disease, is more common in untreated patients or in those receiving inadequate treatment and presents with minimal systemic features or neuritis.[2,3] This contrasts with the features of ENL. The lesions are described as painful and tender red patches that appear on the skin, particularly on the extremities, become purpuric (the color not disappearing on pressure); the center of the purpuric lesion becomes necrotic and ulcerated and finally develops a brown or black crust (eschar) which falls off after a few days to leave a superficial atrophic scar (Figs 5.11 and 5.12).[4] On the legs, the ulceration is larger and more lasting, with jagged edges surrounded by an inflammatory zone. The lesions are frequently described as triangular, polygonal or angular, ulcers.[4] The disorder responds to steroids, or in many cases proper administration of MDT, but significantly not to thalidomide. The evolution of the process from onset to healing takes about fifteen days.

While Rea stated that Lucio's phenomenon is a distinctive reactional state, as judged by clinical, histopathological and therapeutic criteria, he further surmised that those patients have a singularly deficient defence mechanism which permits unhindered multiplication of bacilli, and exposure of bacterial antigen to circulating antibody results in vasculitis, infarction and skin necrosis.[4] The morphology of lesions corresponds with a histology of leukocytoclastic vasculitis superimposed on findings of diffuse lepromatous leprosy. A dense infiltrate of foam histiocytes replaces the dermis and, sometimes, extends to the subcutaneous tissue in the severe ulcerative lesions.

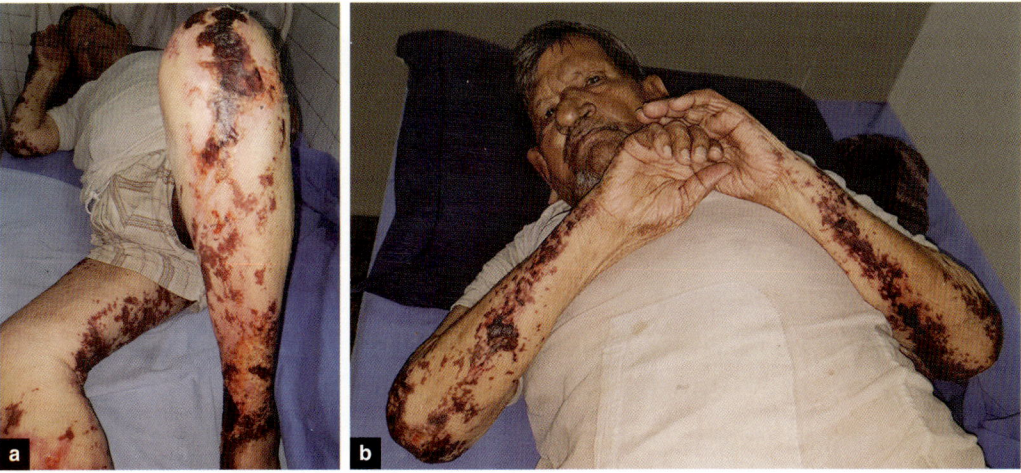

Fig. 5.11: (a) Lucio phenomenon (lower limb) with necrotic lesions with jagged margins; (b) Lucio phenomenon (upper limb)

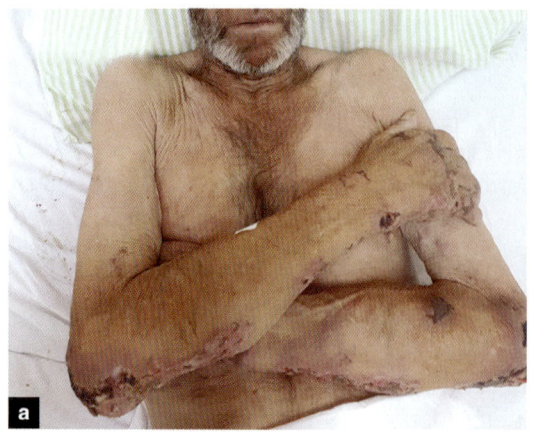
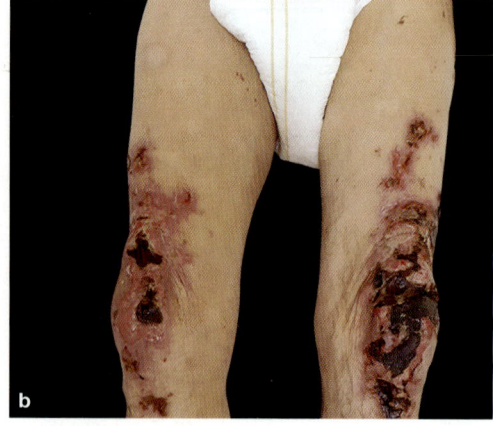

Fig. 5.12a and b: There are extensive, irregular shaped ulcers due to vascular thrombotic epidermal necrosis, mimicking an antiphospholipid antibody syndrome (*Courtesy*: Dr Jaison A Barreto)

The number of acid-fast bacilli is decreased, although they are found in great quantity in the surrounding areas. The ulceration is consequent to endothelial proliferation and thrombosis in the superficial vessels.[5]

Rea and Ridley[5] have compared the histology of these two types of reaction, and distinguish Lucio's phenomenon from ENL by ischemic epidermal necrosis, necrotising vasculitis of small blood vessels in the upper dermis, severe focal endothelial proliferation of mid-dermal vessels, and by the presence of large numbers of bacilli in endothelial cells. Thus, it seems to have a close resemblance to the Arthus reaction, a resemblance strengthened by the fact that neither type of reaction responds to thalidomide (compare ENL in which vasculitis plays a primary role). In fact, the clinical presentation mimics vasculitis and often can progress to digital gangrene with presence of antiphospholipid antibodies.[6]

While some authors believe that Lucio leprosy may be an extension of conventional ENL with severe vasculitis, purists differ and the difference are listed in Table 5.4.

Table 5.4: Difference between Lucio leprosy and ENL	
Lucio reaction	ENL
Seen in Lucio leprosy	Seen in BL and LLs leprosy
Seen in untreated cases or a few years after onset of disease	Usually patient is on treatment
Purpuric vasculitic lesions that may ulcerate and heal stellate scars	Nodules which are painful, generalized and occasionally necrotic
No general symptoms	Systemic features with fever seen
No neuritis	Neuritis may be marked
Superficial leukocytoclastic vasculitis and necrosis seen on histopathology	Superficial and deep leukocytoclastic vasculitis and superficial and deep necrosis seen
Does not respond to thalidomide; Lesions resolve in 15 days	Chronic condition in a proportion of cases and responsive to thalidomide

ACUTE EXACERBATIONS

Acute exacerbation of the disease is seen mainly in very advanced lepromatous patients with nodular and plaque-like lesions. Clinically the lesions undergo ulceration, that mimic a reaction but are exemplified by a lack of associated systemic features which are seen in ENL[8] (Fig. 5.13a and b). Histologically, there are small localized areas of necrosis in the middle of a large sheet of macrophages eliciting a localized infiltration of neutrophils. Vasculitis is rarely seen. The macrophages contain a relatively large load of AFB with many solid staining organisms which helps to differentiate acute exacerbation from ENL. It seems that there is a sudden localized burst of bacterial multiplication which outgrows the macrophage population resulting in localized necrosis and acute inflammation. Continuing the MDT seems the most useful measure.

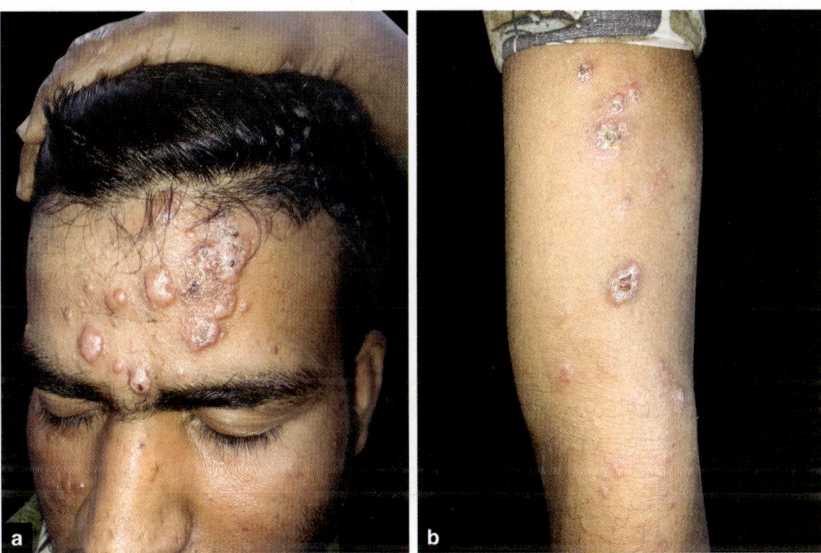

Fig. 5.13a and b: Acute exacerbation in an advanced untreated case of lepromatous leprosy with ulcerating nodules and plaques over face and arm. The slit smear showed a BI of 6+ with globi

REFERENCES

1. Lucio R., Alvarado I. Opusculosobre el mal de San Lazaro o elephantiasis de los Griegos. México: Murguía e Cia; 1852.
2. Saul A., Novales J. Lucio-Latapi leprosy and the Lucio phenomenon. Acta Leprol 1983;1:115–32.
3. Latapi F., Zamora A.C. The "spotted' leprosy of Lucio (la lepra Manchada de Lucio): An introduction to its clinical and histological study. Int JLepr 1948;16:421–30.
4. Rea TH. Lucio's phenomenon: an overview. Lepr Rev 1979;50:107–12.
5. Rea TH, Ridley DS. Lucio phenomenon: A comparative histological study. Int J Lepr 1979;47: 161–6.
6. Nunzie E, Ortega Cabrera LV, Macanchi Moncayo FM, Ortega Espinosa PF, Clapasson A, Massone C. Lucio Leprosy with Lucio's phenomenon, digital gangrene and anticardiolipin antibodies. Lepr Rev 2014;85:194–200.
7. Fogagnolo L, de Souza EM, Cintra ML, Velho PE. Vasculonecrotic reactions inleprosy. Braz J Infect Dis 2007;11:378–82.
8. Ridley DS, Ridley MJ. Exacerbation reactions in hyperactive lepromatous leprosy. Int J. Lepr Other Mycobac Dis 1984;52:384–94.

CHAPTER

6

Drug Resistance in Leprosy

6.1 DRUG RESISTANCE

Mallika Lavania, Utpal Sengupta

INTRODUCTION
Drug resistance is clinically assessed when there is a decrease in the effectiveness of a medication and usually means that the pathogens have "acquired" a mechanism leading to reduced response to a drug.[1–4] Currently, leprosy control is mainly based on World Health Organization (WHO) recommended multi-drug therapy (MDT).[5,6] It has been noted earlier that any therapeutic control measure of disease with antibiotics may lead to emergence of drug resistance.[1–7] Therefore, a surveillance mechanism should be in place for detecting the appearance of drug resistance in the community. Inability to deal with emerging resistance with appropriately tailored drug regimens will defeat the whole purpose of chemotherapy.

Global Epidemiology of Drug Resistance
In 2008 WHO started a surveillance network with six countries where leprosy is endemic (Brazil, China, Colombia, India, Myanmar and Vietnam), and subsequently a total of 19 countries participated in this sentinel surveillance.[5] In a recent WHO report, overall, 8% strains were found to have resistance conferring mutations. The average rate of rifampicin resistance among all leprosy cases was 3.8%, while in relapsed cases the resistance rate was 5.1% (secondary resistance) and in new cases the rate was 2.0% (primary resistance). Similarly, dapsone resistance was seen in 5.3% with secondary and primary resistance rates of 6.8% and 4% respectively. Ofloxacin resistance was seen in 1.3% with secondary and primary resistance rates of 1.7% and 1% respectively.[5] Further, the multi-drug resistance levels were low (20 of 154 resistant cases being resistant to both rifampicin and dapsone, to ofloxacin and dapsone but none to all three drugs or against both rifampicin and ofloxacin).[4,5]

Types of Drug Resistance
Drug resistance in leprosy may be primary or secondary. Primary resistance refers to infection with a strain of *M. leprae* which is already resistant to a drug in a treatment-naïve case. Drug-resistant *M. leprae* mutants in this scenario having been acquired from an infection source containing drug-resistant leprosy.[8] These cases typically present as new cases which are not responding to standard MDT regimen.[9] Secondary

resistance refers to development of resistance in a case on monotherapy or MDT who was initially responsive but later becomes unresponsive or who relapses after completing one or more courses of MDT.[8, 9] Typically, inadequate and irregular treatment has been implicated in the development of secondary drug resistance. Relapse is defined as a patient who completes an adequate course of treatment but subsequently develops new signs and symptoms of the disease either during surveillance period or thereafter[10] and may be caused by either persisters or rarely via reinfection[11] (*also see Chapter 2, Section 2.2*).

Different Mechanisms Involved in Drug Resistance

Antimicrobial resistance (AMR) is not a new phenomenon. In nature, microbes are constantly evolving in order to overcome the antimicrobial compounds produced by other microorganisms. The development of antimicrobial drugs and their widespread clinical use leads to selective pressure that promotes further evolution of resistance. Several important factors can accelerate the evolution of drug resistance. These include the overuse and misuse of antimicrobials, inappropriate use of antimicrobials, sub-therapeutic dosing of antimicrobials, and patient noncompliance to therapeutic regimen. Different resistance mechanisms may be employed by the microorganisms as discussed below and depicted in Fig. 6.1.

a. *Drug Modification or Inactivation*

Resistance genes may code for enzymes that chemically modify an antimicrobial, thereby inactivating it, or destroy an antimicrobial through hydrolysis. Resistance to many types of antimicrobials occurs through this mechanism.

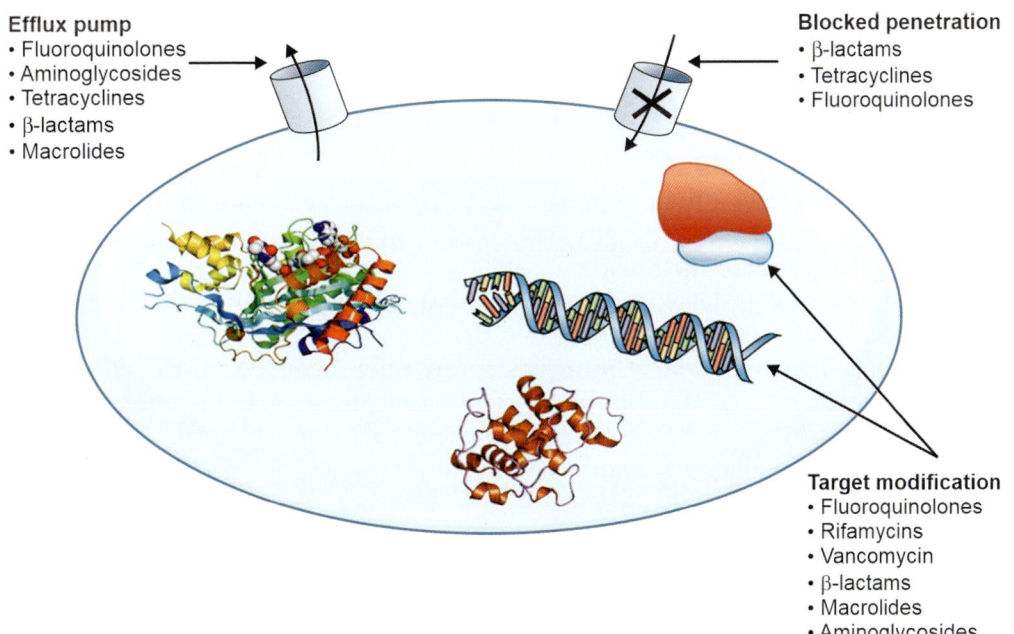

Fig. 6.1: A depiction of different mechanisms involved in drug resistance to antibiotics

b. Prevention of Cellular Uptake or Efflux

Microbes may develop resistance mechanisms that involve inhibiting the accumulation of an antimicrobial drug, which then prevents the drug from reaching its cellular target. This strategy is common among gram-negative pathogens and can involve changes in outer membrane lipid composition, porin channel selectivity, and/or porin channel concentrations.

c. Target Modification

Because antimicrobial drugs have very specific targets, structural changes to those targets can prevent drug binding, rendering the drug ineffective. Through spontaneous mutations in the genes encoding antibacterial drug targets, bacteria have an evolutionary advantage that allows them to develop resistance to drugs. This mechanism of resistance development is quite common.

d. Target Overproduction or Enzymatic Bypass

When an antimicrobial drug functions as an antimetabolite, targeting a specific enzyme to inhibit its activity, there are additional ways that microbial resistance may occur. First, the microbe may overproduce the target enzyme such that there is a sufficient amount of antimicrobial-free enzyme to carry out the proper enzymatic reaction. Second, the bacterial cell may develop a bypass that circumvents the need for the functional target enzyme. Both of these strategies have been found as mechanisms of sulfonamide resistance.

e. Target Mimicry

A recently discovered mechanism of resistance called target mimicry involves the production of proteins that bind and sequester drugs, preventing the drugs from binding to their target.

ANTI-LEPROSY DRUGS AND DEVELOPMENT OF RESISTANCE

Drug Susceptibility Testing[12-19]

Drug resistance is currently determined by *M. leprae* growth pattern in mouse footpad (MFP), several phenotypic methods as well as molecular methods like line probe assay/sequencing. These methods are not easy to use in field settings. Rapid DNA-based assays have been developed for detecting drug resistant *M. leprae* directly from clinical specimens over the past three decades (Fig. 6.2). Even though these assays have been based on molecular techniques, many reference laboratories in leprosy-endemic countries have the capability of utilizing these tools for detecting drug resistance (Fig. 6.3).

The WHO has mandated certain prerequisites for testing for resistance which are given in Table 6.1 and depicted in Fig. 6.4.[19a]

Mouse Foot Pad

Leprosy presents a very special problem for detecting drug resistance because *M. leprae* cannot be cultured axenically. Accordingly, drug susceptibility testing was non-existent until 1962 when Shepard and Chang developed the MFP assay for determining

Drug Resistance in Leprosy

Table 6.1: WHO recommendations for resistance testing in leprosy

New cases Inclusion criteria	Only *smear-positive* MB cases with a bacillary index (BI) >2+ are to be tested as these have a higher chance of a positive PCR
Retreatment cases	To detect secondary resistance, all retreatment leprosy cases have to be tested with the exception of transferred in cases unless they are considered at risk for AMR due to irregular treatment
Testing for drugs	PCR+ sequencing for *folP1*, *rpoB* and *gyrA* gene mutations
Samples	• 2 slit skin smear samples of the lesion with a BI ≥2+ should be taken, with the ear lobe being the preferred sampling site together with the most prominent skin lesion OR • 1 skin biopsy (e.g. 4 mm punch biopsy) should be taken from a prominent lesion with a BI ≥2+

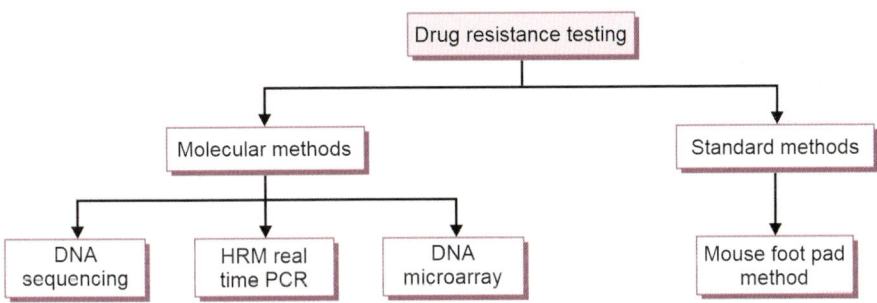

Fig. 6.2: Various techniques used for drug susceptibility testing

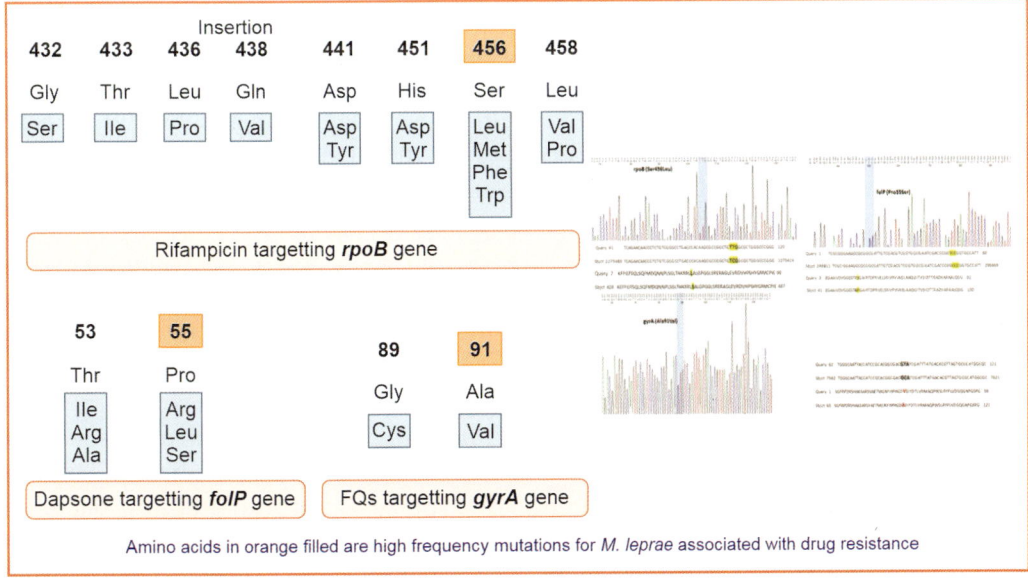

Amino acids in orange filled are high frequency mutations for *M. leprae* associated with drug resistance

Fig. 6.3: A depiction of multi-drug resistance by qPCR

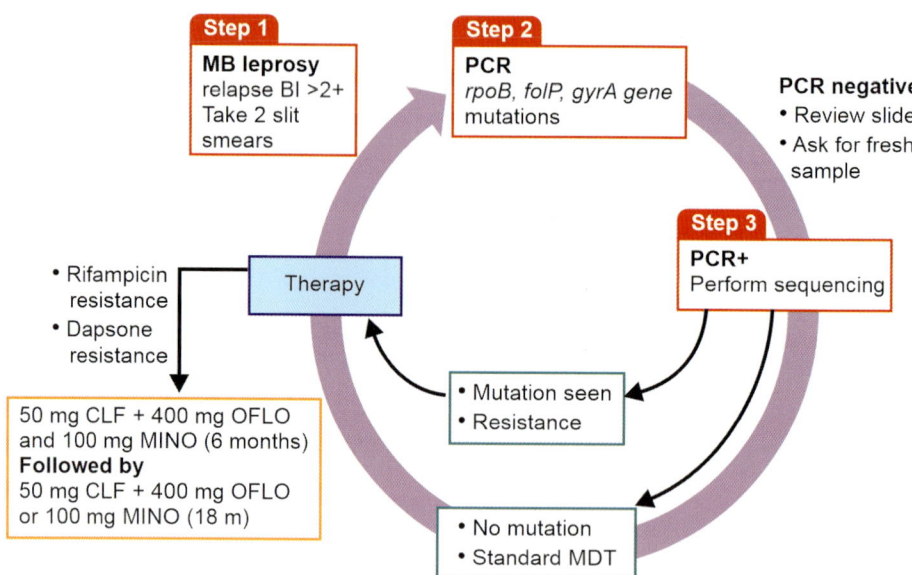

Fig. 6.4: Flow diagram for testing drug resistance in leprosy patients

M. leprae's susceptibility to anti-leprosy drugs.[20] Since its development, the MFP assay has been the 'gold standard' for leprosy drug susceptibility testing. This method requires the recovery of a sufficient number of viable organisms from a patient to inoculate the footpads of 20 to 40 mice (depending on the number of drugs to be tested) with each footpad receiving 5000–10,000 organisms. Infected mice are treated with the appropriate drug(s) orally. Mice are sacrificed after a defined period of time (usually 6 months or longer) and the numbers of bacilli in the footpads of treated mice and untreated mice are compared.

Minimal effective dose (MED) and minimum inhibitory concentration (MIC) are determined using the 'continuous' technique, involving the continuous administration of the drug (starting with the maximum tolerated dose, MTD) from the day of infection. If the drug is active at the maximum tolerated dose (MTD), the MED is determined from groups of mice receiving falling doses of the drug below the MTD, and the MIC is the concentration of the drug as determined in the serum of mice receiving the MED.

The list of drugs with their MICs is given in Table 6.2. Of these only rifampicin was first assessed and established as a powerful antileprosy drug by the mouse footpad technique before being tried in man.[13] The other drugs were tested only after having been first used successfully for the treatment of leprosy patients. The antileprosy drugs used after 1982, were first tested in mouse footpad.

The emergence of drug resistance during treatment (secondary drug resistance) is largely restricted to patients with multibacillary leprosy (BB, BL and LL types). The reason for this is that the frequency of drug-resistant mutants in a bacterial population is never greater than one per million bacteria, and bacterial populations of this size are only present in patients with multibacillary leprosy. Bacteriological proof of the emergence of drug-resistant strains of *M. leprae* as the cause of relapse in treated

Table 6.2: MIC of anti-leprosy drugs

	MED (% in diet)	MIC (µg/ml)	Bactericidal action
Rifampin	0.003	0.3	High
Dapsone (DDS)	0.0001	0.003	Low
Clofazimine	0.0003	NT	
Ofloxacin	0.025	0.2	High
Minocycline	0.01	0.2	High
Clarithromycin	0.01	0.125	High

NT: Estimate of MIC is not possible because of deposition of drug in tissues.

patients is dependent on the application of the MFP technique for identifying multiplication of bacteria in treated mice receiving doses of the drug in excess of the MED for the respective drug. By this method, the first bacteriological proof of drug resistance was reported to dapsone by Pettit and Rees in 1964.[14] Primary dapsone resistance refers to the patient who has never received dapsone but presents with a dapsone-resistant infection, having been infected with a dapsone-resistant strain of *M. leprae* and the first case of primary dapsone resistance was diagnosed in Ethiopia by Pearson et al (1977).[15] In the laboratory, dapsone-resistant *M. leprae* is defined as strains that multiply in mice receiving 0.0001% or more dapsone in the diet. Furthermore, with dapsone there are degrees of resistance ranging from low, intermediate or high depending on the growth of bacilli in mice who are administered 0.0001%, 0.001% or .0.01% dapsone in their diet. Thus, resistance to dapsone involves a multistep mutation.[16] Rifampicin resistant strains were discovered initially in 1976 by Jacobson and Hastings[17] followed by Grosset et al in 1989[18] and here there is a single step mutation with a median time to relapse of 9 years (1–12 years).[18] Unlike other drugs, the repository characteristic of clofazimine appears, to have delayed the development of resistance and the first clofazimine-resistant strain of *M. leprae* reported on further passage in mice was not fully substantiated.[19] Regarding ofloxacin, mutations are seen in the *gyrA* and *gyrB* genes and the first ofloxacin-resistant *M. leprae* was described in 1994.

Mutation Detection by PCR-DNA Sequencing

Drug susceptibility testing by MFP is cumbersome, time-consuming, not applicable to many strains and does not provide comprehensive data to monitor global level of resistance. In this regard, mutation detection by PCR-DNA sequencing is advantageous. Globally, researchers are using this method for mutation detection.[1, 5–7, 21, 22] The method requires bacilli scrapped from active lesion or ear lobes in 70% ethanol vial and transported to laboratory for DNA extraction. The drug mutations lie in one or several codons located within short stretches of DNA in each target gene, referred to as the drug resistance determining regions (DRDRs). Further DRDRs are amplified by PCR targeting genes *rpoB*, *folP* and *gyrA* responsible for resistance to rifampicin, dapsone and ofloxacin respectively (Table 6.3). PCR amplified products are sequenced. Samples with known missense mutations within a limited region in these genes are checked.

Table 6.3: Mutations within anti-leprosy drug target genes that confer resistance to *M. leprae*		
Drug susceptibility MFP assay[1]	Amino acid mutation[2]	Number of resistant isolates
R	Thr53Ala	14
NC	Thr53Ala; Pro55Leu	1
R	Thr53Arg	7
R	Thr53Ile	15
R	Thr53Val	3
R	Pro55Arg	21
R	*Pro55Leu*	27
R	Pro55Ser	1
R	Gln438Val	1
R	Phe439 (Lys + Phe insert) Met440	1
NC	Asp441Tyr	2
NC	Asp441Asn	1
NC	Asp441Asn; Leu458Pro	1
R	His451Asp	2
R	His451Asp; Gly432Ser	1
R	His451Tyr	20
R	*Ser456Leu*	70
R	Ser456Met	1
R	Ser456Met; Leu458Val	1
R	Ser456Phe	2
NC	Ser456Trp	1
NC	Gly89Cys	1
R	*Ala91Val*	12

[1]R: Resistant in mouse footpad assay. NC: Not confirmed in mouse footpad assay.
[2]Amino acid substitution in drug target protein; Mutant amino acids in bold and italics are high frequency mutations for *M. leprae* drug resistance.

Probe-based Drug Susceptibility Testing

Analysis of mutations is generally performed by sequencing the target genomic region, amplified by PCR, although the implementation of sequencing is not easy in many developing countries. Therefore, a simple and rapid method which can be carried out without any special equipment such as sequencer, has been developed. In microarray, a series of oligonucleotides probes corresponding to each mutation detected in the *folP*, *rpoB* and *gyrA* genes are selected and fixed on glass slide as capture probes. Probes are hybridized with the denatured samples of leprosy patients and further result analyzed in the form of dots/signal on slides.[23]

Another method—GenoType Leprae DR involves probes to capture wild type and mutants coated on a strip. PCR products for the above mentioned genes are amplified, denatured, then hybridized and coloration is performed.

Real-time PCR-based High Resolution Melting Analysis

Real-time PCR-based high resolution melt (PCR-HRM) analysis is a novel simple post-PCR step that exploits thermal characteristics of the amplicons for detection of sequence variants. Emerging real-time PCR technologies can eliminate post-PCR procedures for genotyping any *M. leprae* genomic target of interest, particularly those suitable for leprosy epidemiology applications. In HRM analysis, amplified DNA is denatured in precise temperature increments to produce melt curves with features that are dependent upon nucleotide sequence. Curves with similar shapes are derived from the same DNA sequence and can be clustered together, allowing researchers to analyze genetic variants post-PCR. This technique proved inexpensive and convenient for the preliminary screening of DNAs and rapid classification of clinical strains into wild type or variant clusters, which carry some of the known mutations in the DRDRs.[24]

CONCLUSION

Although mouse footpad studies are recommended for confirmation of drug resistance in leprosy, these facilities are not available freely, forcing clinicians to rely on clinical features alone. Drug resistance may itself be a reason for relapse and it is important to differentiate the two, as outlined in Table 6.4.[25]

Results obtained from drug resistance testing could be used to develop point of care tests and also determine strategies for effective leprosy eradication programmes. The information on resistant cases should become an integral component of an overall public health strategy and help in better patient care in future. In addition, it can provide monitoring of the spread of drug-resistant *M. leprae*.

Table 6.4: Drug-resistant leprosy versus relapse

Drug-resistant leprosy	*Relapse*
Because of primary or secondary drug resistance	Mainly due to persisters
Initial amelioration followed by halt or worsening	Recurrence after release from MDT
Appearance of new lesions	Appearance of new lesions over old lesions
Patient downgrades	Patient rarely downgrades

REFERENCES

1. Honore N, Cole ST. Molecular basis of rifampin resistance in *Mycobacterium leprae*. Antimicrob. Agents Chemother 1993;37:414–8.
2. Ebenezer GJ, Norman G, Joseph GA, Daniel S, Job CK. Drug resistant *Mycobacterium leprae*—results of mouse footpad studies from a laboratory in South India. Indian J Lepr 2002;74: 301–12.
3. Williams DL, Gillis TP. Molecular detection of drug resistance in *Mycobacterium leprae*. Lepr Rev 2004;75:118–30.
4. Matsuoka M, Budiawan T, Aye KS, Kyaw K, Tan EV, Cruz ED, Gelber R, Saunderson P, Balagon V, Pannikar V. The frequency of drug resistance mutations in *Mycobacterium leprae* isolates in untreated and relapsed leprosy patients from Myanmar, Indonesia and the Philippines. Lepr Rev 2007;78:343–52.
5. Cambau E, Saunderson P, Matsuoka M, Cole ST, Kai M, Suffys P, et al. WHO surveillance network of antimicrobial resistance in leprosy. Antimicrobial resistance in leprosy: Results of the first

prospective open survey conducted by a WHO surveillance network for the period 2009–15. Clin Microbiol Infect. 2018;24:1305–10.

6. Lavania M, Nigam A, Turankar RP, Singh I, Gupta P, Kumar S, Sengupta U, John AS. Emergence of primary drug resistance to rifampicin in *Mycobacterium leprae* strains from leprosy patients in India. Clin Microbiol Infect 2015;21:e85–6.
7. Lavania M, Singh I, Turankar RP, Ahuja M, Pathak V, Sengupta U, Das L, Kumar A, Darlong J, Nathan R, Maseey A. Molecular detection of multidrug-resistant *Mycobacterium leprae* from Indian leprosy patients. J Glob Antimicrob Resist 2018;12:214–9.
8. Williams DL, Gillis TP. Drug-resistant leprosy: Monitoring and current status. Lepr Rev 2012,83:269–81.
9. Global leprosy programme. Drug resistance in leprosy. Worl Health Organisation. Available from: http://www.searo.who.int/entity/global_leprosy_programme/top-ics/drug_resistance/en/. Accessed on 20th september 2019.
10. Kaimal S, Thappa DM. Relapse in leprosy. Indian J Dermatol Venereol Leprol 2009;75:126–35.
11. Ramu G. Clinical features and diagnosis of relapses in leprosy. Indian J Lepr 1995;67:45–59.
12. Jacobson RR. Treatment of leprosy. In: Hastings RC, editor. Leprosy. New York: Churchill Livingstone; 1994. p. 317–49.
13. Rees RJW, Pearson JMH, Waters MFR. Experimental and clinical studies of rifampin in treatment of leprosy. British Medical Journal 1970,1:89.
14. Pettit JHS, Rees RJW. Sulphone resistance in leprosy. An experimental and clinical study. Lancet 1964;2:673–4.
15. Pearson JMH, Haik GS, Rees RJW. Primary dapsone-resistant leprosy. Leprosy Review 1977;48:129–32.
16. Meade TW, Pearson JMH, Rees RJW, North WRS. The epidemiology of sulphone-resistant leprosy. International Journal of leprosy 1973;41:684.
17. Jacobson RR, Hastings RC. Rifampin-resistant leprosy. Lancet 1976;2:1304–5.
18. Grosset JH, et al. Study of 38 documented relapses of multibacillary leprosy after treatment with rifampicin. International Journal of Leprosy 1989;51:607–14.
19. Levy L. Clofazimine resistant *M. leprae*. International Journal of Leprosy 1986;54:137–40.
19a. Leprosy. In Sardana K, Sinha S, Rani S. Compendium of Dermatology for Examinations. CBS Publishers & Distributors Pvt Ltd., 1st Edn, 2020, 325.
20. Shepard CC, Chang YT. Effect of several anti-leprosy drugs on multiplication of human leprosy bacilli in footpads of mice. Proc Soc Exp Biol Med 1962;109:636–8.
21. Honoré N, Roche PW, Grosset JH, Cole ST. A method for rapid detection of rifampicin-resistant isolates of *Mycobacterium leprae*. Lepr Rev 2001;72:441–8.
22. Lavania M, Jadhav RS, Chaitanya VS, Turankar R, Selvasekhar A, Das L, Darlong F, Hambroom UK, Kumar S, Sengupta U. Drug resistance patterns in *Mycobacterium leprae* isolates from relapsed leprosy patients attending The Leprosy Mission (TLM) Hospitals in India. Lepr Rev 2014; 85:177–85.
23. Matsuoka M1, Aye KS, Kyaw K, Tan EV, Balagon MV, Saunderson P, Gelber R, Makino M, Nakajima C, Suzuki Y. A novel method for simple detection of mutations conferring drug resistance in *Mycobacterium leprae*, based on a DNA microarray, and its applicability in developing countries. J Med Microbiol 2008;57:1213–9.
24. Li W, Matsuoka M, Kai M, Thapa P, Khadge S, Hagge DA, Brennan PJ, Vissa V. Real-time PCR and high-resolution melt analysis for rapid detection of *Mycobacterium leprae* drug resistance mutations and strain types. J Clin Microbiol 2012;50:742–53.
25. Desikan KV. Relapse, reactivation or reinfection? Indian J Lepr 1995;67:3–11.

6.2 CLINICAL RELEVANCE OF RESISTANCE

Kabir Sardana, Ananta Khurana

While resistance testing methods are discussed in detail in another chapter, our aim here is to dwell on two aspects relevant to the practicing clinicians, namely when to suspect and test for resistance and most importantly the therapeutic relevance of resistance in the real world scenario.

While the WHO protocol recommends[1] that resistance testing may be performed for new cases, re-treatment (including re-treatment after loss to follow-up, relapse, transferred in and other retreatments), most of the data on resistance focusses on relapse. The data on resistance varies worldwide; a WHO study noted that of the 1932 cases studied (1143 relapse and 789 new), 8.0% had *M. leprae* strains that were found to have mutations conferring resistance.[2] The therapeutic implications are that the alternative leprosy drugs are to be administered only in cases of rifampicin resistance which was seen in 5.1% of relapse case but ominously was also seen in 2% of new cases. Post-dating this study, another work showed antimicrobial resistance (AMR) in 11.3% of cases from France and 43.24% from the Brazilian Amazon.[3,4] The data from other parts of the world like India also reports this trend though the level of AMR is markedly less with an initial study showing an incidence of only 3.6% with respect to rifampicin resistance.[5–8]

Here it is relevant to appreciate that resistance is not a common "suspect" in all relapse cases as in the latter persisters are probably a commoner cause than AMR. While reaction and relapse can be differentiated on clinical grounds (*see Chapter 2, Section 2.2*), there is a need to suspect resistance in nonresponders and those on irregular treatment in both relapses and certain reactions.[1,8a] A patient, especially multibacillary (MB), whose morphological index (MI) does not fall even after 6 weeks of regular MDT may be a good working definition of a nonresponder as clinical activity may not necessarily correlate with the treatment efficacy. An ideal scenario would be to inoculate and confirm growth in mouse footpad, but this is not a technically feasible option and moreover requires at least 10,000 bacilli as an inocula which may not be possible in all cases—specially paucibacillary (PB) cases. A more important relevant association is with reactions. We have seen documented cases of ENL—recurrent and chronic—and also type 1 reactions (downgrading) with proven resistance by molecular confirmation.[9,10] While it may be theorized that mere presence of resistant bacilli does not mean that it is the overbearing cause of a reaction, salutary response to alternative leprosy therapy (ALT) has been seen, thus translating this important aspect into clinical practice.[9,10] In a recent symposium, a center in Chhattisgarh,[11] India, used reactions as a criterion for resistance testing and included recurrent reactions—both type 1 lepra reaction after release from treatment (RFT) and type 2 lepra reaction. Interestingly, all patients (100%) with recurrent type 1 reaction or relapse after RFT were prone to develop drug resistance followed by patients with recurrent type 2 reaction (75%). Drug resistance in defaulters was seen in only 3% of cases.[11]

It has been believed that the immune response in reactions is towards dead bacilli but two studies have shown that, both in type 1 reaction, and late reaction, viable *M. leprae* have a role.[12,13] Notably, even smear negative BT patients manifesting as late reversal reactions had viable bacilli on mouse footpad inoculation. One plausible explanation for viability even after MDT is possibly resistance. Recently, a late reaction case which was being treated with steroids was found to have resistant bacilli thus highlighting the perils of administering steroids or immunosuppressive drugs.[14]

The treatment implications and outcomes in patients with resistance has not been adequately studied. It is established that resistance to dapsone does not require any change in therapy of multibacillary disease and clofazimine is a good replacement of dapsone in PB MDT. Ofloxacin resistance again is not a cause of worry as it is not part of the conventional MDT. While rifampicin resistance is treated with ALT, published data on long-term relapses is not available. In reactions, though the majority of the work has focused on cytokines and methods to suppress the immune response, surprisingly no thought has been spent on the possibility of resistance as a trigger for reactions. This is surprising as most of cytokine response is directed at the antigen- largely *M. leprae*, and there is good reason to believe that more the load of live bacilli, more persistent would be the reaction. More important is the fact that most immunosuppressive drugs suppress the immune response, and by extension the cytokines that protect against *M. leprae*, and thus the use of such drugs would also possibly prolong the viability of *M. leprae*.

It seems that the therapy of reactions is largely directed at the effect and not the cause. We have seen documented cases of reactions who were unresponsive to high doses of steroids, immunosuppressive and even thalidomide but responded within weeks of starting ALT,[10,11] which accounts for the relevant "clinical outcome" data in a subset of reactions, which needs to be further explored. Conversely, in a case of late reaction with resistance, the patient's lesions subsided on steroids before resistance was confirmed, but we added the modified regimen,[14] this has major therapeutic implications as such cases can be a source of resistant bacilli transmission of which has been documented in a recent paper.[15]

Thus, it is time to modify the WHO criterion for suspecting resistance with a wider inclusion criterion that includes certain reactions, in addition to relapses. This may make the implications of resistance more clinically relevant. Pertinently, to make it clinically useful, an attempt should be made to delineate scenarios where resistance can be suspected and also look at whether modified treatment affects the outcomes and reduce transmission characteristics of leprosy.

REFERENCES

1. A guide for surveillance of antimicrobial resistance in leprosy: 2017 update ISBN: 978 92 9022 619 2 © World Health Organization 2017.
2. Cambau E, Saunderson P, Matsuoka M, Cole ST, Kai M, Suffys P, et al. Antimicrobial resistance in leprosy: Results of the first prospective open survey conducted by a WHO surveillance network for the period 2009–2015. Clin Microbiol Infect 2018;24:1305–10.
3. Chauffour A, Lecorche E, Reibel F, Mougari F, Raskine L, Aubry A, Jarlier V, Cambau E; CNR-MyRMA. Prospective study on antimicrobial resistance in leprosy cases diagnosed in France from 2001 to 2015. Clin Microbiol Infect 2018;24:1213.e5–1213.
4. Beltrán-Alzate C, López Díaz F, Romero-Montoya M, Sakamuri R, Li W, Kimura M, Brennan P, Cardona-Castro N. Leprosy Drug Resistance Surveillance in Colombia: The Experience of a Sentinel Country. PLoS Negl Trop Dis 2016;10:e0005041.
5. Lavania M, Singh I, Turankar RP, Ahuja M, Pathak V, Sengupta U, et al. Molecular detection of multidrug-resistant *Mycobacterium leprae* from Indian leprosy patients. J Glob Antimicrob Resist 2018;12:214–9.

6. Vedithi SC, Malhotra S, Das M, Daniel S, Kishore N, George A, Arumugam S, Rajan L, Ebenezer M, Ascher DB, Arnold E, Blundell TL. Structural Implications of Mutations Conferring Rifampin Resistance in *Mycobacterium leprae*. Sci Rep 2018;8:5016.
7. Hasanoor Reja AH, Biswas N, Biswas S, Lavania M, Chaitanya VS, Banerjee S, et al. Report of rpoB mutation in clinically suspected cases of drug-resistant leprosy: A study from Eastern India. Indian J Dermatol Venereol Leprol 2015;81:155–61.
8. Lavania M, Jadhav RS, Chaitanya VS, Turankar R, Selvasekhar A, Das L, et al. Drug resistance patterns in *Mycobacterium leprae* isolates from relapsed leprosy patients attending The Leprosy Mission (TLM) Hospitals in India. Lepr Rev 2014;85:177–85.
8a. Kamat D, Narang T, Ahuja M, et al. Multidrug Resistant *Mycobacterium leprae* in a Case of Smear Negative Relapse. Am. J. Trop Med, Hyg. 2020, Feb 10.
9. Sinha S, Sardana K, Agrawal D, Malhotra P, Lavania M, Ahuja M. Multidrug resistance as a cause of steroid-nonresponsive downgrading type I reaction in Hansen's disease. Int J Mycobacteriol 2019;8:305–8.
10. Arora P, Sardana K, Agarwal A, Lavania M. Resistance as a cause of chronic steroid dependent ENL: A novel paradigm with potential implications in management. Lepr Rev 2019;90:201–05.
11. Turankar RP, Lavania M, Singh I, Ahuja M, PAthank VK, Singh V, et al. Relapse and Drug Resistance in Leprosy: Present Scenario and Critical Issues. Indian J Lepr 2018;90:79–93.
12. Shetty VP, Wakade A, Antia NH. A high incidence of viable *Mycobacterium leprae* in post-MDT recurrent lesions in tuberculoid leprosy patients. Lepr Rev 2001;72:337–44.
13. Save MP, Dighe AR, Natrajan M, Shetty VP. Association of viable *Mycobacterium leprae* with Type 1 reaction in leprosy. Lepr Rev 2016;87:78–92.
14. Sardana K, Mathachan SR, Agrawal D, Lavania M, Ahuja M. Late reversal reaction with resistant *Mycobacterium leprae*: An emerging paradigm. Trop Doct 2019 Nov 9:49475519884421.
15. Avanzi C, Busso P, Benjak A, Loiseau C, Fomba A, Doumbia G, Camara I, LamouA, Sock G, Drame T, Kodio M, Sakho F, Sow SO, Cole ST, Johnson RC. Transmission of Drug-resistant Leprosy in Guinea-Conakry Detected Using Molecular Epidemiological Approaches. Clin Infect Dis 2016;63:1482–4.

CHAPTER 7

Chemotherapy

7.1 TREATMENT OF LEPROSY

Kabir Sardana, Premanshu Bhushan, Ananta Khurana

INTRODUCTION

The introduction of WHO multi-drug therapy (MDT) in 1982 was meant to sufficiently treat leprosy patients and while it has been a largely successful, there has been of late the emergent need for a second line drug therapy in view of drug resistance. An important finding of the Marchoux chemotherapy study was to assess the long-term efficacy of MDT, where it was found that relapses were significantly more frequent among the patients with BI ≥4 before MDT or ≥3 at the end of MDT.[1] That rifampicin (RMP) or clofazimine (CLO) resistance was not demonstrated among the strains of *M. leprae* isolated from relapsed patients, and that relapse was closely correlated with the bacterial load of the patient, suggest that the relapses were not caused by the emergence of drug resistance, but by viable *M. leprae* ("persisters") that had survived treatment. Thus, these patients would respond to a second course of MDT. While resistance to dapsone (DDS) has been known, it is largely a secondary resistance. The treatment modification is however definitely needed in case of rifampicin resistance. While this is one major area of interest, the MDT itself can have issues including adverse drug reactions (ADR) which might need modification of the treatment regimen. Further, adherence to the long treatment regimens is another important issue and completion needs to be ensured for both treatment efficacy and prevention of relapses. Patients on paucibacillary MDT (PB-MDT) must complete their course of 6 doses within 9 months and those on multibacillary MDT (MB-MDT) are expected to complete 12 doses within 24 months. A uniform 3-drug regimen for both PB and MB cases (uniform MDT or U-MDT) is a step in easing some complexities associated with the current WHO MB-MDT and PB-MDT regimens (discussed later). One of the goals of disease control is prophylaxis, which is an issue that has bothered leprosy workers for ages. Even though it is difficult to find an ideal prophylactic regimen for a disease like leprosy with a long incubation period, single dose rifampicin (SDR) has been recommended for chemoprophylaxis and is undergoing further trials in different endemic areas to overcome the scientific issues that some experts feel affects its universal applicability *(see Chapter 7, Section 7.2)*.

The aim of this chapter would be to dwell on the basis of chemotherapy of leprosy, its rationale and the principles that involve new drug discovery.

Rationale of MDT Therapy[2,3]

The aim of MDT is to kill all viable bacilli, both the resistant and susceptible, with the secondary aim to avoid relapses.

Drug resistant mutants: The principle employed is the rule of genetic independence of mutation, which defines that bacilli resistant to one drug remain sensitive to another if it has a mechanism of action different from the former. In a patient with multibacillary (MB) leprosy, the maximal number of acid-fast bacilli (AFB) could be 100 billion (10^{11}) or 1 trillion (10^{12}), of which on an average only 1% (10^9 or 10^{10}) are viable.[3,4] It is estimated that of these, 1 in 10^7 are resistant to rifampicin while 1 in 10^6 each are resistant to dapsone or clofazimine. Thus, a patient with MB leprosy harbors, at most, 10^9 drug-susceptible organisms, 10^3 rifampicin-resistant mutants, and 10^4 dapsone-, clofazimine- or thioamide-resistant mutants (Fig. 7.1). Further, a two-drug combination of rifampicin with either dapsone or clofazimine will likely have a resistant strain in 1 of 10^{13} bacilli, which is beyond the total number of bacilli in the patient. Similarly, resistance to the combination of three drugs (rifampicin, clofazimine and dapsone) is likely in a proportion of 1 in 10^{19}, which is way more than the biological load of bacilli in the patients (Table 7.1). Thus, while in theory, even a two-drug combination is enough, this three-drug

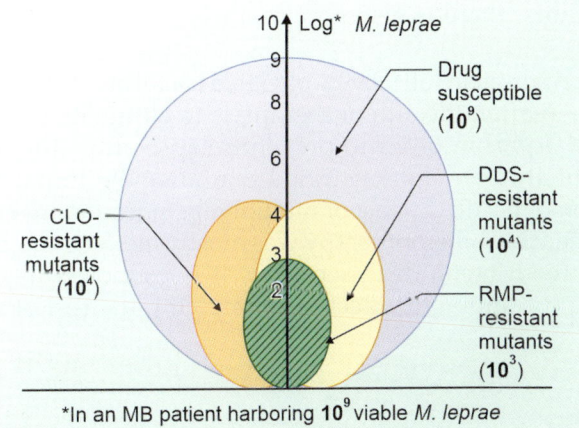

Fig. 7.1: Bacillary population in multibacillary leprosy with resistant mutants, out of the total viable bacilli

Table 7.1: Drug-resistant mutants in a sample population of *M. leprae*		
	Resistant mutants*	
Drug(s)	%	Total no.
Rifampin (RMP)	1 per 10^7	10^3
Dapsone (DDS)	1 per 10^6	10^4
Clofazimine (CLO)	1 per 10^6	10^4
RMP + DDS	1 per 10^{13}	10^{-3}
RMP + CLO	1 per 10^{13}	10^{-3}
DDS + CLO	1 per 10^{12}	10^{-2}
RMP + DDS + CLO	1 per 10^{19}	10^{-9}

*In all MB patient harboring 10^{10} viable *M. leprae*

combination is recommended to take care of the possibility of primary and secondary dapsone resistance[5] (Fig. 7.2).

Dapsone, being poorly bactericidal, must be given at a daily dose of 100 mg in adults while clofazimine, also poorly bactericidal, has to be given daily at a dose of 50 mg with a monthly supplement of 300 mg. For rifampicin, a single dose of 600 mg kills more than 99% of the susceptible organisms present at the start of treatment, that is as much as 3 to 6 months of daily treatment with the combination dapsone plus clofazimine (Fig. 7.2).[2, 3, 6] Since daily treatment with rifampicin did not demonstrate a greater bactericidal activity than monthly treatment,[7] there is no need to give rifampicin daily, even during the initial phase of chemotherapy. By definition, mutants resistant to dapsone and clofazimine are fully susceptible to rifampicin and are killed by the first dose(s) of rifampicin; whereas it takes a much longer duration of daily administration of dapsone and clofazimine to get rid of rifampicin-resistant mutants. The duration of this is *not* defined and hence these two are given throughout the treatment period. Similarly, while in paucibacillary (PB) cases the total number of bacilli is about 10^6 and chance of resistance is low, but in view of primary dapsone resistance, at least two drugs are recommended.

Drug sensitive bacilli: During the initial phase of MDT, in addition to the killing of drug-resistant mutants, there is also an extremely rapid killing of drug-susceptible organisms (Fig. 7.3).

The first doses of rifampicin kill 99.99% of viable bacilli and thus, reduce their number from 10^{10} to 10^5. Thereafter, the aim of therapy is to eliminate these remaining viable drug-susceptible *M. leprae* in order to prevent relapse after stopping treatment. The Bamako-Chingleput study[3, 7] demonstrated that after the initial rapid killing of *M. leprae*, the proportion of bacilli capable of multiplying in mice remained constant during the 2 years of treatment and chemotherapy was mostly ineffective against the remaining organisms despite them being drug-sensitive. It is proposed that after initial rapid killing (due to the post-antibiotic effect of rifampicin), the rest of the doses maintain

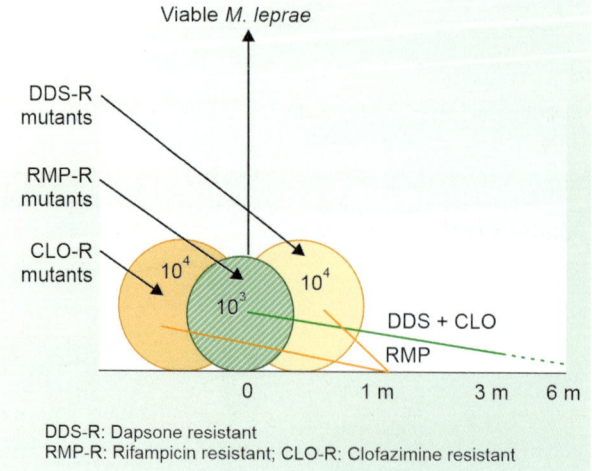

Fig. 7.2: Outcome of drug-resistant mutants in patients on combined chemotherapy (MDT) RMP is able to kill the CLO- and DDS-resistant mutants in addition to RMP susceptible mutants, within a short span. DDS + CLO however would take a much prolonged time to kill RMP-resistant mutants

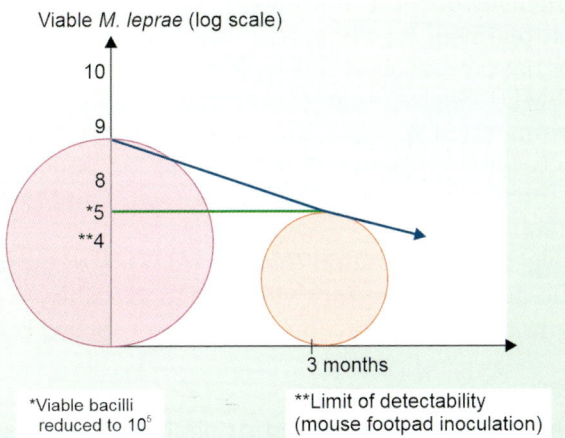

Fig. 7.3: Outcome of drug-susceptible *M. leprae* with MDT—a rapid fall in viable bacilli within a small duration of time (estimated to be 3 months)

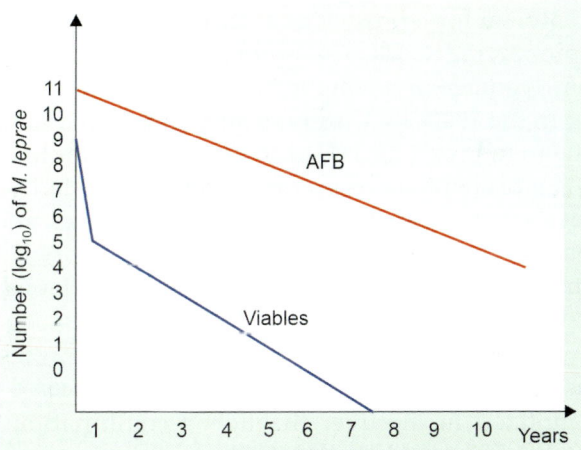

Fig. 7.4: A depiction of decrease in the bacillary load in a MB case (0.62 log per year). While the population of viable bacilli reduces rapidly initially, with initiation of MB-MDT (a fall from about 10^{11} to 10^5 bacilli within a short span), further fall is gradual and parallels the fall in slit skin smears

the remaining organisms in their dormant state so that the clearing mechanisms of the host can eliminate them progressively. Based on existing data, the time required to clear 10^5 *M. leprae* at a speed of 0.62 log per year is about 7–8 years for a MB case of leprosy with maximal bacterial load (Fig. 7.4). This is, more or less, the time necessary for a MB patient with a bacterial index (BI) of 4 to 5 + to reach skin-smear negativity, and may be shorter in cases with lower initial BI. It has been shown that the relapse rates are higher in patients with higher initial BI (≥4), very short-course MDT and those who have received <3 doses of rifampicin; thus accounting for the longer duration of treatment which should ideally be optimized based on the bacillary load of individual patients.

Even after 6-month course of MDT in PB cases, about 4–28% cases[8] have active lesions, but they usually subside after stopping MDT. In addition, reversal reactions may happen after stopping treatment[9] and cause nerve damage.[9] Because of the relatively low frequencies of these findings, it is not recommended to extend the 6-month duration of treatment for PB leprosy. Even among MB cases of leprosy, less than 1% of relapses have been observed within the first 5 years of follow-up after completion of WHO-MDT. Such a finding is a strong evidence of the potent bactericidal activity of the recommended regimen and of its capacity to cope with persisters. Another finding of crucial importance is that, among MB patients who relapsed after an extremely short course of MDT containing rifampicin,[10] the bacilli were sensitive to a repeat course of treatment.

Based on the above, a fixed duration therapy (FDT) is recommended, but certain clinicians prolong the duration in certain MB cases to, possibly, avoid relapses. This is admittedly contrary to the U-MDT recommendation proposed by WHO (*see below*).

Common Drugs Used

While we are detailing the commonly used drugs below, details of these and other drugs are provided in the formulary (*see pages 257 to 277*).

1. DAPSONE (DDS—4,4'-DIAMINODIPHENYL SULFONE)

The first effective treatment for leprosy was a sulfone named Promin (glucosulphone sodium), and this pioneering work was reported from Carville, USA in 1943.[11] It however had the disadvantage of having to be administered intravenously. Dapsone was introduced later in the 1940s by Cochrane and Muir in India, Lowe and Davey in Nigeria and Souza Lima in Brazil. The history of dapsone prior to the development of bacterial resistance is a brilliant success story covering a period exceeding 20 years. When we realize that the ingestion of one tablet of 100 mg gives, after about 4 hours, a peak blood level that is 500–600 times the minimum inhibitory concentration (MIC: 0.003 µg/mL) and measurable amounts can be found in the blood 10 days later, we need not be surprised that it had such a long unbroken reign. Dapsone acts by inhibiting folate metabolism in *M. leprae*.[12] Dosage is 6–10 mg/kg of body weight per week, adults over 50 kg receiving 100 mg/day, while those under 50 kg receive 50 mg/day.

Dapsone is metabolized in the liver through a combination of hydroxylation [cytochrome P450 (CYP450) dependent], into hydroxylamines which are toxic and implicated in the hematological side-effects of the drug, and *acetylation* (N-acetyl-transferase dependent) into monoacetyldapsone which is *nontoxic*.[13,14]

Side-effects of Dapsone

1. Effects on Blood

Hemolysis of red blood cells is the most important side-effect of dapsone and should be suspected in any patient developing anemia while on treatment. Mild hemolysis with a drop in hemoglobin of 1–2 g/dL occurs in *most* patients at a standard therapeutic dose. Hydroxylated metabolites of dapsone cause oxidation of glutathione, which in its reduced state plays an important role in maintaining erythrocyte cell membrane integrity.[14] These hydroxylamine derivatives (DDS-NHOH) are known to be the main metabolite responsible for the hematologic toxicity of dapsone. DDS-NHOH can make changes in the erythrocyte membrane proteins causing hemolysis and, when it reacts to hemoglobin in the presence of oxygen, methemoglobin and nitroso-dapsone are produced.

A study of the hemolytic effect of dapsone in normal men, and in men with deficiency of glucose-6-phosphate dehydrogenase (G6PD), confirmed that the latter were more susceptible to hemolysis and there was a direct relationship between dosage and the extent of hemolysis in both groups.[15] The main risk factors for *hemolysis* are G6PD deficiency, dosage of dapsone, and age. Clinical *suspicion* occurs in patients with fatigue, dyspnea, weakness and the diagnosis is confirmed by laboratory exams presenting anemia, a decrease of haptoglobin and increased reticulocytes, lactate dehydrogenase (LDH) and indirect bilirubin. Dapsone is unrelated to iron deficiency anemia, so the only justification for giving iron with dapsone is that the iron will be useful in countering iron deficiency from other causes. Iron is not indicated in the treatment of hemolytic anemia as it is liberated by the hemolyzed red cells and retained in the body and stored for future use. Hemolysis is usually mild and symptomless on therapeutic dosages.

Methemoglobinemia causes headache, shortness of breath, lethargy and a bluish discoloration of lips and fingertips (which will disappear spontaneously or on reduced dosage; and on its own it is not an indication to interrupt therapy). Cimetidine can reduce methemoglobin levels by inhibition of CYP450, which reduces synthesis of the toxic hydroxylated metabolites. Another option is to administer. Vitamin C 500 mg twice daily for 1 month. More severe cases may require treatment with oxygen and IV methylene blue 1% solution to restore the iron in hemoglobin to its reduced oxygen carrying state.[13, 14]

Agranulocytosis is a rare side-effect due to a direct toxic effect of hydroxylated metabolites and occurs in about 1:10,000 prescriptions. It is usually gradual in onset, occurring within 2–16 weeks of starting therapy, but may be sudden. It may also arise late in the course of treatment. A significant drop in neutrophil count can present with fever, mouth ulcers and sore throat. It may be accompanied by thrombocytopenia.[13,14] The first report of agranulocytosis in treating leprosy appeared in 1986[16] and the circumstances were tragic, not only because the patient died, but because he was being treated for indeterminate leprosy. Further reports have appeared,[17] but it is not a common side-effect.

Thrombocytopenia is usually not severe enough to cause symptoms.

2. Effects on Skin

A sensitivity reaction to dapsone is rare and takes the form of asymmetrical maculopapular rash sparing the face (exanthematous skin reaction), and it is fortunate that hypersensitivity skin reactions are rarer still for they include exfoliative dermatitis, toxic epidermal necrolysis, Stevens-Johnson syndrome, and 'DDS syndrome' ("sulphone syndrome").

DDS syndrome usually takes the form of DRESS (drug reaction [or rash] with eosinophilia and systemic symptoms) type reaction.[18] While this was described in the early years of dapsone's use when dangerously large doses were sometimes used; it disappeared during the decades when low dosage was in vogue, only to reappear in recent years. It is estimated to occur in approximately 1% of patients. The onset is usually within 4–6 weeks of starting therapy but may be delayed up to 6 months. Patients present with fever, a morbilliform rash that progresses to exfoliative dermatitis, lymphadenopathy, hepatitis with elevated liver enzymes, peripheral eosinophilia and atypical lymphocytes. If not recognized, the condition deteriorates and there is a significant risk of death. The drug should be withdrawn immediately and corticosteroids may be of benefit in controlling it.[13, 14]

Fixed drug eruption may complicate treatment with dapsone after the drug has been well-tolerated by the patient for months or even years; it begins with one or more raised, erythematous, sharply demarcated, round or oval plaques which heal and become brown or black. The pathogenesis is obscure.

3. *Other Side-effects*

Liver involvement manifests either as true toxic hepatitis or obstructive jaundice and is not fatal and almost *always* reversible with discontinuance of the drug and remarkably does not consistently recur on initiation of dapsone. This could be possibly as liver damage is seen in doses >100 mg.

Peripheral neuropathy usually takes the form of a motor neuropathy with bilateral weakness of limbs and tendon reflexes may be weak or absent.[19] This side-effect has been recorded by dermatologists using doses larger than those used in leprosy. The neuropathies involve distal axonal degeneration and are seldom, if ever, painful. The most commonly involved nerves are the ulnar and median nerves. These are *dose* related and are *reversible*.

Psychosis is not uncommon in leprosaria where it has an incidence of about 10%, and as many factors are responsible, it is very difficult to assess the role of dapsone; but rare cases have been reported in outpatients who have recovered on stopping the drug. Symptoms have included insomnia, irritability, delusions, and disordered thought and speech. A small minority of patients taking 100 mg/day complain that, an hour or two after taking the tablet, they feel temporarily 'woolly-headed' and unable to think clearly. This symptom improves if dosage is reduced, but before doing so it is worthwhile to try the effect of taking the 100 mg tablet—on going to bed at night.

Erythema nodosum leprosum (ENL) and other manifestations of type 2 reaction may be precipitated by dapsone (as by other antileprosy drugs), but these are not toxic effects as they are due to the killing of *M. leprae* and the release of antigen.

Pregnancy (FDA Category C)

Should a pregnant woman take dapsone? The answer to this question is that no doctor likes giving drugs in the first trimester, but having regard to the importance of treating the patient's leprosy, and to the fact that countless numbers of pregnant women have taken dapsone without trouble, any theoretical risk can be ignored. Another advantage of treating the pregnant woman is that, in untreated lepromatous leprosy (LL), viable leprosy bacilli are present in breast milk. Thus, treatment during pregnancy will ensure that any bacilli in breast milk will be granular (dead).

Dapsone has been used safely with no evidence of teratogenicity since its introduction in 1947. Folic acid 5 mg daily should be given to females who are pregnant. The greatest risk is in the last trimester when it may lead to neonatal hemolysis and methemoglobinemia.

Lactation

Dapsone is secreted in breast milk and absorbed by the infant, giving rise to mild hemolytic anemia but this risk to the infant is considered small unless he/she has G6PD deficiency.

Children

Dapsone has been used safely in infants and children at doses of 1–2 mg/kg/d. Serious effects of accidental overdose of dapsone have been reported, especially in children, and the importance of treatment with activated charcoal has been stressed.[20]

2. CLOFAZIMINE (LAMPRENE; B663)

This red iminophenazine dye, first used by Browne and Hogerzeill in the treatment of leprosy, is another drug that has proved its worth. Although the exact mechanism of antimycobacterial action is unclear, with renewed interest in the drug in view of its utility in treatment of drug resistant tuberculosis, some recent research has been conducted on this aspect. A possible important mechanism which has emerged is generation of a reduced clofazimine (with involvement of the mycobacterial respiratory chain where it competes with menaquinone for electrons) which undergoes spontaneous oxidation, resulting in the generation of damaging antimicrobial reactive oxygen species such as superoxide and hydrogen peroxide.[21] Apart from this, a membrane disruptive role is also postulated.[21] It is put up in capsules of 50 mg and 100 mg, and dosage is 300–350 mg/week, preferably administered as a daily capsule of 50 mg.

In the 2nd edition of this book, mention was made of its additional property of being effective as an anti-inflammatory agent in controlling the two types of lepra reaction; but this view has been challenged and must now be reconsidered. The present balance of opinion is that clofazimine is ineffective in type 1 reaction, and unacceptably large doses are required over a long period of time to control ENL. While some clinicians still maintain that it is useful in ENL, it has no effect on acute episodes but might be effective in chronic ENL. A pertinent paper has showed in a randomized study protocol that clofazimine 100 mg per day or placebo, showed no benefit in reducing ENL frequency or severity.[22] The reputation of clofazimine for causing serious gastro intestinal side-effects and the cosmetically unpleasing pigmentation is largely a consequence of the high doses and it is not warranted in all cases of reactions.

Side-effects

These are red-brown *pigmentation* of skin and conjunctivae, with darkening of skin lesions to mauve, slate-grey or black, thus highlighting the lesions more; red coloration of urine, stools, sputum, sweat and tears; dryness of skin, particularly of forearms and lower legs, which may progress to typical ichthyosis; and, less commonly, irritation or burning discomfort in skin lesions.

A reddish blue hue is seen in patients within 2 weeks of taking the drug and the dark brown pigmentation of the skin develops a few months later. It remains as long as the patients take the drug and discontinuance of the drug leads to clearance of most of the pigment within 6–12 months, although traces have been seen as long as 4 years or more. The postulated cause is a drug-induced reversible ceroid lipofuscinosis with some contribution from the presence of the drug in tissues.[23] Job et al concluded that the reddish blue tinge of the tissues is due to clofazimine accumulation in the lesions while the dark brown pigmentation is a drug-induced ceroid lipofuscinosis.[23]

Gastrointestinal (GI) adverse effects are common, affecting up to 50% of patients, and include nausea, vomiting, abdominal pain and diarrhea. Rarely, a severe painful and sometimes fatal enteropathy can occur due to the formation of clofazimine crystals in the tissues (sometimes referred to as clofazimine crystal storing histiocytosis). Lymphadenopathy and splenic infarction may occur. Clofazimine should be discontinued immediately if patients develop severe GI symptoms.

Pregnancy and Lactation (FDA Category C)

Clofazimine crosses the placenta and appears in breast milk in relatively large amounts. Breast milk may turn pink and nursing infants of mothers taking clofazimine have developed skin discoloration. The drug is safe for the pregnant woman, but more studies of infant mortality will have to be made now that there has been a report of three neonatal deaths in 15 pregnancies.[24]

3. RIFAMPICIN: RMP (RIFAMPIN: RMP)

A semisynthetic derivative of rifamycin B, one of a group of antibiotic compounds produced by *Streptomyces mediterranei*. A forerunner of rifampicin was rifamycin SV, introduced by Opromolla in Brazil in 1963,[25] and early publications on its successor, rifampicin, appeared in 1970. Since then, this antibiotic has become established as a highly potent bactericidal drug, and it acts by inhibiting the bacterial DNA dependent RNA polymerase. Rees and his colleagues reported in 1970[26] that it had a rapid action in human leprosy, the morphological index (MI) of bacilli in skin reaching 0 in 5 weeks as against 5 months in controlled lepromatous cases on dapsone; and they found it to be effective against dapsone-resistant bacilli. They gave 600 mg rifampicin daily in a single dose before breakfast and reduced the daily dose to 450 mg for patients weighing less than 35 kg. No toxic effects were encountered and lepra reaction was a minor problem.

Since then, the rapid action of rifampicin in rendering bacilli in human skin non-infective to mice has been demonstrated in several trials. A dosage of 600 mg daily was able to do this within 14 days[27] in one trial and a similar result was obtained within 5 days in a later trial with a single dose of 1200 mg.[28] The advantages of having an antibiotic that will do this, and at the same time render the patient non-infectious, make it the corner stone of therapy. Unfortunately, however, rifampicin is no more capable than is dapsone in eradicating the lepromatous infection, for it has been shown that even after 5 years of continuous treatment, persister bacilli still survive in favored tissues.[29] Rifampicin has a particularly rapid effect in relieving nasal symptoms in lepromatous leprosy and in healing leg ulceration resulting from breaking down nodules. Most leprologists who have used rifampicin find that lepra reaction is neither more common nor more severe.

Dosage

The choice lies between daily or monthly treatment. Generally, the second alternative is preferred because it is well tolerated and effective, monthly dosage can be supervised and there is a great saving in cost. Rifampicin is put up in capsules of 150 mg and 300 mg; and the usual daily dose is 600 mg. A monthly dosage of 1200 mg is ideal,[30] but 600 mg is a satisfactory alternative and has been recommended by the WHO study group as part of multi-drug therapy. Persons weighing less than 35 kg can receive 450 mg doses. It should be given at least 30 min before food if it is to have its full effect.

Before the era of blister packs of MDT, special techniques were described for storing tablets and capsules, but are not of much importance now.

Side-effects

1. Side-effects of Daily or Intermittent Administration

Mild effects consist of red coloration of urine, transient rash, gastrointestinal symptoms, drowsiness, weakness and dizziness. Serious side-effects are uncommon, and include hepatitis, thrombocytopenia, psychosis, osteomalacia and hypersensitivity reactions (Stevens-Johnson syndrome, porphyria cutanea tarda and pemphigus vulgaris).

2. Side-effects confined to Intermittent Administration

These may occur with once weekly or twice-weekly administration, but are very unlikely with once monthly treatment, and include: (1) "Flu "syndrome" characterized by episodes of fever and malaise which begin 1–2 hours after each treatment and last up to 8 hours; (2) shock, dyspnea, hemolytic anemia and renal failure.

3. Further Side-effects

A unique side-effect of rifampicin is that the effectiveness of steroids will be reduced if given to a patient taking this antibiotic. This is caused by rifampicin's capacity to stimulate the production of hepatic microsomal enzymes which increase the metabolic degradation of steroids. While it has been stated in the 5th edition of this book that dosage of steroid should 'at least' be doubled,[31] this applies particularly to daily treatment. These observations also apply to oral contraceptives.

Rifampicin monotherapy has resulted in the development of resistant strains of *M. leprae*, first reported in 1976, and is a single-step mutant type.[32]

NEWER DRUGS

The newer drugs were primarily discovered for shortening the duration of MDT but now have importance as they are useful in drug-resistant *M. leprae* (*see Chapter 6, Sections 6.1 and 6.2*) which is increasingly being reported (Box 7.1).[33, 34] It is clear that the three new drugs ofloxacin (OFLO), minocycline (MINO) and clarithromycin (CLARI) are individually and in combination much more active than dapsone and clofazimine.[34] Other drugs that have been tested and found to have a profound bactericidal activity include moxifloxacin, rifapentine and linezolid (*see drug formulary, pages 257–277*).[35–37]

Principles of Choosing a New Drug and Regimen[38–40]

The ideal properties of newer drugs are listed in Box 7.2. Existing data shows that, while the efficacy of OFLO, CLARI and MINO is largely similar, they are less potent than rifampicin but significantly more active than dapsone or clofazimine. Moxifloxacin (MOXI) has been shown to be more potent than OFLO, CLARI or MINO and as potent

---

 Box 7.1: Rationale for newer drugs in leprosy

- For reducing the *duration* of MB-MDT
- To circumvent the *compliance* issues of patients
- With skin smears being the weakest link in the programs, a *common* regimen would be useful for both PB and MB cases
- Special regimens needed for patients who *cannot* take clofazimine or rifampicin
- Treatment of cases with bacilli *resistant* to one or more of the primary anti-leprosy drugs.

Box 7.2: The ideal characteristics of a new anti-leprosy drug

1. It should be administered orally
2. It should be bactericidal and should not antagonize rifampicin in combination
3. It should not have debilitating side-effects
4. The drugs should be first tested in the laboratory
5. The bactericidal effects should be studied in clinical trials
6. Long-term relapse rates should be assessed.

as rifampicin. Rifapentine (RPT) has been found to be more potent than rifampicin. RPT is a long lasting rifamycin derivative, the serum half-life of which is three times longer than that of the parent compound rifampicin. The MIC of RPT against *M. tuberculosis* is similar or one dilution inferior to that of rifampicin. Since there is cross-resistance between RPT and other rifamycin derivatives, the advantage of RPT as previously mentioned, over rifampicin lies only in its pharmacokinetic properties.

Thus, of all the drugs tested, two drugs have been found to be of potential use, and this was based on a trial conducted on the premise that RPT can replace rifampicin and MOXI can replace OFLO in single dose ROM (R: Rifampicin, O: Ofloxacin, M: Minocycline) combination.[35,36] Using the proportional bactericidal test[41] with single-dose therapy of individual drugs and various combinations, promising results were found (Table 7.2):

a. A single dose of 10 mg/kg RPT killed 20 times more *M. leprae* than a single dose of 10 mg/kg rifampicin.
b. A single dose of 150 mg/kg MOXI, equipotent to 400 mg in man, killed 5 times more *M. leprae* than 150 mg/kg OFLO, and as much as 10 mg/kg rifampicin.
c. A single dose of the three-drug combination RPT, MOXI and MINO (PMM) killed 50 times more *M. leprae* than a single dose of ROM.

Thus, one potential method of shortening the present treatment duration is to consider a daily dose regimen with rifampicin/MINO/OFLO or RPT/CLARI/MINO.[42]

While many drug regimens have been tried including intermittent and monthly schedules, none has been approved yet by WHO, except the protocol for resistant cases (*see below*). This is as serial mouse footpad (MFP) inoculation, despite being the accepted method of assessing a drug's efficacy, has an important limitation that the

Table 7.2: Results of comparison of newer drugs versus rifampicin[34,40]

Drugs	% bacilli killed by treatment
Moxifloxacin > Ofloxacin	92.1% > 60.2%
Rifapentine > Rifampicin	99.6 > 92.1%
Moxifloxacin = Rifampicin	92.1%
MOXI + MINO	93.7%
RIF + OFLO + MINO	95%
RPT + MOXI + MINO	99.9%

OFLO: Ofloxacin 150 mg/kg; MOXI: Moxifloxacin 150 mg/kg; RIF: Rifampicin 10 mg/kg; RPT: Rifapentine 10 mg/kg; MINO: Minocycline 25 mg/kg.

number of *M. leprae* that can be recovered from skin biopsies and inoculated into a MFP is small and often inadequate. Also, this technique can only demonstrate 99.99% of killing and in a MB case with 10^{10} bacilli, failure to demonstrate bacilli at the end of therapy may not mean that all the viable bacilli are killed. Non-isolation may just mean that the bacilli cannot be isolated from the MFP. Thus, relapse rate is the "gold standard" for assessing the results of a new drug combination, for which a follow up of up to 7 years may be needed—an argument against the recommendation of the U-MDT and the newer drug regimens in leprosy.[38, 43]

ADVERSE DRUG REACTION (ADR)

As with any drug combination, ADRs are seen with MDT and ALT (alternative leprosy therapy) drugs, but in clinical practice they do not warrant discontinuation in most cases. However, it is important to bear in mind that with such long courses of treatment, as required for leprosy, default rates are high (reported to be as high as 30–60% in some series from India[44] and Philippines[45]) and monitoring for adverse effects to drugs becomes an important part of follow-up. The serious side-effects of dapsone include hemolytic anemia, agranulocytosis, methemoglobinemia, hepatitis and dapsone syndrome.[46,47] Serious ADR to rifampicin are thrombocytopenia, hepatitis, and acute renal failure.[47] Clofazimine-induced side-effects are generally mild, and include skin discoloration, ichthyosis and mild gastrointestinal discomfort, which rarely necessitate modification of MDT.

Several studies on adverse events from MDT have reported an adverse event rate between 37% and 45%, but with a smaller percentage actually requiring a change in MDT regimen in view of these (ranging from 5 to 24%).[48–50] A recent study[51] found that a quarter (24%) of patents on MDT had ADR that needed modification of MDT, the most *common* ADR being hemolytic anemia (12.7%) followed by hepatitis (9.3%). The most serious ADR was agranulocytosis (2%). The most frequent recorded cause of medication intolerance as reported by Dupnik et al was anemia (cause of change in drug regimen in 58.2% of all who needed it) followed by headache (in 4.2% patients).[52] Similary, a study from India also reported headache and the "nervous side-effects" (insomnia, headache, vertigo) of dapsone in about 20% of leprosy and 27% of non-leprosy patients taking the drug.[53] In the series by Deps et al, about 43.85% of all side-effects were attributable to dapsone, 12.3% to rifampicin and 9.25% to clofazimine.[54] Byrd et al reported that hemoglobin level decreased an average of 2 g/dL after 1 month of dapsone therapy for leprosy, and that 87% of women and 83% of men had a decrease in hemoglobin of 1 g/dL or more, while 3% of women and 21% of men had a hemoglobin decrease of 3 g/dL or more.[55] Another study reported that women and younger patients had greater risk of medication intolerance and medication intolerance related to anemia.[52] Adverse effects were more common (72%) during the initial 2 months of MDT compared to later months, which suggest that observant monitoring, with 2 weekly testing, is warranted in the *first 2 months* of therapy.

A study where patients were administered the alternate anti-leprosy therapy (ALT), for side-effects or in case of relapses, found that mild and transitory side-effects occurred in 33.3% of patients and were attributed largely to ofloxacin and included abdominal pain, nausea, vomiting, headache, and insomnia.[56]

THERAPEUTIC REGIMENS

MDT as Recommended by the WHO Study Group[57]

Treatment of Multibacillary Leprosy

The proposed regimen is designed for all categories of multibacillary patients: Those freshly diagnosed, those who have responded satisfactorily to previous dapsone therapy; and those who have relapsed. The regimen is detailed in Table 7.3.

While the last edition recommended a duration of at least 2 years and continuation of treatment, if possible, up to smear negativity; now a reduced fixed duration of 12 months is recommended by WHO.

Treatment of Paucibacillary Leprosy

The standard regimen is given in Table 7.4. Recent WHO publication recommends that PB leprosy cases should also be treated with the same three-drug regimen that is used in MB cases, but for a duration of six months.[58] However, this has not been universally accepted.

Table 7.3: MB-MDT for MB cases			
	Dapsone	*Rifampicin*	*Clofazimine*
Adult 50–70 kg	100 mg given daily	600 mg given once a month under supervision	50 mg daily and 300 mg given once a month under supervision
Child 10–14 years*	50 mg given daily	450 mg given once a month under supervision	50 mg alternate day and 150 mg given once a month under supervision

*Adjust dose appropriately for child less than 10 years. For example, dapsone 25 mg daily, rifampicin 300 mg given once a month under supervision, clofazimine 50 mg given twice a week, and clofazimine 100 mg given once a month under supervision. Alternately, prescribe weight based doses: Rifampicin 10 mg/kg once a month; Clofazimine 1 mg/kg daily and 6 mg/kg once a month; Dapsone: 2 mg/kg daily.

Table 7.4: PB-MDT for PB cases		
	Dapsone	*Rifampicin*
Adult 50–70 kg	100 mg given daily	600 mg given once a month under supervision
Child 10–14 years*	50 mg given daily	450 mg given once a month under supervision

*Adjust dose appropriately for child less than 10 years. For example, dapsone 25 mg daily and rifampicin 300 mg given once a month under supervision. Alternately, weight based dosing as mentioned in Box 7.1.

Alternate Regimens

Various alternate regimens have been tried in trials, but none is in wide use as yet (Table 7.5). It is known that a long duration of treatment is probably necessary in leprosy to effectively kill the slow growing *M. leprae* and very short duration regimens have been associated with high relapse rates.[59,60] There have also been high relapse rates after the WHO sponsored 4-week course of MDT.[59]

Table 7.5: Alternative regimens tried for leprosy		
S. No.	Regimen	Remarks
1.	Single dose ROM vs MDT for PB disease[61]	ROM *less* effective than MDT
2.	Multiple dose ROM vs MDT for MB disease[61]	Some encouraging results in small studies; plus advantage of fewer adverse effects; however not enough information to substantially conclude on the efficacy over MB-MDT; larger trials needed
3.	Six-week regimen consisting of: Daily rifampicin 600 mg, ofloxacin 400 mg and clofazimine 100 mg with weekly minocycline 100 mg[60]	*High* relapse rates; cannot be recommended
4.	Moxifloxacin based regimens	Small series report rapid clearance of bacilli and clinical resolution with short courses of moxifloxacin (400 mg at day 0, days 8 to to 56), later followed by MDT.[62] Trials to evaluate its role as an additional bactericidal agent in rifampicin/rifampin based regimens are warranted for possible shorter regimens and more effective bacterial clearance
		A combination of rifapentine, moxifloxacin and minocycline (PMM regime) was proposed to be taken up for trials, but further trials are awaited. Animal experiments showed that the combination killed 99.99% of viable *M. leprae*, and was slightly more bactericidal than was rifapentine alone, indicating an additive effect[35]
5.	Daily rifampicin and ofloxacin (RO) for one month[63]	Compared with standard MDT (12 and 24 months) and MDT plus ofloxacin for initial 1 month.
		High relapses (38.8%) in RO group versus 0–5% in others
		Addition of ofloxacin to MDT did not increase its efficacy

SPECIAL SITUATIONS

1. Resistance

In the initial studies that documented[64–66] rifampicin-resistant *M. leprae*, the patients were subjected to a drug regimen wherein, in the first 2–3 months, daily 400 mg ofloxacin, 500 mg clarithromycin, 100 mg minocycline and 100 mg clofazimine was administered. During the following 6 months, treatment given was daily 500 mg clarithromycin, 100 mg minocycline and 50 mg clofazimine and then, up to smear negativity, either 100 mg minocycline and 50 mg clofazimine or 50 mg clofazimine alone, or 100 mg minocycline alone. This formed the basis of the present WHO regimen for resistant cases of leprosy (Table 7.6).[2, 64]

Table 7.6: Treatment of drug-resistant leprosy (WHO)		
	Treatment	
Resistant type	First 6 months (daily)	Next 18 months (daily)
Rifampicin resistance	Ofloxacin 400 mg* + minocycline 100 mg + clofazimine 50 mg Ofloxacin 400 mg* + clarithromycin 500 mg + clofazimine 50 mg	Ofloxacin 400 mg* or minocycline 100 mg + clofazimine 50 mg
Rifampicin and ofloxacin resistance	Clarithromycin 500 mg + minocycline 100 mg + clofazimine 50 mg	Clarithromycin 500 mg or minocycline 100 mg + clofazimine 50 mg

*Ofloxacin 400 mg can be replaced by levofloxacin 500 mg or moxifloxacin 400 mg.

It has been recommended that all patients who start MDT and are found to have resistance to rifampicin alone or in association with resistance to dapsone, shall *restart* a full course of second-line treatment, regardless of clinical outcomes with MDT. The above-mentioned treatment regimen is mandatory for patients harboring *both* rifampicin- and dapsone-resistant *M. leprae*. In India, the number of cases of quinolone resistance appears to equal the number of cases of dapsone resistance,[64] highlighting the need to limit the use of quinolones to persons with clear indications only. Because fluoroquinolones are active against TB, leprosy patients starting a second-line regimen should be investigated for signs and symptoms of TB, to ensure that persons with TB are treated with an appropriate regimen effective against both diseases, to avoid emergence of drug-resistant TB.[64]

It is compulsory to report treatment outcomes of leprosy patients detected with drug resistance and to send it to the National Leprosy Programme so that the information can be entered in the drug resistance register. Thus, to reiterate the three salient principles of therapy for resistance are listed below:

1. If the results show a **sensitive strain**, MB-MDT treatment is to be continued.
2. For patients who are reported to be resistant to **dapsone** only, standard MB-MDT can be continued, but the patient should be followed at the end of treatment and regularly examined for possible relapse.
3. For patients with resistance only to **quinolones**, MDT should be continued.

2. Treatment of Leprosy during Pregnancy and Lactation

Leprosy is exacerbated during pregnancy, so it is important that the standard multi-drug therapy be continued during pregnancy. Standard MDT regimens are considered safe, both for the mother and the child, and therefore, should be continued unchanged during pregnancy. It is important that all who oversee these programmes should keep notes on the progress of pregnant patients and should publish their observations. A small quantity of anti-leprosy drugs is excreted through breast milk, but there is no report of adverse effects as a result of this, except for mild skin discoloration of the infant due to clofazimine. It must be noted though that 3 neonatal deaths in 15 pregnancies have been associated with clofazimine treatment during pregnancy.[24]

3. Treatment of Patient with Concomitant Active Tuberculosis[2,5,57]

For such patients, it is necessary to treat both infections at the same time. Rifampicin is common to both regimens and it must be given in the doses required for tuberculosis. MDT, as appropriate for leprosy, should be given except rifampicin (which should continue as recommended for tuberculosis).

4. Treatment of Patients with Concomitant HIV Infection[2,5,57]

The management of a leprosy patient infected with HIV is the same as that of any other patient. The information available so far indicates that the response of such a patient to MDT is similar to that of any other leprosy patient and management, including treatment of reactions, does not require any modifications.

5. MDT with Immunosuppressive Agents

One challenge in treating transplant recipients with leprosy is the potential for drug interactions, particularly between rifampicin and cyclosporine. For this reason, leprosy in this patient group may require the use of alternative antimycobacterial agents (e.g. minocycline, clarithromycin, ofloxacin). In addition, the duration of therapy in these patients is in question, because it is unclear if this group should receive a prolonged treatment course considering their immunocompromised state.

6. ADR or Drug Intolerance with MDT

For adult patients who are unable to tolerate the recommended agents, alternative agents are available. Fluoroquinolones have been used successfully in early clinical trials and are a continued focus of research in the treatment of both tuberculosis and leprosy. The fluoroquinolones inhibit bacterial DNA replication by inhibiting DNA gyrase or topoisomerase, and several agents in this class appear to be bactericidal against *M. leprae*.

a. **Clofazimine intolerance:** Based on clinical data, ofloxacin (400 mg/day) is used most commonly as a substitute for clofazimine,[47] although other drugs (minocycline, 100 mg daily and moxifloxacin 400 mg,) also appear to be effective in the treatment of leprosy.[47,68,69]

   Thus, WHO recommends the following schedule[46,47] wherein clofazimine in the normal 12-month multi-drug therapy may be *replaced* by: Ofloxacin, 400 mg daily for 12 months, *or* minocycline, 100 mg daily for 12 months.

b. **Dapsone intolerance/short supply:** For minor side-effects, including hemolysis, the drug can be temporarily stopped and restarted at a lower daily dose (50 mg) and the patient usually tolerates the full dose (100 mg) subsequently.[51] If dapsone produces severe toxic effects in any leprosy patient, either with paucibacillary or multibacillary leprosy, dapsone must be immediately stopped.

Fluoroquinolones and other alternative agents like minocycline (100 mg/day) can be used in place of dapsone.[47,57] According to WHO, in MB patients there is no need to substitute a new drug, while in the PB cases, dapsone should be replaced by clofazimine.[47] Here it is pertinent to point out that some national recommendations differ and do not advise a two-drug regimen for MB in such situations and in Brazil, the health ministry recommends replacing dapsone with minocycline or ofloxacin in MB regimens.

c. **Rifampicin intolerance:**[47] Special treatment regimens are required for individual patients who cannot take rifampicin because of side-effects or intercurrent diseases, such as chronic hepatitis, or who have been infected with rifampicin-resistant *M. leprae*. Alternative regimen with clofazimine, ofloxacin and minocycline for 6 months followed by clofazimine and ofloxacin for 18 months can be administered (Table 7.6).

d. **Hepatitis:** Liver dysfunction is often seen, and the first step is to rule out other causes of hepatitis. Elevation of serum aminotransferases to more than twice the upper limit of normal is usually an indication to withhold therapy. Herein, both dapsone and rifampicin can be the causative drugs. Once the LFT returns to normal, rifampicin can be re-introduced first, and LFT is repeated three days later. It has been noted that the increased enzymes may be transient and return to the normal range despite continuing the drug. If LFT derangement recurs, rifampicin is discontinued permanently, and patient is started on an alternative regimen. If the LFT remains normal, dapsone can be restarted initially at a lower dose with weekly monitoring of LFT, increasing gradually to the full dose.

7. Uniform Multi-drug Therapy (U-MDT)

The WHO guidelines development group[58] concluded that changing to a 3-drug regimen with a duration of 6 months for PB leprosy might be associated with improved clinical outcomes and potential advantages with regard to implementation in the field. For MB leprosy though, there was *insufficient* evidence to recommend a decrease in the duration of the current 3-drug regimen for MB leprosy from 12 to 6 months.

The results of an open label randomized Clinical Trial of Uniform Multi-drug Therapy conducted in Brazil (U-MDT/CT-BR),[71] concerning: (i) Frequency of reactions; (ii) trends of bacteriological index (BI) during treatment and follow-up; (iii) disability progression; and (iv) relapse rates with U-MDT versus standard MDT was recently reported. U-MDT group showed a higher rate of relapses (over five years) as well as a higher rate of disability progression, though these did not reach statistical significance. The fall in BI was greater with MDT, although this again did not reach statistical significance. Development of reactions was similar between the two groups. A large non-randomized study reported zero relapses.[72] Another study found a 6-month regimen associated with a trend towards worse clinical outcomes compared with a 2-month regimen (good clinical response at 24 months (25 *vs* 77%).[73]

There are other practical issues with U-MDT. One is that giving 3 drugs to all patients would add to the side-effects, especially as clofazimine pigmentation is a common reason for patients to stop or dispense with taking the therapy regularly. Secondly, U-MDT disregards the established data on the requirement of longer duration of MDT (up to 2 years) in patients with higher BI. Most importantly, longer durations of follow-up are ideally needed to assess whether U-MDT impacts favorably on leprosy relapses.

8. Late Reactions

After completing the multi-drug therapy regimen for leprosy, patients may have a lepra reaction (either type 1 or type 2) or may develop neuritis. These patients should be treated with oral prednisolone as if they have developed lepra reactions during MDT. There is a small risk of relapse in these patients since corticosteroids are known to accelerate the multiplication of organisms located in dormant foci and may cause disseminated reactivation. Thus, it is recommended that clofazimine 50 mg daily, should be given as a prophylactic measure if the duration of corticosteroid therapy is expected to exceed 4 months.[57] Clofazimine should be continued until corticosteroid therapy is stopped.

9. Management of Relapse, Defaulters (lost to Follow-up), Referred Cases and Change in Classification (WHO Recommendations)[46,47,58]

All cases with suspected relapse (*see Chapter 2, Section 2.2*) after a full course of appropriate MDT should be thoroughly examined and investigated to differentiate from delayed reaction as well as possible resistance.[74] Unless resistance is suspected, relapse cases should be reassessed to classify as PB or MB and given a new full course of appropriate MDT.

Patients who have interrupted treatment for a total of 3 or more months (if PB) or a total of 6 or more months (if MB) were previously defined as "defaulters" but term has been changed to "lost to follow-up" to use a non-derogatory language towards persons affected by leprosy. These patients should, similarly, be reassessed for current classification and disability status and started on the treatment as a fresh case, but registered as re-entered patient (other cases) and not a new case. Patients who have been started on PB-MDT but develop new lesions during therapy, leading to reclassification as MB, should also be given a full course of MB-MDT. However, referred cases who have completed part treatment from another center, should receive remaining treatment of the initial MDT regimens.

DRUG FORMULARY

The aim of the drug details is to enable a quick summary of the various drugs used in leprosy. While various aspects of the drugs used for leprosy and its complications are mentioned in the text previously; herein, aspects that have either been missed or not covered are stated.

The drugs range from conventional and newer drugs used in leprosy, drugs used for reactions and adjuvants. While we have not covered all the drugs, with some notable drugs like NSAIDs, colchicine and apremilast, this is as either they have no special consideration in leprosy or do not have sufficient data to recommend their use. We have on the contrary detailed others like methotrexate which is being studied in erythema nodosum leprosum (ENL), though we feel, the effect of drugs like methotrexate on cytokines has a dose-dependent effect and is largely limited by the levels of implicated cytokines, a consideration that has been probably overlooked in using these drugs in ENL. Also there are intrinsic aspects of this drug which should be understood in any indication.

1. Clofazimine

■ **Drug class**	• Antimycobacterial • **MIC:** Unknown, multiplication of *M. leprae* is inhibited by feeding mice 0.0001 g% clofazimine in their diet

■ **Mechanism of action/ pharmacokinetics**	• Unknown; Postulated mechanisms (acts on outer membrane):
	  – Interaction with respiratory chain → redox cycling → oxidation of reduced clofazimine → reactive oxygen species (ROS), H_2O_2 → interference with ATP production → cell death.
	  – Interaction with membrane phospholipids → antimicrobial lyso-phospholipids → interference with K^+ transport → interference with ATP production → cell death.
	  – It is weakly bactericidal against *M. leprae* and antimicrobial activity can be demonstrated in humans only after continuous exposure for about 50 days.
	• 70% absorbed after oral administration, t½ = 70 days, serum levels 0.5 µg/mL (exact half-life is difficult to determine because the drug seems to be excreted more rapidly from some tissues than others); excretion is via sebum, sweat, feces and urine.
	• *Resistance*: Only inconclusive isolated reports of resistance so far.

■ **Dosage**	• **Leprosy treatment:** 300 mg once a month, to be administered under supervision and 50 mg daily, to be self-administered • **ENL:** 100 mg 3 times a day for one month, subsequent dose reductions are required; may take 4–6 weeks to attain full effect. A recent RCT has found that the drug's role in ENL might be overrated.
■ **Drug interaction**	None of significance
■ **Side-effects**	• **GIT:** Nausea, abdominal pain, appetite ↓, weight ↓ Side-effects seen only with >100 mg (in 25% of such patients), sub-acute intestinal obstruction if 100 mg TDS given for >3 months • **Eye:** Dry eye, eye discoloration • **Skin:** Hair color changes (reversible), xerosis (due to anticholinergic action), skin discoloration (including areas exposed to light) due primarily to a drug-induced reversible ceroid lipofuscinosis (localized to lesions; disappears on stopping the drug in 6–12 months), red discoloration of body fluids • **Others:** Headache, lymphadenopathy, splenic infarction, depression or suicide.
■ **Pregnancy**	Category C; MDT continued • Clofazimine crosses the placenta, though the kinetics remain to be elucidated. • Hyperpigmentation of the neonate that resolves gradually is reported in humans. • Three neonatal deaths reported. Rodent studies are generally reassuring, revealing no evidence of teratogenicity despite the use of doses higher than those used clinically, embryotoxicity and intra-uterine growth retardation were noted.

■ **Lactation**	• MDT continued • Clofazimine is excreted in breast milk, with milk levels of 1.33 mg/L with an average infant daily dose of 0.2 mg/kg/d. • Hyperpigmentation of the newborn resolving over 5 months is reported.
■ **Patient advise**	• Avoid if persistent abdominal pain and diarrhea • May discolor soft contact lenses
■ **Reference**	*Journals* • Holdiness MR. Clin Pharmacokinetics of clofazimine: A review. Clin Pharmacokinet 1989;16:74–85. • Lopes VG, Sarno EN. Rev Assoc Med Bras 1994;40:195–201. • Kar HK, Bhatia VN, Harikrishnan S. Combined clofazimine- and dapsone-resistant leprosy. A case report. Int J Lepr Other Mycobact Dis 1986;54:389–91. • Warndorff-van Diepen T. Clofazimine-resistant leprosy, a case report. Int J Lepr Other Mycobact Dis 1982;50:139–42. *Books* • British National Formulary (BNF 78), September 2019. • Jacobson RR. Treatment of Leprosy. In: Hastings RC, Editor. Leprosy. New York: Churchill Livingstone, 1994; p. 342. • Systemic Drugs in Dermatology. Sardana K, Editor, New Delhi, Jaypee Publishers, 2016.

2. Dapsone

■ **Drug class**	• Antimycobacterial • *MIC*: 0.003 µg/mL
■ **Mechanism of action/ pharmacokinetics**	• Bactericidal/bacteriostatic; competes with para-aminobenzoic acid and inhibits folic acid synthesis • *Resistance*: Stepwise mutation (Hastings, 1977); rapid acetylators are less likely to develop sulfone resistant disease (Shepard et al, 1976) • *Absorption*: 90% absorbed, equilibrium is set up between dapsone and its monoacetyl derivative (MADDS); secreted in the urine, peak serum concentration of approximately 2 µg/mL; $t_{1/2}$ = 28 hours
■ **Dosage**	• 100 mg tablets; Inj acedapsone 225 mg every 11 weeks • Adult (body weight up to 35 kg): 50 mg daily; alternatively 1–2 mg/kg daily, self-administered • Adult (body weight 35 kg and above): 100 mg daily; self-administered • Glucose-6-phosphate dehydrogenase (G6PD) deficiency—start at 25 mg twice weekly; increase every 3–4 weeks to 50–100 mg daily.
■ **Drug interaction**	Rifampicin lowers dapsone levels 7- to 10-fold by enhancing plasma clearance (usually with daily dose).
■ **Side-effects**	'DDS syndrome': Agranulocytosis, hepatitis, peripheral neuropathies, methemoglobinemia and hypoalbuminemia. Other less common side-effects: Headache, nervousness and insomnia. • *DDS syndrome*: About 6 weeks after the start of therapy; presents with erythroderma, other skin rashes, generalized lymphadenopathy, hepatosplenomegaly, fever and hepatitis.

	• *Hemolytic anemia:* Reticulocyte count 2–5% range, usually with a mild drop in hemoglobin and hematocrit. • Dose-dependent methemoglobinemia may supervene during the 2nd week treatment. • *Agranulocytosis*: 1:10000, fever, ulcerating pharyngitis (sore throat), pallor, or purpura. • *Peripheral neuropathies*: Motor—ulnar/median, distal axonal degeneration, dose related, reversible. • *Liver*: Toxic hepatitis or jaundice, reversible.
■ Pregnancy	Category C; MDT continued • Transfer across the human placenta likely, as there are reports of neonatal methemoglobinemia after maternal dapsone. Dapsone appears unassociated with fetal abnormalities in humans. Animal studies have revealed no evidence of teratogenicity.
■ Lactation	• MDT continued • Dapsone is excreted in breast milk in substantial amounts, achieving a relative infant dose of 6.3–22.5%. Dapsone may be compatible with breastfeeding, but caution is advised. Dapsone should be avoided in infants at risk for G6PD deficiency or hyperbilirubinemia.
■ Monitoring	• Complete blood count (CBC) and reticulocyte count • Urea, electrolytes and creatinine • LFTs • G6PD in patients from ethnic groups at risk of deficiency.
■ Patient/physician advise	• Avoid in acute porphyrias, cardiac disease, G6PD deficiency, pulmonary disease, patients susceptible to hemolysis. • Patients should be told how to recognize signs of blood disorders and advised to seek immediate medical attention if symptoms such as fever, sore throat, rash, mouth ulcers, purpura, bruising or bleeding develop.
■ Reference	*Journals* Bhargava P, Kuldeep CM, Mathur NK. Int J Lepr Other Mycobact Dis 1996; 64:457–8. *Books* • 78 British National Formulary (BNF), September 2019. • Jacobson RR. Treatment of Leprosy. In: Hastings RC, Editor. Leprosy. New York: Churchill Livingstone, 1994; p. 342. • Systemic Drugs in Dermatology. Sardana K, Ed. New Delhi; Jaypee Publishers; 2016.

3. Rifampicin (RMP)/Rifapentine (RPT)*

■ Drug class	• Antimycobacterials • *MIC*: 0.3 µg/mL
■ Mechanism of action/pharmacokinetics	• Inhibits DNA-dependent RNA polymerase • Resistance develops with a single step mutation (Gacobs and Hastings, 1976)

*RPT has a pharmacokinetic superiority over RMP and a single dose of RPT is significantly more bactericidal than RMP; though it is also believed that the inherent anti-*M. leprae* activity of RPT may be greater than that of RMP because RPT exhibited lower MICs against various cultivable mycobacteria. A single dose of the combination rifapentine, moxifloxacin and minocycline (PMM) killed 99.9% of the viable *M. leprae*, significantly more than the combination rifampicin, ofloxacin, minocycline (ROM), which killed 95.0%.

- *Absorption*: Rapidly and completely absorbed if taken on empty stomach.
- *Metabolism*: Hepatic, peak concentration of 7 μg/mL in 2–4 hrs, t½ of 3 hours, excretion via GIT.

■ Dosage

- Adult (body weight up to 35 kg): 450 mg once a month, supervised administration.
- Adult (body weight 35 kg and above): 600 mg once a month, supervised administration.

■ Drug interaction

- Due to its interaction with various metabolic enzymes and transporters, rifampicin is known to alter the plasma level of a large number of drugs. Clinical significance limited in leprosy as use is only once monthly.
- May ↑ metabolism of the following drugs: Antiarrhythmics (e.g. disopyramide, mexiletine, quinidine, tocainide), anticonvulsants (e.g. phenytoin), antifungals (e.g. fluconazole, itraconazole, ketoconazole), barbiturates, β-blockers, calcium channel blockers (e.g. diltiazem, nifedipine, verapamil), cardiac glycoside preparations, chloramphenicol, clofibrate, corticosteroids, cyclosporine, dapsone, diazepam, doxycycline, fluoroquinolones (e.g. ciprofloxacin), haloperidol, levothyroxine, methadone, narcotic analgesics, nortriptyline, oral anticoagulants, oral hypoglycemic agents (sulfonylureas), oral or other systemic hormonal contraceptives, progestins, quinine, tacrolimus, tricyclic antidepressants (e.g. amitriptyline, nortriptyline), theophylline, and zidovudine.
- Women using oral or other systemic hormonal contraceptives should be advised to change to non-hormonal methods of birth control.
- May increase the requirements for coumarin-type anticoagulant drugs. It is recommended that a PT or INR be performed frequently.
- Ketoconazole and rifampicin: ↓ the serum concentrations of both.
- Enalapril: ↓ concentrations of enalaprilat, the active metabolite of enalapril.
- Antacid use may ↓ the absorption of rifampicin. The daily dose of rifampicin should be given at least 1 hour before the antacid.
- Probenecid and cotrimoxazole may increase the blood level of rifampicin.
- Rifampicin concentrations may be decreased if taken with food.

■ Side-effects

i. Common or very common: Nausea, thrombocytopenia, vomiting
ii. Uncommon: Diarrhea, leukopenia
iii. Others: Renal failure, shock, hepatotoxicity, hemolytic anemia, thrombocytopenia, leukopenia, elevated LFTs, interstitial nephritis, nausea/vomiting, diarrhea, anorexia, headache, fatigue, dizziness, abdominal pain, pruritus, rash, dyspnea, ataxia, visual changes and urticaria.
- Patients should be warned that treatment may produce reddish discoloration of urine, tears, saliva and sputum and that contact lenses may be irreversibly stained.
- Toxicity appears to be uncommon after the first year of therapy
- Hepatotoxic: If SGOT/SGPT rises 2–3 times upper limit of normal—stop.

iv. *Intermittent therapy (relevant in leprosy)*
- Flu-like syndrome: Chills, fever, headache, myalgia, bone pain rarely thrombocytopenia.
- Serious immunological reactions, resulting in renal impairment, hemolysis, or thrombocytopenia can be seen in patients who resume taking rifampicin after a prolonged delay of treatment. In this situation, it should be immediately withdrawn. Temporary oliguria, dyspnea and hemolytic anemia have also been reported. These reactions *subside* when *daily* dosage is substituted.

■ **Pregnancy**	Category C; MDT continued • No conclusive evidence of increased risk of congenital malformations with intake during pregnancy.
■ **Lactation**	• MDT continued • 0.05% of drug transferred to infant via breastfeeding; thus potential dose of 0.45 to 0.735 mg/kg/day (about 2.2–7.3% of infant therapeutic dose of 10–20 mg/kg/day). • Monitor the infant for adverse effects (fever, nausea, vomiting, increased liver enzymes)
■ **Monitoring**	• Renal function should be checked before treatment. • Hepatic function should be checked before treatment. If there is no evidence of liver disease (and pre-treatment liver function is normal), further checks are only necessary if the patient develops fever, malaise, vomiting, jaundice or unexplained deterioration during treatment. However, liver function should be monitored on prolonged therapy. • Blood counts should be monitored in patients on prolonged therapy. • In adults, those with alcohol dependence should have frequent checks of hepatic function, particularly in the first 2 months. Blood counts should also be monitored in these patients.
■ **Reference**	*Journals* • Ji B, Grosset J. Combination of rifapentine-moxifloxacin-minocycline (PMM) for the treatment of leprosy. Lepr Rev 2000 Dec;71 Suppl:S81–7. • Ozturk Z, Tatliparmak A. Leprosy treatment during pregnancy and breastfeeding: A case report and brief review of literature. Dermatol Ther 2017;30(1). • Tran JH, Montakantikul P. The safety of antituberculosis medications during breastfeeding. J Hum Lact 1998;14:337–40. *Books* • 78 British National Formulary (BNF), September 2019. • Jacobson RR. Treatment of Leprosy. In: Hastings RC, Editor. Leprosy. New York: Churchill Livingstone, 1994; p. 342. • Systemic Drugs in Dermatology. Sardana K, Editor. New Delhi; Jaypee Publishers; 2016.

4. Ofloxacin

■ **Drug class**	Fluoroquinolones
■ **Mechanism of action/ pharmacokinetics**	• Inhibits topoisomerase IV and DNA gyrase • Daily ofloxacin for 1 month is considered as capable as 2 years of dapsone plus clofazimine in killing the rifampicin-resistant mutants. • Correlation between ofloxacin resistance and missense mutation in the gyrA gene has been confirmed at positions 91 (Ala91Val) and 89 (Gly89Cys). • Peak serum level 2.9 µg/mL; serum half-life of 7 hours; excreted via kidneys.
■ **Dosage**	*Indications* • Treatment of patients with multibacillary leprosy, who cannot take rifampicin/resistance to rifampicin.

Chemotherapy

	• Treatment of patients with multibacillary leprosy, who refuse to take clofazimine. *Dose* 400 mg is bactericidal against *M. leprae*, although less than a single dose of rifampicin; **28** daily doses killed **99.99%** of the viable organisms.
■ Drug interaction	• Quinolones form chelates with alkaline earth and transition metal cations. • Use of quinolones with antacids containing calcium, magnesium, or aluminum; with sucralfate; with divalent or trivalent cations such as iron; with multivitamins containing zinc; or with didanosine chewable/buffered tablets or the pediatric powder for oral solution may substantially *interfere* with the absorption of quinolones, resulting in systemic levels considerably lower than desired. These agents should *not* be taken within 2 hours before or after ofloxacin. • ↑ serum levels of cyclosporine were reported with concomitant use of cyclosporine and some other quinolones. • Most quinolones inhibit CYPs, which may lead to a ↑ level for some drugs metabolized by this system (e.g. cyclosporine, theophylline/methylxanthines, warfarin). • Use with NSAIDs may increase the risk of CNS stimulation and convulsive seizures. • Steady-state theophylline levels may increase when used with ofloxacin. • Because disturbances of blood glucose, including hyperglycemia and hypoglycemia, are reported in patients treated with quinolones with antidiabetic agent, careful monitoring of blood glucose is recommended. • May produce false positive urine screening results for opiates using commercially available immunoassay kits.
■ Side-effects	Vaginitis, photosensitivity, pseudomembranous colitis, seizures, increased intracranial pressure, headache, psychosis, nausea/vomiting, diarrhea, abdominal pain, dyspepsia, dizziness, insomnia, agitation, tendonitis, arthralgias, and elevated LFTs.
■ Pregnancy	Category C Less than 4% of maternal ofloxacin crosses the isolated perfused human placenta.
■ Lactation	The relative infant dose approximates 3%. Even with 100% oral absorption, breastfeeding mothers who take ofloxacin will expose their infants to lower concentrations than used in the pediatric population.
■ Hepatic	Dose adjustments: Manufacturer advises maximum 400 mg daily in hepatic failure (risk of decreased elimination).
■ Renal impairment	Dose adjustments: Usual initial dose, then use half normal dose if eGFR 20–50 mL/minute/1.73 m^2; 100 mg every 24 hours if eGFR less than 20 mL/minute/1.73 m^2
■ Patient/physician advise	• Caution-hepatic or renal dysfunction, seizure disorder, CNS abnormalities, diabetes mellitus, dehydration, sun exposure • Patients with hepatic or renal impairment may require reduced dosage • Ofloxacin should be administered cautiously to patients with epilepsy since seizures may be precipitated • Ensure adequate fluid intake since crystalluria may occur • Quinolones, such as ofloxacin, have been shown to cause arthropathy (degenerative changes in weightbearing joints)

- Risk factor for QT interval prolongation.
- Driving and skilled tasks may affect performance of skilled tasks (e.g. driving); effects enhanced by alcohol.

■ **Reference**	*Journals* • Ji B, Grosset J. Combination of rifapentine-moxifloxacin-minocycline (PMM) forthe treatment of leprosy. Lepr Rev 2000 Dec; 71 Suppl: S81–7. • Loebstein R, Addis A, Ho E, et al. Antimicrob Agents Chemother 1998; 42:1336–9. • Muanda FT, Sheehy O, Bérard A. Br J Clin Pharmacol 2017; 83:2557–71. *Books* • Systemic Drugs in Dermatology. Sardana K, Editor. New Delhi; Jaypee Publishers; 2016. • Jacobson RR. Treatment of Leprosy. In: Hastings RC, editor. Leprosy. New York: Churchill Livingstone, 1994; p. 342.

5. Moxifloxacin

■ **Drug class**	Fluroquinolones
■ **Pharmacokinetics**	Peak concentration achieved rapidly—within 2 hours; t½ about 12 hours.
■ **Dosage**	• 400 mg • Potent anti-*M. leprae* activity; potential use in shortening anti-leprosy regimens. • Combination of rifapentine, moxifloxacin and minocycline (PMM regime) proposed to be taken up for clinical trials. • Animal experiments showed that the combination killed 99.99% of viable *M. leprae*, and was slightly more bactericidal than was rifapentine alone, indicating an additive effect.
■ **Drug interaction**	• Coadministration with rifampicin reduces serum concentration of moxifloxacin. • Caution with simultaneous use of other drugs causing increased QT interval.
■ **Side-effects**	• Idiosyncratic hypersensitivity reactions • Mild ALT elevations, idiosyncratic acute liver injury • Prolongation of the QT interval and isolated cases of torsades de pointes reported; cautious use with hypokalemia and in arrhythmic states.
■ **Pregnancy and lactation**	Pregnancy category C; selective short term use only • No information is available on the use of moxifloxacin during breastfeeding but is likely safe with monitoring of infant for possible effects on GI flora such as diarrhea or candidiasis (thrush, diaper rash). • Fluoroquinolones have traditionally not been used in infants because of concern about adverse effects on the infants' developing joints. However, recent studies indicate little risk.
■ **Reference**	*Journals* • Gillespie SH. The role of moxifloxacin in tuberculosis therapy. Eur Respir Rev 2016;25:19–28.

- https://pubchem.ncbi.nlm.nih.gov/compound/Moxifloxacin.
- Ji B, Grosset J. Combination of rifapentine-moxifloxacin-minocycline (PMM) for the treatment of leprosy. Lepr Rev 2000;71:S81–7.
- Padberg S, Wacker E, Meister R, et al. Observational cohort study of pregnancy outcome after first-trimester exposure to fluoroquinolones. Antimicrob Agents Chemother 2014;58:4392–8.
- Pardillo FE, Burgos J, Fajardo TT, Dela Cruz E, Abalos RM, Paredes RM, Andaya CE, Gelber RH. Powerful bactericidal activity of moxifloxacin in human leprosy. Antimicrob Agents Chemother 2008; 52:3113–7.

6. Clarithromycin	
■ Drug class	Macrolides*
■ Mechanism of action/pharmacokinetics	The drug acts by linking to the 50S ribosomal subunit, thus inhibiting bacterial protein synthesis. Potent bactericidal activity against *M. leprae*, but less than rifampicin.
■ Dosage	<ul><li>500 mg daily</li><li>Kills 99% of *M. leprae* by **28** days and **99.99%** by 56 days</li><li>Peak serum level: 1 µg/mL, serum half-life of 6–7 hours.</li><li>Tissue concentrations are higher than those in the serum.</li><li>Active component 14OH-clarithromycin.</li><li>Though some synergism between minocycline and clarithromycin was demonstrated in a mouse model, the combination of 100 mg minocycline and 500 mg clarithromycin was not more active in man than each component alone, perhaps because the potency of each individual drug was too strong.</li></ul>
■ Drug interaction	<ul><li>May ↑ plasma theophylline concentrations.</li><li>May ↑ plasma concentrations of carbamazepine.</li><li>Simultaneous oral administration of clarithromycin and zidovudine to HIV-infected adult patients causes ↓ zidovudine steady-state concentrations.</li><li>May potentiate the effects of the oral anticoagulants.</li><li>May ↑ digoxin levels, producing clinical signs consistent with toxicity, including potentially fatal arrhythmias.</li><li>There have been postmarketing reports of drug interactions and CNS effects (e.g. somnolence and confusion) with the concomitant use of triazolam.</li><li>May ↑ concentrations of HMG-CoA reductase inhibitors (e.g. lovastatin, simvastatin).</li><li>There are reports of CYP3A-based interactions of clarithromycin with alfentanil, bromocriptine, carbamazepine, cilostazol, cyclosporine, disopyramide, ethylprednisolone, quinidine, rifabutin, and tacrolimus.</li></ul>
■ Side-effects	Side-effects include anaphylaxis, Stevens-Johnson syndrome, arrhythmia, pseudomembranous colitis, diarrhea, nausea, abdominal pain, dyspepsia, headache, and rash.

*HMR 3647 (RU 66647, telithromycin) (HMR) is a ketolide, a new class of macrolides possessing a 14-membered ring and is more bactericidal than clarithromycin.

Pregnancy	Category C
• Clarithromycin crosses the human placenta to a greater degree than other macrolides (6% maternal dose).
• There is no evidence that any of the macrolides are human teratogens, and no teratogenic effects are noted in most studies of rats, rabbits, and monkeys. However, there are reports of a modest increase in cardiovascular malformations and cleft palate in certain rodent strains.
Lactation	Clarithromycin enters human breast milk, reaching levels as high as 75% of the maternal concentration, but it is acceptable in nursing mothers.
Reference	• Consigny S, Bentoucha A, Bonnafous P, Grosset J, Ji B. Bactericidal activities of HMR 3647, moxifloxacin, and rifapentine against *Mycobacterium leprae* in mice. Antimicrob Agents Chemother 2000 Oct;44(10):2919–21.
• Einarson A, Phillips E, Mawji F, et al. Am J Perinatol 1998; 15:523–5.
• Gilljam M, Berning SE, Peloquin CA, et al. Eur Respir J 1999; 14:347–51.
• Jacoby EB, Porter KB. Am J Perinatol 1999; 16:85–8.
• Jover-Diaz F, Robert-Gates J, Andreu-Gimenez L, Merino-Sanchez J. Infect Dis Obstet Gynecol 2001; 9:47–9.

7. Minocycline (MINO)

Drug class	Tetracyclines
Mechanism of action/ pharmacokinetics	MINO binds reversibly at the 30S unit of the ribosome, blocking the binding of aminoacyl transfer RNA to the messenger RNA-ribosomal complex, thereby inhibiting protein synthesis.
Dosage	*Indications*
• Treatment of multibacillary patients who cannot take rifampicin.
• Treatment of multibacillary patients who refuse to take clofazimine.
• Standard dose is 100 mg daily, with a blood level of 2–4 μg/mL (above the apparent MIC for *M. leprae* of 0.2 μg/mL).
• More than 99% and 99.9% of the viable *M. leprae* killed by **28** and **56** days of treatment, respectively.
• Definite clinical improvement is seen in some patients as early as 14 days after beginning treatment, improvement in all patients by 1 month, and marked improvement in all patients by 2 months.
Drug interaction	• Patients on anticoagulants may require a lower dose of their anticoagulant because tetracyclines can depress plasma prothrombin activity.
• It is advisable to avoid using tetracycline with penicillin because bacteriostatic drugs may interfere with the bactericidal action of penicillin.
• May cause fatal renal toxicity when used with methoxyflurane.
• Minocycline may render oral contraceptives less effective.

- Isotretinoin should be avoided shortly before, during, and shortly after minocycline therapy as each drug alone has been associated with pseudotumor cerebri.
- There is an increased risk of ergotism when ergot alkaloids or their derivatives are given with tetracyclines.

Side-effects

- *Rare or very rare*: Acute kidney injury, hearing impairment, respiratory disorders, tinnitus.
- *Frequency not known*: Alopecia, antibiotic associated colitis, arthralgia, ataxia, breast secretion, conjunctival discoloration, drug reaction with eosinophilia and systemic symptoms (DRESS), dyspepsia, hyperbilirubinemia, hyperhidrosis, polyarteritis nodosa, abnormal sensation, tear discoloration, tongue discoloration, vertigo.

Pregnancy

Category D

There are no adequate reports or well-controlled studies in human fetuses. It is unknown whether minocycline crosses the human placenta. It is unlikely the maternal systemic concentration will reach a clinically relevant level if applied topically for acne.

Lactation

It is unknown whether minocycline enters human breast milk. Milk discoloration is reported. No harm of short-term use of minocycline.

Monitoring

If treatment continued for longer than 6 months:

Monitor every 3 months for hepatotoxicity, pigmentation and for systemic lupus erythematosus—discontinue if these develop or if pre-existing systemic lupus erythematosus worsens.

Reference

- Hunt MJ, Salisbury EL, Grace J, Armati R. Br J Dermatol 1996;134:943–5.
- Ji B, Grosset J. Combination of rifapentine-moxifloxacin-minocycline (PMM) for the treatment of leprosy. Lepr Rev 2000;71 Suppl:S81–7.
- Loo WJ, Dean D, Wojnarowska F. Clin Exp Dermatol 2001;26:726–7.

8. Prednisolone

Drug class

- Anti-inflammatory
- Dose equivalence of different steroids: Cortisol 20 mg = prednisone 5 mg = prednisolone 5 mg = methylprednisolone 4 mg = dexamethasone 0.75 mg.

Mechanism of action/ pharmacokinetics

- *Genomic effects*—interact with proinflammatory transcription factors (NF-κB, AP-1, etc.) that have bound to DNA, ↓ production of proinflammatory molecules. Genomic effects develop at small doses of ≤30 mg/day as well and develop after a latency of >30 minutes.
- *Nongenomic effects*—at higher doses of ≥30 mg/day of prednisone; as a result of binding of the steroid molecule to membrane glucocorticoid receptors on lymphocytes and monocytes leading to anti-inflammatory effects.
- *Innate immune system*: ↓ production of prostaglandins, (–) NF-κB which suppresses COX-2 synthesis, ↓ phagocytosis and cytokine production, neutrophilia, eosinopenia.

- *Adaptive (acquired) immune response*: Lymphopenia, (–) T-helper [Th1 > Th2] and Th17 cytokine production, B cells less affected than T cells, immunoglobulin production preserved unless prolonged (>1 year) use at nonphysiologic doses (>12.5 mg/day prednisone).
- *Leprosy reactions*: There is marked variation in responsiveness; its effect on cytokines (IFN-gamma, IL-12 and iNOS) takes 28 days which can revert to increased levels on stopping steroids.

■ Dosage

- Type 1 reaction and ENL
  - Individualized dosing; with a period of about 12 to 20 weeks or more, initial dose: 40 mg tapered by 5 mg every two weeks.
  - Longer periods of use are needed in chronic ENL, where adjuvants are advised
- $t^{1/2}$ is 2.1–3.5 hours; so effect wanes in 5 half lives; splitting the dose of high-dose prednisone to twice a day when treating severe disease manifestation is useful.
- The maximum effect on lymphocytes by redistribution and genomic effects occurs at a single dose of 20 to 30 mg; therefore dose of 20 to 30 mg once a day is more immunosuppressive than a split dose regimen of 10 to 15 mg twice daily.

■ Drug interaction

- Barbiturates, phenytoin, ephedrine, and rifampicin, which induce liver microsomal drug-metabolizing enzyme activity, may enhance metabolism and require that the dose of prednisolone be increased.
- Increases activity of both cyclosporine and corticosteroids with concurrent use.
- Estrogens may decrease the liver metabolism of some corticosteroids, thus increasing their effect.
- Ketoconazole decreases the metabolism of some corticosteroids by up to 60%, leading to an increased risk of corticosteroid side-effects.
- May decrease the response to warfarin; clotting indices should be monitored closely.
- Use with aspirin (or other NSAIDs) increases the risk of GI side-effects.
- Observe patients closely for hypokalemia if used with potassium-depleting agents (i.e. diuretics, amphotericin B).
- The routine administration of vaccines or toxoids should be deferred until corticosteroid therapy is discontinued if possible. (Vaccinations: Live vaccines safe if on <20 mg/day for adults or <2 mg/kg per day if child weighs <10 kg. Response to vaccines: Less response if on >40 mg/day).
- Dose adjustment of hypoglycemic agents.

■ Side-effects

- Even with short-term use of prednisone (<30 days), up to 20% of patients will experience an adverse event particularly with higher doses or split doses of steroids.
- Glucose intolerance and increased triglycerides attributable to insulin resistance (>10 mg/day).
- Skin disorders (bruising, striae, delayed wound repair, hirsutism).
- Peptic ulcer disease (doses >10 mg/day with nonsteroidal anti-inflammatory drugs [NSAIDs] increases risk 3×).
- Weight gain (>5 mg/day). Up to 25% of patients get cushingoid on >7.5 mg/day.

Chemotherapy

- Infection (doses >20–25 mg/day/≥0.3 mg/kg) causes unacceptable risk.
- Mycobacterial (especially *Mycobacterium tuberculosis*) risk increases at >10 to 15 mg/day for a month.
- *Pneumocystis jiroveci* infection increased risk at >15 to 20 mg/day for >3 to 4 weeks.
- Anergy can occur within 2 to 4 weeks on prednisone 30 mg/day.
- Hypertension (doses >10 mg/day).
- Mental disturbance (≥20–30 mg/day): Rare in children.
- Osteoporosis (≥5 to 7.5 mg/day for 3 months).
- Osteonecrosis (risk at dose >20 mg/day for 1 month).
- Muscle weakness (>10–20 mg/day)
- Abnormal menstruation (↓follicle-stimulating hormone and luteinizing hormone) and depressed hormone levels (thyroid-stimulating hormone, testosterone).
- Adrenal suppression: >20 mg of daily prednisone for >3 weeks, or on ≥5 mg/day for >1 year; patients with a fasting morning plasma cortisol <5 to 10 μg/dL should be considered to have a potentially suppressed HPA axis; recovery takes 6 to 9 months after stopping.
- Ophthalmologic: Posterior subcapsular cataract formation (risk even at 5 mg/day), glaucoma (>10 mg/day), and central serous choroidopathy (any dose).

■ **Pregnancy**	Category C: • Prednisone and its metabolite, prednisolone, cross the human placenta which metabolizes prednisolone back to prednisone, reducing fetal exposure to about 10% of the maternal level. • Collaborative Perinatal Project followed women treated during the first trimester found no increase in congenital malformations. Only risk is possibly clefting.
■ **Lactation**	Minor amounts of prednisolone are secreted into human breast milk (1.5–5%). The long clinical experience suggests prednisolone therapy is compatible with breastfeeding. Some advise waiting for 4 hours after intake of prednisolone.

■ **Investigation/ monitoring**	• Urine analysis, hemoglobin, complete blood count, erythrocyte sedimentation rate, lipid profile, HIV, chest X-ray (if clinical suspicion of TB), blood sugar, BP, stool examination for ova and cysts for protozoal and parasite worms.
	  – A strongly positive Mantoux or a positive interferon gamma release assay (IGRA): Prophylactic isoniazid should be initiated.
	  – Gut infection by strongyloidiasis, can cause severe disease; for which a single dose albendazole to anyone starting steroids is advised.
	• Mini-mental status examination.

■ **Patient/physician advise**	• Prescribe corticosteroids at the lowest possible dose and taper the dose as soon as the disease activity permits. • Encourage physical activities and avoid immobilization (helps prevent myopathy). • Osteoporosis management – Prescribe dietary and supplemental calcium to achieve intake of 1000 to 1500 mg/day.

- Supply vitamin D at a minimum of 1000 IU/day.
- Consider bisphosphonate therapy implementation (if >7.5 mg/day for >3 months)
- Regular exercise (30 minute, 3–5 times/week): Aerobic, strength, flexibility, and balance.
- Limitation of alcohol consumption to ≤2 drinks/day.
- Limitation of caffeine consumption to ≤2 servings/day.
- Smoking cessation.
- Fall prevention, avoid high impact/twisting motion

■ **Reference**

Journals
- Lockwood DN. Steroids in leprosy type 1 (reversal) reactions: Mechanisms of action and effectiveness. Lepr Rev. 2000;71 Suppl: S111–4.
- Manandhar R, Shrestha N, Butlin CR, Roche PW. High levels of inflammatory cytokines are associated with poor clinical response to steroid treatment and recurrent episodes of type 1 reactions in leprosy. Clin Exp Immunol 2002;128:333–8.
- Negera E, Walker SL. The Effects of Prednisolone Treatment on Cytokine Expression in Patients with Erythema Nodosum Leprosum Reactions. Front Immunol 2018;9:189.
- Rao PSSS, Sugamaran DST, Richard J, Smith WCS. Multi-centre, double-blinded, randomized trial of three steroid regimens in the treatment of type 1 reactions in leprosy. Lepr Rev 2006;77:25–33.

Books
- Drugs for Pregnant and Lactating Women. 3rd Edition, Carl Weiner.
- British National Formulary (BNF 78), September 2019.
- Systemic Glucocorticoids in Rheumatology. https://expertconsult.inkling.com/read/hochberg-rheumatology-2-vol-set-7e/chapter-64/(last accessed 5/1/2020).
- Systemic Drugs in Dermatology. Sardana K, Editor. New Delhi; Jaypee Publishers; 2016.

9. Thalidomide

■ **Drug class**	Immunomodulatory and anti-inflammatory activity.
■ **Mechanism of action/ pharmacokinetics**	• No bactericidal or bacteristatic effect on *M. leprae*. • Mechanism in ENL not clearly known; decreased TNF-α levels likely important but contradictory evidence exists at present. • Stimulatory and inhibitory activities on IL-10 and IL-12 levels respectively may play a role. • Absorption: Slow and extensive after a single oral dose of 200 mg. • Time to peak concentration: 3–4 hour; plasma t½: 6 hours. • Multiple dosing at 200 mg/d caused no accumulation or change in the pharmacokinetics.
■ **Dosage**	**ENL**—first used by Sheskin (1965) 1. *Steroid naïve case* • Acute cases: Start 100 mg 3–4 times daily (controls ENL in 48 hours); taper—50 mg decrements every 2 to 4 weeks; can stop in 3–4 weeks. • Chronic cases: 100 mg 3–4 times daily; start dose tapering once control achieved; reduce by 50 mg decrements every 2–4 weeks; to 100 mg OD/alternate day/BD; duration of treatment: 3–6 months.

Chemotherapy

2. *Steroid dependent case*
- Steroid should be reduced to alternate day dose and tapered until the reaction recurs. Thalidomide is started at that time at a dose of 100 mg 4 times daily, and after control, prednisone can be discontinued and thalidomide tapered to a maintenance level. Every 6 months, an attempt should be made to discontinue it as outlined above.
- Another option is to initiate thalidomide at 50 mg BD and gradually increase to 50 mg TDS; in a proportion of cases effective control is achieved after which steroids can be tapered (based on a similar response in prurigo nodularis). Interestingly Japanese experience mirrors this regimen and a dose of 50–100 mg can be effective in ENL with less side-effects.

ENL unresponsive to thalidomide: May be due to:
- The reaction may not be ENL.
- BL case where both type 1 downgrading and type 2 reactions appear to be occurring simultaneously.
- ENL occurring in borderline cases may not respond to thalidomide.

■ **Drug interaction**	• May enhance the sedative activity of barbiturates, chlorpromazine, ethanol, and reserpine. • Effective contraception is essential during thalidomide treatment and any disturbaces thereof must be kept in mind. Thus, as concomitant use of carbamazepine, griseofulvin, certain herbal supplements such as St. John's wort, HIV protease inhibitors, modafinil, penicillins, phenytoin, rifabutin, or rifampicin with hormonal contraceptive agents may reduce the effectiveness of contraception during and up to 1 month after discontinuation of these concomitant therapies, women on thalidomide requiring treatment with one or more of these drugs must use two other effective or highly effective methods of contraception or abstain from heterosexual–sexual contact while taking thalidomide.
■ **Side-effects**	• Birth defects, peripheral neuropathy, toxic epidermal necrolysis, seizures, bradycardia, hypertension, orthostatic hypotension, headache, Stevens-Johnson syndrome, drowsiness, dizziness, rash, diarrhea, fever, chills, increased appetite, weight gain, confusion, amnesia, mood changes, photosensitivity, neutropenia, and increased HIV viral load. • Most frequent adverse drug reaction encountered: Drowsiness (in 13.5%), constipation (in 13.4%) and dizziness (in 6.8%).
■ **Pregnancy**	• Category X; also excreted in semen; thus treated males should wear a condom during coitus. • Limb abnormalities after first-trimester exposure, perhaps by creating a pro-oxidant balance. Even a single 50 mg dose can cause this defect.
■ **Lactation**	Considering the size of the molecule and the lack of protein binding, it is likely to be excreted into breast milk; may cause sedation in infant but exact effects not known
■ **Hepatic**	Use with caution
■ **Renal**	Use with caution

■ Investigation/ monitoring	• Effective contraception obligatory from **1 month** before starting, during treatment, and until **1 month** after therapy; document negative hCG test 24 hours prior to initiating thalidomide.
• Men should use condoms during treatment, during dose interruption, and for at least **1 week** after stopping if their partner is pregnant or is of childbearing potential and not using effective contraception.
• Monitor white blood cell count (including differential count) and platelet count (reduce dose or interrupt treatment if neutropenia or thrombocytopenia develop—consult product literature).
• Monitor for arterial or venous thromboembolism.
• Monitor patients for signs and symptoms of peripheral neuropathy.
• Hepatic disorder: Liver function should be monitored, particularly when there is history of, or concurrent, viral liver infection, or when thalidomide is combined with drugs known to be associated with liver dysfunction (e.g. paracetamol).
■ Patient/physician advise	• Advised about symptoms of thromboembolism and advised to report sudden breathlessness, chest pain, or swelling of a limb.
• Advise on risk of neutropenia (fever, sore throat) or of thrombocytopenia (such as bleeding)
• Warn about reporting any symptoms of peripheral neuropathy such as paresthesia, abnormal coordination, or weakness develop.
• Thalidomide Education and Risk Management System (TERMS) is advised.
■ Reference	*Journals*
• Ishii N, Ishida Y, Okano Y, Ozaki M, Gidoh M, Kumano K, Goto M, NogamiR, Hatano K, Yamada A, Yotsu RR [Japanese guideline on thalidomide usage in the management of erythema nodosum leprosum.] Nihon Hansenbyo Gakkai Zasshi 2011;80:275–85.]
• Mahmoud M, Walker SL. A systematic review of adverse drug reactions associated with thalidomide in the treatment of erythema nodosum leprosum. Leprosy review 2019;90(2):142–16.
• Matsuki T, Okano Y, Aoki Y, Ishida Y, Hatano K, Kumano K. [Effectiveness of thalidomide for erythema nodosum leprosum (ENL): Retrospective study of 20 Japanese cases in National Sanatorium Oku-Komyo-En]. Nihon Hansenbyo Gakkai Zasshi 2014;83:1–6.
• Sardana K. An observational analysis of low dose thalidomide in recalcitrant prurigo nodularis. Clin Exp Dermatol 2020;45(1):92–96.
• Sheskin J. Thalidomide in the treatment of lepra reactions. Clinical Pharmacology and Therapeutics 1965;6:303–6.
• Teo S, Resztak KE, Scheffler MA, Kook KA, Zeldis JB, Stirling DI, Thomas SD. Thalidomide in the treatment of leprosy. Microbes Infect 2002;4:1193–202.

Books
• Systemic Drugs in Dermatology. Sardana K, Editor. New Delhi; Jaypee Publishers; 2016.
• British National Formulary (BNF 78), September 2019.
• Jacobson RR. Treatment of Leprosy. In: Hastings RC, Editor. Leprosy. New York: Churchill Livingstone, 1994; p. 342. |

10. Azathioprine (AZA)

Drug class	Immunosuppressants
Mechanism of action/ pharmacokinetics	• Well absorbed after oral administration • Extensive metabolism with many active metabolites • AZA is a prodrug converted to 6-mercaptopurine, which is then converted to thiopurine nucleotides 6-thioguanine, which decrease *de novo* synthesis of purine nucleotides with resultant inhibition of DNA, RNA, and protein synthesis. • The metabolism is by xanthine oxidase (XO) and thiopurine methyltransferase (TPMT) which leads to inactive metabolites (those with intermediate activity of TPMT have GI side-effects, but also 50% of those, who have neutropenia, have normal TPMT levels.) • AZA causes ↓ in numbers of circulating B and T lymphocytes (particularly suppressor T cells and CD8+ T cells) immunoglobulin M (IgM) and IgG synthesis, and interleukin-2 (IL-2) secretion. • Onset of action is slow (8 weeks).
Dosage	• *Dosage*: 50 to 200 mg/day (1–2.5 mg/kg per day). Start 25 to 50 mg/day and increased by 25 to 50 mg every 1 to 2 weeks to desired dose. • It has been tried both in ENL and type I reaction but its results are better in combination with prednisolone.
Drug interaction	• Sulfasalazine, ACE inhibitors and trimethoprim/sulfamethoxazole increase the risk of leukopenia. • AZA may cause warfarin resistance. • Patients more likely (3×) to get a rash if co-treated with ampicillin or amoxicillin.
Side-effects	• *Common or very common*: GI intolerance, including nausea and diarrhea, bone marrow depression (dose-related), increased risk of infection, leukopenia, thrombocytopenia. • *Uncommon*: Anemia, hepatic disorders (liver enzymes mildly increased in 33%, or isolated hyperbilirubinemia; severe toxicity is rare), hypersensitivity (rash, fever, hepatitis, renal failure within first 2 weeks of use), pancreatitis. • *Rare or very rare*: Agranulocytosis, alopecia, bone marrow disorders, diarrhea, gastrointestinal disorders, neoplasms, photosensitivity reaction, pneumonitis, severe cutaneous adverse reactions (SCARs). • *Frequency not known*: Nodular regenerative hyperplasia, sinusoidal obstruction syndrome.
Pregnancy	Category D • Most pregnancies treated with azathioprine end successfully, even in transplant patients. • Azathioprine is teratogenic in rodents treated with human-equivalent doses, producing a constellation of malformations that are both skeletal and visceral.
Lactation	Most experts consider breastfeeding as acceptable up to 3.5 years of age. Avoid feeding for 4 hours after a dose.
Hepatic	Use with caution

■ Renal	Use with caution
■ Investigation/ monitoring	• TPMT: Some practitioners routinely order the TPMT test prior to administration of AZA or 6-MP, but this has not been universally adopted. With a lack of cost-effective data and optimal clinical circumstances for which the test should be ordered, other practitioners do not routinely check TPMT and elect for slow dose escalation with close monitoring of the blood counts. • CBC, platelet count, every 2 weeks during dose escalation and every 4 to 6 weeks after dose stability. (If leukopenia or thrombocytopenia occurs, the dose should be reduced by 50% or the drug discontinued. Patients developing macrocytosis require closer monitoring once alternative causes have been excluded.) • Liver transaminases should be checked every 6 to 8 weeks during therapy.
■ Patient/physician advise	Bone marrow suppression: Patients and their care givers should be warned to report immediately any signs or symptoms of bone marrow suppression e.g. inexplicable bruising or bleeding, infection.
■ Reference	*Journals* • Durães SM, Salles Sde A, Leite VR, Gazzeta MO. Azathioprine as a steroid sparing agent in leprosy type 2 reactions: report of nine cases. Lepr Rev 2011;82:304–9. • Lockwood DN, Darlong J, Govindharaj P, Kurian R, Sundarrao P, John AS. AZALEP a randomized controlled trial of azathioprine to treat leprosy nerve damage and type 1 reactions in India: Main findings. PLoS Negl Trop Dis 2017;11:e0005348. • Marlowe SN, Hawksworth RA, Butlin CR, Nicholls PG, Lockwood DN. Clinical outcomes in a randomized controlled study comparing azathioprine and prednisolone versus prednisolone alone in the treatment of severe leprosy type 1 reactions in Nepal. Trans R Soc Trop Med Hyg 2004;98:602–9. *Books* Chapter 67: Immunosuppressive agents: Cyclosporine, cyclophosphamide, azathioprine, mycophenolate mofetil, and tacrolimus. https://expertconsult.inkling.com/read/hochberg-rheumatology-2-vol-set-7e.

11. Methotrexate (MTX)

■ Drug class	Immunosuppressant, anti-cancer
■ Mechanism of action/ pharmacokinetics	Polyglutamation of MTX, leads to immunomodulating effects and long duration of action (4 to 6 weeks). • MTX (–) AICAR transformylase which leads to ↑ in the intracellular concentration of its substrate AICAR, which → release of adenosine. Adenosine is a tissue protective retaliatory metabolite with potent anti-inflammatory properties, including counter-regulation of neutrophils and dendritic cells, downregulation of macrophages, cytokine modulation, and inhibition of collagenase synthesis. • The time required for intracellular accumulation and elimination of the active MTX polyglutamates explains why a drug with a serum

half-life of 8 hours is effective when administered weekly and why it takes 4 to 6 weeks for a clinical response or flare to be observed with dose changes.

- Cytokine (Gerard et al, Funk et al)
  - While in rheumatoid arthritis, T cells isolated from methotrexate-treated patients have ↓ capacity to produce the cytokines characteristic of type 1 and type 2 T helper cells (namely IFN-γ, IL-4 and IL-13), as well as reduced production of granulocyte macrophage colony-stimulating factor, the effect on cytokines like TNF-α is *not* consistent and with high levels the response is poor. Hence, the response in ENL may *not* be consistently seen.
  - Also normalizes T regulatory (Treg) cell function
- Inhibits Janus kinase (JAK)/signal transducer and activator of transcription (STAT) signaling as well.

■ Dosage

- *Indication*: While MTX has been tried in ENL, a trial is underway using 15 or 20 mg of oral MTX each week for 48 weeks and prednisolone 40 mg per day, reducing to zero over 20 weeks.
- *Dose*: 7.5 to 25 mg orally, subcutaneous, or intramuscular weekly. The absorption of oral and parenteral MTX is equivalent at doses <15 mg/week. At higher doses, parenteral MTX gives serum levels 30% higher than oral MTX. Also at oral doses above 15 mg/week, better absorption is obtained if the oral dose is split (within a 24-hour period) or the parenteral form is used.
- Folic acid 1 mg/day should always be given with MTX, and the dose can be increased to 2 to 5 mg/day if symptoms of toxicity (mouth sores) develop. Folinic acid (leucovorin) 5 mg given as one dose, 8–24 hours after weekly dose of MTX can sometimes help mouth sores even if folic acid fails.

■ Drug interaction

- Use of some NSAIDs with high-dose methotrexate has been reported to elevate and prolong serum methotrexate levels. Caution is indicated whenever NSAIDs and salicylates are administered with lower doses of methotrexate. (In rheumatoid arthritis, concurrent use of constant-dosage regimens of NSAIDs, without apparent problems have been seen but the doses used in rheumatoid arthritis (7.5–15 mg/week) are somewhat lower.)
- Toxicity may be increased by the displacement of methotrexate by certain drugs such as phenylbutazone, phenytoin, salicylates, and sulfonamides.
- Oral antibiotics (e.g. chloramphenicol, tetracycline, nonabsorbable broad-spectrum antibiotics) may ↓ intestinal absorption of methotrexate or interfere with the enterohepatic circulation by inhibiting bowel flora and suppressing metabolism of the drug by bacteria.
- Penicillins may ↓ the renal clearance of methotrexate and increase serum concentrations with resultant hematologic and GI toxicity.
- May ↓ the clearance of theophylline; theophylline levels should be monitored closely.
- Vitamin preparations containing folic acid or its derivatives may↓ the response to methotrexate.

■ Side-effects	The most common toxicities associated with low-dose weekly MTX are anorexia, nausea, vomiting, and diarrhea. • *Oral ulcers*: Give folic acid (as above) or add vitamin A 8000 IU/day. • *Photosensitivity*. • *Hepatic toxicity*: Folic acid and subcutaneous dosing may reduce this side-effect. Concern has lessened with further experience, and routine liver biopsy is not recommended. (Obesity and diabetes mellitus increase fat in the liver and chance of MTX hepatotoxicity.) • *Hematologic toxicity*: This includes leukopenia, thrombocytopenia, pancytopenia, and megaloblastic anemia. (This is less likely to occur if renal function is normal.) • *Pneumonitis*: With pneumonitis, it is critical to eliminate infectious causes such as *Pneumocystis jiroveci* pneumonia, if MTX is the cause it must be stopped and not restarted. Symptoms are shortness of breath, cough (82%), and fever. • *Flu-like symptoms*: These include nausea, fatigue, fever, chills, myalgias, and are called "MTX flu". Some patients may have less of these symptoms if dextromethorphan 30 mg given with MTX and 30 mg 8 to 12 hours later. • Worsening nodulosis (5%) and leukocytoclastic vasculitis. • *Lymphomas*: When a patient on MTX is diagnosed with Epstein-Barr virus positive lymphoma, the treatment of the lymphoma is to stop the MTX. The lymphoma may resolve completely without chemotherapy in some patients. • Nonspecific central nervous system effects (e.g. dizziness, headache, mood alteration, memory impairment).
■ Pregnancy	Category X
■ Lactation	Contraindicated in case of high dose–low dose MTX may be considered, if needed, if breastfed 24 hours after weekly low dose.
■ Renal	MTX should not be used in patients on dialysis or who have a CrCl <30 mL/minute. The dose should be reduced by 25% and 50% for CrCl <80 mL/minute and <50 mL/minute, respectively.
■ Investigation/ monitoring	*Before starting* • CBC with platelets, hepatitis B and C serologies, aspartate aminotransferase (AST), alanine aminotransferase (ALT), albumin, and creatinine (CrCl) should be obtained. • Chest X-ray should be performed if the patient has not had one in the past year. *On therapy* • Monitor CBC, creatinine, and liver transaminases every 2 to 4 weeks for the first 3 months then every 2 to 3 months for the next 3 to 6 months, and then every 12 weeks. • Liver biopsy: Routine baseline or periodic liver biopsies in patients receiving MTX are not recommended. If LFTs are deranged, dose is ↓ and if still ↑, stop MTX and therapy is switched. • High-risk patients, defined as those with diabetes, obesity, abnormal liver test results, or significant alcohol intake, routine surveillance liver biopsies are still recommended with long-term use.

■ **Patient/physician advise**	• Should also avoid or limit (less than three to five drinks per week) alcohol (hepatoxicity) and trimethoprim-sulfamethoxazole (decreases excretion). • MTX should be stopped for 3 months in both men and women before planning a pregnancy. This corresponds to the timeframe of spermatogenesis and washout of MTX from tissues following cessation of drug administration. • Polymorphisms of reduced folate carrier (RFC), ATP-binding cassettes (ABC) proteins, and folylpolyglutamyl synthase (FPGS) account for variations in efficacy and toxicity of MTX among patients.
■ **Reference**	*Journals* • Funk RS, Chan MA, Becker ML. Cytokine Biomarkers of Disease Activity and Therapeutic Response after Initiating Methotrexate Therapy in Patients with Juvenile Idiopathic Arthritis. Pharmacotherapy, 2017; 37:700–711. • Gerards AH, de Lathouder S, de Groot ER, Dijkmans BA, Aarden LA. Inhibition of cytokine production by methotrexate. Studies in healthy volunteers and patients with rheumatoid arthritis. Rheumatology (Oxford) 2003;42:1189–96. • Hossain D. Using methotrexate to treat patients with ENL unresponsive to steroids and clofazimine: A report on 9 patients. Lepr Rev 2013;84: 105–12. • https://clinicaltrials.gov/ct2/show/NCT03775460. • Rahul N, Sanjay KS, Singh S. Effectiveness of methotrexate in prednisolone and thalidomide resistant cases of type 2 lepra reaction: Report on three cases. Lepr Rev 2015;86:379–82. *Books* • Chapter 66: Methotrexate: https://expertconsult.inkling.com/read/hochberg-rheumatology-2-vol-set-7e3

REFERENCES

1. Jamet P, Ji B. Relapse after long-term follow up of multibacillary patients treated by WHO multidrug regimen. Marchoux Chemotherapy Study Group. Int J Lepr Other Mycobact Dis 1995;63: 195–201.
2. Guidelines for the diagnosis, treatment and prevention of leprosy ISBN: 978 92 9022 638 3© World Health Organization 2018.
3. Ji B, Levy L, Grosset JH. Chemotherapy of leprosy: Progress since the Orlando Congress, and prospects for the future. Int J Lepr Other Mycobact Dis 1996;64:S80–8.
4. Shepard CC. Recent developments in the chemotherapy and chemoprophylaxis of leprosy. Leprologia (Argent) 1974;19:230–36.
5. WHO study group. Chemotherapy of leprosy for control programmes. Geneva: World Health Organization, 1982. Tech. Rep. Ser. 675.
6. Levy L, Shepard CC, Fasal P. The bactericidal effect of rifampicin on *M. leprae* in man: (a) Single doses of 600, 900 and 1200 mg; and (b) daily doses of 300 mg. Int J Lepr 1976;44:183–7.
7. THELEP subcommittee on clinical trials of the chemotherapy of leprosy (THELEP) scientific working group of the UNDP/WORLD BANK/WHO special programme for research and training in tropical diseases. Persisting *Mycobacterium leprae* among THELEP trial patients in Bamako and Chingleput. Lepr Rev 1987;58:325–37.
8. Boerrigter G, Ponnighaus JM, Fine PE. Preliminary appraisal of a WHO-recommended multiple drug regimen in paucibacillary leprosy patients in Malawi. Int J Lepr 1988;56:408–17.

9. Katoch K, Ramanathan U, Natrajan M, Bagga AK, Bhatia AS, Saxena RK et al. Relapses in paucibacillary patients after treatment with three short-term regimens containing rifampicin. Int J Lepr 1989;57458–64.
10. Marchoux chemotherapy study group. Relapse rates in multibacillary leprosy patients after stopping treatment with rifampin-containing regimens. Int J Lepr 1992;60:525–35.
11. Faget GH, Pogge RC, Johansen FA, Dinan JF, Prejean BM, Eccles CG. The Promin treatment of leprosy: a progress report. Int J Lepr Other Mycobact Dis 1966;34:298–310.
12. Seydel JK, Richter M, Wempe E. Mechanisms of action of the folate blocker diamino-diphenylsulfone (dapsone, DDS) studied in comparison to sulfonamides· International Journal of Leprosy 1980;48:18–29.
13. Sardana K. Miscellaneous Drugs. Dapsone. In: Sardana K, Ed. Systemic Drugs in Dermatology. Jaypee, New Delhi 2018; page 707–15.
14. Wakelin SH, Maibach HI. Dapsone in Systemic Drug Treatment in Dermatology. Second Edition© Taylor & Francis Group, LLC, 2015.
15. Degowin RL, Eppes RB, Powell RD, Carson PE. Haemolytic effect of diaminodiphenylsulfone (DDS) in normal subjects and in those with glucose-6-phosphate-dehydrogenase deficiency. Bulletin of the World Health Organization 1966;35:165–79.
16. Barss P. Fatal dapsone agranulocytosis in a Melanesian. Leprosy Review 1986;57:63–6.
17. Fernandes TRMO, Jesus BN, Barreto TT, Pereira AA. Dapsone-induced agranulocytosis in patients with Hansen's disease. An Bras Dermatol. 2017;92:894–7.
18. Agarwalla A, Agrawal S. Dapsone hypersensitivity syndrome: a clinical-epidemiological review. J Dermatol 2005;32:883–9.
19. Sebille A, Cordoliani G, Raffalli MJ, Nebout M, Chevallard A. Dapsone-induced neuropathy compounds Hansen's disease nerve damage: An electrophysiological study in tuberculoid patients. Int J Lepr Other Mycobact Dis 1987;55:16–22.
20. Reigart JR, Trammel HL (Jr), Lindsey JM. Repetitive doses of activated charcoal in dapsone poisoning in a child. Journal of Toxicology and Clinical Toxicology1982-1983;19:1061–6.
21. Cholo MC, Mothiba MT2, Fourie B3, Anderson R4. Mechanisms of action and therapeutic efficacies of the lipophilic antimycobacterial agents clofazimine and bedaquiline. J Antimicrob Chemother 2017;72:338–53.
22. Maghanoy A, Balagon M, Saunderson P, Scheelbeek P. A prospective randomised, double-blind, placebocontrolled trial on the effect of extended clofazimine on Erythema Nodosum Leprosum (ENL) in multibacillary (MB) leprosy. Lep Rev 2017;88:208–16.
23. Job CK, Yoder L, Jacobson RR, Hastings RC. Skin pigmentation from clofazimine therapy in leprosy patients: A reappraisal J Am Acad Dermatol 1990;23:236–41.
24. Farb H, West b. P, Pedvis-Leftick A. Clofazimine in pregnancy complicated by leprosy. Obstetrics and Gynaecology 1982;59:122–3.
25. Opromolla DVA. First results of the use of rifamycin in the treatment of lepromatous leprosy. International Journal of Leprosy 1963;31:552.
26. Rees RJW, Pearson JMH, Waters MFR. Experimental and clinical studies on rifampicin in treatment of leprosy. British Medical Journal 1970;1:89–92.
27. Shepard CC, Levy L, Fasal P. Further experience with the rapid bactericidal effect of rifampin on *Mycobacterium leprae* in man. American Journal of Tropical Medicine & Hygiene1976;23:1120–4.
28. Levy L, Shepard CC, Fasal P. The bactericidal effect of rifampicin on *M. leprae* in man: (a) Single doses of 600, 900 and 1200 mg; and (b) daily doses of 300 mg. International Journal of Leprosy 1976;44:183–7.
29. Rees RJ, Waters MF, Pearson JM, Helmy HS, Laing AB. Long-term treatment of dapsone-resistant leprosy with rifampicin: Clinical and bacteriological studies. Int J Lepr Other Mycobact Dis 1976;44:159–69.
30. Opromolla DV, Tonello CJ, McDougall AC, Yawalkar SJ. A controlled trial to compare the therapeutic effects of dapsone in combination with daily or once monthly rifampicin in patients with lepromatous leprosy. Int J Lepr Other Mycobact Dis 1981;49:393–7.

31. McAllister WA, Thompson PJ, Al-Habet SM, Rogers HJ. Rifampicin reduces effectiveness and bioavailability of prednisolone. Br Med J (Clin Res Ed). 1983;286:923–5.
32. Jacobson RR, Hastings RC. Rifampin-resistant leprosy. Lancet 1976;(11):2:1304–5.
33. Sehgal VN, Sardana K, Dogra S. The imperatives of leprosy treatment in the pre- and post-global leprosy elimination era: Appraisal of changing the scenario to current status. J Dermatolog Treat. 2008;19:82–91.
34. Grosset JH. Newer drugs in leprosy. Int J Lepr Other Mycobact Dis 2001;69:S14–8.
35. Ji B, Grosset J. Combination of rifapentine-moxifloxacin-minocycline (PMM) for the treatment of leprosy. Lepr Rev 2000;71:S81–7.
36. Consigny S, Bentoucha A, Bonnafous P, Grosset J, Ji B. Bactericidal activities of HMR 3647, moxifloxacin, and rifapentine against *Mycobacterium leprae* in mice. Antimicrob Agents Chemother 2000;44):2919–2.
37. Burgos J, de la Cruz E, Paredes R, Andaya CR, Gelber RH. The activity of several newer antimicrobials against logarithmically multiplying *M. leprae* in mice. Lepr Rev 2011;82:253–8.
38. Ji B. Prospects for chemotherapy of leprosy. Indian J Lepr 2000;72:187–98.
39. Ji B, Jamet P, Perani EG, Sow S, Lienhardt C, Petinon C, Grosset JH. Bactericidal activity of single dose of clarithromycin plus minocycline, with or without ofloxacin, against *Mycobacterium leprae* in patients. Antimicrob Agents Chemother 1996;40:2137–41.
40. Ji B, Sow S, Perani E, Lienhardt C, Diderot V, Grosset J. Bactericidal activity of a single-dose combination of ofloxacin plus minocycline, with or without rifampin, against *Mycobacterium leprae* in mice and in lepromatous patients. Antimicrob Agents Chemother 1998;42:1115–20.
41. Colston MJ, Hilson GR, Banerjee DK.. The proportional bactericidal test, a method for assessing bactericidal activity of drugs against *M. leprae* in mice. Lepr Rev 1978;49:7–15.
42. Arumugam S, Joseph P, Ponnaiya J, Richard J, Das M, Chaitanya VS, Ebenezer M. Evaluation of New Antibacterial Drugs and their Combinations in a Murine Model to Identify Short Duration Alternative Chemotherapy for Leprosy. Indian J Lepr 2016;88:159–76.
43. Ji B. Relapse of multibacillary leprosy after treatment with daily rifampin plus ofloxacin for four weeks. Int J Lepr Other Mycobact Dis 1998;66:391–2.
44. Rao PS. A study on nonadherence to MDT among leprosy patients. Indian J Lepr 2008;80:149–54.
45. Honrado ER, Tallo V, Balis AC, Chan GP, Cho SN. Noncompliance with the World Health Organization multi-drug therapy among leprosy patients in Cebu, Philippines: Its causes and implications on the leprosy control program. Dermatol Clin 2008;26:221–29.
46. Chemotherapy of leprosy: Report of a WHO study group. WHO, Technical Report Series 847, 1994.
47. WHO Expert Committee on leprosy. Eighth report. WHO, Technical Report Series 968, 2012.
48. Deps PD, Nasser S, Guerra P, Simon M, Birshner Rde C, Rodrigues LC. Adverse effects from multi-drug therapy in leprosy: A Brazilian study. Lepr Rev 2007;78:216–22.
49. Singh H, Nel B, Dey V, Tiwari P, Dulhani N. Adverse effects of multi-drug therapy in leprosy, a two years' experience (2006–2008) in tertiary health care centre in the tribal region of Chhattisgarh State (Bastar, Jagdalpur). Lepr Rev 2011;82:17–24.
50. Goulart IM, Arbex GL, Carneiro MH, Rodrigues MS, Gadia R. Adverse effects of multi-drug therapy in leprosy patients: A five-year survey at a Health Center of the Federal University of Uberlandia. Rev Soc Bras Med Trop 2002;35:453–60.
51. Ambooken BE, George S, Azeez N, Asokan N, Xavier TD. Adverse Drug Reactions (ADR) necessitating modification of multi-drug therapy (MDT) in Hansen's disease: A retrospective study from Kerala, India Leprosy review 2017;88:197–207.
52. Dupnik KM, Cardoso FJ, De Macêdo AL, De Sousa IL, Leite RC, Jerônimo SM, et al. Intolerance to leprosy multi-drug therapy: More common in women? Lepr Rev 2013;84:209–18.
53. Kannan G, Vasantha J, Rani NV, et al. Drug usage evaluation of dapsone. Indian Journal of Pharmaceutical Sciences 2009;71:456–60.

54. Deps PD, Nasser S, Guerra P, Simon M, Birshner Rde C, Rodrigues LC. Adverse effects from multi-drug therapy in leprosy: A Brazilian study. Lepr Rev 2007;78:216–22.
55. Byrd SR, Gelber RH. Effect of dapsone on haemoglobin concentration in patients with leprosy. Lepr Rev 1991;62:171–78.
56. Maia MV, Cunha Mda G, Cunha CS. Adverse effects of alternative therapy (minocycline, ofloxacin, and clofazimine) in multibacillary leprosy patients in a recognized health care unit in Manaus, Amazonas, Brazil. An Bras Dermatol 2013;88:205–10.
57. WHO model prescribing information: Drugs used in leprosy Geneva: World Health Organization; 1998.
58. WHO Guidelines for the Diagnosis, Treatment and Prevention of Leprosy 2018 (available at: http://nlep.nic.in/pdf/WHO%20Guide-lines%20for%20leprosy.pdf)
59. Lockwood DN, Cunha Mda G. Developing new MDT regimens for MB patients; time to test ROM 12-month regimens globally. Lepr Rev 2012;83:241–4.
60. Pattyn S, Grillone S. Relapse rates and a 10-year follow-up of a 6-week quadruple drug regimen for multibacillary leprosy. Lepr Rev 2002;73:245–47.
61. Setia MS, Shinde SS, Jerajani HR, Boivin JF. Is there a role for rifampicin, ofloxacin and minocycline (ROM) therapy in the treatment of leprosy? Systematic review and meta-analysis. Trop Med Int Health 2011;16:1541–51.
62. Pardillo FE, Burgos J, Fajardo TT, Dela Cruz E, Abalos RM, Paredes RM, Andaya CE, Gelber RH. Powerful bactericidal activity of moxifloxacin in human leprosy. Antimicrob Agents Chemother 2008;52:3113–7.
63. Cunha Mda G, Virmond M, Schettini AP, Cruz RC, Ura S, Ghuidella C, Viana Fdos R, Avelleira JC, Campos AA, Filho bofloxacin multicentre trial in MB leprosy. FUAM—Manaus and ILSL—Bauru, Brazil. Lepr Rev 2012;83:261–8.
64. A guide for surveillance of antimicrobial resistance in leprosy, 2017 update (https://www.who.int/lep/resources/9789290226192/en/)
65. Grosset JH1, Guelpa-Lauras CC, Bobin P, Brucker G, Cartel JL, Constant-Desportes M, et al. Study of 39 documented relapses of multibacillary leprosy after treatment with rifampin. Int J Lepr 198;57: 607–14.
66. Ji B, Jamet P, Perani EG, Bobin P, Grosset JH. Powerful bactericidal activities of clarithromycin and minocycline against *Mycobacterium leprae* in lepromatous leprosy. J Infect Dis 1993;168: 188–90.
67. Pardillo FE1, Burgos J, Fajardo TT, Dela Cruz E, Abalos RM, Paredes RM, et al. Powerful bactericidal activity of moxifloxacin in human leprosy. Antimicrob Agents Chemother 2008;52:3113–7.
68. Pardillo FE, Burgos J, Fajardo TT, Dela Crux E, Abalos RM, Paredes RM, et al. Rapid killing of *M. leprae* by moxifloxacin in two patients with lepromatous leprosy. Lepr Rev 2009;80:205–9.
69. Jacobson RR. Treatment of Leprosy. In: Hastings RC, editor. Leprosy. New York: Churchill Livingstone, 1994; p. 342.
70. Moet FJ, Pahan D, Oskam L, Richardus JH; COLEP Study Group. Effectiveness of single dose rifampicin in preventing leprosy in close contacts of patients with newly diagnosed leprosy: Cluster randomized controlled trial. BMJ 2008;336:761–4.
71. Penna GO, Bührer-Sékula S, Kerr LRS, Stefani MMA, Rodrigues LC, de Araújo MG, Ramos AMC. Uniform multi-drug therapy for leprosy patients in Brazil (U-MDT/CT-BR): Results of an open label, randomized and controlled clinical trial, among multibacillary patients. PLoS Negl Trop Dis 2017;11:e0005725.
72. Butlin RC, Pahan D, Kya A, Maug J, Withington S, Nicholls P, et al. Outcome of 6 months MB-MDT in MB patients in Bangladesh preliminary results. Lepr Rev 2016;87:171–82.
73. Rao PN, Suneetha S, Pratap DV. Comparative study of uniform—MDT and WHO MDT in pauci- and multibacillary leprosy patients over 24 months of observation. Lepr Rev 2009;80:143–55.

7.2 CHEMOPROPHYLAXIS, IMMUNOPROPHYLAXIS AND IMMUNOTHERAPEUTICS IN LEPROSY

Ananta Khurana, Kabir Sardana

New case detection rate is decreasing slowly and is suggestive of continued transmission of infection and thus chemo- and immunoprophylaxis are needed to reduce new case detection rate (NCDR). Chemoprophylaxis as a means to reduce transmission of leprosy is logistically a more feasible concept than vaccination and was originally researched in 1960s.[1-8] In the 1960s and 70s, long courses of dapsone (2–3 years) or acedapsone (every 10 weeks for 7 months) were attempted and resulted in an overall reduction of the leprosy NCDR of 40% (with dapsone) and 51% (with acedapsone) in contacts.[1,2,7,8] However, owing to the cumbersome treatment schedules, these regimens were not widely implemented.

While certain programmes have inculcated postexposure prophylaxis (PEP), there are important aspects of this that warrant analysis before its implementation (Box 7.3).

In 1988, single dose rifampicin (SDR) chemoprophylaxis (25 mg/kg) was first studied in the Southern Marquesas Islands in a non-controlled trial.[9,10] Of the 2786 inhabitants, 2751 (98.7%) were treated. In addition, 3144 South Marquesas living elsewhere in French Polynesia were administered the same chemoprophylaxis. Follow-up survey 10 years later suggested a 70% effectiveness of chemoprophylaxis, with only 5 new cases being detected in treated population, as against the expected number of 17.[11] However, over the same period, a 50% reduction in the NCDR was observed in the non-treated population of French Polynesia as well. Therefore, the true effectiveness of SDR was estimated to be only 35–40%.[11] In the mid-1990s, chemoprophylaxis was introduced on different pacific islands where the leprosy NCDR had remained very high.[12] Over two cycles, with a 1-year interval, 70% of the population was screened for leprosy and treated prophylactically. Healthy adults received rifampicin, ofloxacin and minocycline (ROM), while children under 15 years received SDR. In 1999, a substantial reduction in the NCDR was observed.

Subsequent to this, a few large scale trials have been conducted with robust methodology. These are summarized in Table 7.7.[13-20] While some positive impact was reported, a glaring finding is that the maximum protection was to *contacts* not directly related to the index patient. Paradoxically, the further the contacts were physically removed from the index case, the more pronounced was the effect of SDR in protecting against leprosy. This is probably due to a *lower* exposure rate and hence

 Box 7.3: Important aspects of PEP that deserve attention

- What type of intervention works best in different epidemiological settings?
- Cost effectiveness of PEP.
- Quality of diagnosis performed by local village workers.
- Why does the closest contact receive the *least* benefit of PEP?
- Why does the benefit of single dose rifampin end after 2 years?
- COLEP—study was not powered for subanalysis (effect on contacts of MB index case).
- Drug donation will be needed for mass coverage.

Table 7.7: Major clinical trials on single dose rifampicin (completed and ongoing)

Trial/authors	Place	Participants	Intervention	Results	Remarks
COLEP trial (Moet et al, 2004)[13]	Bangladesh	21,711 close contacts of 1037 patients with newly diagnosed leprosy	SDR or placebo given to close contacts (household, first and second neighbor and social contacts) in second months of starting the index case on treatment	• 91/9452 contacts in placebo group and 59/9417 in SDR group developed leprosy • Overall a 57% reduction in incidence of leprosy using SDR in the first 2 years. There was no additional effect after 4 and 6 years.[14] However, total difference in incidence between the 2 arms remained statistically significant showing that no apparent excess cases were observed in the SDR arm within 6 years after the intervention • Number needed to treat (NNT) to prevent a case of leprosy among contacts was 297 • Protective effect for BCG (given at infancy) was 56% in the placebo arm and 53% in the rifampicin arm	SDR mainly effective in contacts of paucibacillary leprosy and contacts: 1. Who were not closely related to the index patient; (maximum benefit in neighbor of neighbor and social contact group rather than household contacts) and had lowest risk profile as per intake data 2. Female contacts 3. Who were seronegative for *M. leprae* specific PGL-1 antibodies at intake 4. Without a BCG scar 5. Ages 10–14 and 20–29 The combined effect of SDR with BCG given at infancy showed a protective effect of 80%
MALTALEP (Richardus et al, 2019)[16] (To assess prevention of new leprosy cases among contacts in the first year after BCG vaccination)	Bangladesh	14,988 contacts (household and next door neighbors) of 1552 new leprosy patients randomized into the SDR– arm (n = 7379) and the SDR + arm (n = 7609)	SDR+ arm: BCG vaccination followed by SDR 8–12 weeks later. SDR– arm: BCG vaccination alone given	• SDR+ arm: 19 new leprosy cases in first year and 29 in second year • SDR– arm: 27 new in first year and 24 in second year • Reduction in incidence of leprosy in SDR+ compared to SDR– was 42% (nonsignificant; p = 0.148) in the first year	• To what extent SDR suppresses excess leprosy cases after BCG vaccination is difficult to establish because many cases appeared before the SDR intervention. • Thus, BCG vaccination followed by SDR cannot be recommended as a routine intervention in leprosy control

(Contd.)

Table 7.7: Major clinical trials on single dose rifampicin (completed and ongoing) (Contd.)

Trial/authors	Place	Participants	Intervention	Results	Remarks
				• No additional effect of SDR on 2nd year • 33.6% cases appeared within 8–12 weeks of BCG, the window period between BCG and provision of CDR	
Bakker et al, 2005[17] (Contact versus mass chemopophylaxis with 2 doses of rifampicin)	Indonesia	A total of 3,965 participants in three groups (over 5 islands) 1. Control group: An island where no chemoprophylaxis given (n = 1252) 2. Contact group: Island on which chemoprophylaxis given to contacts of leprosy patients (comprising household and neighbor contacts) (n = 1633) 3. Blanket group: 3 islands where chemoprophylaxis given to all eligible persons (n = 1080)	2 doses of rifampicin 600 mg for adults and 300 mg for children (6–14 years old) with approximately 3.5 months between doses	• The cumulative incidence after 33.5 months follow-up was significantly lower in the blanket group compared with the control group, while no difference was found between the contact and control groups • The effectiveness of blanket supply of prophylaxis based on the adjusted hazard ratio was 74.6% (90.9% if consider only those who received at least one dose supervised)	• Population-based prophylaxis was associated with a reduced leprosy incidence in the first three years • In an area of high endemicity, rifampicin prophylaxis for spatially defined contacts only does not influence leprosy incidence

(Contd.)

Table 7.7: Major clinical trials on single dose rifampicin (completed and ongoing) (Contd.)

Ongoing trials	Place	Participants	Intervention	Primary outcome measure	Other outcome measure
PEP+++[18] (2017–2022)	India and Brazil	• Close contacts who test positive for antibodies against ND-O-LID conjugate are given PEP++ • Negative contacts receive SDR	1. SDR PEP 2. PEP++: A multi-dose regimen comprising three doses of 600 mg rifampicin + moxifloxacin 400 mg given at four weekly intervals	To compare the efficacy of an enhanced chemoprophylaxis regimen (PEP++) with that of SDR PEP	
PEP4LEP[19] (2018–2022)	Mozambique, Ethiopia and Tanzania	Household contacts of index case	1. Community based, using skin camps to screen around 100 contacts of leprosy patients and provide them with SDR when eligible 2. Health centre-based, inviting household contacts to be screened and given SDR when eligible	• To compare the effectiveness of a skin camp prophylaxis intervention to a health centre-based prophylaxis intervention in terms of the rate of leprosy patients detected and delay in case detection • To compare the feasibility of the two chemoprophylaxis interventions in terms of cost effectiveness and acceptability	• To assess the acceptability of a common skin diseases approach and the use of the SkinApp • To compare the capacity of health workers in diagnosing leprosy and other neglected infectious diseases that manifest with skin lesions before the start of the study with their capacity in the third year

a *lower* bacterial load of these further distanced contacts, rendering a single dose of rifampicin more effective.[14] Further, the protection seen so far is largely for *paucibacillary* leprosy and *single lesion* leprosy and not multibacillary (MB) leprosy and lasted for only **2 years**.[13] This again suggests that SDR provides protection only when patients have a low bacillary load. It is also not yet clear whether the intervention only causes a delay in the development of leprosy or a complete clearance of infection and interruption of transmission. This aspect needs a longer follow-up to be clarified. However, as only PB disease is prevented, the transmission with MB cases would continue unabated.

The recently published results of the MALTALEP trial examined the effect of SDR on the increased risk of PB leprosy in the first months after BCG vaccination. The authors found an unexpectedly high proportion of PB cases developing after BCG vaccination before the proposed time of SDR administration. The overall protection offered by SDR was 42%, less than the 57% reported in COLEP trial involving the same population. A possible reason is exclusion of second neighbors and social contacts who were included under COLEP.

While WHO document provides a *conditional recommendation* for SDR "for contacts of leprosy patients, in adults and children 2 years of age and above, after excluding leprosy and TB disease and other contraindications, by programmes that can ensure adequate management of contacts and upon agreement of the index case to disclose his/her disease".[21] The document lays stress on ensuring high coverage of contact screening by leprosy programmes implementing SDR and on obtaining patient consent before going ahead with contact tracing. The Indian programme—National Leprosy Eradication Programme (NLEP) also recommends SDR for "a person who has been living/working/having social activities for more than three months and 20 hours/week with a newly detected case of leprosy in the last one year".[22] However, studies evaluating feasibility and effectiveness of SDR for leprosy chemoprophylaxis are still underway, including the leprosy post-exposure prophylaxis (LPEP) study, which began in 2015 and is expected to be completed soon.[23] The study involves numerous endemic regions, including India, Indonesia, Myanmar, Nepal, Sri Lanka and Tanzania. As a part of this, feasibility and efficacy of blanket SDR administration in a high endemicity isolated Indonesian island community (Lingat village on the Indonesian Selaru island) was recently reported.[23] On the same lines, the WHO guidelines development group (GDG) (2018) also noted that blanket approach might be more feasible in areas of high endemicity and concomitant high population density.[21] In most other study areas, LPEP programme has targeted specific contact groups rather than the blanket approach utilized in Lingat village. The blanket approach may possibly be favorable in the context of high stigma and discrimination associated with leprosy as under this approach disclosure of index cases may not be required. Stigma may form an important hindrance in implementation of SDR in endemic regions, as also seen in the COLEP trial.[13] Another advantage of the blanket approach would be ability to cover the farther distanced contacts, whom are actually most likely to benefit from SDR (as shown in the COLEP trial) and may be missed in programmes only involving the household contacts. But, the feasibility in field settings has not been studied outside Indonesia and in more open communities.[24]

Idema et al examined the cost effectiveness of SDR for contacts of newly diagnosed leprosy patients (participants of the COLEP trial) and observed that in total, $6,009 incremental cost was invested and 38 incremental leprosy cases were prevented, resulting in an incremental cost effectiveness ratio (ICER) of $158 per one additional prevented leprosy case.[25,26] However, SDR was most cost-effective in neighbors of neighbors and social contacts (ICER $214) and slightly less cost-effective in next door neighbors (ICER $497) and least cost-effective among household contacts (ICER $856).[25] Prevention of disabilities, patients' costs and costs caused by loss of production due to absence from work could not be taken into account because no reliable data were available. It is notable that contact tracing is not included in all leprosy programmes and incremental costs thereof must also be considered. Also, the implementation costs would vary from country to country, as does the proportion of PB (more likely to be prevented) and MB cases and the proportion of new cases who are household contacts of a known leprosy case, and hence individual scenarios need to be clarified before implementing the SDR approach widely. The results of LPEP study from different countries would likely clarify these aspects.[23]

The possibility of inducing rifampicin resistance in *M. leprae* and *M. tuberculosis* has been estimated to be very low with the use of single doses of rifampicin, though the

Box 7.4: Single dose rifampicin prophylaxis: Concerns and future directions[42]

- Understanding leprosy endemic areas and mapping hidden case prevalence
- Focusing on including active case finding and contact screening in all national programmes and improving the efficiency of these measures in community where they are already being done
- Development of field-friendly, point-of-care rapid diagnostic test for field workers
- Role of additional supplementation after 2 years
- Use of other drugs and regimens
- Study of ideal vaccine useful in combination with SDR

risk increases with repeated doses.[27] But, in areas with a known high prevalence of primary MDR-TB, caution is needed because exposure to rifampicin in such areas may provide an advantage for already drug-resistant *M. tuberculosis*.[28] Rifampicin prophylaxis also assumes and relies on rifampicin sensitivity of the circulating *M. leprae* strains. Regular sampling and molecular monitoring for mutations associated with rifampicin resistance in *M. tuberculosis* as well as in *M. leprae* would need to be considered in areas where SDR is given to contacts of leprosy patients.[27]

While there are numerous unanswered questions which are yet to be factored in to make SDR, a concept worthy of universal emulation, some concerns are listed in Box 7.4 and can help the clinician make a learned decision regarding implementation of SDR and its hurried implementation may not yet impact on the transmission dynamics of leprosy.

IMMUNOPROPHYLAXIS IN LEPROSY

Even though MDT has been successful the NCDR is not decreasing substantially and there is a need to eliminate transmission for which chemo- and immunoprophylaxis are needed. The ideal vaccine for leprosy is one which can induce a strong, long-lasting T cell response against *M. leprae* antigens and provide immunological memory and sustained protection (Box 7.5).

The potential applications of a leprosy vaccine include:[42]
1. Treatment shortening for paucibacillary (PB) treatment.
2. PEP in leprosy contacts.

Bacillus-Calmette-Guérin (BCG)

BCG was thought of as a vaccine for preventing leprosy after it was demonstrated that it led to lepromin conversion. There is consistent evidence that BCG protects against leprosy, although the reported degree of protection varies widely. Merle et al (2010) performed a review of published literature and reported that the magnitude of protection with BCG is estimated to be approximately 41% from trials and 60% from observational studies.[29] A more recent meta-analysis found the protective effect to be about 26% and again noted an overestimation of the protective effect by observational studies.[30] The protection was noted to be better for MB forms of leprosy compared

Box 7.5: The ideal properties of a leprosy vaccine[42]

- Safety in patients and healthy individuals
- Ability to induce a specific and sustained immune response
- Ability to be used in contacts, with or without SDR, to inhibit transmission and disease progression

with PB forms. Similarly, Schuring et al also observed a statistically significant lower BCG frequency among MB patients compared to PB patients, possibly implying that BCG protects against the development of MB leprosy.[31]

There is limited data on the effects of age on the efficacy of BCG vaccination. The observational studies indicate a reduced protective efficacy with increasing age but none such decrease is observed in experimental studies.[30] BCG offers more protection among household contacts compared with other contacts, although the difference was not found to be significant.[30] WHO recommends that BCG at birth is effective in reducing the risk of leprosy disease and its use should be maintained at least in all leprosy high-burden countries.[21]

For preventing leprosy among contacts of leprosy cases, BCG re-vaccination is used as an approach.[32–34] Brazil officially recommends BCG revaccination (up to 2 life-time doses of BCG) for contacts without signs or symptoms of leprosy upon examination, regardless of whether the index case is PB or MB. However, literature regarding the effect of re-vaccination is contradictory. Cunha et al found no additive protection of revaccination in a randomized controlled trial (RCT) of almost 100,000 Brazilian school children who received their first vaccination at birth.[32] However, another RCT done in Malawian infants and adults showed that a second BCG vaccination afforded an additional 49% protection compared with no revaccination. A paradoxical increase in leprosy cases within a 2–10 months of vaccination in contacts has been noted. The risk is highest among those vaccinated with no previous scar, and assumed not to have received BCG in infancy. In the MALTATEP trial, as mentioned before, this occurred even earlier at about 8–12 weeks after BCG vaccination (Table 7.7). An accelerated pro-inflammatory Th1 immunity to *M. leprae* antigens revealing incipient forms of PB leprosy was proposed as a likely cause. Duppre et al observed that the number of cases detected however declined substantially after the first year, and in the following years the protection rate reached 80%.[34]

The WHO position paper on BCG vaccination notes that there is minimal or no evidence of any additional benefit of repeat BCG vaccination against leprosy.[35] Therefore, BCG re-vaccination is not recommended even if the tuberculin skin test (TST) reaction or result of an interferon-γ release assay (IGRA) is negative. Further, it states that the absence of a BCG scar after vaccination is not indicative of lack of protection and is not an indication for re-vaccination. Although BCG vaccination has proven to be only partially effective, this important vaccine must be maintained and kept available for applications in both TB and leprosy, at least for the foreseeable future.

Other Vaccines

Two inactivated vaccines for *M. leprae* have potential: **MIP**, a whole-cell vaccine of heat-killed mycobacteria (*M. indicus pranii* previously known as *Mycobacterium w*); and **LepVax**, based on a multivalent recombinant protein formulated. The latter contains an antigenic protein adjuvant that has been used in more than a dozen vaccine candidates and is a safe and effective inducer of durable T cell responses.

An immunoprophylaxis trial conducted in South India among 1,71,400 volunteers evaluated four vaccines: (i) A combination of BCG and heat killed *Mycobacterium leprae* **(HKML)**, (ii) the **ICRC bacillus** (a killed vaccine), (iii) *Mycobacterium w* (*Mw*)/*M. indicus pranii* (*MIP*), and (iv) BCG, and employed normal saline as a placebo. The protective efficacies of the vaccines were: BCG + HKML, 64%; the ICRC vaccine, 65.5%; *Mw*, 25.7% and

BCG, 34.1% protection.[36] The "negative effect" of disease induction was also reported here and was similar to other vaccine trials. It was 7.6% with BCG + HKML, 6.9% with ICRC, 11.5% with *Mw* and 28.7% with BCG. However, despite the maximum protection shown in this trial, wider use of ICRC vaccine has not been reported. ICRC is a cultivable mycobacteria belonging to *M. avium intracellulare* complex and shares several antigens with *M. leprae*.

On the other hand, *Mw/MIP* was later tested in a large-scale, double-blind trial in Uttar Pradesh, India. The vaccine consisted of 1×10^9 heat-killed *Mw* bacilli for the first dose, with a second, half dose, given 6 months later.[37] A total of 24,060 household contacts were vaccinated with *Mw* or placebo. When only contacts received the vaccine, *Mw* vaccine showed a protective efficacy of 68.6% at the end of first, 59% at the end of the second and 39.3% at the end of the third follow-up survey. When both patients and contacts received the vaccine, the protective efficacy observed was 68%, 60% and 28% at the end of the first, second and third surveys, respectively. When patients, and not the contacts, received the vaccine, a protective efficacy of 42.9% in the first, 31% in the second and 3% in the third survey was shown. Thus, vaccination of contacts was more valuable in achieving the objective of immunoprophylaxis than that of patients. The protective effect was sustained for a period of about 7–8 years after which the authors suggest a booster vaccination for the sustained protection. Experimental data suggests that macrophages recognize and respond to *MIP* through a TLR2, NOD2 and an MyD88-dependent pathway and its cell wall fraction strongly potentiates protective Th1 activity.[39] Though the vaccine is commercially available ("Immuvac"), it has not yet been tested in other leprosy-endemic regions. Further trials on the vaccine are ongoing in five districts of high endemicity in India.[40,41] Immediate contacts of the patients will be immunized with two doses of *MIP*, with a 6-month interval between inoculations. Also, autoclaved *MIP* would be administered to leprosy patients in conjunction with MDT.

Mycobacterium vaccae and *Mycobacterium habana* have been tested in limited trials but wider use has not ensued.

LepVax: Comprises a hybrid recombinant protein, linking four *M. leprae* antigens: ML2531, ML2380, ML2055, and ML2028 (LEP-F1), formulated in a stable emulsion with a synthetic, TLR4 agonist (GLA-SE) as adjuvant. The four antigens were selected on the basis of immune recognition by paucibacillary leprosy patients and *M. leprae*-exposed individuals. The results of a phase I trial were recently reported and LepVax was found to be safe and immunogenic in healthy subjects. The vaccine induced an LEP-F1-specific antibody response and Th1 cytokine secretion (IFN-γ, IL-2, TNF).[42] A previous study demonstrated that administration of LepVax to already infected armadillos delays the onset of nerve conduction deficits and reduces their severity.[43] LepVax will now enter into phase 2 evaluations in Brazil this year.[44]

IMMUNOTHERAPEUTICS IN LEPROSY

Immunotherapy has been attempted in leprosy in order to achieve a faster and more efficient killing of the bacilli, thus reducing durations of treatment, reactions and relapses.

Mw/MIP immunotherapy has been reported to be efficacious as an adjunct to multi-drug therapy multibacillary regimen in leprosy patients with high bacillary index in various reports from India.[45–53] The vaccine has been administered every 3–6 months along with standard WHO MDT. *Mw* has been reported to produce a faster clinical response, more rapid clearance of granulomas on histopathology and earlier attainment of smear negativity in comparison with MDT alone.[45] A comparison of *Mw* with BCG, given in the same protocol of 3 monthly injections with MDT, showed a slightly better and faster effect on bacteriological clearance and clinical improvement with BCG.[46] A higher incidence of reversal reactions has been reported in a few studies on *Mw* immunotherapy, while the incidence of type 2 reactions has been shown to be similar to control groups or lower.[43,48]

Mw is reported to be well tolerated except for formation of a blister or nodule at injection site after 3–4 weeks which heals on its own in another 6–8 weeks and regional lymphadenopathy. Rare adverse effects include a generalized granulomatous dermatitis reported in 2 patients with lepromatous leprosy.[54] Similarly, disseminated cutaneous BCG infection has been reported with the vaccine's use for immunotherapy of lepromatous leprosy.[55]

While the *MIP* vaccine is undergoing further evaluations in India, the LepVax candidate will enter into Phase 2 evaluations in Brazil this year and these in addition to BCG, bring to the fore three potential vaccine candidates for use in a zero leprosy campaign. Like any other chemotherapeutic aspect in leprosy, the vaccine trials needed to objectively evaluated based on safety and efficacy endpoints, including changes in neurological function and should have well defined targets; including shortening the duration of treatment for PB disease and disease prevention in contacts.[56]

REFERENCES

1. Wardekar RV. DDS prophylaxis against leprosy. Lepr India 1967;39:155–9.
2. Noordeen SK. Chemoprophylaxis in leprosy. Lepr India1969;41:247–54.
3. Noordeen SK, Neelan PN. Chemoprophylaxis among contacts of non-lepromatous leprosy. Lepr India 1976;48:635–42.
4. Noordeen SK. Long term effects of chemoprophylaxis amongcontacts of lepromatous cases. Results of 8 1/2 years follow-up. Lepr India 1977;49:504–9.
5. Noordeen SK, Neelan PN. Extended studies on chemoprophylaxisagainst leprosy. Indian J Med Res 1978;67:515–27.
6. Otsyula Y, Ibworo C, Chum HJ. Four years' experience withdapsone as prophylaxis against leprosy. Lepr Rev 1971;42:98–100.
7. Neelan PN, Noordeen SK, Sivaprasad N. Chemoprophylaxis against leprosy with acedapsone. Indian J Med Res 1983;78:307–13.
8. Neelan PN, Sirumban P, Sivaprasad N. Limited duration acedapsone prophylaxis in leprosy. Indian J Lepr1986;58:251–6.
9. Cartel JL, Chanteau S, Moulia-Pelat JP, Plichart R, Glaziou P, Boutin JP, et al. Chemoprophylaxis of leprosy with a single dose of 25 mg per kg rifampin in the Southern Marquesas; results after four years. Int J Lepr Other Mycobact Dis 1992;60:416–20.
10. Cartel JL, Chanteau S, Boutin JP, Taylor R, Plichart R, Roux J, et al. Implementation of chemoprophylaxis of leprosy in the Southern Marquesas with a single dose of 25 mg per kg rifampin. Int J Lepr Other Mycobact Dis 1989;57:810–16.
11. Nguyen LN, Cartel JL, Grosset JH. Chemoprophylaxis of leprosy in the Southern Marquesas with a single 25 mg/kg dose of rifampicin. Results after 10 years. Lepr Rev 2000;71:S33–5.

12. Blanc LJ. Summary of leprosy chemoprophylaxis programs in the Western Pacific Region. Int J Lepr Other Mycobact Dis 1999;67:S30–31.
13. Moet FJ, Pahan D, Oskam L, Richardus JH. COLEP Study Group. Effectiveness of single dose rifampicin in preventing leprosy in close contacts of patients with newly diagnosed leprosy: cluster randomised controlled trial. BMJ 2008;336:761–4.
14. Feenstra SG, Pahan D, Moet FJ, Oskam L, Richardus JH. Patient-related factors predicting the effectiveness of rifampicin chemoprophylaxis in contacts: 6 year follow-up of the COLEP cohort in Bangladesh. Lepr Rev 2012;83:292–304.
15. Schuring RP, Richardus JH, Pahan D, Oskam L. Protective effect of the combination BCG vaccination and rifampicin prophylaxis in leprosy prevention. Vaccine 2009;27:7125–8.
16. Richardus R, Alam K, Kundu K, Chandra Roy J, Zafar T, Chowdhury ASet al. Effectiveness of single dose rifampicin after BCG vaccination to prevent leprosy in close contacts of patients with newly diagnosed leprosy: Cluster randomized controlled trial. Int J Infect Dis. 2019 Sep 6; pii: S1201-9712(19)30365–0.
17. Bakker MI, Hatta M, Kwenang A, Van Benthem BH, Van Beers SM, Klatser PR, Oskam L. Prevention of leprosy using rifampicin as chemoprophylaxis. Am J Trop Med Hyg 2005;72:443–8.
18. https://nlrinternational.org/news/pep-an-enhanced-regimen-for-leprosy/(last accessed 29/11/2019)
19. https://www.trialregister.nl/trial/7294 (last accessed 29/11/2019).
20. https://clinicaltrials.gov/ct2/show/NCT03662022 (last accessed 29/11/2019).
21. WHO Guidelines for the Diagnosis, Treatment and Prevention of Leprosy 2018 (available at: http://nlep.nic.in/pdf/WHO%20Guidelines%20for%20 leprosy.pdf)
22. http://nlep.nic.in/pdf/OG_PEP_F.pdf (last accessed 29/11/2019)
23. Barth-Jaeggi T, Steinmann P, Mieras L, van Brakel W, Richardus JH, Tiwari A, et al. Leprosy Post-Exposure Prophylaxis (LPEP) Programme: Study protocol for evaluating the feasibility and impact on case detection rates of contact tracing and single dose rifampicin. BMJ Open 2016;6:e013633.
24. Tiwari A, Dandel S, Djupuri R, Mieras L, Richardus JH Population-wide administration of single dose rifampicin for leprosy prevention in isolated communities: A three-year follow-up feasibility study in Indonesia. BMC Infect Dis 2018;18:324.
25. Idema WJ, Majer IM, Pahan D, Oskam L, Polinder S, Richardus JH. Cost-effectiveness of a chemoprophylactic intervention with single dose rifampicin in contacts of new leprosy patients. PLoS Negl Trop Dis 2010;4:e874.
26. Bakker MI, Hatta M, Kwenang A, Van Benthem BH, Van Beers SM, Klatser PR, Oskam L. Prevention of leprosy using rifampicin as chemoprophylaxis. Am J Trop Med Hyg 2005;72:443–8.
27. Mieras L, Anthony R, van Brakel W, Bratschi MW, van den Broek J, Cambau E, Cavaliero A, Kasang C, Perera G, Reichman L, Richardus JH, Saunderson P, Steinmann P, Yew WW. Negligible risk of inducing resistance in *Mycobacterium tuberculosis* with single-dose rifampicin as post-exposure prophylaxis for leprosy. Infect Dis Poverty 2016;5:46.
28. Warren RM, Victor TC, Streicher EM, Richardson M, Beyers N, Van Pittius NC G, et al. Patients with active tuberculosis often have different strains in the same sputum specimen. Am J Respir Crit Care Med 2004;169:610–14.
29. Merle CS, Cunha SS, Rodrigues LC. BCG vaccination and leprosy protection: review of current evidence and status of BCG in leprosy control. Expert Rev Vaccines 2010;9:209–22.
30. Setia, et al. The role of BCG in prevention of leprosy: A meta-analysis. Lancet Infect Dis 2006;6:162–70.
31. Schuring RP, Richardus JH, Pahan D, Oskam L. Protective effect of the combination BCG vaccination and rifampicin prophylaxis in leprosy prevention. Vaccine 2009;27:7125–8.
32. Cunha SS, Alexander N, Barreto ML, Pereira ES, Dourado I, Maroja Mde F, et al. BCG revaccination does not protect against leprosy in the Brazilian Amazon: A cluster randomised trial. PLoS Negl Trop Dis 2008;2(2).
33. Karonga Prevention Trial Group. Randomised controlled trial of single BCG, repeated BCG, or combined BCG and killed *Mycobacterium leprae* vaccine for prevention of leprosy and tuberculosis in Malawi. Lancet 1996;348(9019):17–24.
34. Düppre NC, Camacho LA, da Cunha SS, Struchiner CJ, Sales AM, Nery JA, et al. Effectiveness of BCG vaccination among leprosy contacts: A cohort study. Trans R Soc Trop Med Hyg 2008;102(7):631–8.
35. World Health Organization. BCG vaccines: WHO position paper—February 2018. Weakly Epidemiol Rec 2018;93(8):73–96.

36. Gupte MD. South India immunoprophylaxis trial against leprosy: Relevance of findings in the context of leprosy trends. Int J Lepr Other Mycobact Dis 2001;69(2 Suppl):S10–3.
37. Sharma P, Mukherjee R, Talwar GP, Sarathchandra KG, Walia R, Parida SK, Pandey RM, Rani R, Kar H, Mukherjee A, Katoch K, Benara SK, Singh T, Singh P. Immunoprophylactic effects of the anti-leprosy *Mw* vaccine in household contacts of leprosy patients: Clinical field trials with a follow-up of 8–10 years. Lepr Rev 2005;76:127–43.
38. Pandey RK, Sodhi A, Biswas SK, Dahiya Y, Dhillon MK. *Mycobacterium indicus pranii* mediates macrophage activation through TLR2 and NOD2 in a MyD88 dependent manner. Vaccine 2012 Aug 24;30(39):5748–54.
39. Saqib M, Khatri R, Singh B, Gupta A, Bhaskar S Cell wall fraction of *Mycobacterium indicus pranii* shows potential Th1 adjuvant activity. Int Immunopharmacol 2019;70:408–16.
40. Kumar S. India resurrects forgotten leprosy vaccine. Science 2017;356:999.
41. Sharma P, Misra RS, Kar HK, Mukherjee A, Poricha D, Kaur H et al. *Mycobacterium w* vaccine, a useful adjuvant to multidrug therapy in multibacillary leprosy: a report on hospital based immuno-therapeutic clinical trials with a follow-up of 1–7 years after treatment. Lepr Rev 2000;71:179–92.
42. Duthie MS, Frevol A2, Day T2, Coler RN3, Vergara J2, Rolf T2, et al. A phase 1 antigen dose escalation trial to evaluate safety, tolerability and immunogenicity of the leprosy vaccine candidate LepVax (LEP-F1 + GLA-SE) in healthy adults. Vaccine. 2019 Dec 30.
43. Duthie MS, Pena MT, Ebenezer GJ, Gillis TP, Sharma R, Cunningham K, Polydefkis M, Maeda Y, Makino M, Truman RW, et al. LepVax, a defined subunit vaccine that provides effective pre-exposure and post-exposure prophylaxis of M. leprae infection. NPJ Vacc 2018;3:12.
44. https://zeroleprosy.org (last accessed 29/11/2019).
45. Kamal R, Natrajan M, Katoch K, Arora M. Clinical and histopathological evaluation of the effect of addition of immunotherapy with *Mw* vaccine to standard chemotherapy in borderline leprosy. Indian J Lepr 2012;84:287–306.
46. Narang T, Kaur I, Kumar B, Radotra BD, Dogra S. Comparative evaluation of immunotherapeutic efficacy of BCG and *Mw* vaccines in patients of borderline lepromatous and lepromatous leprosy. Int J Lepr Other Mycobact Dis 2005;73:105–14.
47. Kaur I, Dogra S, Kumar B, Radotra BD. Combined 12-month WHO/MDT MB regimen and *Mycobacterium w* vaccine in multibacillary leprosy: A follow-up of 136 patients. Int J Lepr Other Mycobact Dis 2002;70:174–81.
48. De Sarkar A, Kaur I, Radotra BD, Kumar B. Impact of combined *Mycobacterium w* vaccine and 1 year of MDT on multibacillary leprosy patients. Int J Lepr Other Mycobact Dis 2001;69:187–94.
49. Sharma P, Kar HK, Misra RS, Mukherjee A, Kaur H, Mukherjee R, Rani R. Induction of lepromin positivity following immunochemotherapy with *Mycobacterium w* vaccine and multi-drug therapy and its impact on bacteriological clearance in multibacillary leprosy: Report on a hospital-based clinical trial with the candidate anti-leprosy vaccine. Int J Lepr Other Mycobact Dis 1999;67:259–69.
50. Zaheer SA, Beena KR, Kar HK, Sharma AK, Misra RS, Mukherjee A, Mukherjee R, Kaur H, Pandey RM, Walia R, et al. Addition of immunotherapy with *Mycobacterium w* vaccine to multi-drug therapy benefits multibacillary leprosy patients. Vaccine 1995;13:1102–10.
51. Zaheer SA, Mukherjee R, Ramkumar B, Misra RS, Sharma AK, Kar HK, Kaur H, Nair S, Mukherjee A, Talwar GP. Combined multi-drug and *Mycobacterium w* vaccine therapy in patients with multibacillary leprosy. J Infect Dis. 1993;167:401–10.
52. Kamal R, Natrajan M, Katoch K, Arora M. Clinical and histopathological evaluation of the effect of addition of immunotherapy with *Mw* vaccine to standard chemotherapy in borderline leprosy. Indian J Lepr 2012;84:287–306.
53. De Sarkar A, Kaur I, Radotra BD, Kumar B. Impact of combined *Mycobacterium w* vaccine and 1 year of MDT on multibacillary leprosy patients. Int J Lepr Other Mycobact Dis 2001;69:187–94.
54. Khullar G, Narang T, Nahar Saikia U, Dogra S. Generalized granulomatous dermatitis following *Mycobacterium w* (*Mw*) immunotherapy in lepromatous leprosy. Dermatol Ther 2017;30(2).
55. Khullar G, Narang T, Sharma K, Saikia UN, Dogra S. Disseminated cutaneous BCG infection following BCG immunotherapy in patients with lepromatous leprosy. Lepr Rev 2015;86:180–5.
56. Scollard D. Leprosy research is a necessity. Lepr Rev 2019; 90:232–236.

CHAPTER 8

Other Aspects of Treatment

8.1 NEURAL INVOLVEMENT AND ITS MANAGEMENT

Kabir Sardana, Premanshu Bhushan

Leprosy is primarily a neural disorder and most of the common deformities that result are consequent to nerve damage. New patients often present with some level of nerve function impairment (NFI), which varies between 2% and 55%, with the lower figures for PB cases.[1–4] A major consequence is that inspite of adequate treatment, 2.4–29% of the patients develop neuropathy during or after treatment. Though early assessment of NFI is crucial to identify such patients (*see Chpater 10*), it is also important to know the various stages of nerve affliction and the clinical consequences to understand the correct mode of intervention to effect maximal therapeutic response.[5–7]

Pathomechanism of Nerve Damage in Leprosy (*also see Section 4.4*)

The pathomechanism of nerve involvement in leprosy is multifactorial and incompletely understood, but major considerations are summarized in Table 8.1.

Table 8.1: Key considerations in patho-mechanism of nerve damage in leprosy	
Consideration	*Details*
I. How *M. leprae* reach the nerves?	a. Via lymphatics and blood stream to vasa nervorum (perineural and endoneural blood vessels), endothelial cells and thence to Schwann cells (this mode seems more likely). b. Via dermal nerves as an ascending infection (*schwannian relay* like fish swimming upstream).
II. Why *M. leprae* especially affect the nerves?	Schwann cells are the main target cells of *M. leprae*. The special selectivity is explained by relatively specific binding of mycobacterial antigens [phenolic glycolipid 1 (PGL-1) and laminin-2-binding protein (LBP21)] to the G domain of the laminin α_2-chain which is expressed on the Schwann cell surface and this complex subsequently binds to the $\alpha\beta$-dystroglycan (DG) in the basal lamina of the Schwann cell leading to endocytosis into the Schwann cells. This process may be helped by other binding molecules as well.

(Contd.)

Other Aspects of Treatment

Table 8.1: Key considerations in patho-mechanism of nerve damage in leprosy *(contd.)*	
Consideration	Details

III. How *M. leprae* infection leads to nerve damage?	Many mechanisms, *typically in different combinations, at different times, in same or different patients,* including:
	1. **Obstruction of vasa nervorum:** Via endothelial proliferation (*leprous vasculitis*),[7] and more so during reactions when edema shuts off the obliquely passing perineural vessels leading to anoxic damage.
	2. **Interference with Schwann cell metabolism:** For example, *nitrotyrosine*, an end product of the metabolism of nitric oxide leads to demyelination while *M. leprae* cell wall proteins interfere with host cell metabolism.
	3. **Biochemical changes:** Such as hypophosphorylation of axonal neurofilaments making it unable to support the neuron.
	4. **Immunologic mechanisms**
	   a. Nerves typically do not express major histocompatibility complex II (MHC-II) on their surface and are protected from immune attacks. The leprosy infected Schwann cells start expressing leprosy antigens with MHC-II and thus invite the immunological damage.
	   b. Cell-mediated immune attack during type 1 reaction
	   c. Immune complex mediated damage during type 2 reaction
	   d. Cytokine mediated damage from infiltrating cells in leprous granuloma
	   e. Autoimmune damage caused by autoantibodies against nerves as damaged nerves release antigens.
	5. **Pressure effect:** Leprosy granuloma in nerves with increased edema during reactions with a relatively nonexpanding perineurium produces damage to nerve fibers, especially in fibro-osseous canals.
	6. **Fibrosis:** Eventually all damaged nerve fibers are replaced by endoneural fibrosis leading to irreversible nerve damage.

IV. What are the terminal features of leprous nerves?	Three main features: a. Segmental (patchy) demyelination b. Neuronal degeneration c. Fibrosis
V. What are traditional types of leprous neuritis?	Three types:[8] a. Intrafascicular (resulting from Schwann cell involvement) b. Extrafascicular (resulting from reactional inflammation) c. Extraneural (resulting from compression in the fibro-osseous canals due to swelling and edema of the nerve).
VI. What are the main sites of nerve involvement?	Terminal nerve fibers in skin lesions and nerve trunks where they are superficially located (colder), in the fibro-osseus grooves (easily compressed), in trauma-prone sites (repeated trauma) and when a skin lesion is overlying the nerve trunk.
VII. Which modalities are affected?	Sensory (thermal followed by pain) followed by autonomic and motor functions.
VIII. How is leprous neuropathy typically described?	*"Mononeuritis multiplex"*: Inhomogenous but widespread

Risk Factors

There are many factors that predict the extent of nerve damage, but the *delay* in diagnosis is probably the most important and commonest cause.[9] The twin principles that dictate the management remain—recognizing onset of nerve damage and early treatment (Boxes 8.1 and 8.2).

Of the many factors detailed below (Table 8.2), it is important to highlight that none of these have a direct and linear causal relationship. It is more like a matrix of factors where one or more of them may predominate in some patients, at some time, in some nerves.

Box 8.1: Recognizing the onset of nerve damage

- Areas of loss of sweating
- Areas of sensory loss
- Weakness or paralysis of some muscles in a previously normal part of the hand or foot

Box 8.2: Early detection of worsening of nerve damage

Worsening of nerve damage may be indicated by:
- Increase in areas of loss of sweating
- Increase in areas of impaired sensibility
- Increase in severity of sensory loss
- Increase in muscle weakness or paralysis

Table 8.2: Risk factors for nerve damage	
Genetic[10-12]	Ninjurin 1, lncRNA *(also see Chapter 4)*
Type of leprosy	LL > BL > BB > BT > TT
	[Imp: In TT, the dermal nerves are completely destroyed in the lesions while the nerve trunk involvement, though early, is restricted to one or two nerve trunks in close relation to the skin lesion. In LL, the dermal nerves are spared till late and nerve trunk involvement is slow but progressive, leading eventually to more nerve damage than TT]
Sex	More in males
Nerve	• Thickening of a nerve, recurrent neuritis
	• More commonly damaged—ulnar nerve, posterior tibial nerve
	• Early to recover—facial and radial nerve
Treatment	Early treatment reduces the chances of nerve damage
Local factors	Cooler locations, anatomic constrictions, microtrauma, skin lesion overlying or close to a nerve trunk

Stages of Nerve Involvement

The sequential stages of nerve damage have been simplistically depicted in Fig. 8.1 but the stage of involvement can be subdivided into stages of parasitization, host response, clinical involvement and nerve damage, as described below:

i. ***Stage of parasitization:*** This is the initial stage of nerve involvement in leprosy and has been discussed in detailed elsewhere *(see Section 4.4)*.

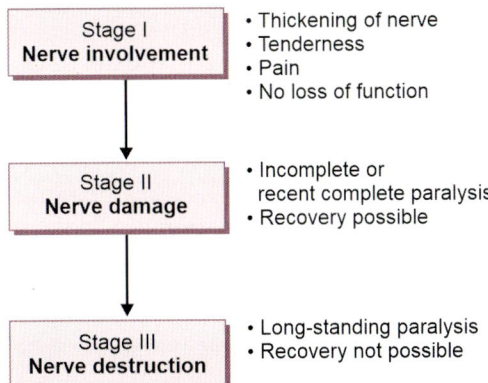

Fig. 8.1: Progression of clinical nerve involvement in leprosy

ii. *Stage of host response:* This stage is characterized by induction of a host immune response which is seen only when there is persistent infection of the nerve. The initial response is nonspecific but can progressively become more defined as a tuberculoid, borderline or lepromatous response. In some cases, especially in borderline leprosy, the host response in the nerve may be more towards lepromatous pole compared to the cutaneous lesion.

iii. *Stage of clinical involvement:* This stage is reached when there is a detectable thickening of the nerve with/without nerve pain and tenderness. While various symptoms and signs can be elicited at this stage, there is no evidence of loss of function, i.e. anesthesia or muscle weakness. The nerve thickening, tenderness and nerve pain may further be graded as mild, moderate and severe though its clinical replicability is questionable.[13]

iv. *Stage of nerve damage:* This is the next stage, characterized by significant damage to neuronal conducting pathways which allows routine clinical examinations to detect nerve function impairments. First to be affected are the small *non-myelinated* C and *thinly-myelinated* Aδ fibers mediating autonomic and sensory functions. Thus, loss of thermal sensations, loss of pain sensations and loss of sweating are seen earlier, either alone or in combinations. The later involvement of *thick* and *myelinated* fibers produces motor function deficits. The INFIR study however found that the order of first affected modality and nerve fiber differs from patient to patient. The clinical signs are listed in Box 8.3.

Here the term "incomplete paralysis" is important as these cases are amenable to timely interventions and to appreciate the clinical manifestations include:
- Sensations are still felt in *some* areas of skin supplied by the affected nerve
- Loss of sensibility is *partial,* affecting only certain *types* of sensations
- *Some* of the muscles supplied by the affected nerve are not completely paralyzed.

 Box 8.3: Stage of nerve damage—clinical presentation

- Loss of sweating
- Loss of sensibility
- Muscle weakness: Paralysis of muscles: Incomplete paralysis or recent (<6–9 months) complete paralysis—recovery possible

v. ***Stage of nerve destruction:*** This is the terminal stage of nerve involvement in leprosy. At this stage, even with treatment, the nerve cannot recover function to any useful degree. This stage is diagnosed when the nerve has been completely paralyzed for at least one year. In this stage, the extent of ultrastructural damage to the nerve varies with the clinical type of leprosy. A single fascicle or only some parts of one fascicle may be involved in tuberculoid leprosy and caseous degeneration may occur leading to formation of a "cold abscess" within the nerve. Conversely, in lepromatous leprosy, nerve gets replaced by fibrosis (collagen deposition which may undergo hyalinization).

Onset and Progression of Nerve Damage

Nerve function impairment in leprosy may present and progress in one of the following four forms (Fig. 8.2):

1. *Quiet nerve palsy (QNP):* It is now accepted that insidious palsy of sensory and motor function in leprosy is a reality and its occurrence is probably a *rule* rather than an exception. The nerve impairment is initially *dissociated*—involving pain and temperature—and becomes complete later on. Loss of sweating parallels the sensory impairment while motor paralysis appears later. This type of palsy has been described in all types except indeterminate leprosy. This form is amenable to resolution if MDT is initiated and, in case of incomplete and/or recent onset palsy, to steroids.
2. *Episodic onset and progression:* This is seen with episodes of reactions with neuritis, easily diagnosed by pain, tenderness and increased swelling of the affected nerve trunk. This may be isolated or may be accompanied by cutaneous activity. In cases of ENL, the microabscess may be seen and this is referred to as a "hot abscess". Nerve abscesses though are more characteristic of type 1 reaction (T1R). Each episode of neuritis may eventually leave a residual defect in the nerve function and repeated such insults may eventually culminate in pronounced damage.

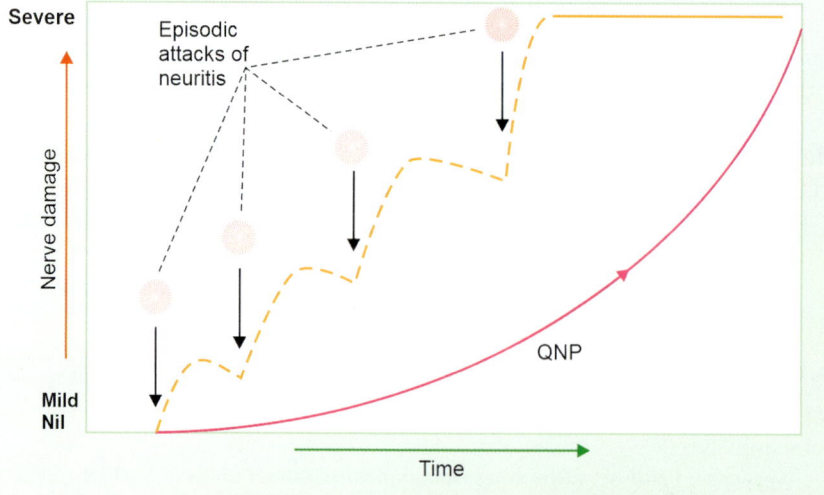

Fig. 8.2: Worsening of nerve damage in acute neuritis or quiet nerve paralysis (QNP)

3. *Catastrophic onset:* This unusual mode results in complete paralysis of a nerve trunk, without acute neuritis, within hours and is possibly consequent to an acute *vascular* lesion involving a major vessel supplying the nerve.
4. *Nerve damage of late onset:* The most troublesome is the late damage that is seen in patients after having completed treatment, wherein the onset is insidious and may be accompanied by positive sensory phenomena, like tingling or burning sensations, as well. These patients have no evidence of relapse of the disease and the nerve trunk is not unduly enlarged or tender. Nerve damage in these cases is attributed to progressive intraneural *fibrosis* and there is no way to predict which patient will develop this kind of nerve damage though it is believed that TGF-β1 may play a role.[15]

Diagnosis and Nerve Function Assessment

Diminished sweat function or blood flow (autonomic), pain, touch, pressure, warmth, cold and vibration sensation (sensory), and muscle strength (motor) can be assessed to detect leprosy neuropathy. Common methods used in the field to detect sensory nerve function impairments are monofilament testing (MFT) and ballpoint testing (BPT); both assess touch sensation on the hands and feet.

While the standard original set of Semmes-Weinstein monofilaments used to contain 20 filaments, a pocket kit of 5 to 6 filaments, with increasing thickness and pressure is more commonly used in leprosy (a typical kit with 6 filaments has green 0.05 g, blue 0.2 g, purple 2.0 g, red 4.0 g, orange 10 g, and pink 300 g filaments).[16–18] This is a reliable and standardized method to test for sensory impairments, in contrast to a BPT for which pressure is not standardized and which can only provide a yes/no outcome, although the low costs and high availability give BPT a huge advantage.

For the detection of motor nerve function impairments, voluntary muscle testing (VMT) is performed and graded by the modified 0–5 MRC scale (Medical Research Council 0–5 grades for voluntary muscle testing) or a simplified 3-point S-W-P (strong, weak, paralyzed) scale which is more suitable for field conditions.[19,20]

The warm detection threshold (WDT) and nerve conduction studies (NCS) are able to detect subclinical neuropathy up to 12 weeks before the clinical neuropathy was noticeable with MFT or VMT,[21] but this is not yet useful for field settings.

Management of Nerve Damage and Neuritis

We would be discussing early paralysis and acute neuritis in this section, while aspects of surgical decompression and nerve abscess are dealt with elsewhere (*see Section 8.3*).

Here, it is pertinent to point that while a NFI of <6 months is amenable to treatment, there is no reliable method to establish the duration of NFI.

1. **Early paralysis:** The term early paralysis includes recent paralysis (which may or may not be complete) as well as incomplete paralysis (which may or may not be recent). As discussed above, quite nerve palsy is eminently amenable to treatment. The therapy depends on status of the disease, treatment (MDT) status and the state of the nerve.
    a. *Untreated case*—anti-leprosy treatment—with appropriate multiple drugs must be instituted and the progress of the nerve damage closely monitored for a few weeks. In many cases, paralysis may regress partially with anti-leprosy treatment

alone. When that does not happen, steroid therapy in immunosuppressive dosage should be started and maintained for 4–6 months (*see below*).
   b. *Relapse:* Start steroid therapy along with antileprosy treatment.
   c. *Quiet nerve palsy:* When quiet nerve paralysis occurs in patients already under proper treatment for leprosy, the only recourse available is steroid therapy.[22] This will be worth trying when there is motor weakness or paralysis because it appears to be beneficial in that situation. But, it is uncertain if steroids are useful in case of sensory affliction alone.

   TRIPOD studies showed that after 12 months, 75% and 51% of the nerves, with mild sensory impairment and long-standing NFI (6–24 months duration) respectively, improved *spontaneously*.[23,24] A similar finding was reported in the AMFES trial in Ethiopia, where acute neuropathy recovered *spontaneously* in 42%.[25] Similarly, a full recovery occurred in 9% patients with untreated motor nerves involvement and 17% of those with untreated sensory nerve involvement.[26] The corresponding figures for partial improvement were 33% and 62% respectively.[26] Thus, it must be appreciated that several studies have reported spontaneous recovery of nerve function impairments, even for chronic impairments.

2. **Acute neuritis:** Acute neuritis of a nerve trunk may or may not be associated with the onset of neural deficit, but because the risk of nerve damage is very much increased by attacks of acute neuritis, it is essential to get the inflammation resolved as rapidly as possible. Pain is the predominant and persistent symptom associated with neuritis in leprosy and unlike other medical conditions it is difficult to justify giving long-term analgesics because of their adverse effects and habit-forming potential. The chances of nerve damage are more in case of upgrading reactions rather than downgrading reactions or ENL.

   Steroids remain the bulwark of therapy with analgesics and sedatives, which can help to reduce the anxiety of patients. In reversal reaction, prednisolone 40–60 mg/day, is required and might be needed for a long duration (up to 6 months in some cases). While steroids act by dispersing intraneural edema, and by doing so, they relieve the pressure on nerve fibers, the mode of action of thalidomide is not clearly known. In T1R, there is an added factor causing pressure on nerve fibers, namely the intraneural granuloma resulting from cellular reaction. Thus, it is important to continue antileprosy drugs as in these cases the intraneural granuloma slowly resolves; and with the removal of the damaging effects of edema and cellular reaction there can be recovery of nerve function.

   Steroids are given in a similar regimen as for T1R, i.e. started at 1 mg per kg of prednisolone per day, then tapered over a period of 20 weeks. If worsening NFI is detected during the monthly review visits, then the dose may be increased. This should only be done twice at the very most, and nerve decompression should be considered in appropriate cases.[27]

   The duration of steroid therapy has however been debated and can range from 12 weeks to 20 weeks or more. At present, it seems that a 20-week course is sufficient to improve nerve function in 78% of patients with recent NFI. WHO recommends a standard 12 weeks tapering course of prednisolone for use in control programs (40 mg, 30 mg, 20 mg, 15 mg, 10 mg, and 5 mg each for 2 weeks).[28] But the dosimetry of steroids, specifically the duration, cannot be dogmatic as sometimes a longer course of steroids may be needed as it seems that the immune response against dead *M. leprae* is sometimes persistent and may not be permanently suppressed by even a 32-week prednisolone course.[29–30a] The neuritis specially in T1R has a definite cytokine basis[30b] and the reason for nonresponders has been explained due to persistently high cytokine levels which precludes to the increased likelihood of relapse of neuritis after steroid withdrawal. Also, one must remember that there are a high proportion of patients experiencing spontaneous nerve function improvement depending of the severity of NFI and the type of nerve (as mentioned before).[24] Thus, pending a placebo controlled trial—which has its own intrinsic ethical issues—it is best to be flexible with steroid dosimetry and look for other options of treatment. These other measures include

   a. *Affected nerve trunk*: Rest (sling, splint, plaster cast), heat or ultrasound treatment of nerves and surgery to relieve compression of nerves
   b. *Affected muscles*: Exercise and splints
   c. *Affected joints*: Massage and splints

3. **Neuropathic pain:** Neuropathic pain is characterized by positive and negative symptoms including pain, hypoesthesia to touch, tingling, electric shocks and pins and needles sensation. The importance of neuropathic pain in leprosy was ignored for long but it is now being increasingly recognized as an important late complication of leprosy. Here, it is important to appreciate that the neuropathic pain in leprosy is as heterogeneous as neuropathic pain of other etiologies and it is not possible to easily differentiate it from other etiologies. About 26% of leprosy patients (mostly post-treatment) from a referral center in Brazil were reported as having neuropathic pain.[31] Similar figures have been reported from Ethiopian (29%) and Indian (21%) studies as well. Symptoms are commonest in distribution of the ulnar nerve.[32,33] These symptoms may often be misdiagnosed as reactions. The pathogenesis of neuropathic pain in leprosy is not well understood but proposed mechanisms include entrapment of nerves, firing of the nervi nervorum, sensitization of nociceptors, axonal damage, and lowered activation thresholds.[31, 34–37]

Steroids are *not* recommended for neuropathic pain in leprosy.[37] Patients should be treated with an analgesic ladder starting with paracetamol, then using a nonsteroidal drug such as ibuprofen. Many patients will need treatment with the antidepressant amitriptyline.[38] Gabapentin can also be used for patients with pain that is not alleviated by other measures.

REFERENCES

1. Croft RP, Nicholls PG, Richardus JH, Smith WC. Incidence rates of acute nerve function impairment in leprosy: A prospective cohort analysis after 24 months (The Bangladesh Acute Nerve Damage Study). Lepr Rev 2000;71:18–33.
2. van Brakel WH. Peripheral neuropathy in leprosy and its consequences. Lepr Rev. 2000;71: S146–53.
3. van Brakel WH,Nicholls PG, Das L, Barkataki P, Suneetha SK, Jadhav RS, Maddali P, Lockwood DN, Wilder-Smith E, Desikan KV. The INFIR Cohort Study: Investigating prediction, detection and pathogenesis of neuropathy and reactions in leprosy. Methods and baseline results of a cohort of multibacillary leprosy patients in north India. Lepr Rev 2005; 76:14–34.
4. Jiang J, Watson JM, Zhang GC, Wei XY. A field trial of detection and treatment of nerve function impairment in leprosy: Report from national POD pilot project. Lepr Rev 1998; 69:367–75.

5. Smith WC, Nicholls PG, Das L, Barkataki P, Suneetha S, Suneetha L, et al. Predicting neuropathy and reactions in leprosy at diagnosis and before incident events—results from the INFIR cohort study. PLoS Negl Trop Dis 2009;3:e500.
6. Srinivasan H. Disability, deformity and rehabilitation. In: Hastings RC (Ed). Leprosy. London: Churchill Livingstone, 1994;p.411–47.
7. Job CK. Pathology and pathogenesis of leprous neuritis; a preventable and treatable complication. Int J Lepr Other Mycobact Dis 2001;69:S19–29.
8. Ridley DS. Pathogenesis of leprosy and related diseases. London: Butterworth and Co. Publishers; 1988.
9. Nicholls PG, Croft RP, Richardus JH, Withington SG, Smith WC. Delay in presentation, an indicator for nerve function status at registration and for treatment outcome—the experience of the Bangladesh Acute Nerve Damage Study cohort. Lepr Rev 2003;74:349–56.
10. Graça CR, Paschoal VD, Cordeiro-Soubhia RM, Tonelli-Nardi SM, Machado RL, Kouyoumdjian JA, Baptista Rossit AR. NINJURIN1 single nucleotide polymorphism and nerve damage in leprosy. Infect Genet Evol 2012;12:597–600.
11. Fava VM, Manry J, Cobat A, Orlova M, Van Thuc N, Moraes MO, et al. A genomewide association study identifies a lncRNA as risk factor for pathological inflammatory responses in leprosy. PLoS Genet 2017;13:e1006637.
12. Orlova M, Cobat A, Huong NT, Ba NN, Van Thuc N, Spencer J, et al. Gene set signature of reversal reaction type 1 in leprosy patients. PLoS Genet 2013;9:e1003624.
13. Rao PN, Jain S. Newer management options in leprosy. Indian J Dermatol 2013;58:6–11.
14. McKnight J. Clinical testing and prognostic markers for the development of leprosy neuropathy, in Infectious and Tropical Diseases. 2010, University of London: London.
15. Petito RB, Amadeu TP, Pascarelli BM, Jardim MR, Vital RT, Antunes SL, Sarno EN. Transforming growth factor-β1 may be a key mediator of the fibrogenic properties of neural cells in leprosy. J Neuropathol Exp Neurol 2013;72:351–66.
16. Anderson, AM and RP Croft, Reliability of Semmes-Weinstein monofilament and ballpoint sensory testing, and voluntary muscle testing in Bangladesh. Lepr Rev 1999;70:305–13.
17. Villarroel MF, Orsini MB, Lima RC, Antunes CM. Comparative study of the cutaneous sensation of leprosy-suspected lesions using Semmes-Weinstein monofilaments and quantitative thermal testing. Lepr Rev 2007;78:102–9.
18. Bell-Krotoski J. "Pocket filaments" and specifications for the Semmes-Weinstein monofilaments. Journal of Hand Therapy 1990;3:26–31.
19. Roberts AE, et al. Ensuring inter-tester reliability of voluntary muscle and monofilament sensory testing in the INFIR Cohort Study. Lepr Rev 2007;78:122–30.
20. Global Leprosy Strategy 2016–2020. Accelerating towards a leprosy-free world. Monitoring and Evaluation Guide. New Delhi: World Health Organization, Regional Office for South-East Asia; 2017.
21. van Brakel WH, Nicholls PG, Wilder-Smith EP, et al. Early diagnosis of neuropathy in leprosy—comparing diagnostic tests in a large prospective study (the INFIR cohort study). PLoS Negl Trop Dis 2008;2:e212.
22. Srinivasan H, Rao KS, Shanmugam N. Steroid therapy in recent "quiet nerve paralysis" in leprosy. Report of a study of twenty-five patients. Lepr India 1982;54:412–9.
23. Van Brakel WH, Anderson AM, Withington SG, Croft RP, Nicholls PG, Richardus JH, et al. The prognostic importance of detecting mild sensory impairment in leprosy: A randomized controlled trial (TRIPOD 2). Lepr Rev 2003;74:300–10.
24. Richardus JH, Withington SG, Anderson AM, Croft RP, Nicholls PG, van Brakel WH, et al. Treatment with corticosteroids of long-standing nerve function impairment inleprosy: a randomized controlled trial (TRIPOD 3). Lepr Rev 2003;74:311–8.
25. Saunderson P, et al. The pattern of leprosy-related neuropathy in the AMFES patients in Ethiopia: Definitions, incidence, risk factors and outcome. Leprosy Review 2000;71:285–308.

26. Croft RP, Nicholls PG, Richardus JH, Smith WC. The treatment of acute nerve function impairment in leprosy: Results from a prospective cohort study in Bangladesh. Lepr Rev 2000;71:154–68.
27. Ebenezer M, Andrews P, Solomon S. Comparative trial of steroids and surgical intervention in the management of ulnar neuritis. Int J Lepr Other Mycobac Dis 1996;64:282–6.
28. WHO Model Prescribing Information: Drugs Used in Leprosy. Available from: https://apps.who.int/medicinedocs/en/d/Jh2988e/7.html. Last accessed 20th Aug, 2019.
29. Wagenaar I, Post E, Brandsma W, Bowers B, Alam K, Shetty V, et al. Effectiveness of 32 versus 20 weeks of prednisolone in leprosy patients with recent nerve function impairment: A randomized controlled trial. PLoS Negl Trop Dis 2017; 11:e0005952.
30a. Shetty VP, Suchitra K, Uplekar MW, Antia NH. Persistence of *Mycobacterium leprae* in the peripheral nerve as compared to the skin of multi-drug-treated leprosy patients. Lep Rev 1992; 63:329–36.
30b. Manandhar R, Shrestha N, Butlin CR, Roche PW. High levels of inflammatory cytokines are associated with poor clinical response to steroid treatment and recurrent episodes of type 1 reactions in leprosy. Clin Exp Immunol 2002;128:333–8.
31. Giesel LM, Pitta IJR, da Silveira RC, Andrade LR, Vital RT, Nery JADC, et al. Clinical and Neurophysiological Features of Leprosy Patients with neuropathic pain. Am J Trop Med Hyg 2018; 98:1609–13.
32. Saunderson P, Bizuneh E, Leekassa R. Neuropathic pain in people treated for multibacillary leprosy more than ten years previously. Lepr Rev 2008;79:270–6.
33. Lasry-Levy E, Hietaharju A, Pai V, Ganapati R, Rice AS, Haanpää M. Neuropathic pain and psychological morbidity in patients with treated leprosy: A cross-sectional prevalence study in Mumbai. PLOS Negl Trop Dis 2011;05:e981.
34. Malaviya GN. Neuropathic pain in leprosy patients. International Journal of Leprosy and other Mycobacterial Diseases 2005;73:34–5.
35. Croft R. Neuropathic pain in leprosy. International Journal of Leprosy and other Mycobacterial Diseases 2004;72:171–2.
36. Haanpää M, Lockwood DN, Hietaharju A. Neuropathic pain in leprosy. Leprosy Review 2004; 75:7–18.
37. Reis FJ, Saadi LM, Gomes MK, Gosling AP, Cunha AJ. Pain in leprosy patients: Shall we always consider as a neural damage? Lep Rev 2011;82:319–21.
38. Raicher I, Stump PRNAG, Harnik SB, de Oliveira RA, Baccarelli R, Marciano LHSC, et al. Neuropathic pain in leprosy: Symptom profile characterization and comparison with neuropathic pain of other etiologies. Pain Rep 2018;3:e638.

8.2 OCULAR COMPLICATIONS AND MANAGEMENT

Kabir Sardana, Ananta Khurana, Margreet Hogeweg

While there are myriad ocular complication described[1-4] (*Section 2.1*) here we intend to focus on the common treatable ocular disorders. In the present era the most important cause of blindness in leprosy patients is not due to leprosy but due to age-related cataract.[3,4] Reasons why these patients have not been operated vary, but important reasons are the stigma towards leprosy, poverty and lack of guardian or transport. Thus, more than "cosmetic surgeries" early diagnosis and treatment of cataract must be encouraged.[3,4]

1. Reactions
- Acute iritis
- Acute episcleritis
- Acute scleritis

We will discuss primarily acute iritis while the other complications are uncommon and are listed in Box 8.4.

Acute Iritis[5,6]

Leprosy-related acute iritis occurs only in multibacillary (MB) patients and is considered to be a surrogate marker of ENL reaction. Acute iritis may recur at any time, unrelated to disease activity or systemic ENL reaction.

In the differential diagnosis of acute red eye in a leprosy patient, all other common conditions causing an acute red eye should be considered. These include acute conjunctivitis (where a topical antibiotic may be used), corneal foreign body and injury, corneal ulcer and acute glaucoma. In addition, the use of high doses of clofazimine for ENL reaction may also cause red eyes (Figs 8.3 and 8.4).

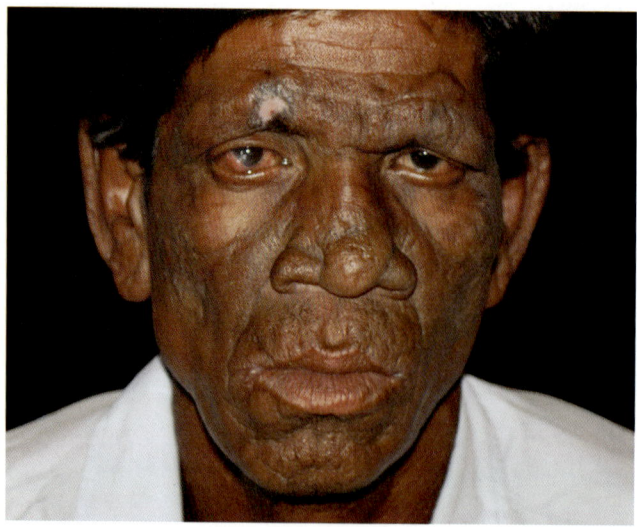

Fig. 8.3: LL Hansen with diffuse infiltration, nodules, madarosis, deformed nose and red eyes (due to clofazimine) (*Courtesy*: Dr Karthikeyan Govindasamy)

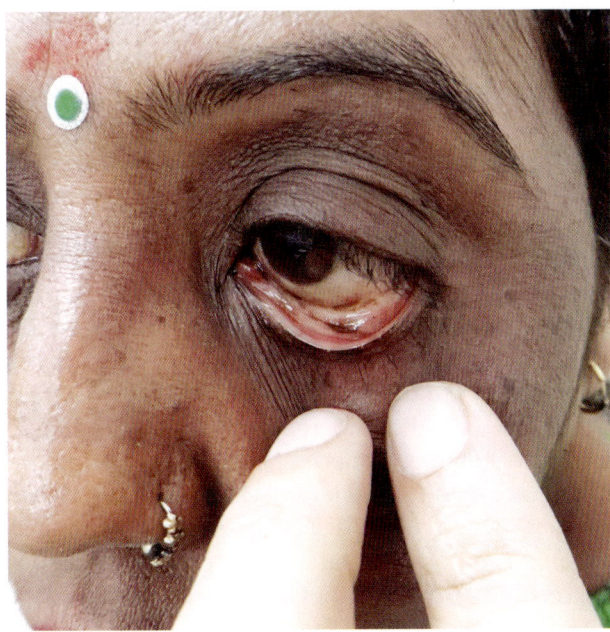

Fig. 8.4: Clofazimine pigmentation of the conjunctiva and sclera

Thus, in leprosy endemic countries, leprosy should be considered as a cause of acute iritis. Patients usually do not offer a history of being treated for leprosy and thus the clinical examination is of importance—including temporal madarosis of eyebrows, early collapse of the nose or nodules on the ear (Fig. 8.3).

Treatment

While various aspects of treatment have been discussed in other chapters (*see Section 8.3.3*) and undoubtedly tarsorrhapy is an important intervention, here we will dwell on the other interventions in ocular leprosy.

Under field conditions, the diagnosis of acute iritis can be confirmed by using a short acting mydriatic eye drop to demonstrate posterior synechiae before instilling atropine. The treatment of iritis largely consists of atropine sulphate 1% twice daily, steroid eye drops 6 times daily and steroid ointment at night time. The rationale of administering eyedrops of 1% homatropine or of 1% cyclopentolate is to keep the pupil as dilated as possible so as to prevent or counter adhesions (synechiae). Systemic steroids are not always required for acute iritis unless there is a concurring severe ENL reaction which then requires systemic prednisolone. This treatment should be continued till the acute phase has subsided and a slit-lamp is of great value in deciding if and when the cellular exudate disappears from the aqueous humour. If the acute phase treatment cannot be followed by slit-lamp examination, treatment should continue for about 6 weeks with a slowly decreasing dosage of topical steroids.

In patients whose eyes have been neglected or incorrectly treated, and posterior synchiae have formed a complete ring round the pupil, Choyce[6] advocated a complete iridectomy; this prevents development of secondary glaucoma resulting from iris bombe, delays the onset of complicated cataract and attacks of acute iridocyclitis become less troublesome.

2. Surgical Management including Cataract Surgery

Cataract surgery is not to be postponed on the basis of a patient being MB, smear positive, on anti-leprosy treatment, on steroid treatment for lepra reactions, in eyes that have had uveitis or scleritis or with concomitant lagophthalmos.[4,7]

In cases of lagophthalmos with healthy corneas, cataract surgery should be followed by a tarsorrhaphy in 1–2 weeks. The patient is to be kept in the hospital till the tarsorrhaphy sutures are removed 2 weeks later. In cases of severe lagophthalmos with ectropion and exposure keratopathy, a temporary tarsorrhaphy can be done until the cornea heals, after which the cataract surgery followed by the definitive lid surgery is done 2–3 weeks later. The visual outcome may not fall within WHO guidelines in these cases but the difference it makes to a previously blind patient, who many might reject as unfit for surgery, is remarkable and the experience extremely rewarding to the surgeon. In patients who have had reconstructive surgery for lagophthalmos (temporalis muscle transfer), it may be necessary to release a tight tendon/graft slip in the upper or lower lid or both lids at the lateral canthus to avoid the patient squeezing the eyelids during surgery which can be disastrous (a peribulbar block will not paralyze the temporalis muscle). A small lateral tarsorrhaphy may be required later.[7]

A summary of the recommendations for cataract surgery in case of leprosy patients is provided in Table 8.3.

3. Glaucoma

Fortunately, glaucoma is a rare complication in leprosy, but if it is suspected because of increase in eyeball pain and tension, acetazolamide (Diamox) should be given in dosage of 250 mg two or three times a day. This acts by interfering with the production of aqueous humour.

Table 8.3: Recommendations for cataract surgery in leprosy patients	
Care management	• Cataract should be removed when it adversely affects patient's visual function • IOL is *not contraindicated* as long as quality of surgery is good and eye is quiet • Chronic lagophthalmos should be treated surgically if cornea is compromised or cosmesis is a problem, regardless of severity of lagophthalmos, by whatever procedure the surgeon does best • New onset lagophthalmos (duration <6 months) should be treated with oral prednisolone *(see Section 8.3.3)* • Acute uveitis should be treated with intensive topical steroid; associated systemic leprosy reaction must be ruled out or treated appropriately if present
Patient education	• At the end of MDT, all patients should be warned that lagophthalmos could develop and understand the risks associated with this outcome. • Patients with residual lagophthalmos must be told about the risk from exposure and specifically warned about development of red eye and decreased vision. • Patients should understand risks to eye during reaction and given explicit instructions on where to report if reaction develops. • All patients should be informed of significance of decreased vision and told to report this to case worker for referral to higher level.

Source: American Academy of Ophthalmology Summary Benchmarks, November 2010 (www.aao.org) ANDICO International Clinical Guidelines Eye Disease in Leprosy (Initial Evaluation and Management)
IOL: Intraocular lens

4. Other Complications

Though in the pre-MDT era numerous other complications were seen (Box 8.4), these are uncommon nowadays.[9]

Box 8.4: Uncommon ocular complications and management

Exposure keratitis, corneal ulcer	• Antibiotic eye ointment and an eye shield. • Do not close an eye which has an exposure ulcer with an eye pad, as the gauze may touch the cornea and cause further damage. It is better to close the eye with a temporary mattress suture. • An exposure ulcer is a definite indication for eyelid surgery.
Scleritis and episcleritis	• Steroids (and atropine, in the case of accompanying acute iritis).

CONCLUSION

The ultimate goal of ocular management is to ameliorate the effect of reactions and also prevent visual impairment and blindness in leprosy. This can be achieved by early diagnosis of leprosy and timely MDT treatment, early recognition of reactions and effective treatment of reactions with systemic steroids, regular eye examination, refraction and treatment of any complications. The two common interventions remain lagophthalmos surgery in patients with a eyelid gap of ≥6 mm and lens extraction with IOL implantation in any leprosy patients who develop blinding cataract.[9]

Acknowledgements

We are thankful to Dr M Hogeweg for her critical comments and review of ocular leprosy in *Sections 2.1 and 8.2*.

REFERENCES

1. Courtright P, Daniel E, Sundar Rao PSS, et al. Eye diseases in multibacillary leprosy patients at the time of their leprosy diagnosis. Finding from the longitudinal study of ocular leprosy (LOSOL) in India, Philippines and Ethiopia. Lepr Rev 2002;73:225–38.
2. Singh L, Malhotra R, Bundela RK, Garg P, Dhillon KS, Chawla S, Lal BB. Ocular disability—WHO grade 2 in persons affected with leprosy. Indian J Lepr 2014;86:1–6.
3. Hogeweg M, Keunen JE. Prevention of blindness in leprosy and the role of the Vision 2020 Programme. Eye (Lond). 2005;19:1099–105. Review Pub Med PMID: 16304590.
4. Hogeweg M. Cataract: The main cause of blindness in leprosy. Lepr Rev 2001;72:139–42.
5. Leprosy and the eye: Teaching set ICEH, 2010.
6. Choyce DP. Diagnosis and management of ocular leprosy. Br J Ophthalmol 1969;53:217–23.
7. Anand S, Neethiodiss P, Xavier JW. Intra- and postoperative complications and visual outcomes following cataract surgery in leprosy patients. Lepr Rev 2009;80:177–86.
8. American Academy of Ophthalmology, Edition 2012–13. Basic and clinical science course: Section 3. San Francisco, 114.
9. Courtright, P. Lewallen S. Prevention of blindness in leprosy, 2nd ed. Available from ICEH as free download,https://www.iceh.org.uk/x/9Y1V.

8.3 DEFORMITIES IN LEPROSY AND THEIR MANAGEMENT

Kabir Sardana, Premanshu Bhushan

With the largely successful experience of MDT in treating leprosy, management of deformities has become a focus area of most leprosy programmes. While management of deformities would involve both surgical interventions and rehabilitation (which is usually not the domain of dermatologists), it is probably the most crucial aspect and a 'missing link' in most programmes where deformity 'grading' is the emphasis and not its treatment. This chapter hence will be in two parts, the first would discuss the various deformities in leprosy and this will be followed by measures that can be employed for their resolution (*Sections 8.3.1 to 8.3.3*).

INTRODUCTION AND OVERVIEW

Leprosy is a disorder that, more than its treatment, is plagued by its perceptions in society. The factors associated with higher perceived stigma include illiteracy, perceived economical inadequacy, need for change of occupation due to leprosy, lack of knowledge about leprosy and perception of leprosy as a severe and difficult to treat disease. Also, visible deformities and ulcers are associated with higher stigma.[1]

A disease may produce changes in the structure and functioning of certain parts of the body.[2] These changes are called *'impairments'*. A *'deformity'* is a visible impairment or a visible consequence of an impairment inside the body. While specific and paralytic deformities are primary impairments, "anesthetic deformities" are secondary impairments. The functional consequence of deformity is known as *'disability'*. A persistently disabled person experiences many disadvantages that limit or prevent that person from fulfilling his or her normal role in the society and these disadvantages are known as *'handicaps'*. Before the multi-drug therapy (MDT) era, often due to lack of adequate treatment, the leprosy patient often would lose social status and becomes progressively isolated from society, family and friends—a process referred to as 'dehabilitation'. *Dehabilitation* is completed when the patient is forced to leave his or her home and settle in a rehabilitation home or in a leprosy colony with other patients. Some patients eventually find themselves completely isolated from all society and become destitutes (without food or shelter). This process is depicted in Fig. 8.5a. An important aim of any leprosy programme is to prevent this progression and correct the deformity before it becomes a disability.[2]

Deformities are seen in approximately 20–25% of leprosy patients and the common cited factors that account for its development include: (1) The *type* of leprosy—incidence higher in MB leprosy, (2) the *duration* of active disease, and (3) the number of *nerve trunks* involved in the patient. Evidently lepromatous and borderline types carry a much greater risk than tuberculoid and indeterminate types. Also, longer the disease and greater the number of nerves involved, more is the propensity of deformities. Reactions and neuritis are another cause for deformities and men are more affected.[3] A delay of more than 3 months between the first noticed symptom by the patient and the first visit to any healthcare provider, is also a major reason for risk of disability among adult leprosy patients.[4]

Deformities are classified into three types: *Specific, paralytic* and *anesthetic* deformities (Table 8.4). Specific deformities are those in which local leprosy-related pathology is

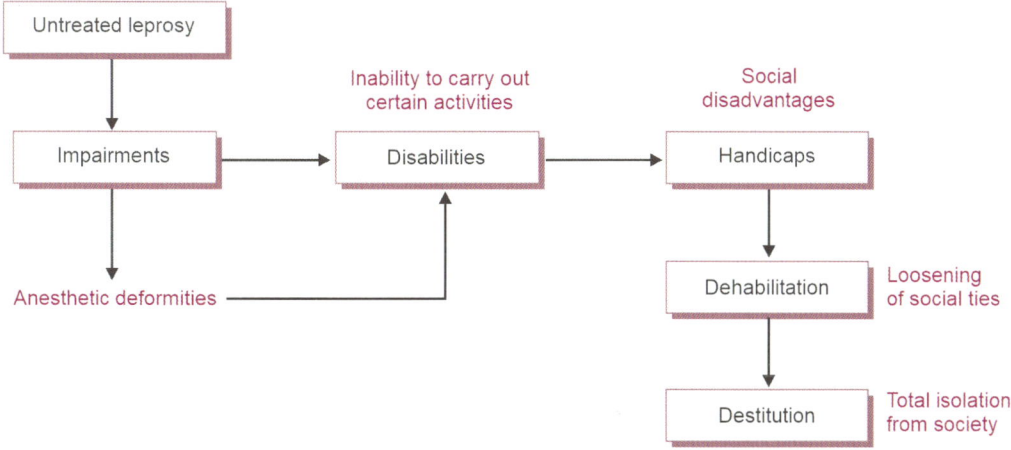

Fig. 8.5a: A depiction of the various consequences of leprosy

Table 8.4: Overview of regional deformities in leprosy			
	Primary impairments		Secondary impairments
	Specific	*Motor paralytic*	*Anesthetic*
Face	• Loss of eyebrows • Premature senility • Sunken nose deformity • Rat bitten ears • Buddha ears—sagging ear lobules	• Lagophthalmos • Facial palsy • Leprous stare	
Hands	• Banana fingers • Nonparalytic clawing and "straight stiff finger" • Intrinsic plus—"swan-neck" deformity • "Reaction hand" or frozen hand • Twisted finger	• Claw hand (intrinsic zero hand) • Drop wrist • Paralyzed thumb	• Shortening of fingers • Mutilation of hand • Disorganization of wrist
Feet	Reaction foot "Intrinsic plus toes"	Claw toes Foot drop	Plantar ulcers Disorganization of foot

responsible for the deformity. Paralytic deformities result from damage to motor nerves. Paralytic deformity is the visible expression of changes in the balance of forces around affected joints. Anesthetic deformities are consequent to damage of the sensory nerves and loss of sensibility. Specific deformitites are the commonest on face, specific and paralytic on hands and anesthetic on feet (Table 8.4).

DEFORMITIES OF HANDS[5-7]

Hands are the most common sites of deformities and we will follow the classification detailed in Table 8.4 in this chapter for uniformity.

A. Specific Deformities

These are either due to direct infiltration of tissues or as a consequence of reactions, most commonly ENL.

i. **Banana fingers:** This is caused by heavy infiltration of the skin and subcutaneous tissue of the fingers followed by atrophy of the skin and deposition of fat under the skin (Fig. 8.5b).

ii. **Reaction hand or frozen hand:** This is the most disabling specific deformity occurring as a consequence of ENL. 'Reaction hand' refers to the severe *edema* of dorsa of hands, arthritis of interphalangeal joints and functional incapacity during bouts of type II lepra reactions.[6] 'Frozen hand' is the result of repeated lepra reaction which leads to *fibrosis* of skin and subcutaneous tissue. This scar-like tissue pulls digits leading to a bizarre deformity. The hand is universally flexed with nails digging into the palm. Often, ring and little fingers show severe *clawing*, *without* any paralysis of intrinsic muscles, with marked *hyperextension* at metacarpophalangeal (MCP) joint which may get dislocated. The deformity is practically impossible to correct.

In the *fully developed state*, it shows:
- Wrist partly flexed and fingers in different postures.
- Skin of the hands, particularly the dorsal skin, shows a hyperpigmented and leathery look and appears as if it is stuck to the deeper tissues.

iii. **Intrinsic plus or "swan-neck" deformity:** The involvement of intrinsic muscles in repeated lepra reactions leads to *fibrosis and contracture of intrinsic muscles* leading to a deformity that appears as the *reverse* of frozen hand, with flexion at basal joint and hyperextension at proximal interphalangeal (PIP) joint, similar to a "swan-neck" (Fig. 8.6) deformity in rheumatoid arthritis.[7] It is often seen in association with 'reaction hand' but may also occur in isolation.

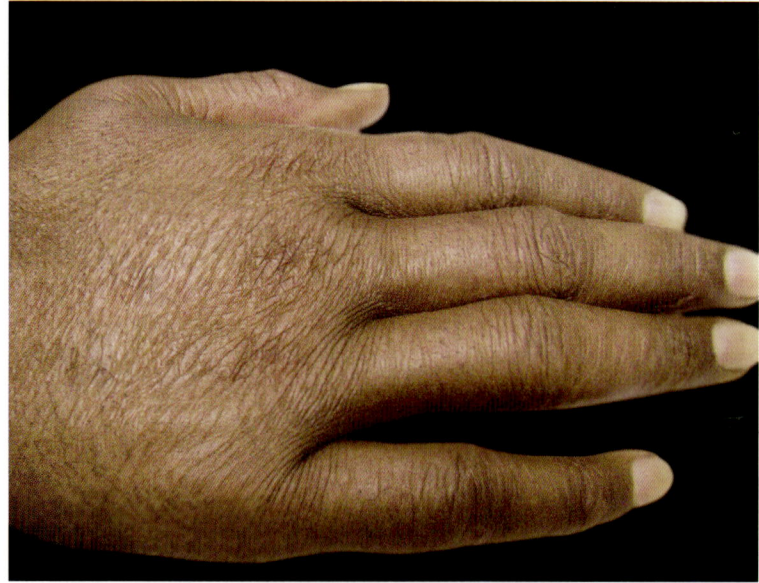

Fig. 8.5b: Banana fingers due to infiltration of the hand

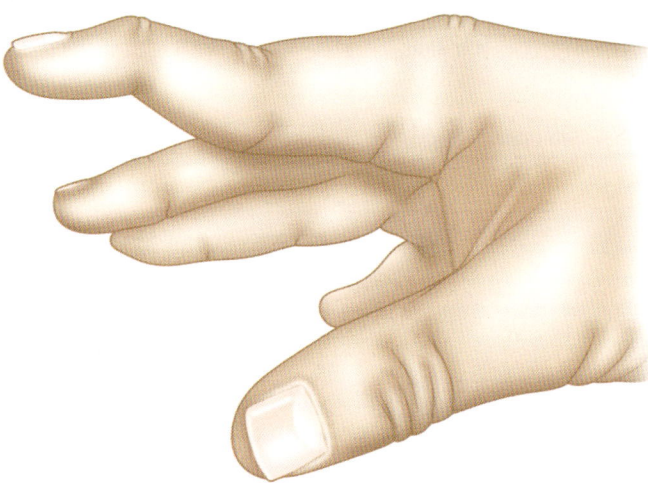

Fig. 8.6: The "swan-neck" deformity with flexion at the DIP joint and hyperextension at the PIP joint. (DIP: Distal interphalangeal; PIP: Proximal interphalangeal)

Another cause is pathological fractures of the juxta-articular zones in small bones of hands which have been decalcified during lepra reactions. When the fractures heal, they produce abnormal tilts (malunion) giving rise to bizarre deformities in which the finger is twisted in any odd direction.[7]

While the prevention of deformities consequent to treatment of reactions have been discussed previously, preliminary radiographs of the hand are of great help in assessing the extent of bone involvement and the risks of a pathological fracture. After the reaction subsides, active movements are gradually added and increased. It should be kept in mind that excessive rest and immobilization will promote stiffness while excessive mobilization will interfere with resolution of the inflammatory process, ultimately leading to stiffness.

B. Motor Paralytic Deformities

Leprosy presents with unique spatio-temporal involvement of nerve trunks in upper limb. The most *common* palsy associated with leprosy is an isolated low ulnar paralysis presenting as ulnar claw hand involving chiefly the little and ring fingers. Ulnar nerve is usually the first and most severely involved followed later by median and less frequently by radial nerve. Isolated median or radial nerve involvement is decidedly uncommon. Sometimes all three are involved (triple palsy). Further, the level of involvement is typically low ulnar (only hand muscles involved with sparing of flexor forearm muscles).

Figure 8.7 depicts the nerve supply and the muscle innervation of the hand that would make the ensuing text easy to understand.

*i. **Ulnar nerve paralysis*** (*intrinsic zero and Z-finger*): The ulnar nerve supplies the following muscles (Fig. 8.7).

In the forearm
- Flexor carpi ulnaris
- Flexor digitorum profundus (ulnar half)

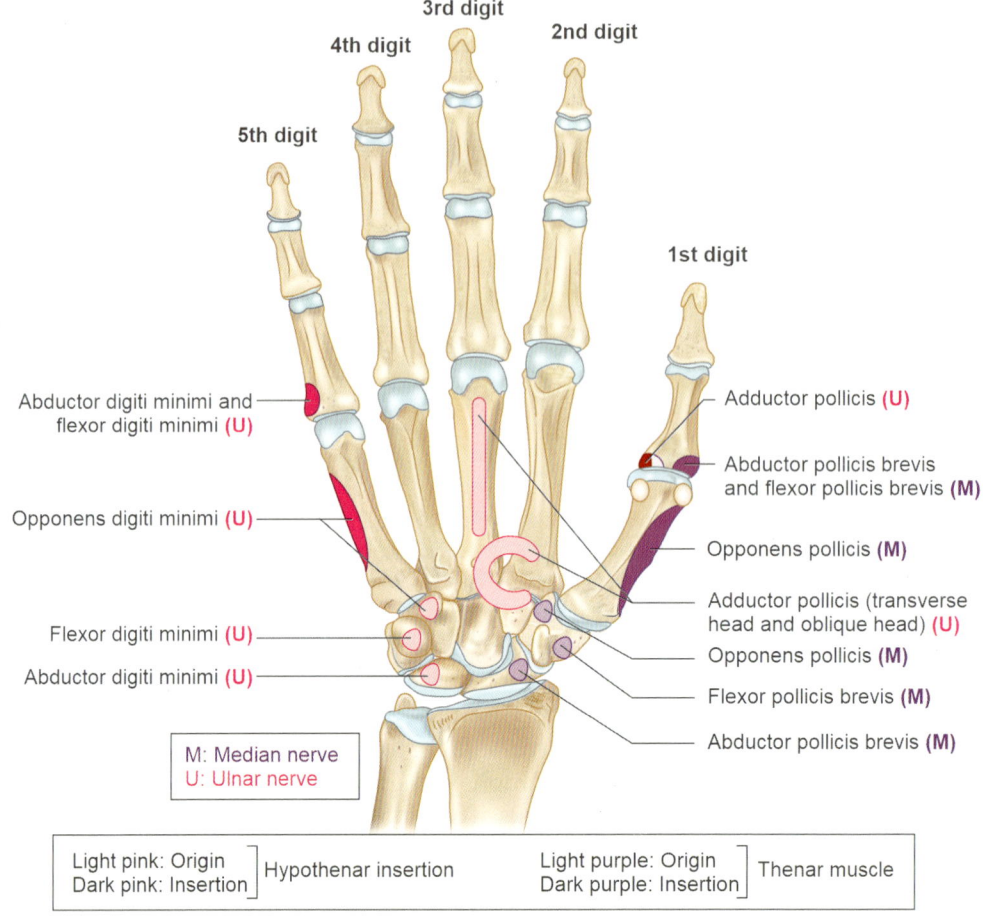

Fig. 8.7: Nerve supply of intrinsic muscles of hand (*Courtesy*: Dr Krishna Garg)

In the hands
- Dorsal and palmar interossei
- Lumbricals of ring and little fingers
- Hypothenar muscles (abductor digiti minimi, flexor digiti minimi brevis, opponens digiti minimi)
- Adductor pollicis of thumb
- Part of flexor pollicis brevis

The visible deformities result from unbalanced motor paralysis around the small joints of the fingers and thumb. The normal finger is acted on by the extrinsic (long extensors and flexors) and intrinsic (lumbricals and interossei) muscles. Intrinsic muscles act as balancing muscles providing flexion force at the MCP joint and extension at the IP joints. When the intrinsic muscles are paralyzed, finger is acted on by extrinsic muscles only.

The *earliest* feature of ulnar palsy is persistent abduction of little finger due to paralysis of adducting third palmar interossei (Fig. 8.8). The digit may also be slightly bent or clawed. The ring and little fingers are completely deprived of functioning intrinsic muscles in ulnar nerve palsy (referred to as '*intrinsic zero*' finger). The deformity caused is a partial "claw hand" (Fig. 8.9). An intrinsic zero finger is mechanically incapable of

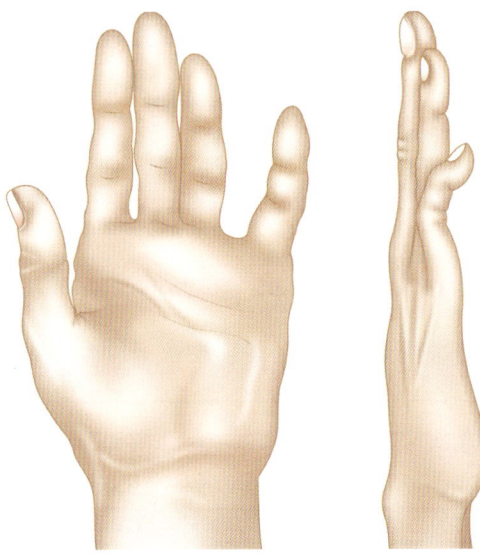

Fig. 8.8: Earliest sign of ulnar nerve palsy is a slight abduction of the little finger (Wartenberg's sign)

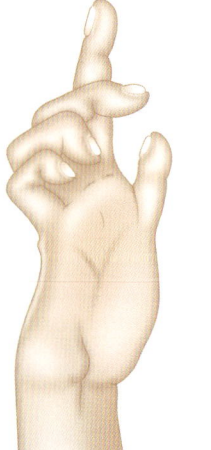 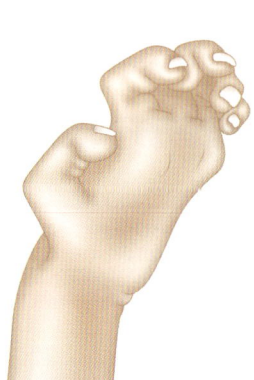 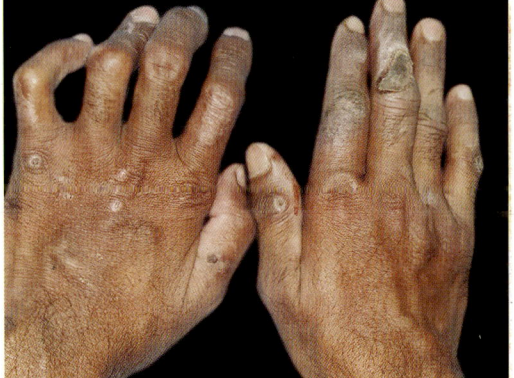

Partial claw hand   Complete claw hand

Fig. 8.9a: Further progression leads to partial (ulnar) claw hand and complete claw hand (when median nerve is also paralyzed)

Fig. 8.9b: A patient with left complete claw hand and trophic changes in the distribution of the median nerve of the right hand

being held straight and on attempting to do so, it collapses into a *zig-zag position* (hyperextension at the basal and flexion at the middle joints) which is the position of equilibrium for such a finger. This is seen as clawing and is also known as the "Z *deformity*". This deformity is also seen in the thumb in ulnar nerve palsy when the MCP-IP joint is "loaded" by a strong pinch (Fig. 8.10a).

An overview of the ulnar nerve deformities is listed in Box 8.5. The resulting disabilities of ulnar paralysis include:
1. Inability to spread the fingers and bring them together. Small objects like coins fall out through spaces between the fingers. Eating rice with hands becomes difficult.

Box 8.5: Deformities due to motor paralysis of the ulnar nerve

- "Clawing" of little and ring fingers. (Middle and index fingers may be normal, mildly clawed or fully clawed).
- Flattening of the hypothenar eminence.
- Wasting of interosseous muscles forming characteristic depression over dorsum of hand. ('Guttering sign' caused by wasting of bulky first dorsal interossei)
- Thenar eminence may show some flattening of the distal part if flexor pollicis brevis is paralyzed (often supplied by the deep branch of ulnar nerve).
- Straightening of thumb at MCP joint so that the proximal phalanx and metacarpal are in a line (if flexor pollicis brevis is paralyzed).
- Flattening of the normally slightly bulging medial border of forearm in case of high ulnar paralysis causing wasting of flexor carpi ulnaris.

2. The ring and little fingers are unable to reach and hold the 'lumbrical position'.
3. Fine work needing delicate manipulation of small objects becomes difficult.
4. Weakening of power grip and awkwardness of precision grip develops.

ii. Median nerve paralysis: The affliction of the median nerve can be of two types either low or high, the former being commoner.

- Low median paralysis: Only intrinsic muscles of hand paralyzed, associated anesthetic sequelae may also be seen (Fig. 8.9b, 8.10a and b).
- High median paralysis (injury above the level of elbow): Both, the intrinsic muscles of hand plus muscles of the front of forearm, are paralyzed. The fingers lose all power of flexion and any movement becomes impossible.

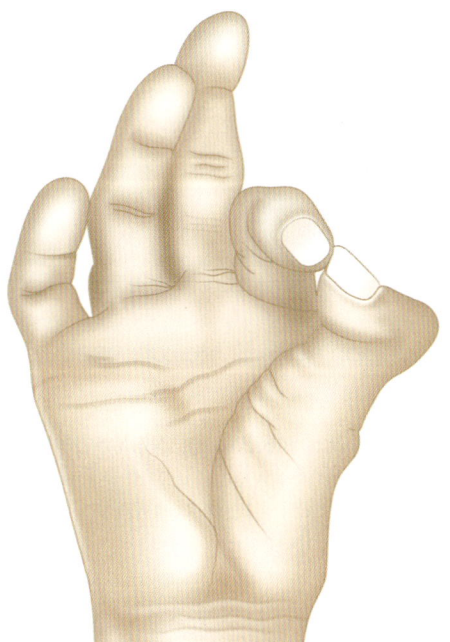

Fig. 8.10a: The Z deformity of the thumb

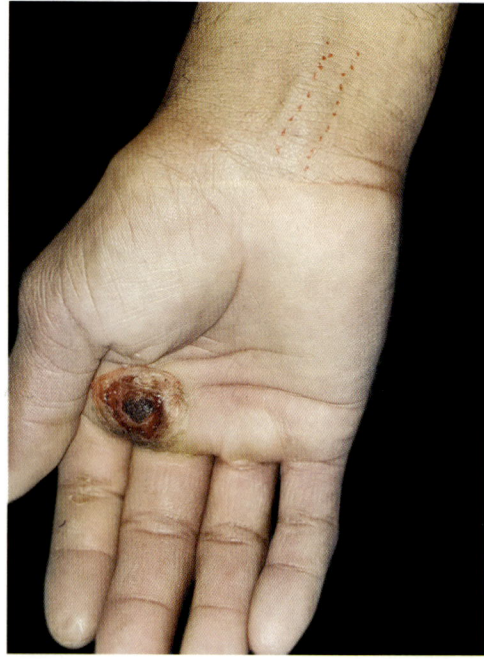

Fig. 8.10b: Enlarged median nerve with trophic ulcer in the nerve distribution

iii. Combined ulnar and median nerve paralysis (total claw hand): A combined ulnar and median palsy causes clawing of all five digits, i.e. all digits become *'intrinsic zero'* (Fig. 8.9a). The thumb comes to lie in the same plane as the other fingers and is also clawed, i.e. it is adducted, hyperextended and externally rotated at the carpometacarpal joint and flexed at the MCP and IP joints. There is flattening of the thenar eminence and the deformity is known as *'Ape thumb'* deformity.

iv. Triple paralysis (ulnar, median and radial paralysis): Radial paralysis is a rare occurrence and when it occurs, its nearly *always* with or after ulnar and median nerve palsy. When the nerve is damaged, it invariably paralyzes only the forearm muscles and triceps paralysis is extremely rare. Clawing due to intrinsic paralysis is not manifest because of the paralysis of digital extensors which normally cause hyperextension of MCP joints. However, once patient tries to keep the wrist and fingers straight with forearm extended outwards and pronated, the wrist drops (dropwrist) because of the paralysis of wrist extensors (Fig. 8.11).[7] However, when only the deep branch of the radial nerve is damaged, wrist extension is possible but active extension of the digits at the metacarpophalangeal joints becomes impossible, because of paralysis of digital extensors. The radial nerve often recovers with treatment and so the patient suffers temporary disability only.

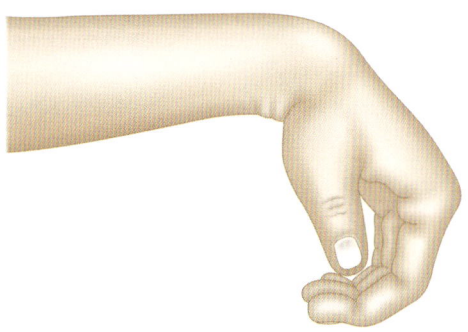

Fig. 8.11: Wrist drop due to radial nerve palsy

DEFORMITIES OF THE FOOT

In the foot, the anesthetic and paralytic deformities are of main concern and specific deformities are uncommon (Table 8.4). Occasionally though, specific ulcers develop because of breaking down of lepromatous nodules or during intense inflammatory response during reaction (ulcerating reaction).

A. Paralytic Deformities of the Foot

i. Claw Toes

Claw toes are nearly as frequent as clawing of fingers, as plantar intrinsic muscles are paralyzed nearly as often as palmar ones,[8] however, they are less obvious and patient may be totally unaware of it. The mechanism of clawing of toes is paralysis of intrinsic muscles (lumbricals, interossei and other intrinsic muscles) of the toes resulting in an imbalance of forces around the metatarsophalangeal and interphalangeal joints. These intrinsic muscles are supplied by the terminal medial and lateral plantar branches of posterior tibial nerve (Fig. 8.12). Superficial digital flexor (digitorum brevis, which is an intrinsic muscle supplied by medial plantar nerve) is the flexor of the middle phalanx that allows firm application of pulp of toes to the ground to avoid slipping. With its paralysis, the toe is curled down by the long flexors, making the tip of the toe to scrape the ground (Fig. 8.13). However, this is not a very reliable indicator of weakness of the muscles in the foot as people who have been habitually wearing closed shoes often have bent toes.

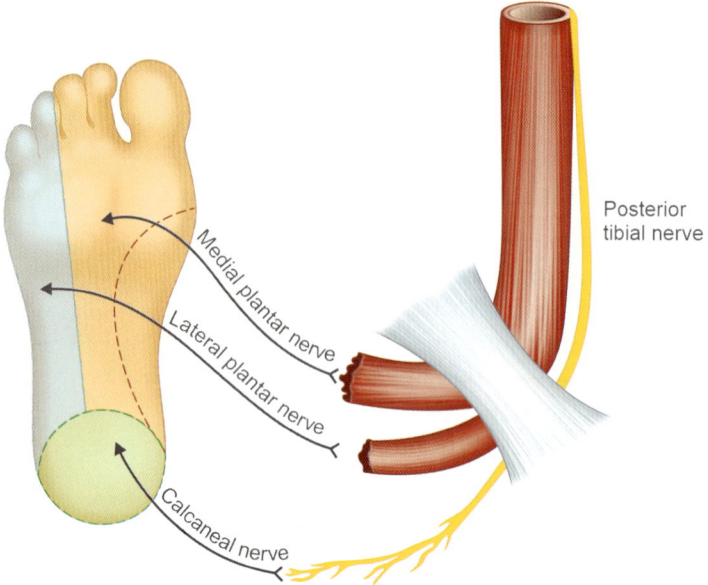

Fig. 8.12: Nerve supply of the foot via the branches of the posterior tibial nerve

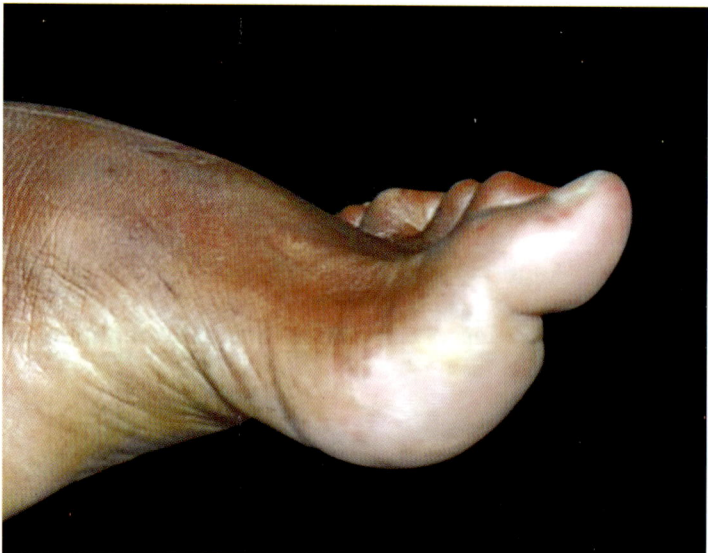

Fig. 8.13: Claw toes

The characteristic deformity of "claw toe" has been defined into the following third degree of severity:[8]
- **Mild (first degree):** Toe can be actively straightened when proximal phalanx is pressed down as the metatarsophalangeal joints and IP joints are mobile.
- **Moderate (second degree):** There is flexion contracture at the PIP joint and toe cannot be actively or passively straightened.
- **Severe (third degree):** Toes cannot even be straightened at the metatarsophalangeal joints because of the stiffness of this joint too (Fig. 8.14). Eventually, there is

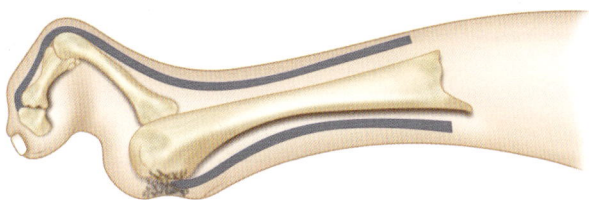

Fig. 8.14: A depiction of severe third degree claw toe due to stiffness and consequent dislocation of the proximal phalanx

dislocation of the proximal phalanx and the severely clawed toe gets high up on dorsum of foot and toe-tip no more touches the ground.

The claw toes may not cause much disability if mild, while in severe cases it may cause toe-tip ulceration and may perpetuate plantar ulceration under the head of the metatarsal.[8]

ii. Drop-foot

Like ulnar nerve, the lateral popliteal nerve (common peroneal) is also commonly involved. The lateral popliteal nerve supplies the anterior group of muscles (tibialis anterior, extensor hallucis longus and extensor digitorum longus) through its deep branch. The lateral group of muscles of the leg (peroneus or fibularis longus and brevis) are supplied by the superficial branch of the common peroneal nerve. Thus, lateral popliteal nerve supplies the dorsiflexors through its deep branch and evertors through its superficial branch. The damage to this nerve, therefore, makes the patient unable to lift up the foot which drops down with its own weight (foot drop). The other manifestations are listed in Box 8.6.

Anesthetic Deformities of the Foot

They are largely characterized by *neuropathic plantar ulcers*, though extra-plantar ulcers can also be seen. The ulcer has its own natural history, independent of that of leprosy. For these reasons the treatment of the ulcer is also independent of that of leprosy. Table 8.5 summarizes the important aspects on pathogenesis and clinical presentation of plantar ulceration in leprosy.

Sites of ulceration: While the sole of foot remains the most common site, the most commonly involved sites on the sole are listed below (Table 8.6):
- Forepart of foot (ball of foot): 70–90% of ulcers involve the forefoot, of which most occur in relation to metatarsal of the big toe (Fig. 8.15a, b and Table 8.6).
- Heel and mid-lateral border (in relation to fifth metatarsal) of sole: 5–10% cases each.
- Toe-tips: 1–5% cases, especially with claw toes.

 Box 8.6: Drop-foot and its consequences

Drop-foot gives rise to:
- High-stepping gait
- Ulceration
- Unstable foot joints
- Twisted and stiff foot

Table 8.5: A précis of the salient aspects of neuropathic plantar ulceration

Pathogenesis	a. External injury with subsequent infection b. Infection through cracks and fissures c. Internal injury caused by walking and other activities of the anesthetic foot (most common)	
Stages of plantar ulcers	Stage of *threatened* ulcer	Tenderness on deep pressure over the metatarsal head, slight puffiness and warmth, splaying of digits
	Stage of *concealed* ulcer	Necrosis occurs, blister forms
	Stage of *overt*, manifest or open ulceration	Visible ulcer underlying bone and muscles may be affected
Types of plantar ulcers	Acute	Acute infection and acute inflammation
	Chronic	Less or scanty discharge, with heaped up hyperkeratotic edges and a hard fibrosed base
	Complicated	Involves the bones, joints and tendon sheaths
	Recurrent	Due to lack of care on the patient's part or other factors (discussed in the subsequent section)

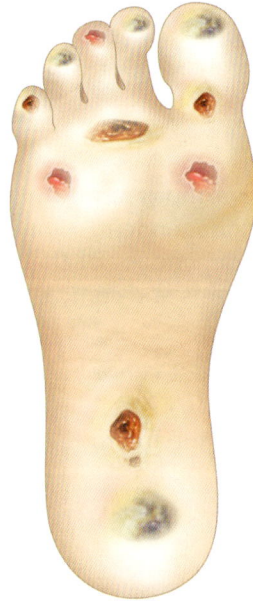

Fig. 8.15a: Different sites of ulceration in the sole of the foot

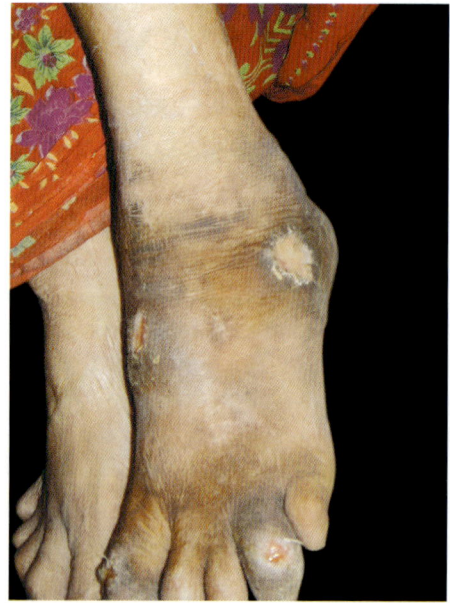

Fig. 8.15b: Leprosy trophic ulcers

An ulcer in the mid-lateral border of the foot may lead to spread of infection to the adjacent cuboid bone and cubometatarsal and calcaneocuboid joints, and is especially dangerous as from there infection may spread to rest of tarsal bones leading to septic disorganization of foot (Table 8.6).[9]

Table 8.6: Different sites of trophic ulceration on feet and their causes[16]

Site of ulceration	Usual causal factor for recurrent ulceration
1. Tips of toes	1st and 2nd degree claw deformity of toes
2. Dorsal knuckle of toes	Claw toes and friction from uppers of shoes
3. Proximal phalanx of big toe	Poor quality of scar
4. Under MTP joints	3rd degree claw-toes deformity, poor quality of scar. Sesamoiditis, scar adherent to sesamoids, severe forefoot deformities, poor quality of scar
5. Middle of sole	Tarsal disorganization with collapse of the longitudinal arch of the foot
6. Front part of heel	Collapse of calcaneum
7. Heel pad	Poor quality of scar. Pathology involving calcaneum
8. Sides of the heel	Chronic osteitis of calcaneum
9. Over lateral malleolus	Chronically infected bursa. Poor quality of scar

Trophic ulceration of leprosy follows the same clinical course and also the same management protocols as any other trophic ulcers *(see Section 8.3.1)*.

DEFORMITIES OF FACE

Characteristic facial deformities caused by leprosy are a leading cause of stigmatization and social prejudices associated with leprosy. Further, facial deformities lead to severe psychological problems in the patients themselves. Most of the facial deformities are caused by heavy infiltration of facial tissue with leprous granuloma and therefore specific deformities are more common on face than the paralytic and anesthetic deformities. Understandably, the specific deformities are seen predominantly in lepromatous type, whereas the paralytic deformities predominate in non-lepromatous leprosy cases.[10]

A. Specific Deformities of Face

These are listed below:
- *Madarosis:* This is loss of eyebrows (supraciliary madarosis) and eyelashes (ciliary madarosis) and is caused by heavy infiltration of skin with lepromatous granuloma resulting in atrophy of hair follicles.
- *Premature senile appearance (sagging face):* Leprous granulomatous infiltrate destroys dermal elastic fibers and on subsidence, skin hangs in redundant folds and results in a deeply wrinkled appearance.
- *Buddha ears*: Similar stretching of the loose skin in the external ear gives rise to this megalobule deformity.
- *'Rat-bitten' ears:* Irregularly scalloped rim of pinna due to ulceration and chondritis during type II lepra reaction.
- *Collapsed pinna:* Rarely the cartilaginous skeleton of the pinna is extensively destroyed and the pinna collapses for want of rigidity.

- *'Sunken nose' deformity:* Nasal septal perforation along with atrophy of anterior nasal spines gives rise to this deformity typical of leprosy. A Korean study noted that nasal septal involvement was the commonest facial deformity in their patients.[11] However, in the present era, nasal deformities should not occur in leprosy patients and in any leprosy program run with reasonable efficiency, a deformity of the nose is indicative of improper treatment, hygiene or myiasis.

B. Paralytic Deformities of Face

The paralytic deformity of face and is caused by involvement of the facial nerve. In leprosy, partial paralysis especially of the upper (zygomatic) branches of facial nerve is more common than lower branch paralysis and total facial paralysis (like Bell's palsy) as damage to the facial nerve trunk is quite rare. The propensity of zygomatic branches to be affected is perhaps related to the superficial cooler location and constriction within the osteofascial tunnels (Fig. 8.16a and b). This upper facial paralysis may produce paralysis of the eyelids (lagophthalmos) or even the upper part of the face. This partial palsy may be mistaken for stroke.[12]

The facial nerve involvement has been associated with skin lesions on face (Fig. 8.16b) with centripetal spread of bacilli from skin to the trigeminal nerves and from there via neural anastomoses to the terminal facial nerve branches.[13] Most cases occur in borderline leprosy with reactions and with prompt and adequate treatment of reactions (with steroids), facial nerve paralysis may be reversed and permanent deformities avoided (Fig. 8.16c).

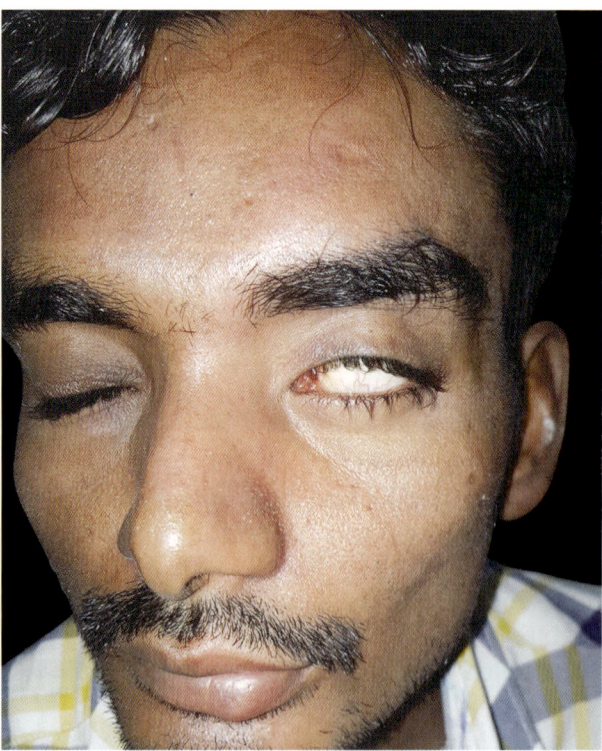

Fig. 8.16a: Left-sided facial palsy with lagophthalmos and Bell's phenomenon

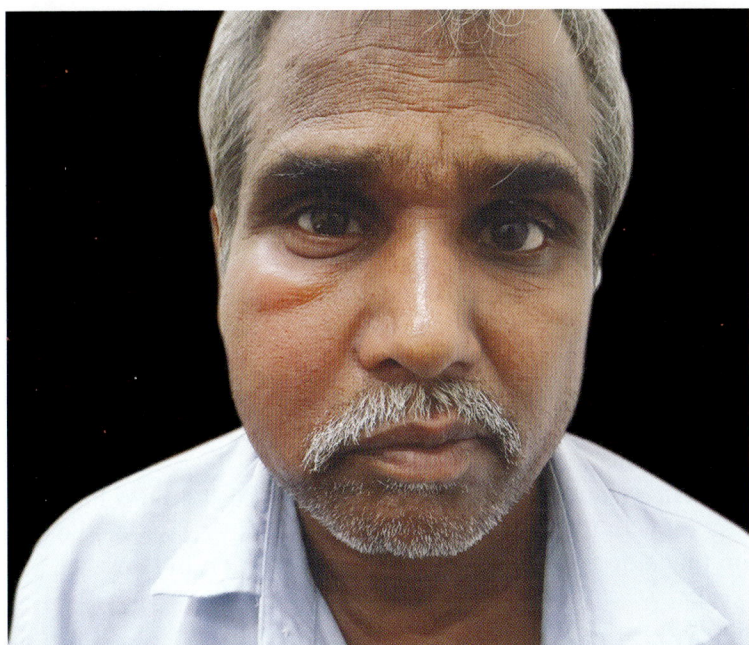

Fig. 8.16b: A case of type 1 reaction with marked edema on the right side of face suggestive of early (right) facial nerve palsy

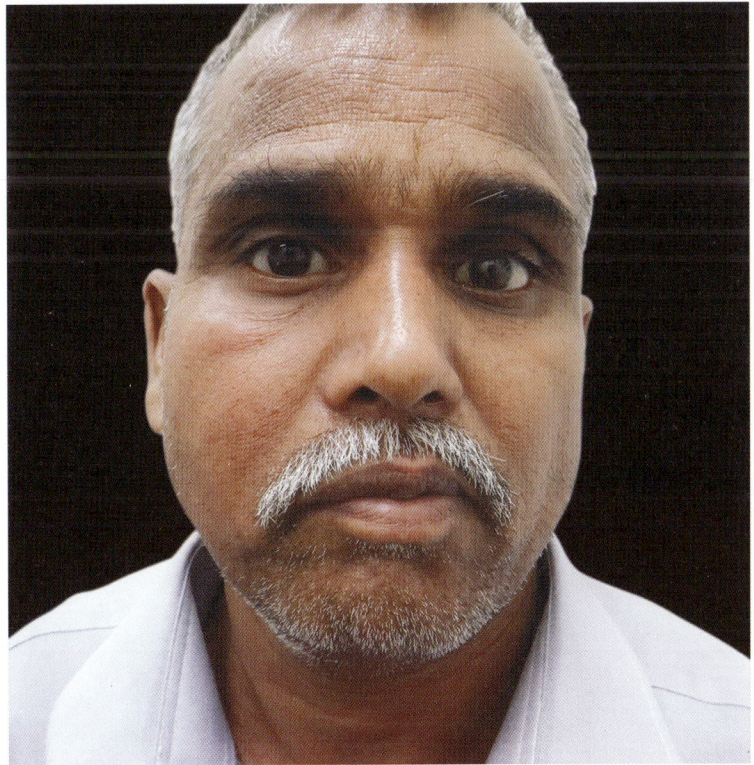

Fig. 8.16c: Near complete improvement with oral prednisolone and physiotherapy (after 7 weeks)

Lagophthalmos or paralysis of the eyelids may range from slight sagging of the lower lid to complete paralysis of both lids. Bilateral lagophthalmos is as common as unilateral paralysis, but is uncommon with pure neuritic leprosy.[14,15] The classic presentation of this is the 'leprous stare' with the white of the eye (sclera) showing above the cornea. This is because of widening of the palpebral fissure caused by the unopposed action of the levator palpebrae superioris muscle (which is innervated by the oculomotor nerve and not by the facial nerve). The flaccid lower lid falls away from the globe (ectropion) and this leads to an overflow of tears (epiphora), which is aggravated by increased lacrimation because of coexistent corneal irritation or conjunctival infection. Voluntary tight closure of the eye becomes impossible and when that is attempted, the only result is that the eyeballs roll upwards and inwards (Bell's phenomenon), leaving the lower part of the cornea uncovered. This exposure, with corneal anesthesia caused by trigeminal nerve involvement, predisposes to keratitis and possible corneal ulceration.

When the facial nerve is completely paralyzed, the affected side of the face is flattened out without any folds in the skin and the mouth is pulled towards the normal side by the muscles on that side (Fig. 8.17), but this is uncommon in leprosy.

OTHER DEFORMITIES

Besides these deformities, some other deformities may also be seen in leprosy. For example, gynecomastia or gynecothelia of male breasts is quite a cosmetic concern. This results from reduced testosterone levels secondary to testicular involvement and with subsiding mastitis during lepra reactions. Complicated cataracts and chronic lymphedema of limbs may also be seen.

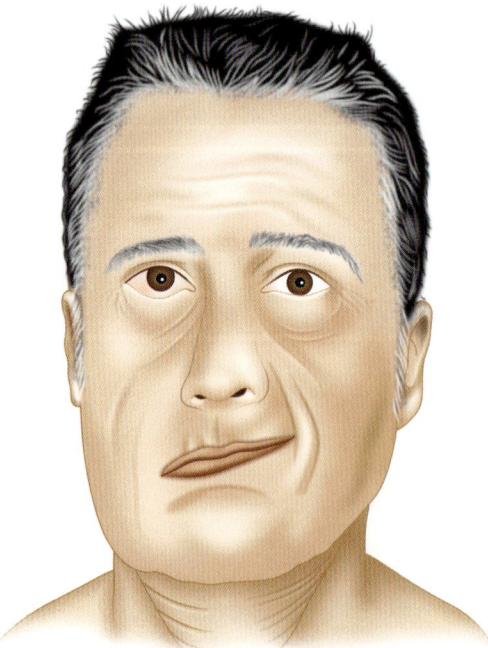

Fig. 8.17: Right facial nerve palsy with the face "pulled up" to the left side

REFERENCES

1. Adhikari B, Kaehler N, Chapman RS, Raut S, Roche P. Factors affecting perceived stigma in leprosy affected persons in western Nepal. PLoS Negl Trop Dis 2014;8:e2940.
2. Srinivasan, H. Prevention of disabilities in patients with leprosy: A practical guide, 1993.
3. de Paula HL, de Souza CDF, Silva SR, Martins-Filho PRS, Barreto JG, Gurgel RQ, et al. Risk Factors for Physical Disability in Patients with Leprosy: A Systematic Review and Meta-analysis. JAMA Dermatol 2019;ISS:1120–8.
4. Srinivas G, Muthuvel T, Lal V, Vaikundanathan K, Schwienhorst-Stich EM, Kasang C. Risk of disability among adult leprosy cases and determinants of delay in diagnosis in five states of India: A case-control study. PLoS Negl Trop Dis 2019;13:e0007495.
5. Srinivasan H. Disabilty, Deformity, Rehabilitation Hastings RC, Editor. Leprosy. New York: Churchill Livingstone, 1994; p. 411–77.
6. Ramu G, Dharmendra. Acute exacerbations (reactions) in leprosy. In: Leprosy. Volume I. Dharmendra, ed. Bombay: Kothari Medical Publishing House, 1978;108–39.
7. Srinivasan H, Dharmendra. Deformities of hands. In: Leprosy. Volume I. Dharmendra, ed. Bombay: Kothari Medical Publishing House, 1978;205–17.
8. Srinivasan H, Dharmendra. Deformities of feet. In: Leprosy. Volume I. Dharmendra, ed. Bombay: Kothari Medical Publishing House, 1978;218–23.
9. Srinivasan H, Dharmendra. Neuropathic ulceration. In: Leprosy. Volume I. Dharmendra, ed. Bombay: Kothari Medical Publishing House, 1978;224–36.
10. Dharmendra. Deformities of face in leprosy. In: Leprosy. Volume I. Dharmendra, ed. Bombay: Kothari Medical Publishing House, 1978;237–44.
11. Kim JH, Lee OJ, Lee JJ, Park CH. Analysis of facial deformities in Korean leprosy. Clin Exp Otorhinolaryngol 2013;6:78–81.
12. Lalla R, Mulherkar RV, Misar PV. Incomplete peripheral facial nerve palsy and ulnar neuropathy due to leprosy mistaken as faciobrachial stroke. BMJ Case Rep 2015;2015: pii: bcr2015210060.
13. Antia N H, Daver BM. Plastic surgery of the face in leprosy. In: Leprosy. Volume I. Dharmendra, ed. Bombay: Kothari Medical Publishing House, 1978;650–57.
14. Jaiswal AK, Subbarao NT. Bilateral lagophthalmos in leprosy: Is it a rare phenomenon? Indian J Lepr 2010;82:201–3.
15. Khan A, Sardana K, Koranne RV, Bhushan P. Bilateral seventh nerve palsy—a manifestation of polyneuritic leprosy. Indian J Lepr 2005;77:140–47.
16. H Srinivasan DD. Palande Essential Surgery. In: Leprosy Techniques for District Hospitals World Health Organization, 1997.

8.3.1 COMMON DEFORMITIES OF HAND AND FEET AND THEIR MANAGEMENT

Karthikeyan Govindasamy, Babu Govindan

This section deals with the common deformities of hands and feet and their nonsurgical management. The facial deformities, surgical interventions, and physiotherapy has been dealt with elsewhere.

COMMON FOOT-RELATED DEFORMITIES IN LEPROSY

1. Foot Drop Deformity

Foot drop is a visible and troublesome deformity caused by involvement of lateral popliteal nerve. If the foot drop is of less than six months, it can be managed conservatively with corticosteroids and appropriate orthosis (Fig. 8.18). If unresponsive in appropriate settings, surgical intervention is needed (*see Section 8.3.2*) (Fig. 8.19a and b).

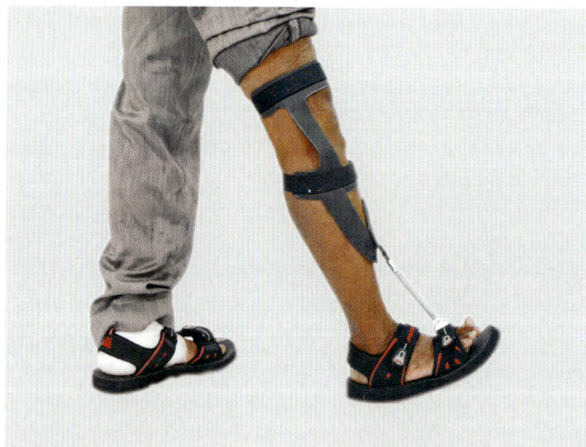

Fig. 8.18: Foot drop spring

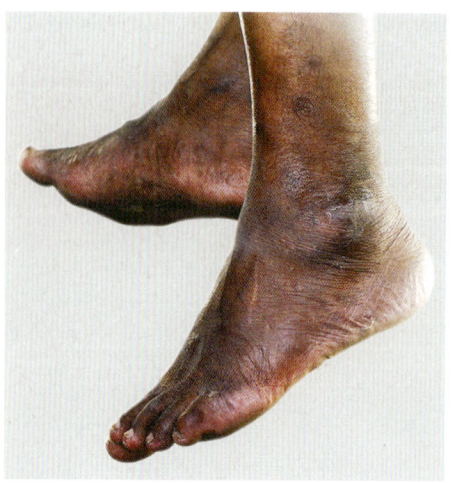

Fig. 8.19a: Before foot drop correction

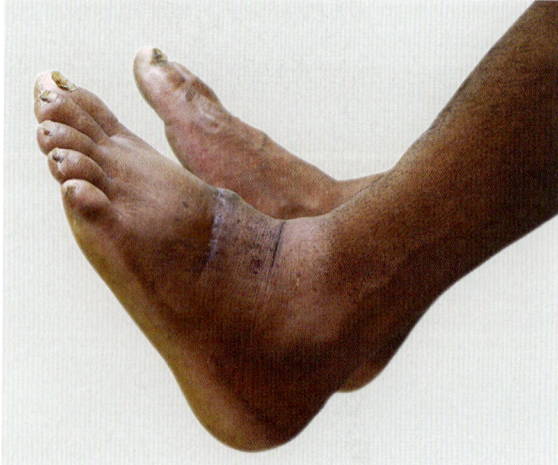

Fig. 8.19b: After foot drop correction surgery

2. Claw Toe Deformities

When the posterior tibial nerve is damaged behind the medial malleolus, it results in paralysis of intrinsic muscles of the foot leading to clawing deformity (Fig. 8.20) of the toes and loss of sensation in the sole. Clawing increases the contact of tip of the toe with the ground and increases the prominence of the heads of the metatarsals, subjecting them to increased shearing forces, resulting in the damage to skin and ulceration.

Here the flexor to extensor transfer surgery straightens out the toes. This is achieved by removing the flexor digitorum longus from its insertion, transferring it to the dorsum of the digits and inserting the tendon into the extensor digitorum. The plaster of Paris (POP) cast or posterior slab is applied to provide rest to the toes after surgery. This procedure provides equal distribution of weight and minimizes the risk of ulceration over the tip of the toes and the metatarsal heads.[5]

3. Plantar Ulcers in Leprosy

Plantar ulceration is a particularly common complication of lepromatous leprosy as even after the arrest of the disease, progressive fibrosis of nerves results in 'glove and stocking' anesthesia. Loss of sensation in the limbs, particularly on the plantar aspect of the foot is one of the commonest impairments in leprosy, occurring in 21 to 63% of newly reported cases.[6,7] The combination of loss of touch and pain and the foot deformity leads to disproportionate weight distribution on the sole of the foot resulting in nonhealing or chronic ulceration.

Acute ulcers present with acute infection and severe acute inflammation.[8] *Chronic ulcers* are long-standing without signs of acute inflammation.[8] *Complicated chronic ulcers* are consequent to spread of infection to deeper structures—underlying bone, joint or tendon sheath *(also see Table 8.6; Section 8.3)*.

1. Acute Ulcer

Diagnosis: The area is swollen, hot and red and there may be an abscess with presence of tender inguinal lymph nodes (Fig. 8.21). Where facilities are available, radiographs (dorsoplantar view for forefoot and mid-foot infections, lateral view for heel infections,

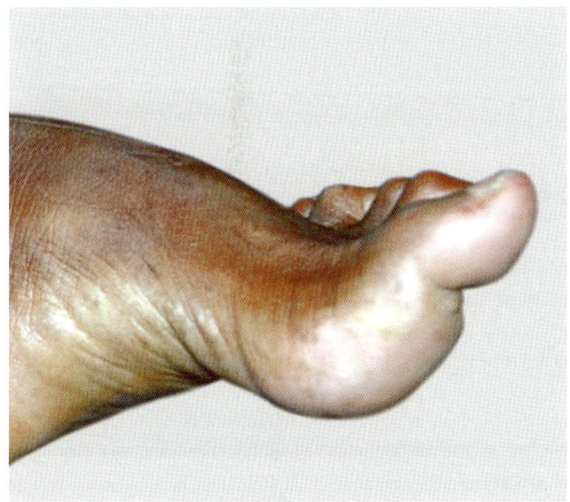

Fig. 8.20: Claw toes

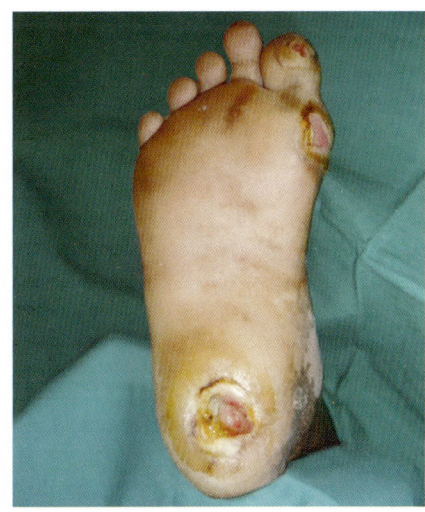

Fig. 8.21: Acute plantar ulcer

dorsoplantar, lateral and oblique views for suspected tarsal infections) should be taken to assess involvement of bones and joints.

Treatment: An overview of the steps of treatment is given in Box 8.7.

Box 8.7: An overview of the steps of treatment

- Advise bedrest, keep the leg and foot raised over pillows or on a Braun splint (for elevation).
- Soak the foot twice a day for 15 minutes in Eusol or irrigate the wound with Eusol using a 20 ml syringe without needle (Eusol: A freshly prepared solution of 12.5 gm of bleaching powder and 12.5 gm of boric acid in 5 L of water).
- Dress the ulcer loosely packing it with ribbon gauze or gauze pieces soaked in Eusol.
- Surgery is confined to drainage procedures to let out the pent-up pus in deep abscesses (incision and drainage).
- Choose a broad-spectrum antimicrobial drug or drug combination since there is likely to be a mixed infection.

Course: The acute inflammation should subside in five to seven days, and in 15–20 days discharge should become minimal and the ulcer should become a clean healing wound.

2. Simple Chronic Ulcer

Diagnosis: This usually presents as a chronic nonhealing ulcer (Fig. 8.22). The ulcer usually has hyperkeratotic heaped up margins and the floor of the ulcer is made up of pale granulation tissue covered with whitish flakes of clotted fibrin. There is minimal discharge and the ulcer is not deep.

Treatment: The aim of treatment of a simple chronic ulcer is to allow it to *heal naturally* on its own by *resting* the part and eliminating walking stresses which damage the growing epithelium and interfere with healing, as well as to protect the epithelium so that it consolidates and does not breakdown during walking.

Steps in treatment of chronic simple ulcer[9] are given in Box 8.8.

Box 8.8: Steps in treatment of chronic simple ulcer

- Wash the leg and foot well with soap and water, mop them dry or soak the foot in water alone.
- Pare the thickened hyperkeratotic margins with a pair of sharp pointed Mayo scissors or scalpel with a No. 10 BP blade without drawing blood.
- Gently scrape the ulcer bed using a Volkmann's curette and remove the superficial unhealthy layer of granulation tissue.
- Wipe the feet dry to avoid maceration of the feet.
- Though optional, an antibiotic cream can be applied over which a layer of Vaseline followed by a few gauze pieces is put. A bandage can be wrapped around the foot 4–5 times to hold the gauze in place. Cut a 1″ piece of the sticking plaster tape and use this to fix the end of the bandage.
- For home care, the above tends to suffice.
- For hospital care, apply a below-the-knee walking plaster cast for six weeks.
- After the cast has dried, which will take 48 hours or longer depending upon the weather, fit a walking device, such as a Böhler iron, to the plaster cast (Fig. 8.23). If a Böhler iron is not available, fit a walking wood, holding it with a few turns of POP bandage.
- In the case of large ulcers (diameter 2 cm or more), epithelialization is hastened by covering the ulcer with split-thickness skin graft and applying a below-the-knee walking plaster cast after the graft has become adherent to the floor of the ulcer.
- Ensure proper foot care advice.

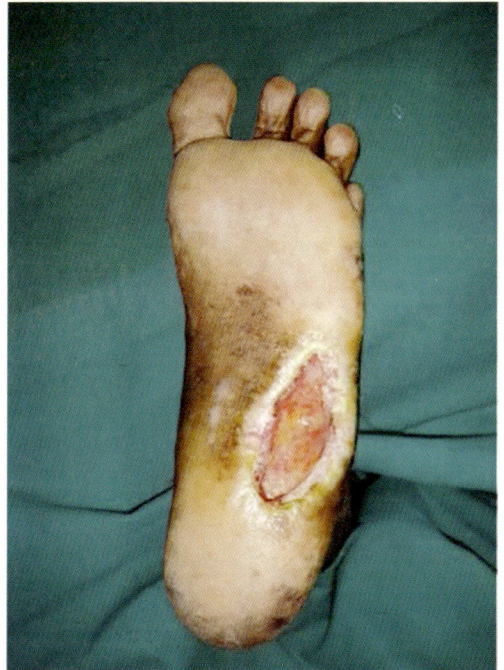

Fig. 8.22: Chronic plantar ulcer

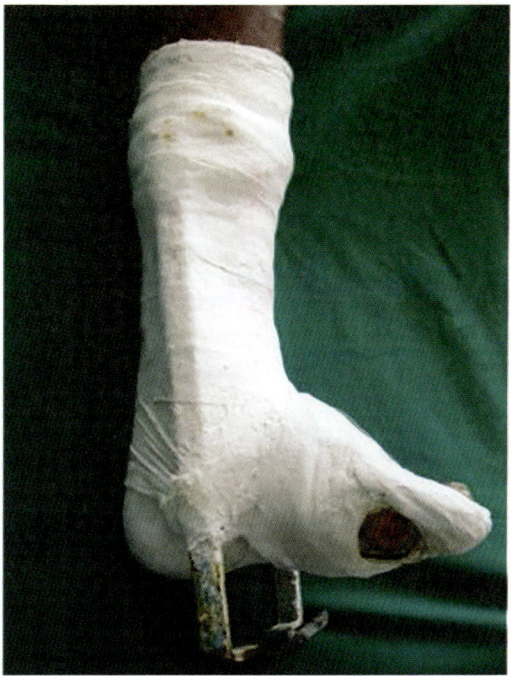

Fig. 8.23: Below knee total contact cast with Böhler iron

Moulded double rocker shoe (MDRS) boot can be used, which provides an effect similar to that of rocker. The cast, shaped like a boot, is applied below the malleoli, but covers entire foot, just like a boot. This technique is contraindicated in the presence of foot drop, stiff claw toes, or heel ulcers. The provision of foot orthosis along with protective footwear using microcellular rubber (MCR) has been used to prevent ulcers as well as to facilitate wound healing.[10] The soft tissue reconstruction of the sole has been used by many to prevent the recurrent ulceration.[5]

It is essential, if recurrence of plantar ulceration is to be avoided, to supply suitable footwear once the plaster has been removed. If this is neglected, a recurrence rate of 40% can be expected.

Other treatment options: Platelet rich fibrin dressings have been used successfully to treat nonhealing trophic ulcers of leprosy.[11,12] Briefly, it involves collecting about 5 ml of blood in a sterile vial without anticoagulant which is then centrifuged at about 2800 rpm for 15 minutes. A natural fibrin matrix gel is obtained at the middle of the tube with RBCs below and plasma above. This fibrin matrix is placed over the ulcer base, covered with a sterile dressing and left *in situ* for 7 days[12] (Fig. 8.24).

3. Complicated Chronic Ulcer

Diagnosis: A complicated chronic ulcer is one which presents with unhealthy granulation and deep sinus tracks that involve the bone, joint or tendon sheath.

Treatment: The aim of treatment in these cases is to eradicate the infection by physically removing all dead, unhealthy and grossly infected tissue, converting the ulcer into a clean, healthy wound and allowing it to heal naturally inside a POP cast.

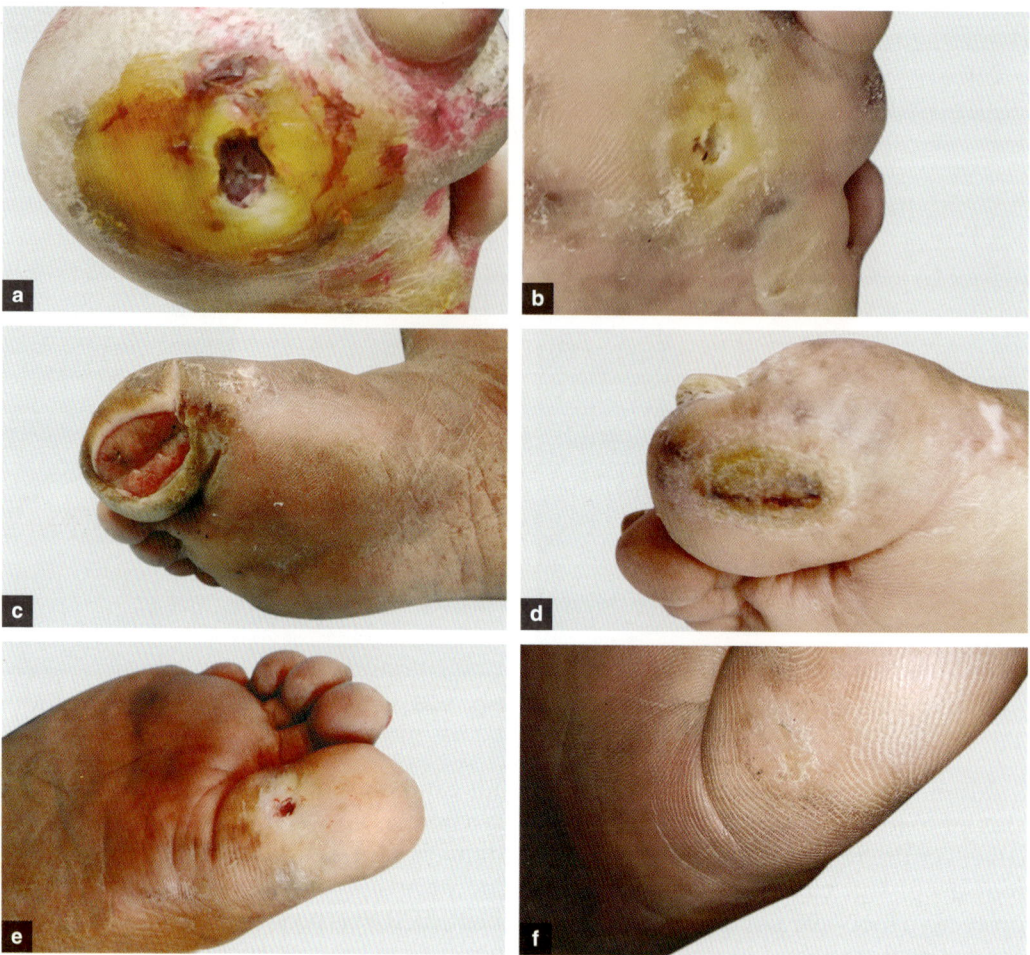

Fig. 8.24: (a) Trophic ulcer on plantar surface at baseline; (b) Trophic ulcer on plantar surface after 4th sitting of PRF; (c) Trophic ulcer on big toe at baseline; (d) Trophic ulcer on big toe after 6th sitting of PRF; (e) Trophic ulcer on big toe at baseline; (f) Trophic ulcer on big toe after 3rd sitting of PRF (*Courtesy*: Dr Konchok Dorjay)

4. Recurrent Plantar Ulceration

While the most common cause for recurrence is lack of use of proper footwear and excessive walking, other implicated causes include: (a) Poor quality of scar and (b) excessive pressures because of a deformity. In some cases, breakdown of the scar and recurrence of ulceration occurs because of circulatory insufficiency and such cases need corrective surgery.

The interventions needed include scar revision and deformity correction. Some cases may need posterior tibial neurovascular decompression which relieves the pressure on the artery, improves the blood flow and brings about the healing of the ulcer. It is important to impress on the patient that corrective surgery for recurrent plantar ulceration is not a substitute for protected use of the foot and that, in fact, the practice of foot care is even more essential after such surgery.

4. Neuropathic Foot

Neuropathic disintegration of the foot is one of the most common and overlooked diagnoses in patients with anesthetic foot in leprosy and is referred to as 'Charcot's foot' or 'hot foot'. The patient usually complains of swelling in the foot but without any pain. On palpation, the foot is warm or hot which is due to strain leading to a fracture or torn ligament. The sequential steps in management of Charcot's foot in leprosy are summarized in Box 8.9.

The neglected hot foot in leprosy can lead to fixed equines, flail foot or rocker bottom foot. This leads to more instability in the foot and inability to maintain the normal gait, leading to recurrent ulcers, particularly in the mid-foot and subsequent amputation. In cases of fixed equinovarus deformity or inversion or flail ankle joints, the ankle joint fusion is achieved by subtalar triple arthrodesis, ankle arthrodesis, subtalar wedge osteotomies and vascularized fibular graft.[5]

Box 8.9: Management for "hot foot/Charcot's foot"

1. Complete bedrest in an elevated position, during the initial few days
2. Immobilization in a non-weight bearing, below knee plaster cast for four to 6 weeks with continued elevation
3. Edema usually subsides after four weeks; total contact plaster is reapplied with a Böhler iron to facilitate ambulation. The immobilization is continued for 4 to 6 months
4. 4th or 5th month—plaster removed, mould taken for customized moulded in sole and fixed ankle brace; then plaster reapplied for another month or till the brace is ready
5. Walking exercise is initiated with the brace and if swelling occurs elastocrepe bandage is applied and foot elevated
6. Brace continued for 12 to 18 months with the regular examination every three months to identify recurrence of hot foot.

5. Other Treatable Foot Problems

With foot deformities, while early treatment is a priority, some consequences are inevitable and neural damage is an often ignored aspect in foot care.[13] Thus, while paralytic deformities are amenable to surgery, one aim should be to prevent trophic ulcers for which certain conditions deserve emergent treatment including:
- Callosities and thickened skin
- Blisters
- Superficial or uncomplicated raw areas
- Recent swelling.

While the management principles of trophic ulcer (as above) can be used to manage most of the problems, a summary of the various interventions is detailed in Table 8.7.

COMMON HAND-RELATED DEFORMITIES

The common conditions that deserve intervention include: (i) Blisters, ulcers, scars, cracks or wounds; deformity; (iii) swelling; and (iv) muscle wasting. While the last aspect has been extensively dealt in a previous chapter, we will discuss the other aspects below.

Table 8.7: Management of common foot problems	
Clinical scenario	Interventions
Callosities	See "Self care" (Section 8.3.5)
Blisters (heat, friction or pressure)	Do not break open or puncture the blister • Clean the part well, but gently, without breaking the skin • Cover the blister with a bulky layer of clean or sterile cloth or gauze • Bandage firmly, preferably with an elastic bandage • Rest at least for 3 days or walk with crutches without bearing weight on the limb with blisters • May need below knee plaster cast with provision for walking made in it after 72 hours. Retain plaster cast for 3 weeks to allow blister to heal
Foot swelling	• Treat the causative factor (infection with inflammation (septic foot); injury with inflammation without infection; and inflammation due to reaction) • Compression bandaging • Elevation • Rest in a splint

1. Blisters or Wounds

While the wounds may be simple or septic, the initial care is similar as in the case of foot wounds. The main principles remain cleaning, covering and rest.

In the hand, the method of covering depends on the type of wound. If it is simple, covering the wound and the surrounding skin with strips of ordinary zinc oxide sticking plaster would suffice. If there are signs of infection, an antiseptic ointment or gauze/cloth soaked in sterile petroleum jelly/liquid paraffin/oil can be applied followed by a few layers of soft clean cloth or clean cotton wool and finally a bandage to keep the dressing in place. One precaution unique to the finger is that one must not tie the bandage at the base of the finger (Fig. 8.25a) but instead, carry the bandage over to the palm and tie it with a knot on the back of the hand (Fig. 8.25b). Alternatively, sticking plaster may be used to secure the bandage.

2. Callus and Corns

The method of treating is similar to that of the foot (*see* above)

3. Swelling

There are three causes of swelling of the hand:
1. Infection and inflammation
2. Injury to a bone or joint
3. Inflammation only, without infection or injury

A management protocol is detailed in Fig. 8.26 and details can be accessed by publications of this topic.[4, 5, 13]

Other Aspects of Treatment

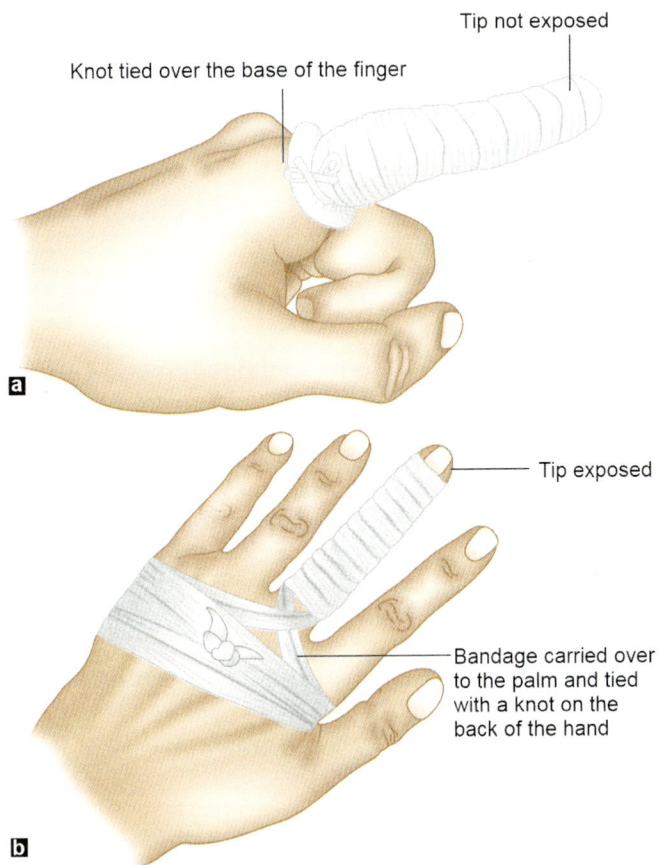

Fig. 8.25: (a) The incorrect and (b) correct way to tie a bandage for covering a wound over a finger.

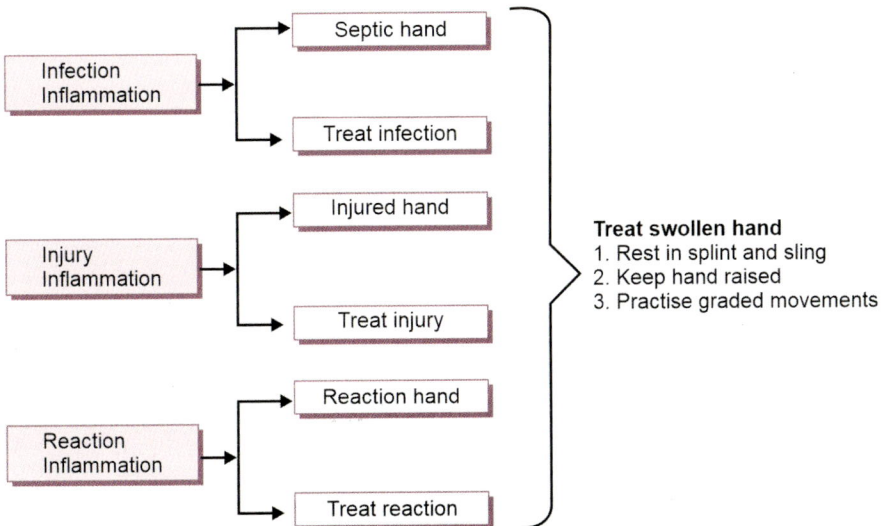

Fig. 8.26: Causes and management of the swollen hand

REFERENCES

1. Andersen JG. Foot drop in leprosy and its surgical correction. Acta Orthop 1963;33:151–71.
2. Srinivasan H, Mukherjee SM, Subramaniam RA. Two-tailed transfer of tibialis posterior for correction of drop-foot in leprosy. J Bone Joint Surg Br 1968;50:623–8.
3. Das P, Kumar J, Karthikeyan G, Rao PSSS. Peroneal strength as an indicator in selecting route of tibialis posterior transfer for foot drop correction in leprosy. Lepr Rev 2013;84:186–93.
4. Paul MSK, Kumar, David Prakash GK. Physical Rehabilitation in Leprosy. In: International Textbook of Leprosy, 2019; p. 1–42.
5. Virmond M, Joshua J, Solomon S, Duerksen F. Surgical Aspects in Leprosy. In: International Textbook of Leprosy, 2019; p. 1–35.
6. Van Brakel WH, Khawas IB. Nerve damage in leprosy: An epidemiological and clinical study of 396 patients in west Nepal—Part 1. Definitions, methods and frequencies. Lepr Rev 1994;65:204–21.
7. Dorairaj A, Reddy R, Jesudasan K. An evaluation of the Semmes-Weinstein 6.10 monofilament as compared with 6 nylon in leprosy patients. Indian J Lepr 1988;60:413–7.
8. Srinivasan H. Atlas of corrective surgical procedures commonly used in leprosy [Internet]. Chennai:2004. Available from: http://www.damienfoundation.in/books/
9. Novartis Comprehensive Leprosy Care Association (NCLCA) IFPMA [Internet]. [cited 2019 Aug 20]. Available from: http://partnerships.ifpma.org/ partnership/novartis-comprehensive-leprosy-care-association-nclca.
10. Cross HA, Sane S, Dey A, Kulkarni VN. The efficacy of podiatric orthoses as an adjunct to the treatment of plantar ulceration in leprosy. Lepr Rev 1995;66:144–57.
11. Nagaraju U, Sundar PK, Agarwal P, Raju BP, Kumar M. Autologous Platelet-rich Fibrin Matrix in Nonhealing Trophic Ulcers in Patients with Hansen's Disease. J Cutan Aesthet Surg, 2017;10:3–7.
12. Vinay K, Sawatkar G, Dogra S, Naranag T. Platelet-rich fibrin dressings in the treatment of non-healing trophic ulcers of leprosy. Lepr Rev 2018;89:158–64.
13. Srinivasan H. Prevention of disabilities in patients with leprosy: A practical guide. [Internet]. Geneva: World Health Organization; 1993. Available from: http://apps.who.int/iris/handle/10665/41226.

8.3.2 SURGICAL CORRECTION OF COMMON DEFORMITIES OF UPPER AND LOWER EXTREMITIES

Anil Dhal, Yasim Khan

INTRODUCTION

Leprosy is a disease known to cause deformities and disabilities. Nerve involvement causes motor, sensory and autonomic dysfunction in the supplied area.[1] Initially the deformities are supple and passively correctable. Sustained neurological deficit over a period of time leads to contracture of soft tissues around the joints and deformities become fixed/irreversible. In so far as deformities are concerned, the primary emphasis is on prevention. In leprosy, we can prevent deformities by diagnosing neurological deficit at the early stage and by counseling and educating patients in advance when they initially present with only skin lesions. Nerve damage can be insidious—quiet nerve palsy—but is also commonly on account of reactions. Patient counseling in detecting signs of nerve damage is crucial and this includes being aware to report numbness in hand or foot, tingling sensation along limbs, weakness in hand or inability to lift the foot.

As discussed previously *(see Section 8.3)*, the affliction of peripheral nerves can manifest with varied clinical presentations. The ulnar nerve involvement causes ulnar claw hand (Fig. 8.27), involvement of both ulnar and median nerves causes total claw hand deformity (Fig. 8.28) and radial nerve involvement causes wrist and finger drop. While common peroneal nerve involvement may lead to foot drop and ulcers over malleoli (Fig. 8.29a), patients with posterior tibial nerve involvement can present with nonhealing ulcers in the sole of the foot due to sensory loss (Fig. 8.30).

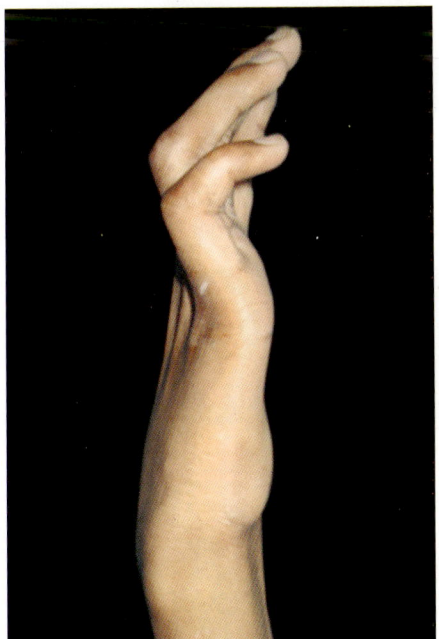

Fig. 8.27: Clawing of little and ring fingers (ulnar claw hand)

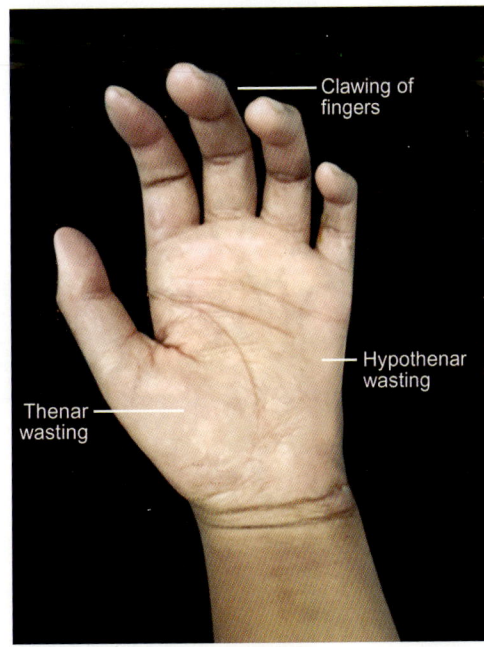

Fig. 8.28: Total claw hand due to ulnar and median nerve involvement

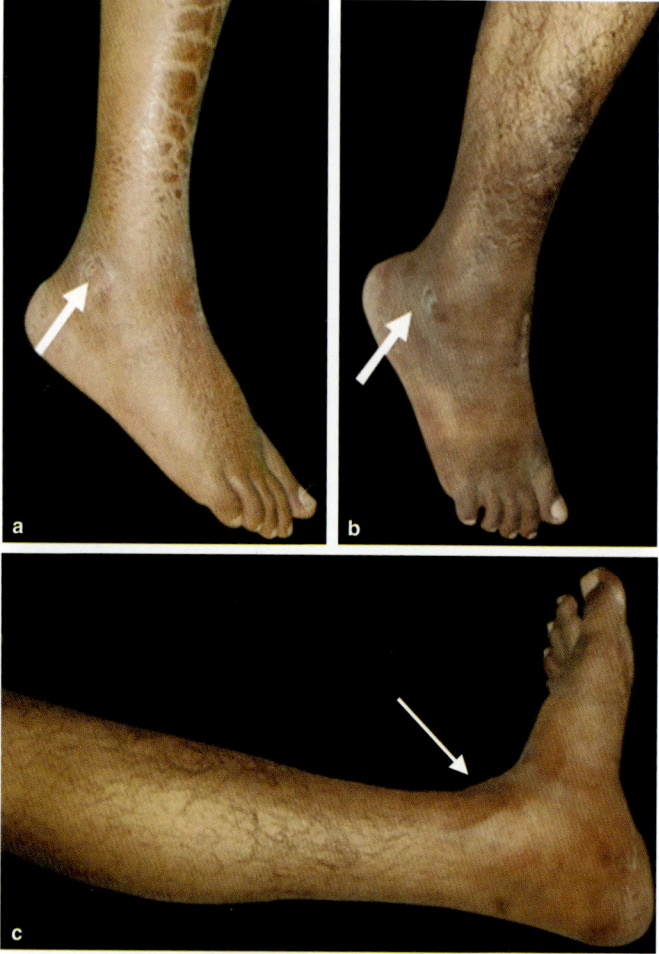

Fig. 8.29: (a) Preoperative photograph showing foot drop, ulcer over lateral malleolus (arrow) and icthyosis of skin; (b) Follow-up photo at 3 months after nerve decompression surgery showing healing of ulcer (arrow) and disappearance of ichthyosis; (c) Follow-up photo at 3 months showing active dorsiflexion and prominence of tibialis anterior muscle tendon (arrow)

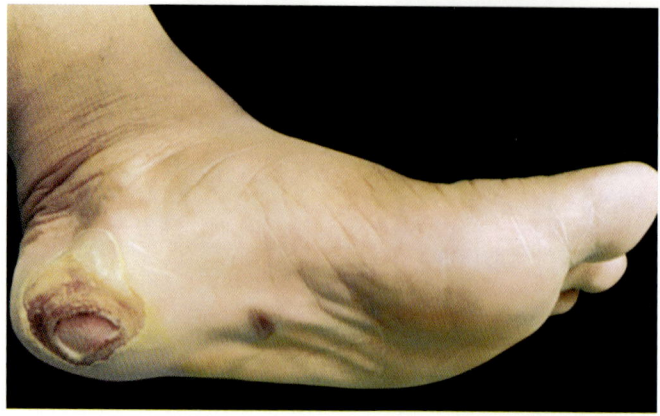

Fig. 8.30: Nonhealing ulcer over heel secondary to involvement of posterior tibial nerve

Evaluation and Investigations

Patients reporting with early neurological deficit should be thoroughly evaluated clinically (*see Chapter 10*). Palpation for nerve thickening can be combined with high-resolution ultrasonography to look for nerve abscess or nerve thickening along the course of nerves (Fig. 8.31a to c). This can also be useful in determining the level of nerve compression.

Management

The medical management of neuritis and early onset nerve function impairment (NFI) has been detailed before (*see Section 8.1*) and here we will focus on the surgical management.

Initial Management

Splintage and passive range of motion exercises can be initiated. A knuckle bender splint for claw hand, a dynamic/static cock-up splint for wrist drop or an ankle foot orthosis for foot drop must be advised depending on the neurological involvement.

In most cases, one will be able to manage acute neuritis satisfactorily with steroids along with the above measures. In case there is a lack of improvement of the functional state of the nerve, surgical intervention by way of surgical decompression of the nerve trunks is indicated (Boxes 8.10 and 8.11).

Surgical Treatment of Neuritis

For the present, in most centers, steroids ("medical decompression") have replaced surgical decompression in the treatment of recent nerve impairment. Surgery is reserved for nerve abscess and unresponsive nerve pain.[2,3] The scientific rationale for surgery in promoting motor and/or sensory recovery is to decompress the nerve at the sites of

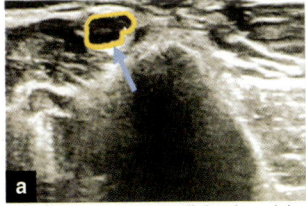
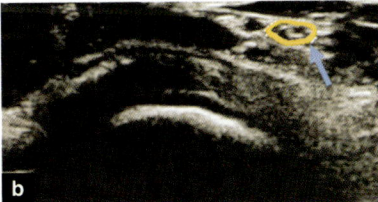
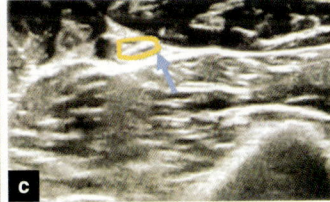

a — Left ulnar nerve at medial epicondyle   b — Left ulnar nerve at wrist joint   c — Left ulnar nerve at mid-forearm

Fig. 8.31: High resolution ultrasonographic image showing: (a) Thickened ulnar nerve behind medial epicondyle with cross-sectional area 0.116 cm² (arrow); (b) Normal ulnar nerve in mid-forearm with cross-sectional area 0.070 cm² (arrow); (c) Thickened ulnar nerve in Guyon's canal with cross-sectional area 0.102 cm² (arrow)

 Box 8.10: Indications of ulnar and median nerve decompression[11]

Main indication: Wherever signs of nerve damage appear or increase while under adequate treatment for acute ulnar neuritis.*

Supplementary indications: Persistence or increase of pain or tenderness of the nerve.

*Steroids in adequate dosage, splinting, physiotherapy for two to three weeks.

Box 8.11: Indications of posterior tibial nerve decompression[11]

Posterior tibial neurovascular bundle decompression may be attempted:
  i. To improve the vascularity of the sole of the foot to get recalcitrant ulcers healed; or
  ii. To arrest and, if possible, reverse nerve damage and restore plantar sensibility in cases of recent plantar anesthesia

---

mechanical compression. This could be supplemented with an epineurotomy or interfascicular neurolysis in order to permit the regenerating axons in the nerve to pass through the 'compressive' area and reach its end organs. For this to be effective, the surgery needs to be performed *before* the skin's sensory end organs or skeletal muscle fibers have irreversibly atrophied. This probably means the patient should have an early nerve decompression and many surgeons would use a rule of less than one year.[2]

While various surgical techniques are elucidated below, it is important to again reiterate the 3 main indications for surgical intervention:
1. Nerve abscess
2. Patients with established irreversible nerve impairment who occasionally suffer from persistent nerve pain many months or years after completing chemotherapy.
3. Lack of improvement of nerve impairment with steroid therapy.

Decompression of nerves and nerve abscess

Even though Cochrane reviews on the subject do not recommend decompressive surgery as this does not show a significant added benefit over steroid treatment alone,[3,4] there is a converse view that the inflamed, swollen nerve is vulnerable to physical trauma, compression, stretch and friction, and hence decompression could be advised as an adjunctive measure to medical therapy.[4] Most published reports show that there is no further deterioration in nerve function after surgical decompression and that in many cases, functional recovery follows the procedure.[5] Two recent studies have in fact found that nerve decompression helped in achieving marked degree of motor recovery[5] and helped to reduce the use of analgesics and corticosteroids.[6] Authors have reported that early, selective surgical nerve decompression results in better functional outcomes.[7]

But it is to be remembered that surgery is deliberate infliction of a wound on a nerve trunk which is already damaged and diseased.[2] Thus, the surgeon should be patient and meticulous in attending to details and should take care to never remove the epineurium around the entire circumference of the nerve trunk, as that is a source of blood supply to the nerve fibers.[2]

Two types of surgical decompression are possible:
  i. *External decompression/neurolysis* in which compression of the nerve trunk by structures external to it is relieved. Anterior transposition or epicondylectomy (resection of the medial epicondyle of the humerus) may be done as part of the external decompression operation in order to eliminate all mechanical stresses on the ulnar nerve consequent to elbow movements. Decompression of the median nerve by dividing the roof of the carpal tunnel is another example of external decompression.

ii. *Internal decompression/neurolysis with epineurotomy*: This is a procedure in which the nerve bundles (fascicles) are released from compression by the epineurium which has become thickened, or fibrosed and constricted.

External and internal neurolysis (achieved via epineurotomy) of ulnar nerve may be performed behind the medial epicondyle (Fig. 8.32). After early surgical nerve decompression, substantial sensory recovery is achieved whereas motor recovery, in terms of improvement in grip strength and restoration of muscle bulk, may also be seen in some patients (Fig. 8.33a and b). Similarly, recovery of dorsiflexion may be achieved following surgical decompression of common peroneal nerve (CPN) in foot drop (Figs 8.34 and 8.29c).

iii. *Nerve abscess* is often a cold abscess occurring due to caseous necrosis and is seen in borderline tuberculoid and tuberculoid leprosy. Hot abscesses may also occur in nerve trunks as part of acute ENL-related neuritis, but they are usually microscopic.

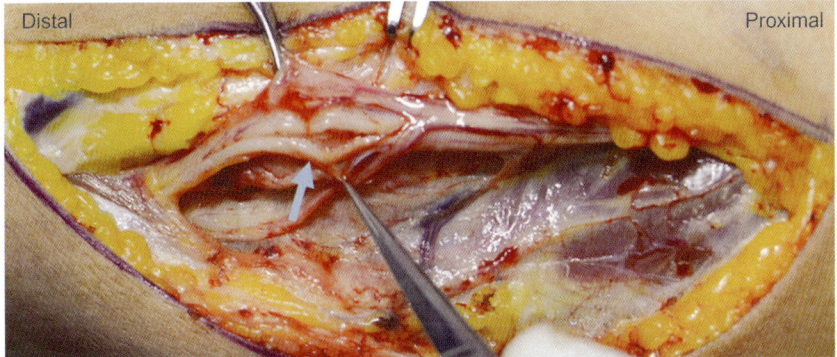

Fig. 8.32: Photograph showing external and internal neurolysis of ulnar nerve behind medial epicondyle

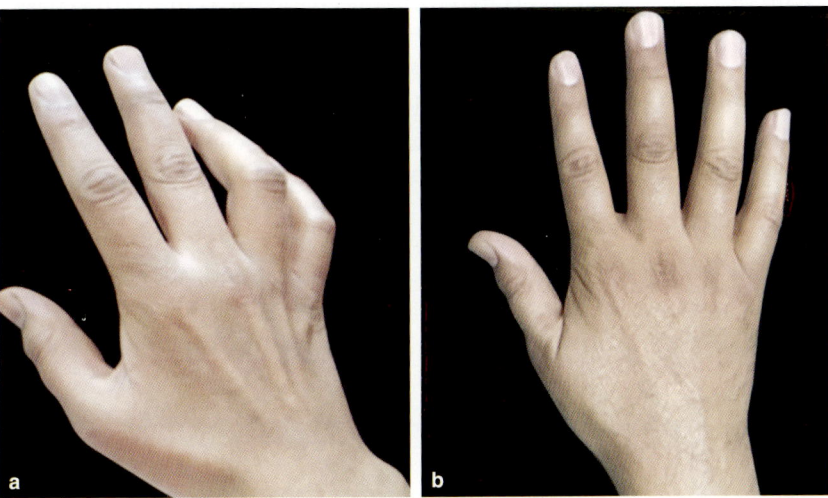

Fig. 8.33: (a) Ulnar claw hand deformity with wasting of first dorsal web space and intermetacarpal spaces; (b) Correction of deformity and restoration of muscle bulk at 2 years follow-up

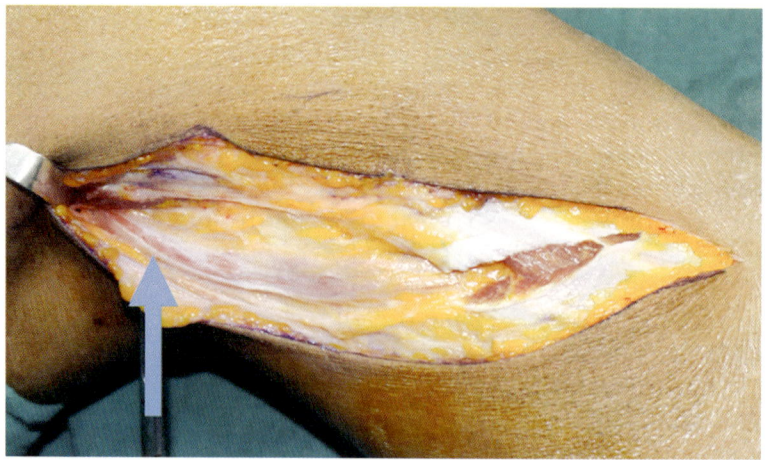

Fig. 8.34: Neurolysis of common peroneal nerve in proximal leg

The swelling will be fluctuant and mobile *transversely* but not longitudinally. The basic principle is that the surgeon should not make the nerve function worse by surgery, nor create a chronic discharging sinus. Thus, the management of a cold abscess in the nerve is governed mainly by the *functional* state of the affected nerve trunk and if the functional state of the nerve is normal, no surgical intervention is needed. If there is a deterioration of nerve function, surgical intervention will be required (Box 8.12).

The various options include:[2,3]

a. *Aspirate* the nerve abscess with a large bore needle, and wait for nerve function to improve.
b. In case of a chronic or recurrent abscess, it can be *surgically exposed* under regional or general anesthesia, the abscess cavity opened and drained and very carefully cleaned of its pseudocapsule wall, without avulsing nerve fascicles. The wound is then closed with separate fascial layers to reduce the chance of a chronic discharging sinus. Under no circumstances should the abscess be surgically excised as this might slice through nerve fascicles that might otherwise have recovered.
c. If the nerve is already completely paralyzed and if it is unlikely to recover (long-standing paralysis, severe atrophy of paralyzed muscles), there is no need to do anything particular for the abscess as such.

Correction of Paralytic Deformities

In long-standing paralysis, surgical reconstruction of hand and feet can be done to restore the lost function. Healing of nonhealing ulcers and relief in neuropathic pain can be expected from delayed surgical nerve decompression also. Nerve trunk

---

 Box 8.12: Indications of surgical management of nerve abscesses[11]

    i. Partial paralysis of the nerve
   ii. Complete paralysis of recent onset (eight weeks or less)
  iii. When the abscess becomes adherent to the overlying skin and threatens to break open to form one or more sinuses.

involvement in leprosy follows a definite pattern. There are certain muscles which are rarely involved in leprosy and hence it makes sense in using such muscles for tendon transfers.[8] Young intelligent patients who are motivated are good candidates for reconstructive surgery.

a. Reconstruction for claw hand deformity (lumbrical replacement operation)[8]

A dynamic or static lumbrical replacement operation can be done. Combined high ulnar and low median palsy results in a nearly useless hand and requires both lumbrical as well as opponens replacement.

Before undertaking lumbrical replacement, it should be confirmed that there is *no joint stiffness* in the proximal interphalangeal joints and that the long extensors and dorsal expansions are intact. This is confirmed by manual assistance to the MCP joint for preventing hyperextension and asking the patient to extend the finger (Bouvier's sign) (Fig. 8.35a). If the patient is not able to extend the affected fingers fully at PIP joint, even when MCP joint is stabilized, then dynamic operations usually fail. If skin is the chief obstacle to extension, then a Z-plasty or a flap of dorsal skin turned volar wards (cross finger flap), may improve extension. Any dorsal hood damage must be repaired prior to lumbrical replacement, failing which arthrodesis of the PIP joint can be undertaken.

Radial nerve palsy when present must be corrected before any other procedure is undertaken for claw hand correction. Staged reconstruction of fingers and thumb should be done with lumbrical replacement preceding opponens replacement. The superficial sores and ulcers should have healed and physiotherapy helps in better postoperative results. Avoid operation during acute phases of disease. Best results are obtained in hands of well-motivated younger persons (15 to 45 years of age), with recent deformity (lesser than 3 years), with no stiffness of finger joints or soft tissue contractures, having no or very little (≤10°) hyperextension at the PIP joints, no or very little (≤15°) ulnar deviation of fingers, and no assisted angle or weakness of forearm muscle.

New muscle tendon units are introduced by rerouting tendons of muscles into the articular joints. The muscles used include the flexor digitorum superficialis (*Bunnel's* operation) (Fig. 8.35b), flexor carpi radialis, palmaris longus (*Antia's* operation), extensor carpi radialis brevis (*Brand's* operation) and extensor digiti minimi (*Fowler's* operation)

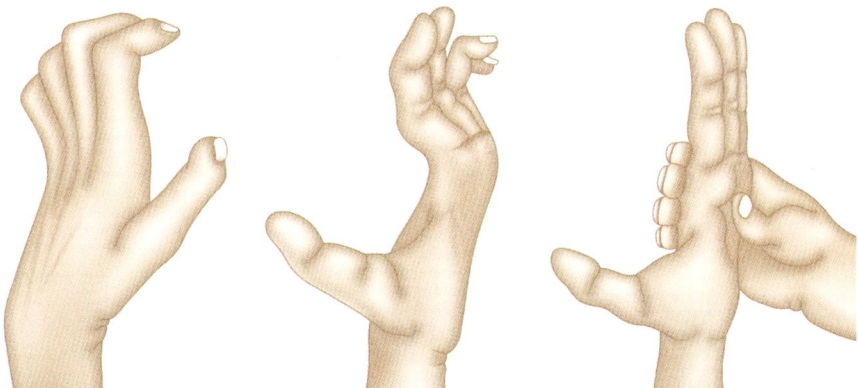

Fig. 8.35a: Illustration of Bouvier's sign, showing extension of interphalangeal joints on flexing metacarpophalangeal joint

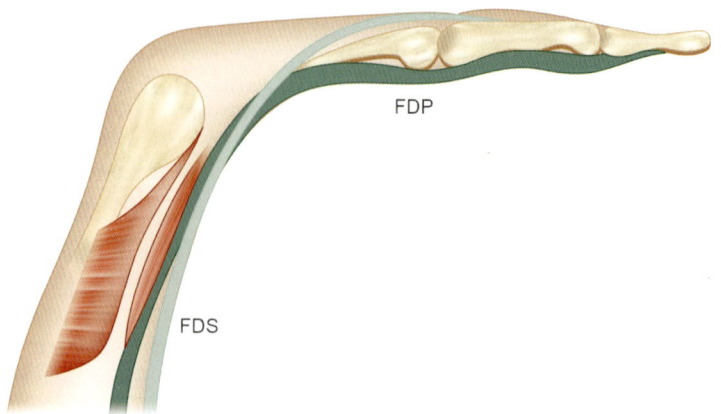

Fig. 8.35b: Diagram showing correction of claw deformity by transferring flexor digitorum superficialis (FDS) slip to the lateral band of extensor expansion

as they are *not* affected in leprosy. These motor tendons can be inserted to any of the following insertion sites—lateral band of dorsal extensor expansion, the proximal annular pulleys of flexor sheath, proximal phalanx and the interosseous tendon.[8,9] A "many-tailed" graft operation that uses palmaris longus or the extensor carpi radialis brevis as the motor muscle can also be used. Presence of palmaris longus should be checked preoperatively by asking the patient to actively flex the wrist with index finger and thumb in opposition. Advantage of using palmaris longus is that it runs a straight course from origin to insertion and provides adequate power.

b. Reconstruction of thumb abduction (opponens plasty)

In combined ulnar and median nerve involvement, there is inability to abduct and oppose the thumb and an instability of the MCP joint. Opponens plasty can be done using the sublimis tendon of the ring finger as motor and rerouting it across the base of palm to insert into dorsal expansion of the thumb. Stability of MCP joint is provided by a Y-insertion across the metacarpal neck and by taking care to route the main tendon accurately across the fulcrum of MCP joint. Alternatively, the extensor indicis proprius (EIP) can be rerouted obliquely across the palm, at the level of the pisiform, to be attached to the insertion of the abductor pollicis brevis tendon, at the base of the proximal phalanx of the thumb (Fig. 8.36a to e). Postoperatively, the thumb is immobilized in abduction for 3–4 weeks followed by opposition exercises. Adequate restoration of thumb abduction and opposition occurs by 3 months.

c. Thumb web space contracture

This can be managed by manual stretching, abduction traction with dynamic splint, serial plastering and transposition of skin flap from the dorsum of the hand.

d. Wrist drop

It can be managed by standard triple tendon transfer of pronator teres to extensor carpi radialis brevis, flexor carpi ulnaris or flexor carpi radialis to extensor digitorum communis and palmaris longus to the rerouted extensor pollicis longus tendon after releasing it from the 3rd extensor compartment of the wrist. Cock up splint should be used pre- and postoperatively.

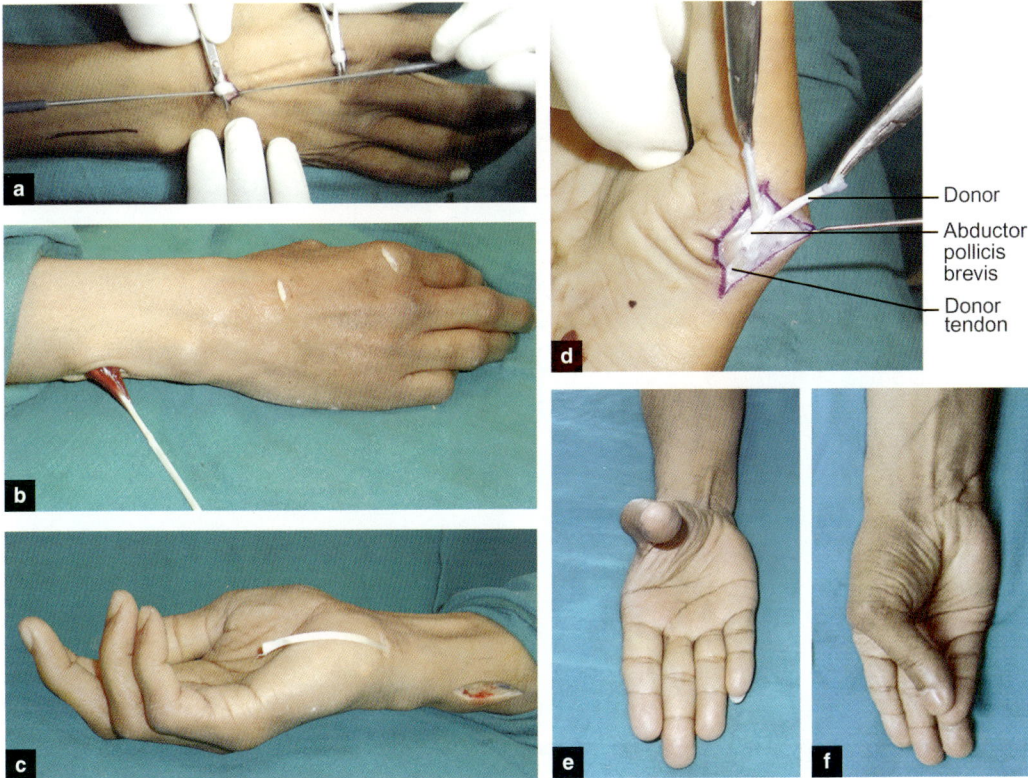

Fig. 8.36a to f: Extensor indicis proprius (EIP) transfer to restore thumb opposition: (a) Tendon being harvested; (b) EIP withdrawn through a dorsoulnar incision, distal forearm; (c) EIP rerouted to exit near pisiform; (d) EIP tendon APB insertion; (e and f) Restoration of thumb abduction and opposition

e. Foot drop deformity

Due to involvement of the common peroneal nerve, foot drop deformity can be surgically managed by tibialis posterior tendon transfer to the dorsum of foot, after proper muscle charting. At least grade 4 power is required in tibialis posterior muscle to achieve good postoperative results. The tendon of tibialis posterior is exposed through a 5 cm medial incision, centred on the navicular bone (Fig. 8.37a). The tendon is divided at its insertion and withdrawn through a second incision over the medial aspect at the junction of proximal two-thirds and distal one-third of the leg (Fig. 8.37b). This tendon is then passed through the interosseous membrane and delivered into an anterior incision 2 cm proximal to the ankle joint (Fig. 8.37c). It is inserted into the base of 3rd metatarsal or the middle cuneiform (Fig. 8.37d). Below knee plaster cast is applied and continued till 6 weeks postoperative followed by an ankle foot arthrosis (AFO) for another 6–8 weeks. Active foot dorsiflexion is initiated after plaster is removed. Adequate dorsiflexion with good power is usually restored by 6 months following tibialis posterior transfer (Fig. 8.37e).

A protocol for appropriate physiotherapy of patients which helps in success of foot drop surgery is given in Table 8.8.

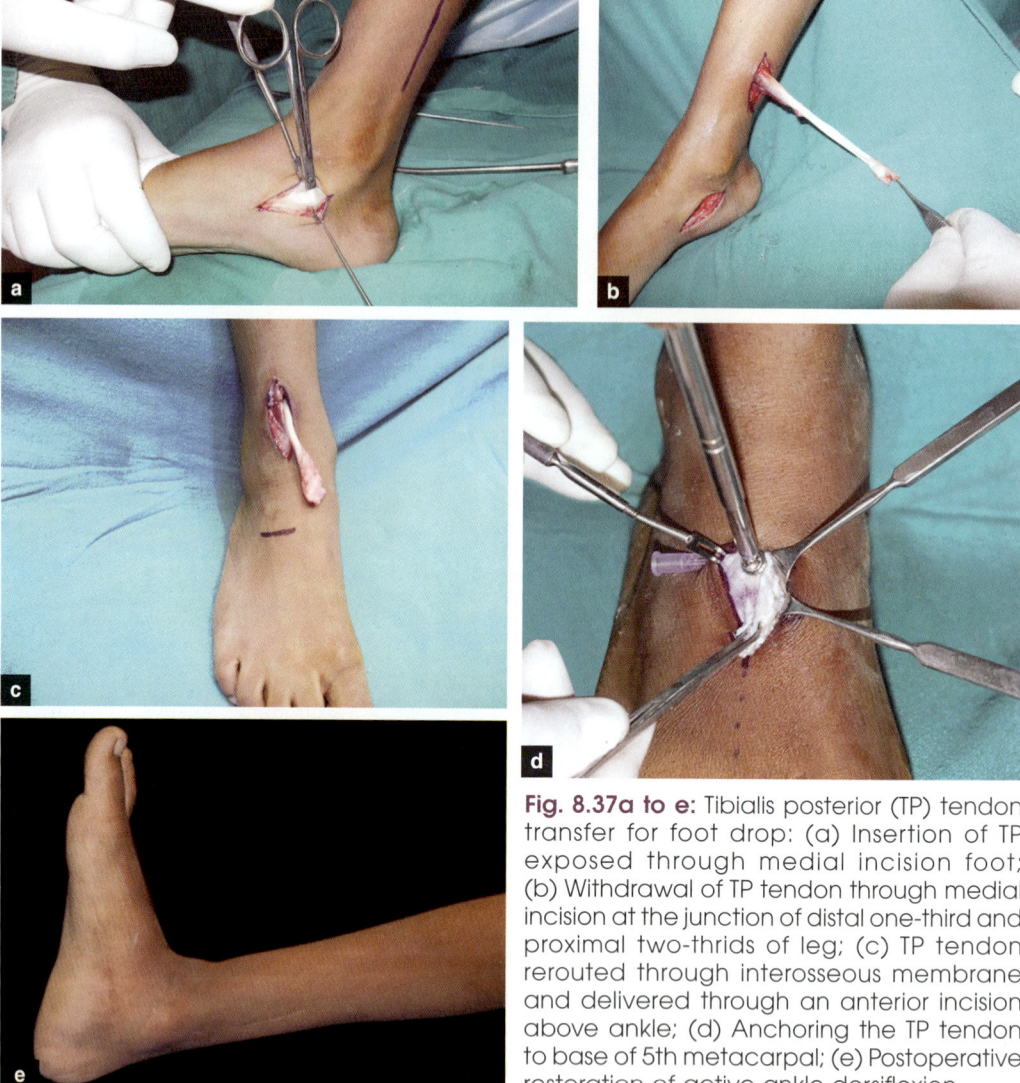

Fig. 8.37a to e: Tibialis posterior (TP) tendon transfer for foot drop: (a) Insertion of TP exposed through medial incision foot; (b) Withdrawal of TP tendon through medial incision at the junction of distal one-third and proximal two-thrids of leg; (c) TP tendon rerouted through interosseous membrane and delivered through an anterior incision above ankle; (d) Anchoring the TP tendon to base of 5th metacarpal; (e) Postoperative restoration of active ankle dorsiflexion

f. Loss of sole sensations

Due to involvement of the tibial nerve, may lead to nonhealing ulcers in the sole or heel. Regular antiseptic dressings usually result in healing. Microcellular rubber (MCR) footwear helps in prevention of ulceration. Nerve decompression/nerve transfers may be considered in such patients or neurovascular island flaps for sensory restoration in the sole.[10]

CONCLUSION

While the aim of the chapter is to delineate the objectives of surgical interventions for deformities of the hand and feet in leprosy, it is to be appreciated that surgical reconstruction is an art that is the need of the hour to ameliorate deformities where

Table 8.8: Outline of pre- and postoperative physiotherapy protocol for foot drop deformity in leprosy

Days	Preoperative physiotherapy protocol
1–7 days before surgery	• Tendo-Achillis stretching • Isolation exercise to tibialis posterior muscle action (inversion and plantar flexion)

Postoperative physiotherapy protocol

Day of surgery	Plaster cast with foot in 65 to 70 degrees dorsiflexion
5th day	Böhler iron is fixed to enable ambulation
6th week	• Plaster is removed and posterior slab continued till weight bearing exercise • Patient practices contraction of tibialis posterior muscle action with gravity reduced position. The foot will now move in dorsiflexion direction
7th week	Contraction of tibialis posterior muscle action in against gravity position. The patient gradually learns to do dorsiflexion at will. If the patient has difficulty in contracting the tibialis posterior muscle, electrical stimulation may help them activate the action
8th week	• Initiate partial weightbearing—standing with the support between the parallel bar • MCR footwear with an appropriate orthosis (mainly to support the medial arch)
9th week	• Full weightbearing exercise with a normal gait, heel-to-toe pattern • Initially walking between the parallel bar and then in other terrain

Courtesy: Dr Karthikeyan Govindasamy

medical therapy does not help. Some excellent text on surgical interventions have been written[2,7–9,11,12] which can be referenced for details and patients may be referred to centers where such surgeries are performed.

REFERENCES

1. Scollard DM. The biology of nerve injury in leprosy. Lepr Rev 2008;79:242–53.
2. Richard. B. Surgical Management of Neuritis. In: Surgical reconstruction and rehabilitation in leprosy and other neuropathies. Schwarz R, Brandsma JW, Kathmandu: Ekta Books Distributors; 2004.
3. Van Veen NH, Schreuders TA, Theuvenet WJ, Agrawal A, Richardus JH. Decompressive surgery for treating nerve damage in leprosy. A Cochrane review. Lepr Rev 2009;80:3–12.
4. Wan EL, Rivadeneira AF, Jouvin RM, Dellon AL. Treatment of Peripheral Neuropathy in Leprosy: The Case for Nerve Decompression. Plast Reconstr Surg Glob Open 2016 Mar 17;4(3):e637.
5. Wan EL, Noboa J, Baltodano PA, Jousin RM, Ericson WB, Wilton JP, Rosson GD, Dellon LA. Nerve decompression for leprous neuropathy: A prospective study from Ecuador. Leprosy Review 2017;88:95–108.
6. Kenedi M, de Freitas Cabral E, Narahashi K. Pain perception and functional limitation, assessed in the years after nerve decompression in leprosy, et al. Leprosy review 2018;89:208–18.
7. Khan Y, Prakash S, Kalra P, Arora S, Dhal A. Functional Outcome of Early, Selective Surgical Nerve Decompression in Leprous Neuropathy. The Journal of Hand Surgery Asia Pacific Volume.
8. Brand PW. The reconstruction of the hand in leprosy. 1952. Clin Orthop Relates. 2002;396:4–11.
9. Anderson GA. The surgical management of deformities of the hand in leprosy. J Bone Jt Surg Br 2006;88:290–4.
10. Agarwal P, Shukla P, Sharma D. Saphenous nerve transfer: A new approach to restore sensation of the sole. J Plast Reconstr Aesthetic Surg 2018;71:1704–10.
11. H. Srinivasan, DD Palande. Essential Surgery. In: Leprosy Techniques for District Hospitals. World Health Organization, 1997.
12. Atlas of Corrective Surgical Procedures Commonly Used in Leprosy H. Srinivasan 2004, Chennai.

8.3.3 CORRECTION OF DEFORMITIES OF FACE IN LEPROSY

Atul Shah, Vinita Puri

The various deformities affecting the face in leprosy have been detailed in Table 8.4 (*see page 307*) and the aim of this chapter will be to address their surgical correction. While there are various deformities that may develop, the most common and clinically important complication in leprosy remains facial palsy and subsequent lagophthalmos, often followed by exposure keratitis. While specialized eye surgery is not a field that is taught in dermatology training, it should be a priority that leprosy patients who need sight restoring cataract surgery have access to it.

LOSS OF EYEBROWS

Loss of eyebrows (supraciliary madarosis) is a specific deformity and is due to the infiltration of facial skin which eventually involves the hair follicles (Figs 8.38 and 8.39). In the early stage, lateral one-third of the eyebrow gets involved and the hairs fall off (Fig. 8.38). At this stage differential diagnoses in absence of other signs, includes hypothyroidism and alopecia areata.[1] The typical timing of intervention or reconstruction is *after* the completion of MDT for lepromatous leprosy.

Reconstructive techniques for supraciliary madarosis are of the following types:

a. *Hair transplant:* Hair from the occipital region can be harvested in the form of follicular unit transplant (FUT) or follicular unit extraction (FUE) in a manner of transplanting hair for alopecia. Hair transplant for the eyebrows needs to take into factor the normal arch of the eyebrow and the direction of the hair.

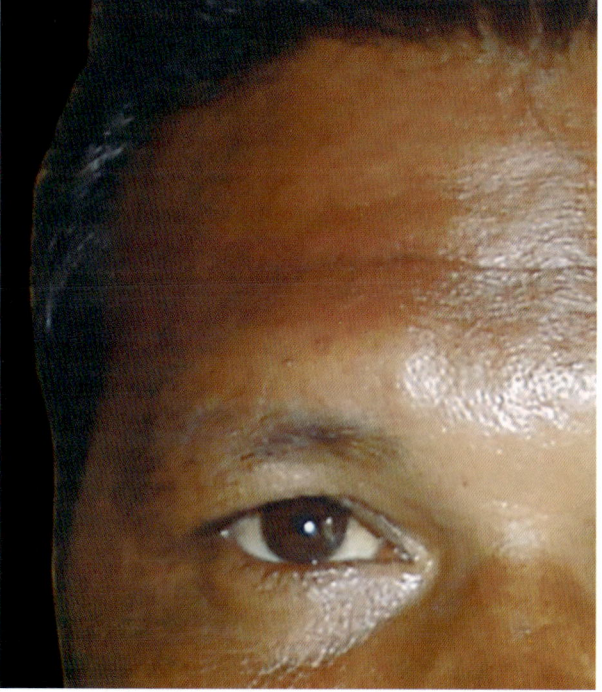

Fig. 8.38: Loss of lateral one-third of eyebrow in an early case of leprosy

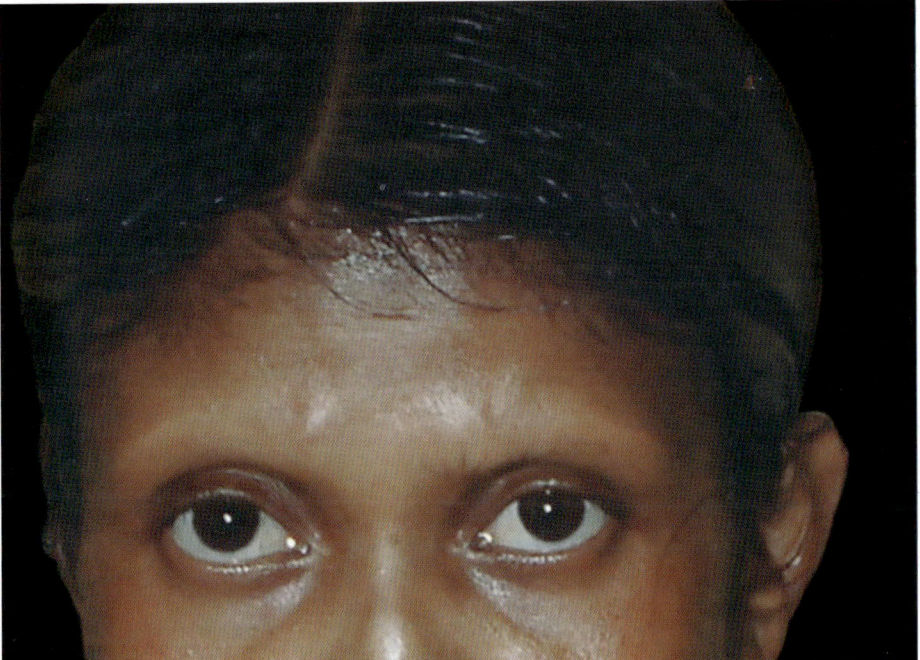

Fig. 8.39: Total loss of eyebrows in lepromatous leprosy

b. *Hairy full thickness free scalp graft:*[2] An elliptical piece of scalp skin, generally from the occipital region is harvested (Figs 8.40 and 8.41). The elliptical area is divided in the center, shaped and then transplanted as eyebrow graft noting the direction of the hair growth like normal eyebrows. Typical regrowth of hairs occurs in about 4 months' time giving an appropriate thin eyebrow hairline. While this is more acceptable in females, males sometimes would like to have bushy eyebrows for which pedicle flap transfer is the solution.

c. *Pedicled flap transfer:* The pedicle is based on the superficial temporal artery. Its course is marked with indelible ink. The pivot point is based just above the tragus and the required length to reach above the medial canthus is marked on the scalp (Fig. 8.42). The flap is elevated in the plane of loose areolar tissue and inset into the defect created by excising the small portion of the skin over the eyebrow. The flap is inserted by exteriorizing the pedicle over the skin between ear and lateral end of the eyebrow insertion.

After 14 days, the flap is divided and the exteriorized portion is discarded. The same procedure can be done for the opposite side. Both sides can be done together or in separate sittings.

When the flap is raised as a visor flap (bipedicle scalp flap), the flap is rotated as a bucket handle and inserted throughout, i.e. even in between the skin of two eyebrows. Subsequently, when eyebrows are adjusted, this excess skin (which is hardly 1 to 2 cm in length and 1 cm in width) is divided and discarded. The result is a bushy eyebrow which may require reshaping by discarding the superior excess skin. It also needs to be trimmed by the patient when hair growth reaches higher proportion.

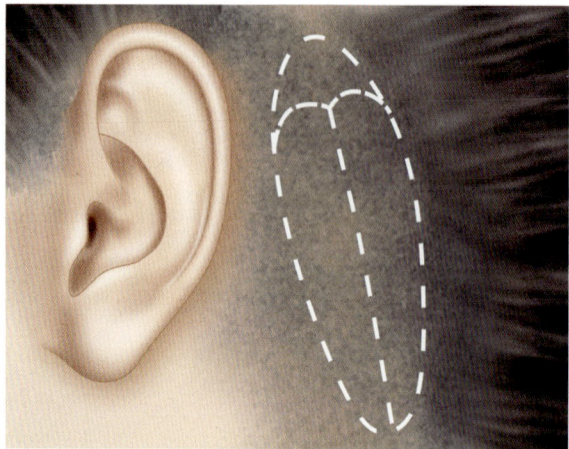

Fig. 8.40: Marking of an ellipse of hair-bearing skin in the retroauricular region of the scalp in a way that when divided in center it will fit both sides of the eyebrow for reconstruction

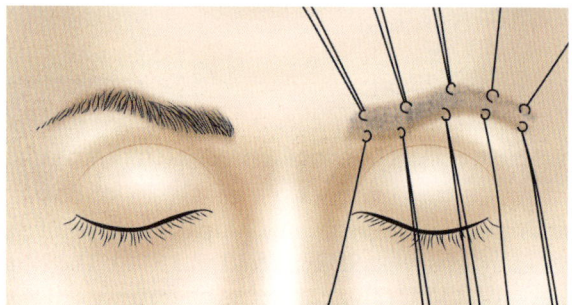

Fig. 8.41: Placement of long tie over sutures through the graft and adjacent skin

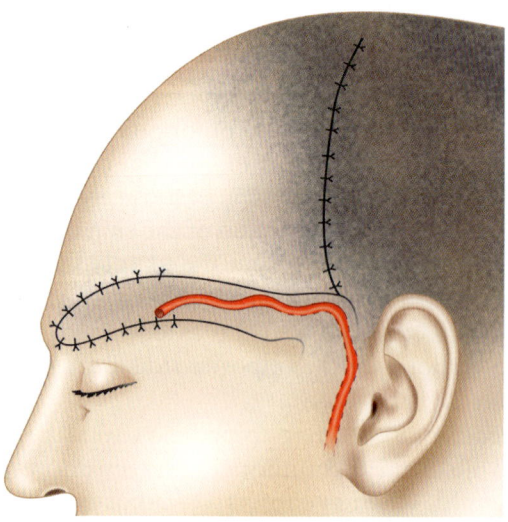

Fig. 8.42: Pedicled flap based on superficial temporal artery raised and rotated towards a defect made in the eyebrow skin and inserted. Note that a dog ear may occur at the point of rotation. A second stage surgery is needed to cut and discard the pedicle which overlies the normal skin

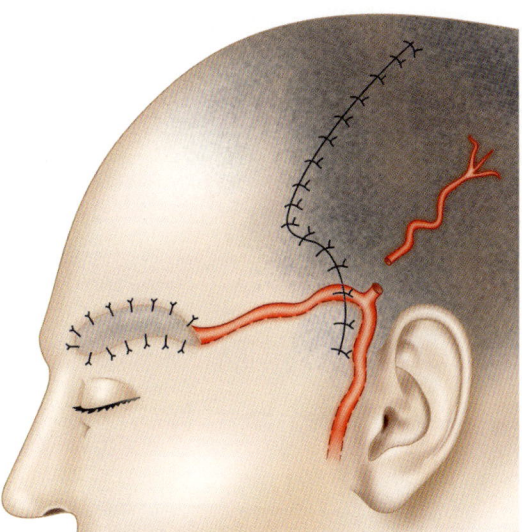

Fig. 8.43: Design of the island pedicle flap based on anterior branch of superficial temporal artery in which the vascular pedicle is tunneled under the skin of temporal region and thus does not require second operation for dividing the pedicle

d. *Island pedicle flap:* The island of anterior scalp hair-bearing skin, supplied by either posterior or anterior branch of the superficial temporal artery, is raised keeping surrounding subcutaneous tissues attached to it and transferred onto the eyebrow area through a tunnel (Fig. 8.43). It is technically difficult and can result in flap necrosis.

NASAL DEFORMITY

Nasal deformity is a source of stigma in leprosy (Figs 8.44 and 8.45) and its correction is crucial as it provides confidence to the leprosy affected person to integrate into the society. It is difficult to establish timing of the surgery as ideally surgery can be done only when mucosa is free from active lesions and there is no infection as seen in nasal smears, thus as with MDT by 6 weeks the MI is zero this would also be as appropriate time to attempt surgery.

Anatomically, skin over the nose remains uninvolved in leprosy and if involved primarily, a differential diagnosis of syphilis or yaws must be considered. Reconstruction primarily aims at replacing the lost nasal lining and the dorsal bridge support. In advanced severe cases, one may need to add skin when there is severe contracture with deficiency of skin and external nasal fistulae due to perforations of skin inside out.

The following are the choices of procedures:

a. *Postnasal epithelial inlay of Gillies[3]/Antia:* It replaces the nasal lining with a split thickness skin graft from the medial aspect of the arm. This procedure is rarely performed nowadays.

b. *Farina's nasolabial flaps:* The procedure is based on the fact that skin besides the nose is an easy and excellent site for providing the lining of the nose. Generally, in these patients, there is loose skin or wrinkling and sagging which can be used to our advantage. The required length of nasolabial flap is marked on either side of the face.

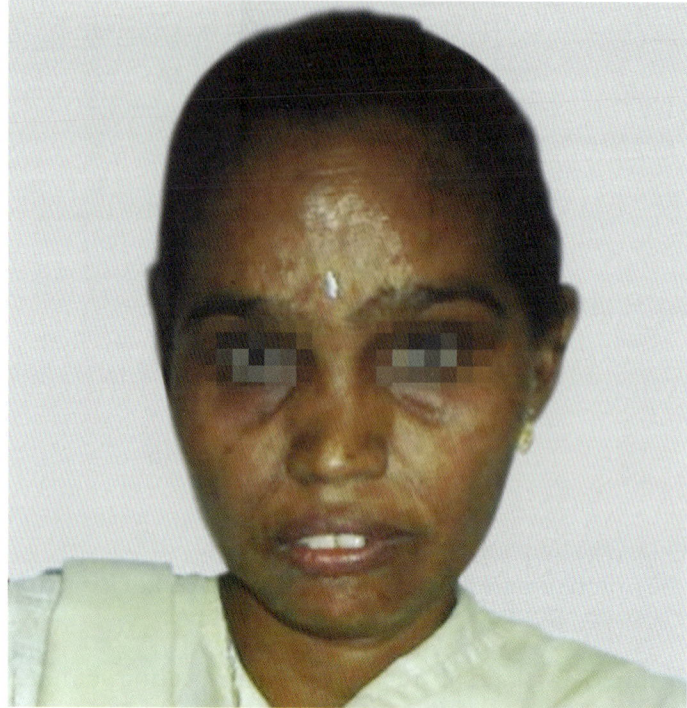

Fig. 8.44: Early "saddle nose" deformity

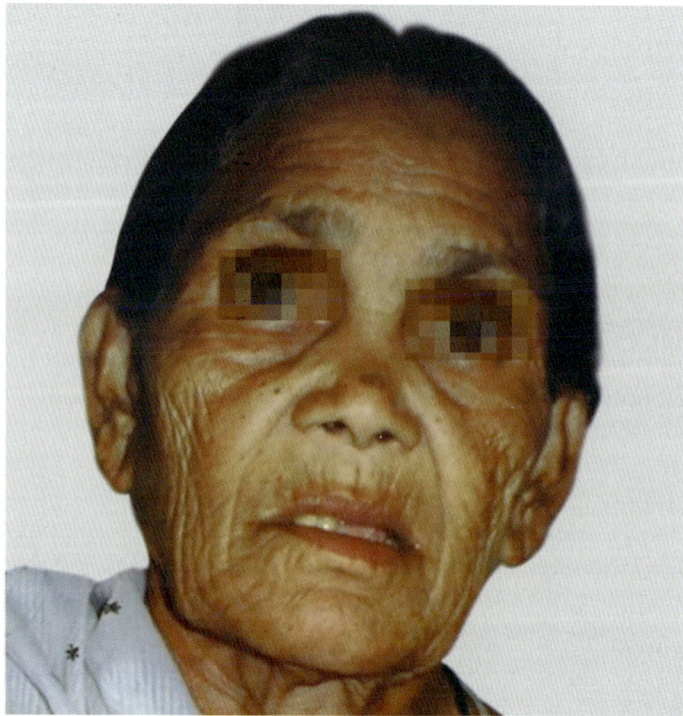

Fig. 8.45: "Saddle nose" deformity along with wrinkled face in a late case

Its width is about 1.5 cm maximum on one side. The columella and one of the sides of the base of nostril is incised and lifted to define the edge of the pyriform margin and a cut is made all around the margin. The flap is pulled in right up to other side and its base is sutured to pyriform margin mucosal remnants. The opposite flap is sutured similarly making a tunnel through which a bone graft is inserted under the nasal skin and above the nasolabial flap lining.

c. *Atul Shah's (author) modification*[4] makes it simpler by using the principle that nasal skin can be sustained on the circulation from the branch of the facial artery entering at the base of the ala. Author uses an inverted U-shaped incision to expose the root of the nose followed by dividing the nasal lining to enter the nasal cavity and dissecting out the pyriform margin till the snarl is released. The nasolabial flaps are now turned over and sutured to the opposite side. Bone graft is kept as a backup plan. Author has used the silastic implant put through routine mid-columellar incision in such a case which provided support for nearly five years before it is extruded. Ancillary procedures include bone or cartilage graft for shaping the dorsum of nose or nasolabial fat transplantation for augmentation of nasal dorsum.

d. *Forehead flap*: In severe deformities with severe scarring, contractures and skin perforations, where there is deficiency of all layers, a combination of procedures needs to be done wherein mucosal lining can be provided with bilateral nasolabial flaps, the framework can be reconstructed with cartilage graft or bone graft and skin cover can be provided with a median or paramedian forehead flap.

SAGGING SKIN OF FACE OR WRINKLING OF FACE

Redundancy and wrinkling of face in leprosy is the result of destruction of collagen and elastic tissue fibers of the dermis and makes a young person look aged. The wrinkling occurs mainly around nasolabial area and on the lips. It may be associated with other deformities like saddle nose or mega ear lobules. Where possible, a standard facelift can be done. But application of rhytidectomy technique of plastic surgery is not effective except in a very young patient with wrinkles around cheek only and hence nasolabial skin excision is advocated in many. This is in the form of excision of crescent shaped area unilaterally from the nasolabial fold (Fig. 8.46) or both sides excision can be combined as a horseshoe-shaped incision.

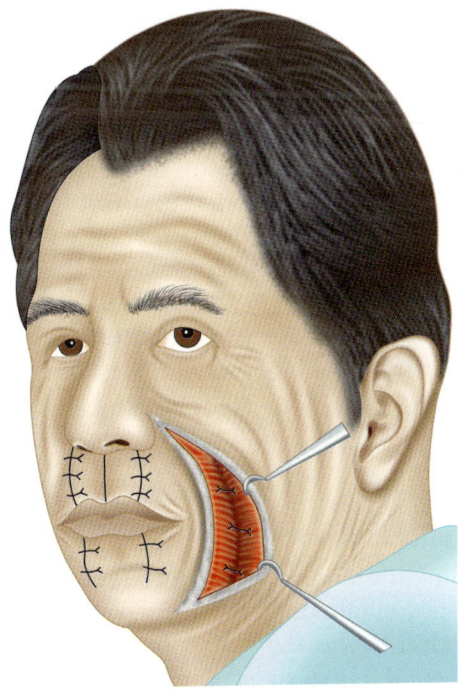

Fig. 8.46: Nasolabial excision for wrinkled face/sagging skin of the face

HANGING EAR LOBES /MEGA LOBULES[5]

The enlarged ear lobe occurs due to stretching of skin by lepromatous granuloma and destruction of the elastic fibers due to the inflammatory process. Once the ear lobe smears are negative or the disease is burnt out, the mega lobules can be corrected. Antia et al[2] advocated M-shaped excision and defect suturing in two incisions; one horizontal and other vertical. A crescent wedge excision from medial lobe can be done. The lateral part is then rotated superiorly, and skin closure is done on both sides of the lobe (Fig. 8.47).

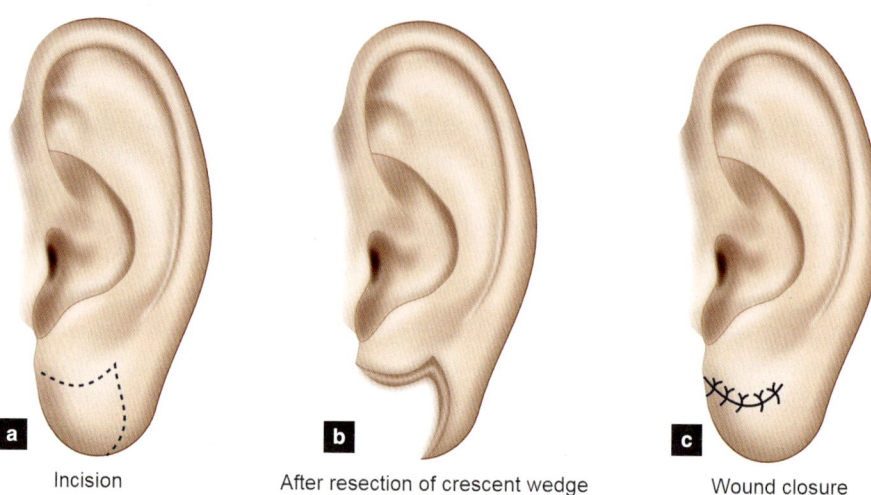

Fig. 8.47: Mega lobules correction. (a) Incision for crescent excision; (b) The defect; (c) The rotation and suturing reducing the hanging mega lobule

LAGOPHTHALMOS[6,9]

Lagophthalmos occurs due to paralysis of the facial nerve or part of the facial nerve supplying orbicularis oculi muscle. The extracranial facial nerve especially zygomatic branch involvement often occurs in leprosy which causes paralysis of the orbicularis oculi muscle. This leads to uninhibited action of the levator palpebrae superioris muscle resulting in an inability to close eye (lagophthalmos). Along with this, when there is loss of corneal sensation, it can cause dryness and exposure keratitis, leading to corneal ulceration and blindness. After early detection, steroids should be initiated followed by surgery.[7]

Treatment of lagophthalmos is dependent on (Box 8.13):
1. *Duration* of the lagophthalmos.
2. *Width* of the eyelid gap, and exposure of the cornea.
3. Presence or absence of *corneal hypoesthesia*.

Surgical Procedures

Three different kinds of procedures are commonly used in the surgical management of lagophthalmos (Box 8.13). They are: (i) Empowering the eyelids by muscle/tendon transfer, (ii) lid tightening procedures, and (iii) other procedures for narrowing the palpebral fissure like tarsorrhaphy or lid-loading. Procedures of the first kind provide active correction of eyelid paralysis while the others aim to protect the cornea or correct ectropion of the lower lid and alleviate epiphora (overflow of tears).

> **Box 8.13:** Guidelines of treatment of lagophthalmos
>
> | Scenario | Treatment |
> |---|---|
> | **Duration** of lagophthalmos <6 months | Systemic steroids as for reversal reaction. |
> | **Duration** of lagophthalmos >6 months and eyelid gap <6 mm (without corneal exposure and with intact corneal sensitivity): will in general not lead to exposure keratitis | Conservative treatment (see Section 8.3.5, on self care*)
Surgery not indicated except sometimes for cosmetic issues |
> | **Duration** of lagophthalmos >6 months and eyelid gap ≥6 mm | **Surgery**
Surgery is also indicated when
1. *Exposure keratitis* is present
2. *Exposed cornea* in sleeping position
3. *Corneal anesthesia*
4. *Bilateral* involvement
5. Continuous *epiphora* or intermittent redness |
>
> *'Think blink': Conscientious and regular strong blinking throughout the day. By making use of the Bell's phenomenon (upward turning of the eyes on attempted closure of the eyelids), the cornea is moistened behind the upper eyelids in a kind of 'reverse blinking'.

Lateral Tarsorrhaphy

In this procedure, the palpebral fissure is made narrow by stitching the lids together for some distance. This is indicated mainly as an *emergency* procedure when there is an imminent danger of damage to the cornea because of exposure keratitis and corneal ulceration (Fig. 8.48). It is *not* recommended as a permanent solution as it leads to a loss of visual field on the temporal side. In addition, a tarsorraphy does not correct any laxity or ectropion of the lower eyelid. McLaughlin tarsorrhaphy (Fig. 8.49) is done by judging the point of closure which will enable the eyelid to close, particularly cornea, when the patient tries to close eyelid normally and not forcefully. It involves excising the skin and eyelashes from that point to lateral canthus while keeping the conjunctival part as such. From the corresponding portion of the upper eyelid, only the conjunctival part is excised. About 5 to 8 mm of excision on both sides is enough. The raw areas are now approximated over a single horizontal suture passed on the skin side through a rubber tube to keep pressure for about 10 days. The result should be a normal looking curve of the upper eyelid.

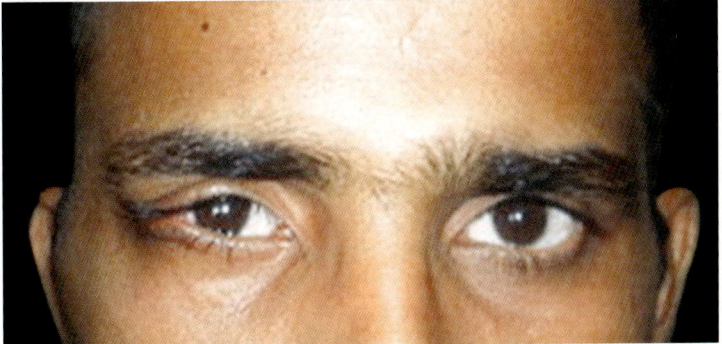

Fig. 8.48: A lateral tarsorrhaphy done on the right eye

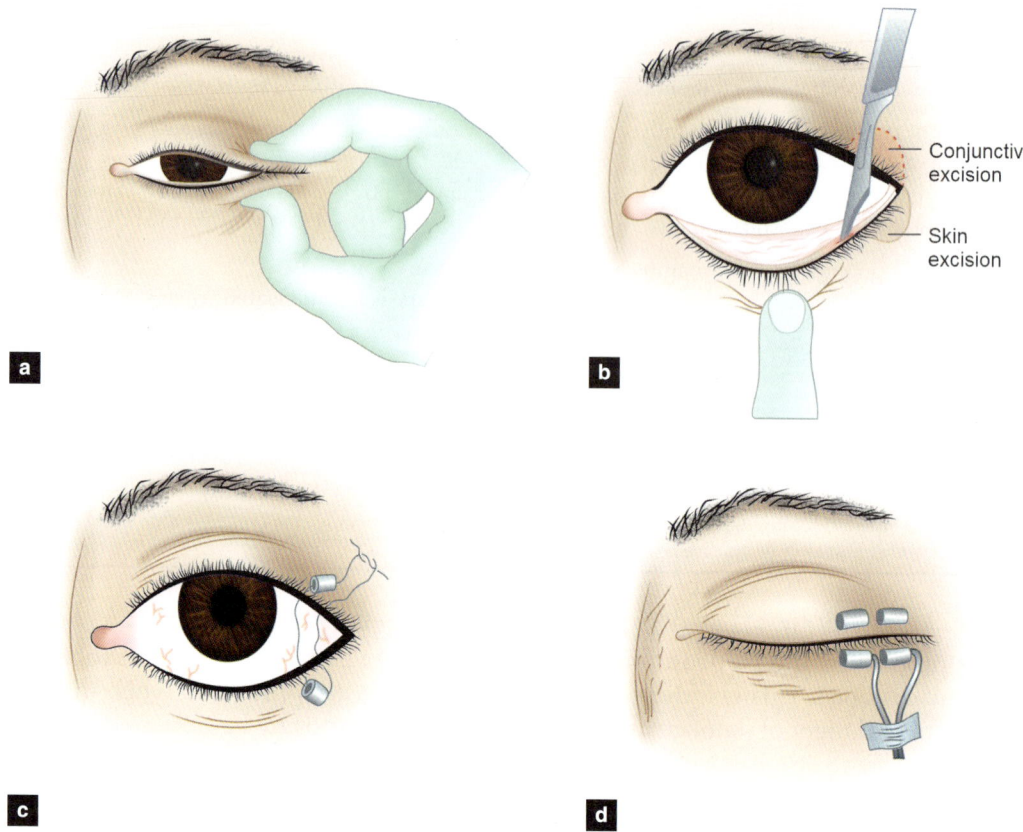

Fig. 8.49: (a) Assess the extent of tarsorrhaphy needed for protecting the cornea. Usually at least one-third of the palpebral aperture will need to be occluded; (b) Incise the lid margin just behind the eyelashes for the required distance, splitting the lid to a little extent; a crescent shaped excision of lower eyelid skin and similar extent of conjunctiva from upper lid is excised; (c) Stitch the lids together using horizontal mattress sutures and tie them over short pieces of small rubber tubing as shown in these figures; (d) Leave the threads long and fix them to the cheek with adhesive tape

Temporalis Transfer

The main dynamic procedure is the *temporalis sling*. For making a sling, either the fascia over the temporalis muscle or an external graft of plantaris/palmaris tendon or a fascia lata strip is used (Fig. 8.50a to d).

An overactivity of the opposing muscle, in this case levator palpebrae superioris, may occur with resultant muscular contracture in absence of the opposing action of orbicularis oculi to close the eye. Weights inserted in the upper eyelid with the help of gravity can effectively allow the eye to close and open like normal person obviating the need of postoperative rehabilitation in the form of liquid diet for 3 weeks and clenching the teeth to close the eye (i.e. to mimic the action of the temporalis muscle). The material found most suitable to insert is 24-carat gold which is generally not rejected, is malleable and holes also can be made easily to fix it to tarsal plate.[8] The implant is sutured to the tarsal plate with monofilament sutures. The possible drawback

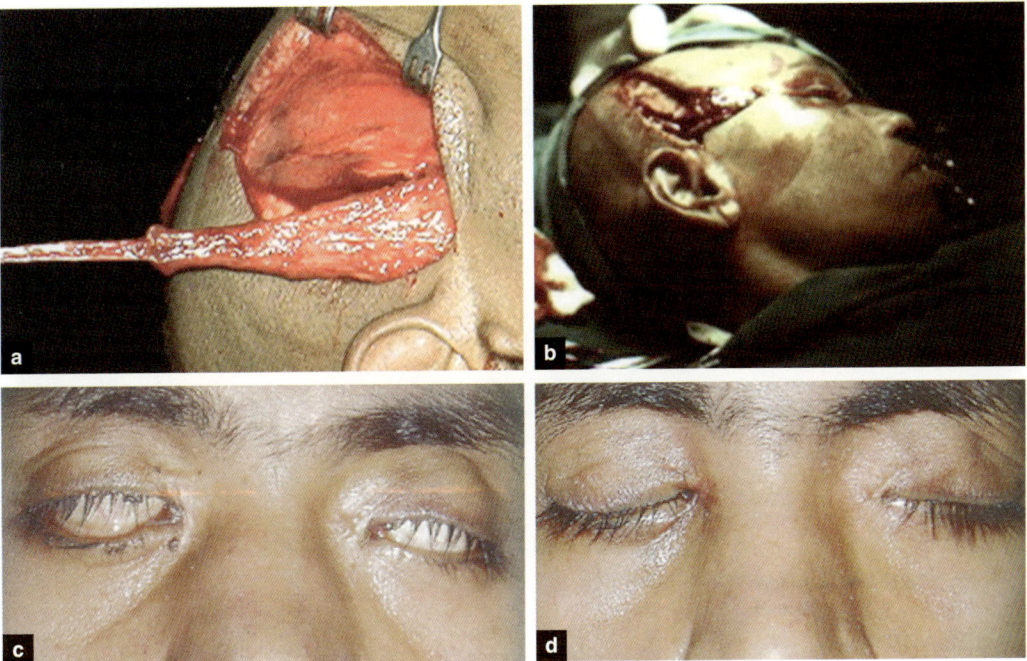

Fig. 8.50: (a) Temporalis muscle with attached fascia; (b) Muscle is turned over the skin and tunnel is marked; (c and d) Before and after temporalis musculofascial sling operation.
((c and d) reproduced from IAL Handbook of Leprosy, Bhusan Kumar et al (Eds) with permission from Bhalani Publishing House, 2018, Mumbai)

is that since in sleeping position gravity does not assist closure, a part of eyelid may remain open. However, that is also the case with all operations mentioned earlier.

FACIAL PALSY

Correction of facial palsy can be done with procedures like those used for post-traumatic palsies. The procedures may be static or dynamic. Dynamic procedures are the procedures of choice and the type of procedure can be chosen according to the time since affection, condition of muscles and treatment status of leprosy. Static procedures may be done in the very elderly or in those found unfit for postoperative rehabilitation required for dynamic procedures.

a. *Static procedures:* They are used to establish symmetry without any motion. A sling is made and proximally attached to the zygoma or temporal fascia and distally attached to the oral commissure, upper lip and nasolabial groove to passively gain position. Slings can be of either autografts like fascia (temporalis fascia, tensor fascia lata or palmaris tendon), or of prosthetic material like allodermic or multivector sutures.

b. *Dynamic procedures:* The major dynamic procedure still remains the temporalis musculofascial transfer (TMT) with which not only the facial deviation but also the lagophthalmos can be corrected.

Pedicled muscle transfer (temporalis, masseter)[10–12]: The temporalis muscle can be used in a retrograde or antegrade manner (Fig. 8.51a and b). The deep temporal fascia or tendon of insertion of temporalis needs to be extended using grafts. It is then tunneled

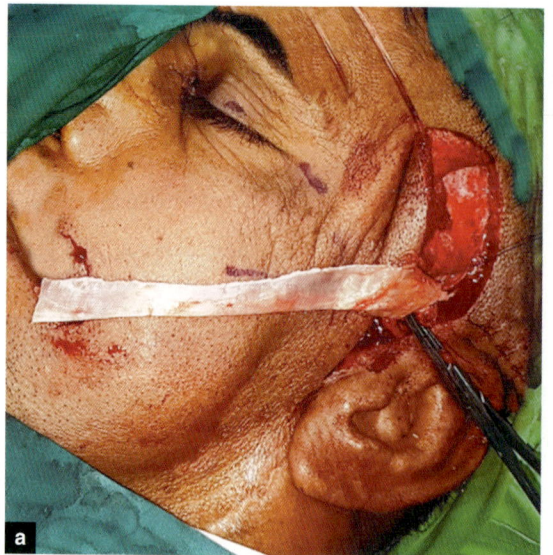 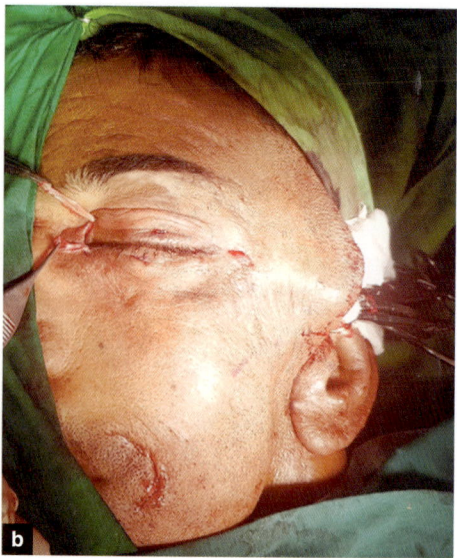

Fig. 8.51a and b: Tendon graft used to extend the temporalis muscle for total correction of facial palsy, i.e. lagophthalmos and drooping angle of the mouth for elevation (*Courtesy*: Dr Venkateshwaran N)

into the face. Facial strips are divided to reanimate the upper and lower eyelids, the commissure and the nose. Overcorrection is done to compensate for muscle tone. Similarly, if the masseter muscle is used, its superficial fibers are detached from their mandibular insertion and inserted in the skin for angle of the mouth reanimation.

c. *Nerve transfer procedures:* Nerve transfers and nerve crossover procedures can be performed for intermediate duration facial paralysis as the native facial musculature is still viable.

Cross facial nerve grafting:[10,11] The procedure can be utilized if the contralateral facial nerve is intact and functional. A branch of the normal side healthy facial nerve is transferred to innervate the affected side muscle. One of the distal branches of the normal facial nerve is used as the donor nerve by extending it to the affected side using a sural nerve graft through the upper lip and coapted to the affected branch. As nerve growth is slow, reinnervation may take 6–8 months or longer and motor recovery is weaker than normal side. A babysitter procedure using the masseteric nerve or hypoglossal nerve (which are spared in leprosy) can be done to maintain motor end plate of facial muscles till nerve growth in cross facial nerve graft has reached to desired level as examined by Tinel's sign. The babysitter procedure is then reversed, and the cross-face graft allowed to innervate the affected nerve.

Masseteric nerve transfer: This is the transfer of choice in bilateral facial nerve palsy. The nerve is anatomically closer to the facial nerve and as it has a shorter course; thus the reinnervation is much quicker.

Hypoglossal nerve transfer: The ipsilateral hypoglossal nerve can also be a donor nerve. As it can cause ipsilateral hemiatrophy of tongue, one can consider using a partial transfer of hypoglossal nerve.

REFERENCES

1. Banerjee S. Reconstruction of facial deformities in leprosy patients. J Indian Med Assoc 2004; 102:700–1.
2. Antia NH, Enna CD, Daver BM. The Surgical Management of Deformities in Leprosy and other peripheral neuropathies. Bombay Oxford University Press, 1992;30–60.
3. Frank McDowell, Carl D Enna Surgical Rehabilitation in Leprosy. Baltimore, The William and Wilkins Company, 1974;56–160.
4. Shah A. Surgery in Leprosy. In: Koticha KK, Editor. Leprosy: A Concise Text, 1st ed. Bombay, Darsan K Koticha,1990;202–14.
5. Srinivasan H, Palande DD. World Health Organization. Action Programme for the Elimination of Leprosy. (1996) Essential surgery in leprosy: Techniques for district hospitals/H Srinivasan, DD Palande, World Health Organization.
6. Hogeweg M, Kiran KU, Suneetha S. The significance of facial patches and type 1 reaction for the development of facial nerve damage in leprosy. A retrospective study among 1226 paucibacillary leprosy patients. Lepr Rev 1991;62:143–9.
7. Srinivasan H. Disability, deformity and Rehabilitation. In Robert C Hastings, Leprosy, 2nd ed. Churchill Livingstone, Longman Group, UK, 1994; p411–48.
8. Shah A, Shah N. Deformities of Face, Hands and Feet, and Their Management. In: IAL Textbook of Leprosy, 1st ed. Jaypee Brothers Medical Publishers, 2010;424–46.
9. Shah A, Shah N. Deformities of face, Hands, Feet, Trophic Ulcers and Their Management. In: IAL Handbook of Leprosy, 1st ed, Bhalani Publishing House, 2018;193–03.
10. Das P, Kumar J, Karthikeyan G, Rao PS. Efficacy of temporalis muscle transfer for correction of lagophthalmos in leprosy. Lepr Rev 2011;82:279–85.
11. Agrawal K. Textbook of Plastic, Reconstructive and Aesthetic Surgery; Vol III, Head and Neck Reconstruction. Thieme Publisher, 2018; 797–812.
12. Mathes Plastic Surgery; The Head and Neck; Vol 3, 2nd edition, Philadelphia: Saunders, 2005; p883–915.

8.3.4 PHYSIOTHERAPY AND ORTHOSES

Atul Shah, Neela Shah

INTRODUCTION

Physiotherapy (physical therapy) plays a major role in the management of deformities and disabilities occurring in leprosy. The sooner physiotherapy is started, the less is the chance of the patient developing complications resulting from long-standing unattended deformities.[1]

Physiotherapy comprises exercises, oil massage, wax baths, hydrotherapy, splinting, electrical stimulation of muscles, short wave diathermy, ultrasonics and acupuncture.

PHYSIOTHERAPY EXERCISES

Physiotherapy is an integral part of management of the visible deformities of leprosy and achieves the goals of ameliorating deformities by varied means:

  i. First and foremost, it helps to *prevent* worsening of the *deformity* as it prevents contractures of the opposing uninvolved muscles and of the skin. For example in foot drop cases, the tendo-Achillis (TA) gets shortened or becomes tight while in total claw hand, the PIP joint needs special attention as the long extensors extend or rather hyperextend the MCP joint and compensatory flexion occurs at the PIP joint. Thus, exercises are aimed at extending the PIP joint and keeping it mobile (Fig. 8.52).

  Also the thumb web often gets contracted due to pull of the adductor fascia as it is constantly lying in the palmar plane. So, holding the thumb with one hand and fingers with the other hand, a stretching force is applied to thumb web while bringing the thumb in abduction position. A thumb spica or thumb web release spring splint is also applied to retain the gain of exercises.

  ii. Another purpose of the preoperative exercises is aimed at the isolation of the action of *donor muscle* to be used in tendon transfer procedure and strengthening it. For example, tibialis posterior when transferred for foot drop deformity would need strong isolated action to dorsiflex the foot. Hence, teaching patient the action

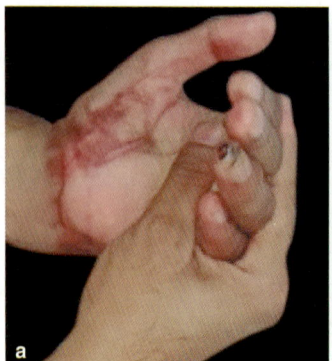
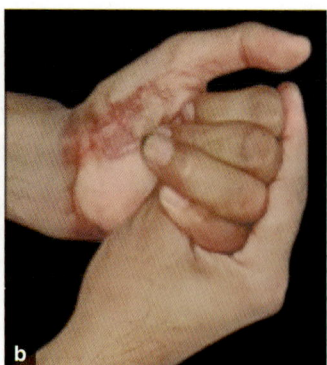
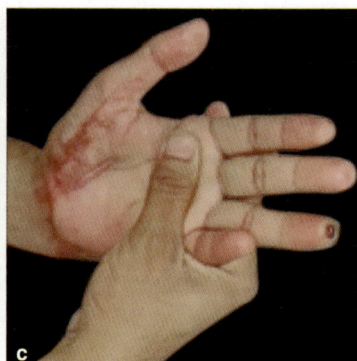

Fig. 8.52a to c: For claw hand, an important exercise is to keep the PIP joint mobile by holding the affected hand with thumb and index finger supporting MCP flexion (a) and carrying out flexion (b) and extension of PIP joint (c) or in bilateral affection taking the support of inanimate object to flex the MCP joint and flexing and extending the PIP joint

of inversion of foot and making it strong with stimulation and lifting of gradually increasing weights tied to foot will hasten its strength thus enabling it to perform dorsiflexion easily postoperatively.

iii. The next and most important aim of exercises is the postoperative *rehabilitation* and re-education exercises. The results of the tendon transfer procedures depend on good postoperative exercises as much as a good technique by surgeon.

In leprosy, exercises aimed in general health care set up are generally preoperative exercises to keep the range of motion of joint as normal as possible. For the field area purpose, health workers visiting patients with deformity need to be trained to teach simple exercises, which can be carried out by patients at home. There are many exercises for the prevention of worsening or bringing about improvement, but it is better to employ "one exercise for each deformity".

Important exercises that are useful and can be explained to the patient for self practice are detailed below.

1. Exercise for the fingers. The patient should keep the knuckles of the fingers firmly bent, using the other hand, as shown in Fig. 8.53a. Alternatively, the hand can be pressed against the thigh or the top of a padded bench, table or stool (Fig. 8.53b). Keeping the knuckles bent in this manner, the patient should open the fingers fully, until the backs of the fingers touch the other hand or surface (Fig. 8.53c and d). This movement should be repeated at least 20 times, twice a day.
2. Exercise for the thumb: The patient should take hold of the affected thumb with the other hand, steadying it and allowing only the tip of the thumb to move, as shown in Fig. 8.54a. Holding the thumb in this manner, the patient should then lift up the tip of the thumb as much as possible (Fig. 8.54b). This exercise should be repeated at least 20 times, twice a day.
3. Important exercises for claw hand deformity are shown in Fig. 8.52.
4. Massage for the fingers. The patient should rest the back of the hand on the top of a padded table, bench or stool, or on the thigh (Fig. 8.55a). The patient should then gently stroke the fingers with the other hand, using the edge or the flat of the palm, and straighten them out as much as possible (Fig. 8.55b). Not much force should be used. The patient should do this at least 20 times, twice a day.
5. Massage for the thumb: The patient should rest the edge of the palm on the top of a padded table, bench or stool or on the thigh. The patient should then grasp the tip of the thumb with the other hand, as shown in Fig. 8.56a and pull on it gently but firmly, so that the end joint of the thumb straightens out (Fig. 8.56b). Not much force should be used, otherwise cracks may develop in the skin in front of the end joint of the thumb. The massage should be repeated at least 20 times, twice a day.
6. For the foot drop, advise to use a suitable material like bath towel or saree or any such long cloth which can be wrapped around the forefoot and pulled with hand to dorsiflex the ankle (Fig. 8.57).
7. **Eye:** For lagophthalmos, pulling of lateral canthal skin obliquely upward to close the eyelid should be done several times in a day (Fig. 8.58). Once skin is pulled, patient cannot actively open the upper eyelid.[2]

All the above exercises can be taught to patients to do regularly at home. Patient is asked to report to the physiotherapy department *only* if he/she needs electrical stimulation therapy, wax bath, oil massage and passive or active exercises under supervision or for postoperative re-education exercises.

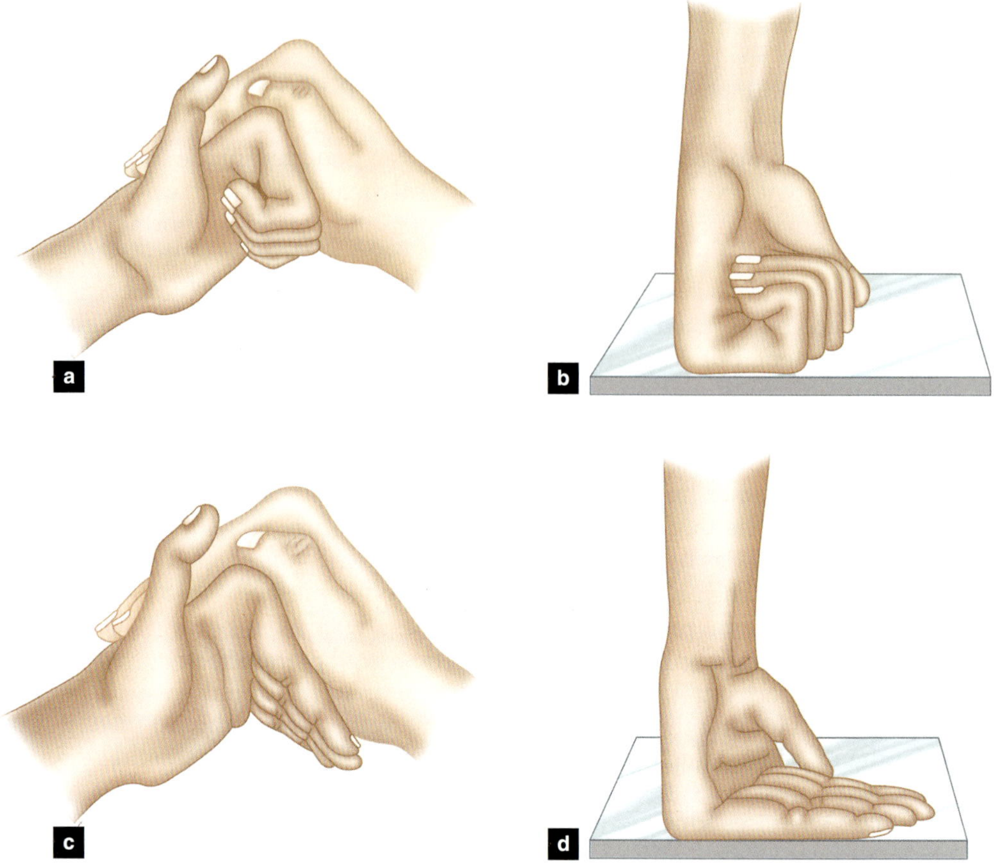

Fig. 8.53a to d: A depiction of various exercises for the fingers (*see* text)

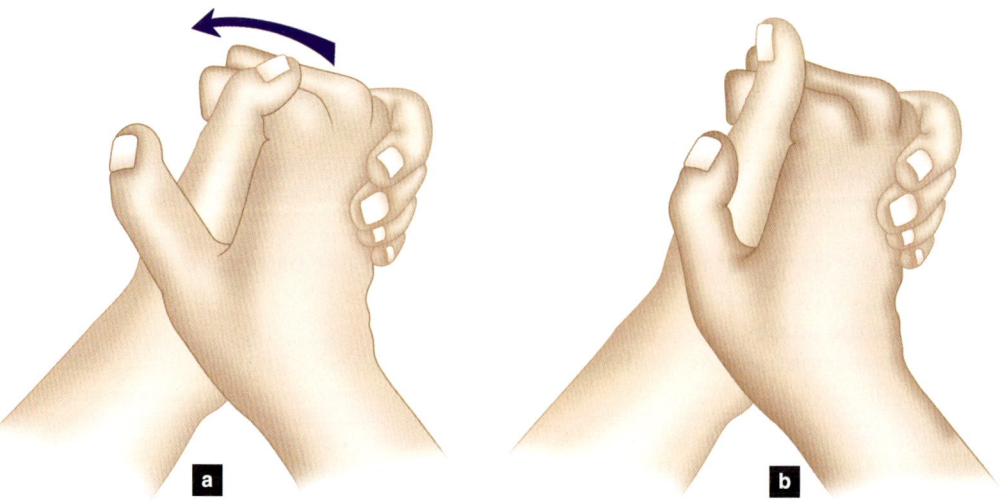

Fig. 8.54a and b: Thumb exercise where the thumb is held down by the other hand and then patient is asked to lift up the tip

Other Aspects of Treatment

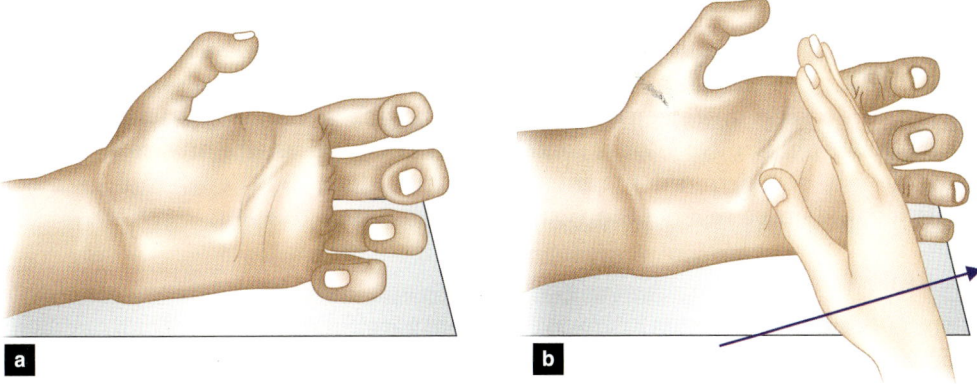

Fig. 8.55a and b: Depiction of massage of fingers to avoid contractures

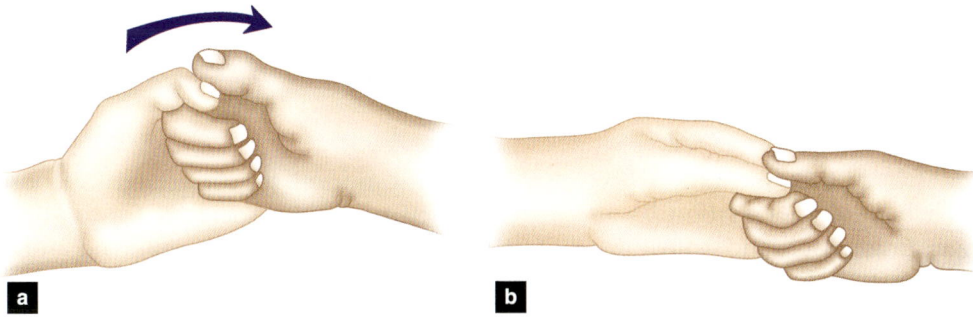

Fig. 8.56a and b: Exercise to avoid thumb contractures

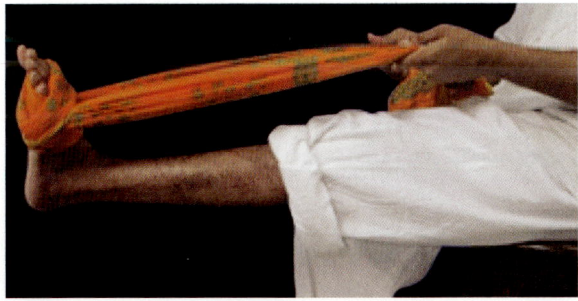

Fig. 8.57: Taking the help of a cloth wrapped around forefoot to pull it up at the ankle for dorsiflexion

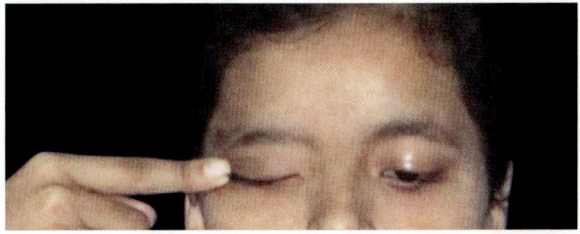

Fig. 8.58: Teaching the passive closure of the eye with fingers pulling the lateral temple skin upwards so that upper eyelid will close the eye. In this position even forcefully, it is difficult to open the eye with the help of only levator palpebrum superficialis (LPS)

ELECTRICAL STIMULATION

With the early identification of weakness arising in the affected muscles, electrical stimulation of muscles supplied by the nerve may be initiated along with passive exercises. The basic aim of electrical stimulation therapy is to know the neural continuity with the aim of allowing at least 90 contractions per day in case the muscle is paralyzed. It is widely believed that if the muscle is kept "alive", i.e. capable of getting re-innervated, the nerve regeneration can allow the muscle function to return.

WAX BATH[3]

In wax bath, a special wooden case is used, where paraffin wax is heated and maintained at 45°C. The brush and wrap methods are used for its application on the patients' hand avoiding burns to his/her anesthetic hands (Fig. 8.59). The heat increases the local circulation, stimulates the sweat glands, softens the skin and loosens the joint stiffness (since the ligaments and joints of the hand are superficial). The net result is a well-insulated, low temperature method of heating tissue. The primary use of wax bath in leprosy is to relieve the PIP joint stiffness.

SPLINTS/ORTHOSES[4,5]

Though in the literature on leprosy, the word "splint" is used, the correct term 'orthoses' which has been classified by modern convention and associated International Organization for Standardization (ISO) standards based on the site involved and the common abbreviations of upper limb orthoses are as follows:
1. Finger orthosis (FgO)
2. Hand orthosis (HdO)
3. Wrist–hand orthoses (WHO)

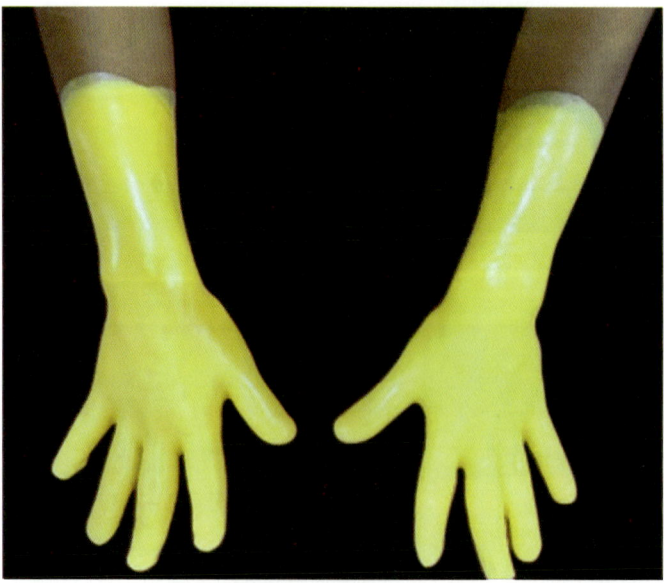

Fig. 8.59: Hands with wax applied (*Courtesy*: Dr Ali Irani, Head, Department of Physiotherapy, Nanavati Super Specialty Hospital)

4. Elbow orthosis (EO)
5. Shoulder orthosis (SO)

Splints in leprosy are recommended for
1. Immobilization
2. Prevention of deformities
3. Correction of deformities
4. Restoration of function
5. Maintaining the improvement made by exercises, massage, wax baths and surgery.

It has been shown that of the four main physiotherapeutic methods of treatment (wax bath, oil massage, exercises and splinting), it is splinting that can sufficiently mobilize moderately contracted joints and tissues. Splinting can often prevent joint deformities from occurring.

They are further divided into "static" and dynamic "orthoses". A *static* splint mainly hold the joints in position not permitting either active or passive movement of the joint, e.g. a plaster of Paris splint. A *dynamic* splint is defined as any splint which incorporates qualities of elasticity or principles of recoil and permits active and/or passive movements/exercising of the joint. Dynamic splints need constant observation and supervision to ensure correct fitting and require technical skill for their manufacture.

The most frequent *indications* of splinting in leprosy are given in Box 8.14.
While we will detail the common splints that are used for leprosy, a comprehensive list of orthoses is provided in Table 8.9 and they are used in specialized centers.

Box 8.14: Common indications of splinting on leprosy

1. Proximal interphalangeal flexion contractures and claw hand
2. Interphalangeal flexion contracture of the thumb
3. Thumb web contracture
4. Paralysis of short muscles of the thumb
5. The reaction hand
6. Open wounds at the finger flexion creases
7. Foot ulcers, foot drop
8. Wrist drop

Table 8.9: Common orthoses for deformities

Deformity	Dynamic splint	Static splint
Claw hand	• Dynamic ulnar nerve palsy splint • Knuckle bender splint • Wrist driven wrist hand orthoses • Hand orthoses with MCP extension stop	• Static ulnar nerve palsy splint • Static WHO (wrist–hand orthoses) splint • Lumbrical bar
Wrist drop	• Dorsal wrist cock up splint with dynamic finger extension • Wrist action wrist hand orthoses • Tenodesis splint	• Static volar wrist cock up splint • Static WHO splint

Splints for the Hand

1. *Ulnar and Median Nerve Palsy*

While physiotherapy centers would generally employ dynamic splints, most leprosy centers use static splints. The hand orthoses used can be either static or dynamic. The former are used when the palsy is mild while the latter is used when the palsy is severe. The static hand orthoses (HdO) also have in addition dorsal and palmar barsto maintain natural concavity and may have components to appropriately position the thumb as a static surface counter for grasping. The static positional wrist–hand orthoses are used for claw hand. These usually have a padding to maximize the surface area of the orthosis and evenly distribute pressure along the forearm and hand. Median nerve palsy in isolation is not seen in leprosy but in case it is seen, the static thumb splint can be re-designed. Some of the splints used for ulnar and median nerve palsy are listed below.

a. **Finger loop splint**—for claw hands without contractures
b. **Gutter splint**—for claw hand *with* contractures
c. **Adductor band**—for abduction deformity of little finger only
d. **Opponens loop splint**—for ape thumb deformity
e. **Dynamic splints**

a. *Finger loop splint* (Fig. 8.60): It allows the exercises of PIP joint to be carried out while holding MCP joint in flexion; thus it achieves external mechanical correction of claw hand. Here it must be ensured that the rubber band should be sufficiently elastic so that it allows the MCP joint to extend before PIP extension is completed. Patient is instructed not to hyperextend the MCP joint while exercising as some patients develop habitual hyperextension at MCP due to long-standing deformity.

The finger loop splint (Fig. 8.60) consists of wrist band with three hooks, so that it can be used on either left or right hand, and four finger loops to be inserted one in each finger and is attached to the wrist band with elastic rubber bands of good quality. At rest, MCP joint is kept in full flexion by the finger loop splint, patient extends the PIP joint from flexed position to straight position. The same action is repeated several times. It results in opening the range of motion at PIP joint, stretching out any mild volar skin contracture and keeps joints mobile till reconstructive surgery is performed. Stabilization of proximal joint, i.e. wrist is not required unless patient has an advanced deformity and has become habituated to flex the wrist while working.

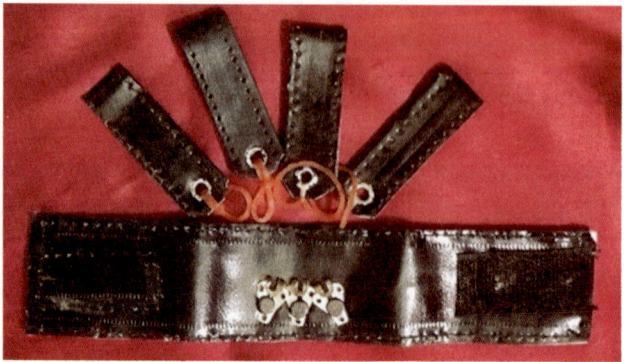

Fig. 8.60: Finger loop splint

b. *Dynamic gutter splint and rigid gutter splint:* Although commonly known as gutter splint indicating that it is a *static* type of splint, the use of elastic hose pipe cut in the center to make a 1.5-, 2- and 2.5-inch length gutter splint (Fig. 8.61) has been found to retain "memory" of elasticity. When one bends it in the center and leaves it, it tends to straighten out, thereby producing its dynamic effect indirectly. It stretches out the skin contracture and helps release joint stiffness.

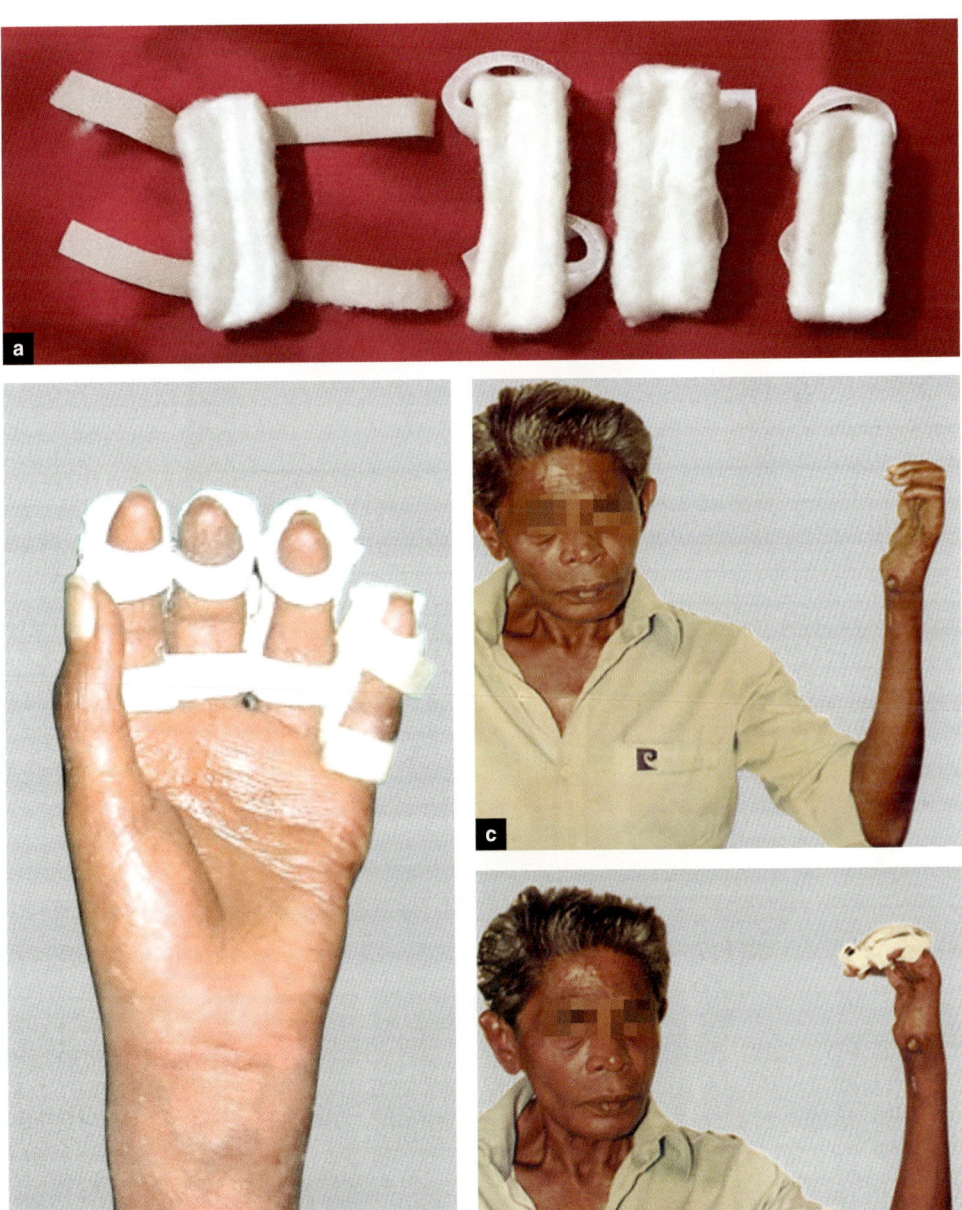

Fig. 8.61: (a) Dynamic gutter splint. Elastic hose pipe cut in vertically half with lint applied on its concave surface and Velcro strips riveted on its convex surface; (b) It is advocated that it be applied on the dorsal side; (c) Deformity; (d) Splint applied

The newer thermoplastic material[5] like Orfit® is commonly used by occupational therapists to make a custom-made static gutter splint quickly. The material is dipped in hot water, made pliable and cool so as to not produce scalds when applied and is fitted into the desired position and allowed to cool. Once hardened, it is retained in position with Velcro straps (Fig. 8.62). The material that is dipped in warm water to make the desired type of splint (but hard one, nonelastic and nonflexible). The self-adhesive Velcro is used to keep it in position.

c. *Adductor band:* It is a simple circular splint made of rexin, felt lining and Velcro at the sides (Fig. 8.63a) and can be wrapped around proximal phalanges keeping all fingers in adduction (Fig. 8.63b). It helps correct early abduction deformity with steroid therapy or after nerve decompression surgery.

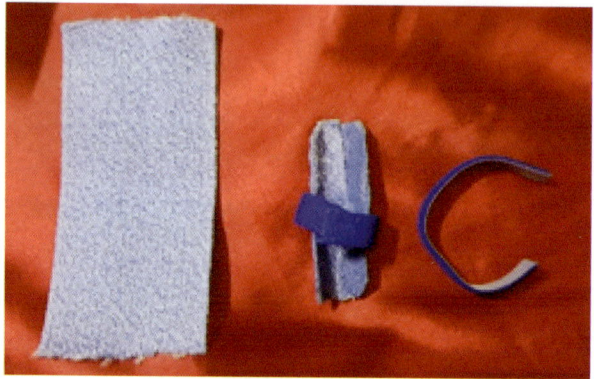

Fig. 8.62: Making splint on the spot with Orfit® material (*Courtesy:* Mr Mukesh Doshi, OT, Nanavati Hospital)

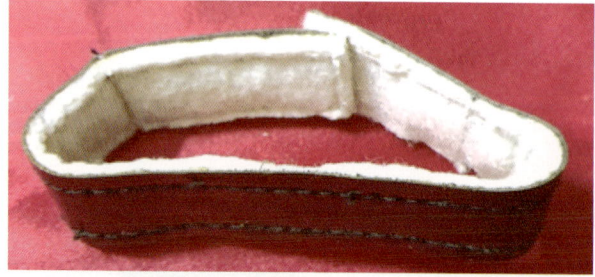

Fig. 8.63a: Adductor band splint to wrap around the base of all four fingers

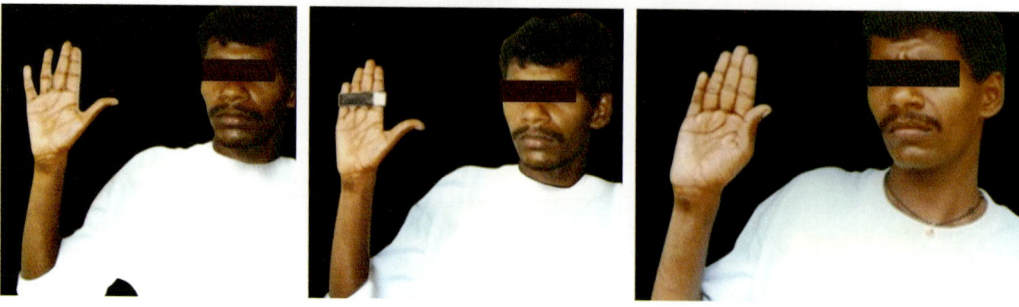

Fig. 8.63b: Early deformity supported with adductor band; with continued therapy helping in recovery

d. Opponens splint or thumb spica: An extended bigger loop-like finger loop can be used to hold the thumb in abduction with rubber band made taut by folding it and attaching it obliquely. Alternately, a ready-made thumb spica[6] (Fig. 8.64) can be used before and after operation of opponens plasty. It stabilizes thumb in abduction and can be removed and reapplied easily for carrying out physiotherapy exercises, which generally consists of opposing thumb to the pulp of donor finger (majority of time—the ring finger). It needs to be worn for at least 6 weeks or till reeducation is complete.

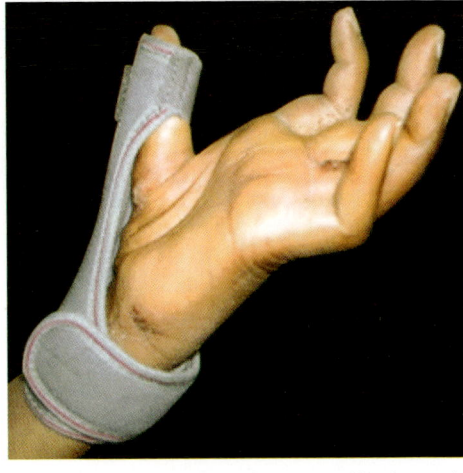

Fig. 8.64: Thumb spica applied post-opponens plasty operation

e. Dynamic splint:[6] The *ulnar nerve palsy splint* holds the MCP joints of the fourth and fifth fingers in slight flexion by a spring coil or the figure-of-eight splint design. The spring coil design assists MCP flexion and permits extension of the MCP joints but blocks hyperextension (Fig. 8.65). A combined splint for both the median and ulnar nerve can also be designed.

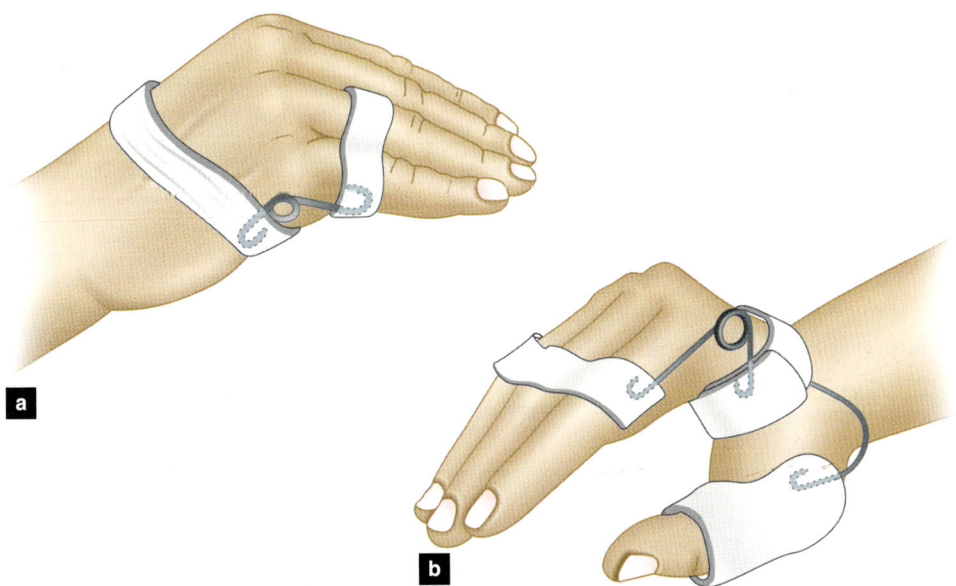

Fig. 8.65a and b: Depiction of combined ulnar median nerve splint

2. Splints for Radial Nerve Palsy[6]

With *radial nerve injuries* distal to the humeral spiral groove, the common presenting condition is wrist drop and finger drop. The goal in this case is to enhance wrist and finger extension. Though the radial nerve involvement in leprosy is uncommon and largely sensory, if there is a high radial nerve palsy, there is a functional loss with

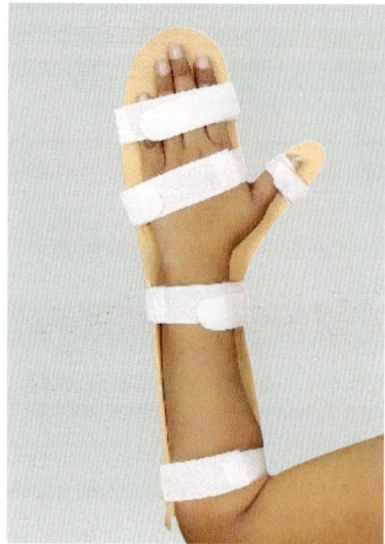
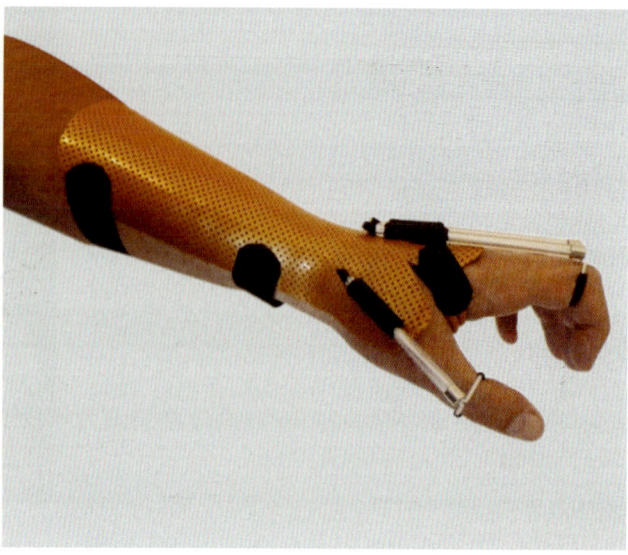

Fig. 8.66: Static volar wrist cock-up splint

Fig. 8.67: Dorsal wrist cock-up with dynamic finger extension splint

inability to stabilize the wrist in extension so that the finger flexors cannot be used normally. Radial nerve palsy often recovers spontaneously; therefore effective splinting may be needed for months during regeneration.

Various splints used include the static volar wrist cock-up splint, dynamic tenodesis suspension splint, and dorsal wrist cock-up with dynamic finger extension splint.[8] Though a "static splint" can be advised (Fig. 8.66), the ideal is a radial nerve palsy splint (Fig. 8.67) which is forearm based with an outrigger that holds the wrist, fingers, and thumb in extension and allows for flexion of the digits.

Splints for the Foot

For foot drop, the various orthoses that have been designed are essentially of two types:[6]
- Custom solid (flexible) ankle–foot orthosis set at 90° for foot drop
- Custom solid (rigid) ankle–foot orthosis set at 90° for plantar spasticity.

The basic idea is to enhance functional use with special footwear that would improve the patients gait and also help in even distribution of pressure on the sole. As these orthoses are used to control the ankle and foot, they are known as ankle–foot orthoses (AFOs) (Fig. 8.68a). These orthoses can be custom-made or prefabricated. If the latter are used, small adjustments

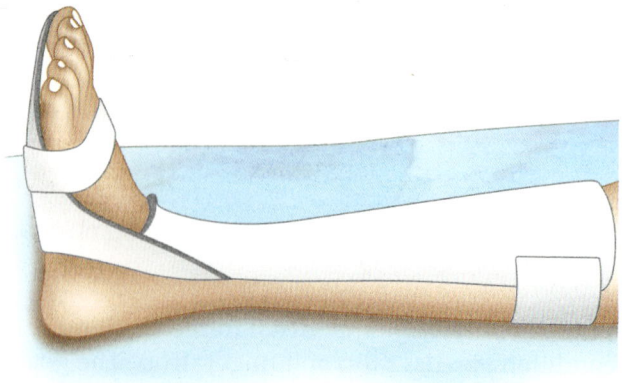

Fig. 8.68a: Ankle–foot orthosis

are usually necessary to make them suitable for the client.

If no prefabricated footwear is available or if there is likely to be much delay in obtaining it, a simple foot-raising device can be made and fitted from locally available materials (Fig. 8.68b). Basically, this consists of a leather leg band which fits just above the ankle, with a strap which is attached to the footwear in such a way that the strap holds up the foot and prevents it from dropping. The leg band should be about 10 cm wide and padded, so that it will not damage the skin. The foot-raising strap should be elastic. Rubber (from old tyres) is often used for the foot-raising strap. It should be hooked onto the footwear at a point between the third and fourth toes, on the upper straps of sandals or the uppers of shoes. Use of the foot-raising device will protect the foot and also abolish the high-stepping gait that identifies the person as having drop-foot due to leprosy.

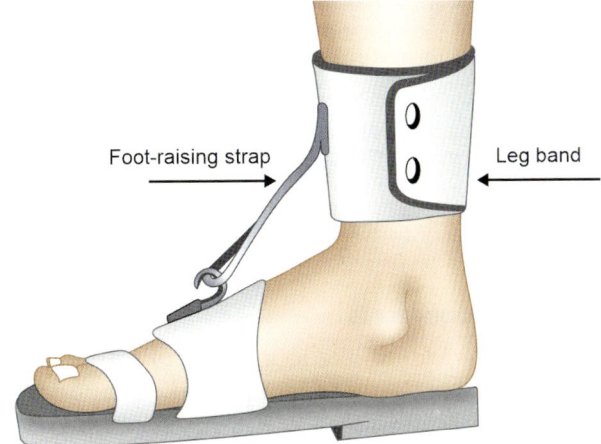

Fig. 8.68b: Ankle–foot-raising device

COMBINATION OF MODALITIES[7]

Combination of modalities achieves a greater effect in claw hand than individual modalities alone. A study initiated by Indian Council of Medical Research found that a combination of splints followed by 10 minutes of electrical stimulation and exercise (which were administered for 2 weeks followed by advise to continue the same at home) achieved greater improvement in grip strength and mean intrinsic muscle strength at 6 months than individual modalities alone (Fig. 8.69a and b).

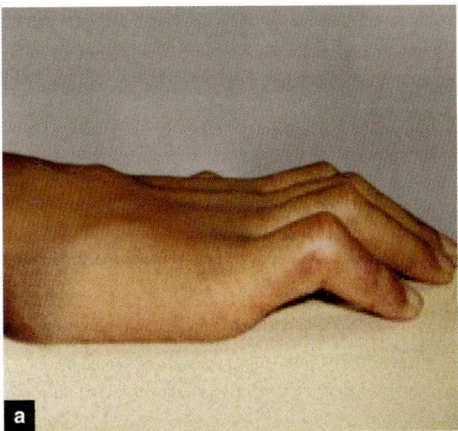
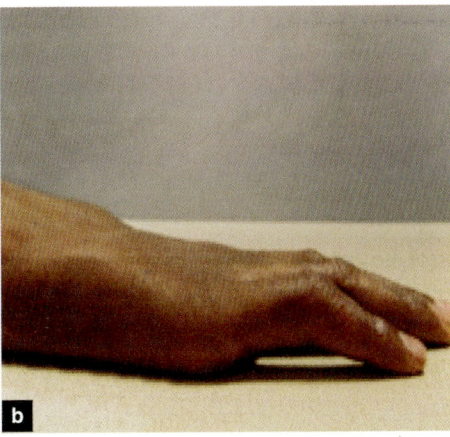

Fig. 8.69a and b: Combination treatment. Photographs of a patient before and after splintage with electrical stimulation therapy (*Courtesy:* Kanchan Mittal, Superintendent of Physiotherapist, Department of Orthopedics–Surgery, All India Institute of Medical Sciences, New Delhi, from her ICMR study)

CONCLUSION

The focus of leprosy work will ultimately shift to disability management as MDT has been largely successful in ameliorating the disease. Thus, rehabilitation and achieving routine activities are important as assistive devices (*see Section 8.3.5*) help in both facilitating mobility and can help in work and employment. It is important to make patients aware of these devices and popularize their use by integrating their production in other assistive device manufacturing facilities, so that benefits of advancements in technology and quality will more likely reach people affected by leprosy.

Acknowledgements

The authors would like to thank Prof Vinita Puri (KEM Hospital, Mumbai) for going through the manuscript and providing inputs, and along with Dr Vivek Gupta, KEM Hospital, Mumbai, and Ms Neela Shah for contributing photographs. The authors would also like to thank the inputs on orthoses by Dr Kabir Sardana.

REFERENCES

1. Antia NH, Enna CD, Daver BM. The Surgical Management of Deformities in Leprosy and other peripheral neuropathies. Bombay Oxford University Press, 1992; p. 30–60.
2. Guidelines for Primary, Secondary and Tertiary Level Care. Central Leprosy Division, Government of India, printed by Novartis Comprehensive Leprosy Care Association, Mumbai, 2012; p.40.
3. Shah A. Physiotherapy—Some Measures. In: Koticha KK, editor, Leprosy: A Concise Text, 1st ed. Bombay, Darsan K Koticha,1990, p.193–200.
4. Shah A. Prevention and Correction of Claw hand by Splintage—A New Approach to Deformity Care. A Comprehensive Leprosy Care Project Training Booklet, Hindustan Ciba-Geigy Limited, 1992.
5. https://expertconsult.inkling.com/read/webster-atlas-orthoses-assistive-devices-5e/chapter-12/design-principles-for-upper limb orthoses-accessed on 28 oct 2019.
6. Upper Limb Orthoses and Lower Limb Orthoses in Braddom's Physical Medicine and Rehabilitation, 5th Edition Authors: David X. Cifu, 2015. Accessed via https://expertconsult.inkling.com/
7. Mittal K. Effect of electrical stimulation and splinting in preventing disability in leprosy patients with claw hand. A study sanctioned by Indian Council of Medical Research, 2014.
8. Hannah SD, Hudak PL. Splinting and radial nerve palsy: A single-subject experiment. J Hand Ther 2001;14:195–201.
9. Assistive devices for people affected by leprosy: Underutilised facilitators of functioning? Borg J, Larsson S. Lepr Rev 2009;80:13–21.
10. Manivannan G, Karthikeyan G, Das P, Babu G. Cost-effective cosmetic prosthesis for lost digits. Lepr Rev 2015;86:117–23.

8.3.5 SELF-CARE, FOOTWEAR AND ASSISTIVE DEVICES

Karthikeyan Govindasamy, Babu Govindan, Neela Shah

PRINCIPLES OF SELF-CARE

All patients with the impairments in eyes, hands and feet need to be educated about self-care to prevent secondary impairments, such as damage to cornea, ulcers, joint contractures, disintegration of bone and shortening of digits/limb. It is estimated that over three million people live with disability due to leprosy, and every year, there is an addition of 30 to 40% of newly diagnosed patients with leprosy presenting with disabilities.[1] Herein lies the role of teaching lifestyle modifications to patients and to encourage them to practice simple self-care procedures regularly to protect their eyes and limbs from being injured. The self-care should be customized to individuals according to their impairments, occupation and environment. The self-care can also be taught in self-care groups where a group of people practice self-care together and provide peer support.[1]

1. Care of Eyes

The loss of sensation in the cornea, absence of blink reflex and lagophthalmos are serious eye-related impairments which if not taken care of may lead to damage to cornea and decreased vision. Although not related to leprosy, self help groups should be aware that the most common cause of poor vision in the elderly (treated) patients is cataract and this is curable by surgery.

a. *Lagophthalmos*

I. In long-standing lagophthalmos (>6 months duration and eyelid gap <6 mm), the following must be taught and practised:
   i. "Blinking exercises" to reinforce the orbicularis function. This involves strong blinking three times daily, with 20 blinks each time.
   ii. 'Think blink': By making use of the Bell's phenomenon (upward turning of the eyes on attempted closure of the eyelids), this exercise leads to moistening of cornea behind the upper eyelids in a kind of 'reverse blinking'.
   iii. Preventing corneal damage: If the patient is unable to close the eye actively, passive exercises are taught to close eyes.

II. Preventing corneal damage in long-standing lagophthalmos

Advise the following simple self-care steps to avoid visual impairment resulting from corneal exposure and damage:
- Wear protective glass (sunglasses) or cover eye with the help of cloth/towel/saree or wide brimmed hat or cap to prevent dust and insects from damaging the eye and prevent dryness on the surface of the eye during the day (Fig. 8.70a).
- While sleeping, cover eyes with the help of towel or bedsheet to prevent damage to the cornea (Fig. 8.70b).
- Wash the eye with clean lukewarm water to flush out dirt (avoid splashing) (Fig. 8.70c). This should be taught to the patient under supervision before they self practise at home. After face washing, inspect the eye in mirror to see early signs of damage such as red eye.
- Avoid rubbing of eye and use soft cloth to wipe the watering.

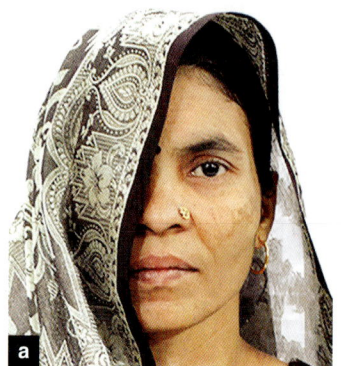 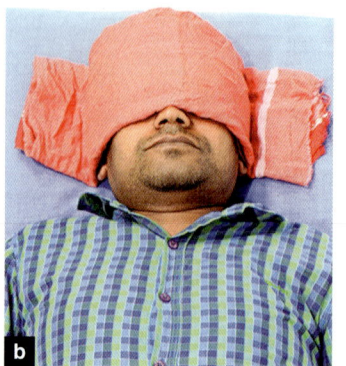 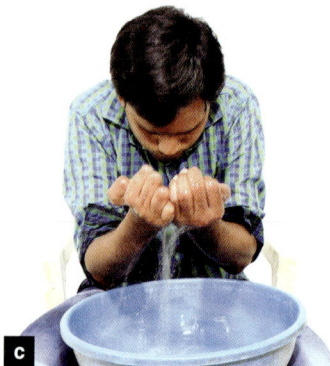

Fig. 8.70a to c: Eye care in long-standing lagophthalmos (*see* text)

Surgical correction of lagophthalmos is indicated in presence of exposure keratitis, severe lagophthalmos (≥6 mm, >6 months) and other conditions as detailed in Box 8.12 of *Section 8.3.4*.

b. Vision Testing

Regularly check vision by looking at the fixed objects as available in the field setting. Also, pay attention to other vision impairing causes as per the patient's age, e.g. presbyopia if >40 years of age.

c. Redness of Eyes

High doses of clofazimine (for type 2 reaction) cause redness of the eyes, which may be confused with a reaction in the eye. This redness will gradually disappear after clofazimine treatment is stopped.

In case of sudden redness or pain, advise patient to seek help at the nearest medical unit, preferably an eye clinic. In case of gradual loss of eye sight in one or both eyes, advise to visit the eye unit, as it may due to cataract and be curable.

2. Care of Hands and Feet

This is a very important aspect of management, as the anesthetic hand or foot may be repeatedly injured by the un-informed patient, and because of the absence of pain, the injured limb is not rested and healing is therefore protracted and often complicated by sepsis.

For those with paralyzed hands, even the simple, yet essential, task of cutting nails becomes difficult, which increases the risk of injuries. Therefore, they need to be taught how to protect their limbs while carrying out essential day-to-day tasks, including work-related activities. The following simple instructions help minimize damage to anesthetic hands/feet:

- The anesthetic hands/feet should be soaked in cool water and scraped thoroughly with stone or commercially available skin scrapers to remove any thickened skin or callosities (Fig. 8.71a and b). The callosities can be scraped with pumice or with a callus file, which is retailed by most chemists. The moisture should then be retained by applying a thin coat of oil or Vaseline while the skin is still moist.
- Advise daily inspection of hands/feet for hot spots, blisters, wounds or swelling.

Other Aspects of Treatment

- Advise to be cautious in handling hot or sharp objects. This can be done by insulating the objects or tools with the help of cloth or soft materials or by use of gloves (Fig. 8.71c and d).
- Rest the wounds to prevent progression. This is especially important for plantar blisters/ulcers. This can be achieved by walking with the help of crutch or canes.
- Advise to perform regular exercise to prevent damage to the joints (contractures).
- Avoid sitting cross legged
- Use of footwear with soft insoles such as microcellular rubber (MCR) and rigid outer soles needs to be worn daily (Fig. 8.71e).
- The footwear needs to be inspected daily for excessive wear and tear or for the presence of any embedded sharp objects.

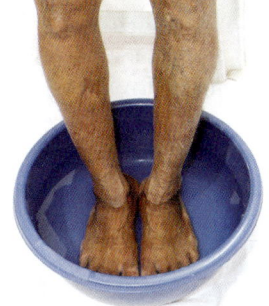
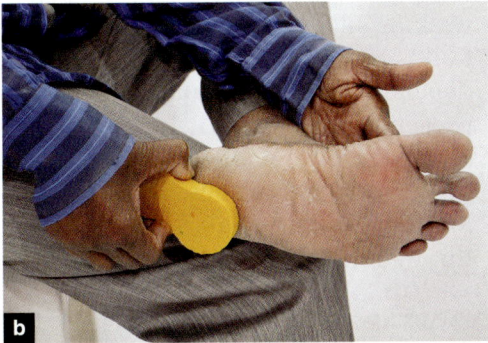
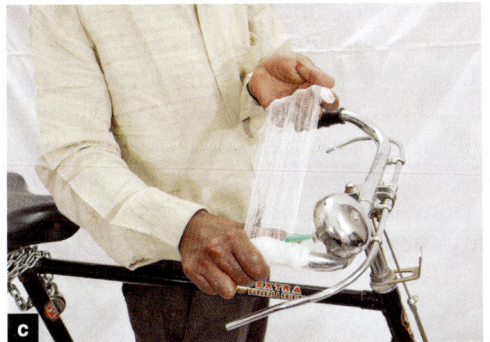
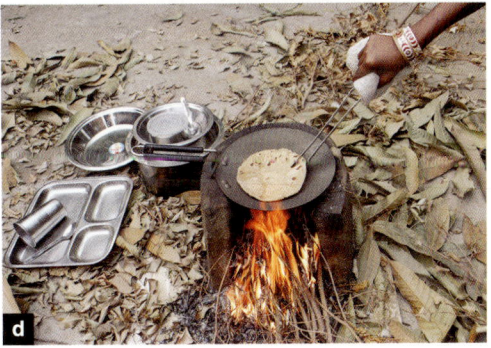
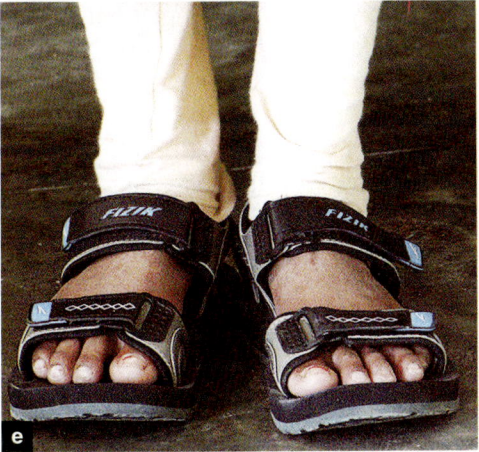

Fig. 8.71: (a) Foot care: Soaking feet in water; (b) Scraping the callosities; (c) Hand care: Protecting anesthetic hands from possible minor injuries by padding of rough surfaces; (d) Hand care: Using tongs to prevent accidental burns while cooking; (e) Foot care using shoes with soft microcellular rubber (MCR) insoles and tough outer soles

> **Box 8.15:** Self-care kit for treating foot ulcers[9]
>
> - The "self-care kit" consists of Savlon bottle of which one "lidful" is used in one liter of water before soaking the feet in it.
> - Next, after 10 minutes, the scrapper included in the kit is used to scrape the dirt and margins of the ulcer if any, while being cautious that ulcer does not bleed.
> - The foot is then wiped dry particularly in between toes to prevent fungal infection.
> - An antiseptic ointment from the kit is applied on the ulcer, and surrounding area is moisturized with Vaseline or any moisturizing ointment included in the kit.
> - The ulcer is then dressed with two small sterile gauzes from the kit and wrapped with bandage.

- To avoid plantar ulceration, the patient must avoid all unnecessary standing and walking, all hurrying or running, and must learn to take short steps while walking. Callosities which often form under the heads of the metatarsals and other sites depending on the impairment in a patient, should be pared down regularly. In the presence of a crack, it is advisable to thin the edges of the crack by rubbing along the line of the edge and not across the edge (as the latter may open it more) (Box 8.15). Patient should wear footwear with off-loading in the insole at the location where the callosities are present. The patient must wear suitable footwear throughout the day—in the house as well as out of doors.

FOOTWEAR

A sandal with a strong stiff sole is ideal in the tropics, and it should be lined by a Plastazote insole which is glued in position to prevent shifting. Alternatively, insoles can be made of microcellular rubber. If shoes are worn, they should be strong, comfortable, free from nails, broad at the toes and without toecap and as with sandals, should be worn throughout the day. Ideally, the tongues should be of extra width, the sole should be of stiff leather and laces should be avoided if the patient has deformed fingers, in which case Velcro is the ideal alternative. Slippers and rubber-soled shoes such as tennis shoes should *never* be worn. The patient must be advised about 'wearing-in' new shoes before they can be worn all day. This means wearing them for an hour a day in the first week 2 hours a day for the second week, and so on. Shoes that are being regularly worn and have become moulded to the shape of the feet should be ranked among the patient's most treasured possessions and can be repeatedly resoled until they literally drop to pieces. Plastazole insoles can play an important part in the prevention of plantar ulceration as they are moulded to the shape of each sole and it is even possible to have shoes made entirely of this material.

Where expertise is available, the podiatry assessment should be done to assess the foot alignment and provide appropriate orthoses along with the footwear. Table 8.10 provides simple guidelines on footwear and orthoses.

Advancement in Protective Footwear

The adherence to protective footwear using MCR has been low due to its cosmetic unacceptability (Fig. 8.72a).[3,4] However, there has been an important advancement in the design of the footwear. The footwear designs, which are at par with designs available in the market, with incorporation of MCR as insole, has been found to improve the adherence to the wearing schedule[5] (Fig. 8.72b and c). Recently, based on the analysis

Other Aspects of Treatment

Table 8.10: Footwear and orthoses specification with indications for insensitive feet due to leprosy

Indication	Footwear and orthoses
Insensitive feet with no deformities	MCR footwear
Insensitive feet with fixed or mobile claw toes and scarring in the forefoot	MCR footwear with a metatarsal rocker
Insensitive feet with pronated subtalar joint	MCR footwear with a tarsal cradle
Insensitive feet with hyperpronated subtalar joint	MCR footwear with a "hatti" pad
Insensitive feet with supinated subtalar joint	MCR footwear with a heel cup or tarsal platform
Insensitive feet with ulcer on the metatarsal head on the supinated foot	MCR footwear with a combination pad (tarsal cradle with plantar metatarsal pad)
Insensitive feet with ulcer on the metatarsal head on a pronated subtalar joint	MCR footwear with tarsal platform with anterior rocker
Insensitive feet with foot drop	MCR footwear with foot drop spring or ankle–foot orthoses (AFO)
Neuropathic foot (Charcot's foot or hot foot)	Moulded insole with fixed ankle brace (FAB)
Shortened foot or severely scarred foot	Moulded insole with patellar tendon bearing (PTB) brace

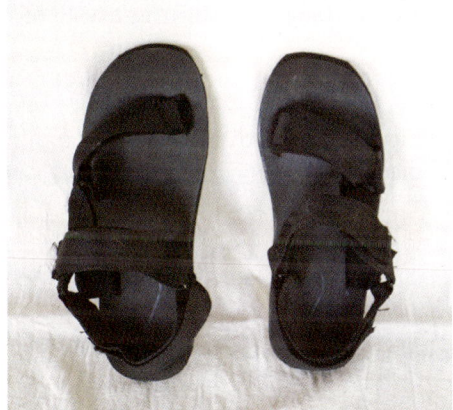 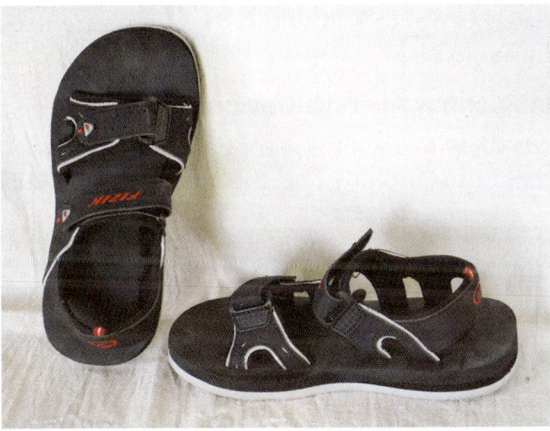

Fig. 8.72a: Old model MCR footwear **Fig. 8.72b:** New model of MCR footwear for male

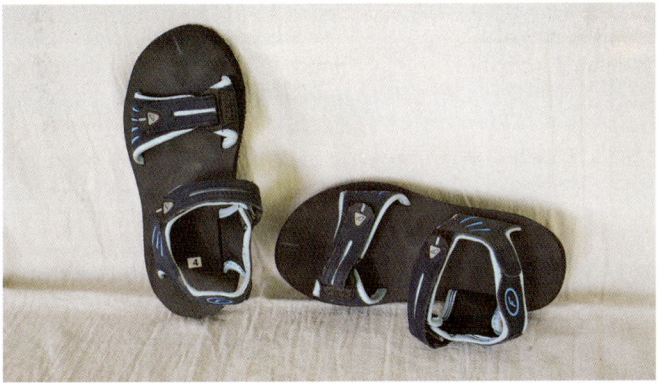

Fig. 8.72c: New model of MCR footwear for female

of plantar pressure using foot scanning technology, customized insoles using computer assisted designing and manufacturing have been tried but their effectiveness needs to be studied with adequate sample size. They provide the advantages of improved fitting, greater patient satisfaction and greater patient compliance than the conventional MCR footwear.

COMMON ASSISTIVE DEVICES USED IN LEPROSY

When patients with impairment have difficulty in performing activities of daily living (ADL) as well as work and leisure related activities, provision of adaptive devices improves their ability to perform the daily activities, such as those related to personal hygiene, brushing, bathing, feeding and dressing. Assistive devices are simple to make and have been found to increase the affected person's sense of satisfaction and independence in carrying out routine activities and participating in social activities. Yet, these methods are least utilized in the rehabilitation of leprosy patients.[6]

Assistive devices can be of two broad types. Firstly, they can be used to prevent impairments and secondary deformities, and secondly they are used to facilitate functioning. Some assistive devices fulfil both preventing and a facilitating role. The assistive devices used for prevention, i.e. protection of the user's body, are listed in Table 8.11 while those that are used for facilitating functioning are listed in Table 8.12.[6]

Indigenous Assistive Devices

Needless to say, it is essential to use the basic principles of assistive devices to make them user-friendly and the same will be detailed below.

Table 8.11: Assistive devices for protection of eyes, hands and feet[6]

Protection of eyes	Eye-glasses, headcloths, hats and caps, pads, cloths, mosquito nets and bed sheets to cover eyes while sleeping
Protection of hands	Adapting tools, splints, gloves, pot holders and cooking gloves, padding around handles, long handles, sticks and prongs
Protection of feet	Footwear, orthoses, splints, foot drop splints, drop-foot supports, crutches, walking sticks

Table 8.12: Assistive devices for facilitation of hand- and foot-related activities[6]

Facilitation of hand-related activities	• Grip-aids (e.g. custom-made Modulan Grip-Aids) • Foam padding for combs, cutlery and pens to increase contact area and decrease pressure • Wrist cuff/straps with holder, e.g. pen, spoon or tool • Velcro straps on shoes instead of buckles or lace
Facilitation of foot-related activities	• Braces • Foot drop splints • Orthoses and prostheses • Crutches • Wheelchairs • Sewing machine pedal spring

A crude way is based on the use of either POP or epoxy resin material and an example is the "Instant" Grip-Aids.[7] The epoxy resin Grip-Aid "Modulan" was made popular by Ciba-Geigy. It consisted of yellow putty of epoxy resin and blue putty of hardener. Both were mixed in equal amount till it turned green. It is applied on the tools used by disabled patients and deformity impression is taken. After a day's waiting, patient can adjust tools in the deformed hand and can work. This could be used for daily activities when it was made part of a "Instant Grip-Aid" kit which included a Velcro strap, which could be wrapped around the palm or amputated hand with a slit to insert the articles of daily activity like spoon, *ring* to hold the glass or a *glass* made with handle with stainless steel strip, a *comb* to enable a patient to do combing after bath as well as *toothbrush* with thin handle which can fit in the slit of the Velcro (Fig. 8.73a to d).

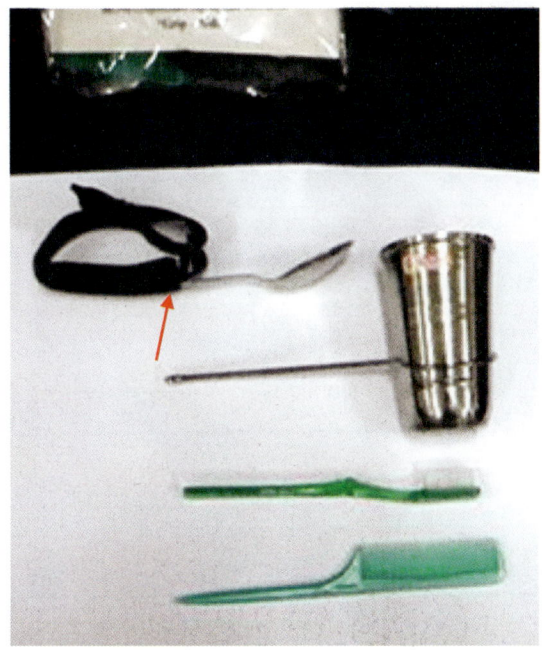

Fig. 8.73a: This shows the design of the Grip-Aid kit and materials offered in the kit. The arrow demonstrates the slit where different tools are inserted as per requirement either by patient or by relative depending on the degree of disability

Various other adapted devices are listed in Table 8.13.

Loss of digits in the hands due to chronic and repeated injuries and resulting absorption are common complications in people affected by leprosy with long-term impairments.

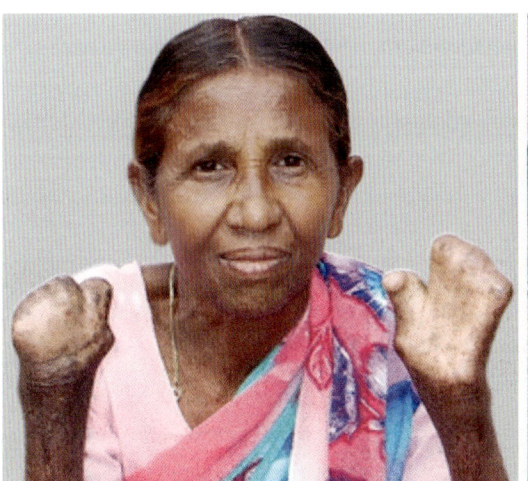 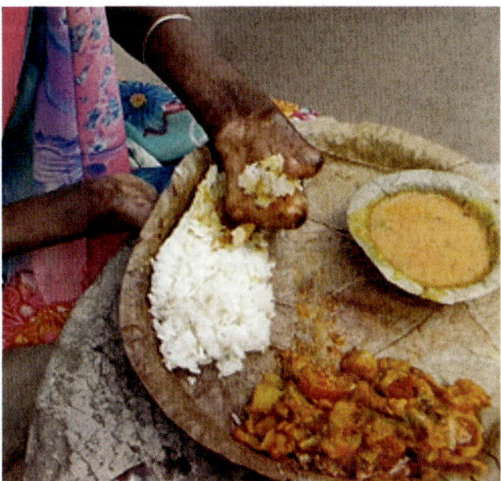

Fig. 8.73b: The image depicts the extreme disability and handicap this lady was facing evident by the way she had to take the food in the hand to eat before a Grip-Aid was provided

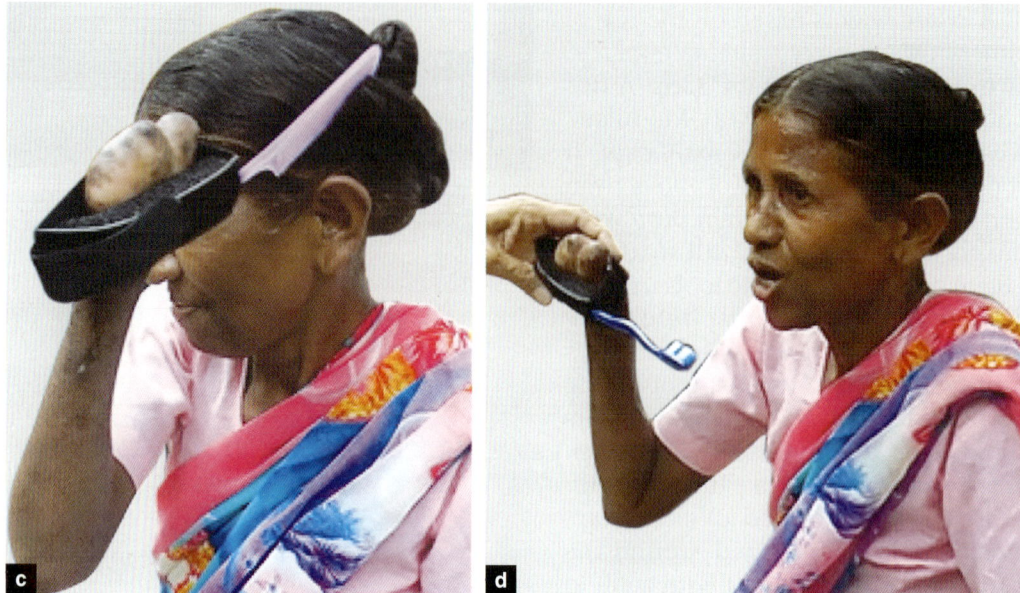

Fig. 8.73: (c) The image shows the patient trying to learn combing hair with comb inserted in the slot of the Grip-Aid; (d) Brushing the teeth with toothbrush applied to the Grip-Aid

Table 8.13: Common adaptive/assistive devices used in leprosy	
Name of the device	Indication
Adapted spoon (Fig. 8.74)	Those with no grasp due to absorbed digits or complete paralysis of hand muscles
Built-up spoon (Fig. 8.75)	Those with some grasp but inability to hold thin items such as spoon or toothbrush during function movement
Nail cutting device (Fig. 8.76)	Those with deformities; clawed fingers and thumb paralysis
Button hook (Fig. 8.77)	Those with difficulty in fine motor activity due to paralysis and/or loss of sensation
Writing aid (Fig. 8.78)	Those with poor prehension (tripod) function with some pinch power
Grip-Aids (Fig. 8.79)	Those with absorbed digits with some grasp/prehension function
Universal cuff (Fig. 8.80a to c)	Those with poor or no grasp due to absorbed digits or paralysis of muscles of the hand. The spoon, toothbrush, comb or razer can be inserted in the cuff to facilitate self-care activities

Aids such as cosmetic prostheses made of latex rubber for absorbed digits and toes restores cosmetic appearance of the limbs (Fig. 8.81a and b). These aids are simple to make and cost-effective as compared to commercially available artificial prosthesis.[8,10,11]

Other Aspects of Treatment

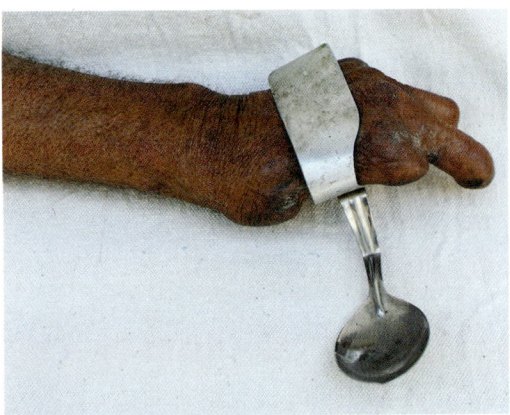

Fig. 8.74: Adapted spoon

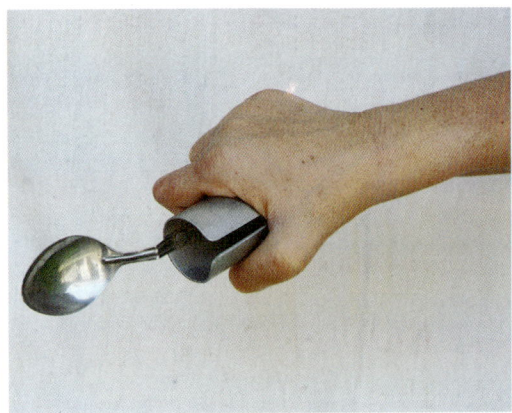

Fig. 8.75: Built up spoon

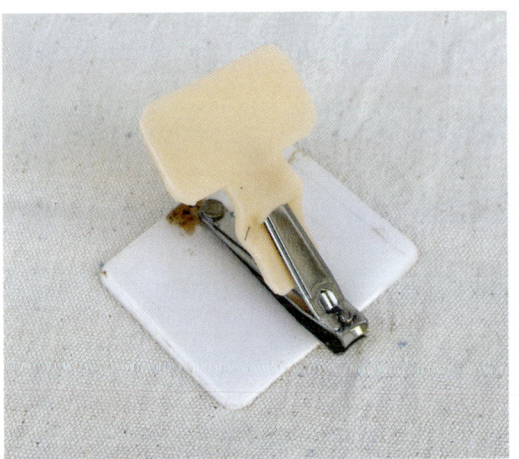

Fig. 8.76: Nail cutting device

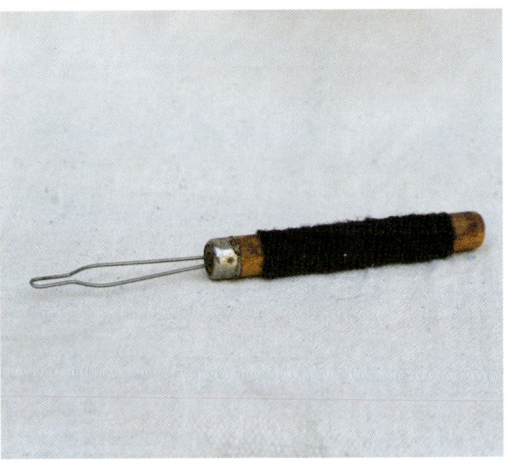

Fig. 8.77: Button hook for buttoning

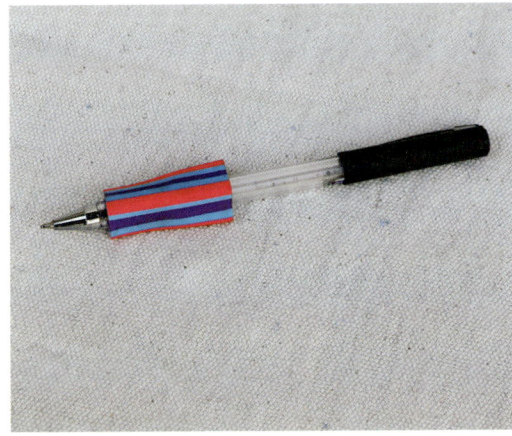

Fig. 8.78: Writing aid

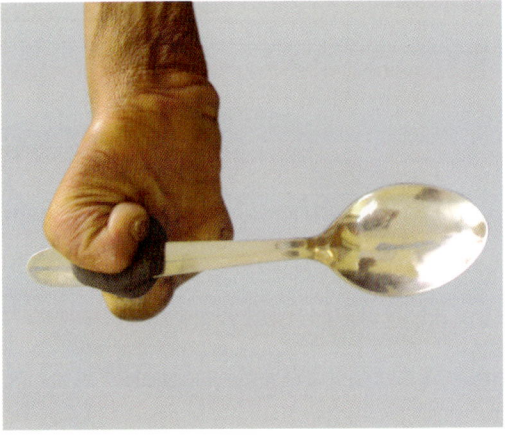

Fig. 8.79: Grip-Aid to hold a spoon

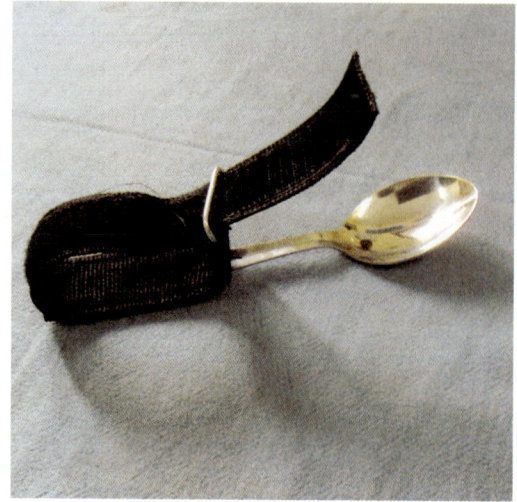

Fig. 8.80a: Universal cuff

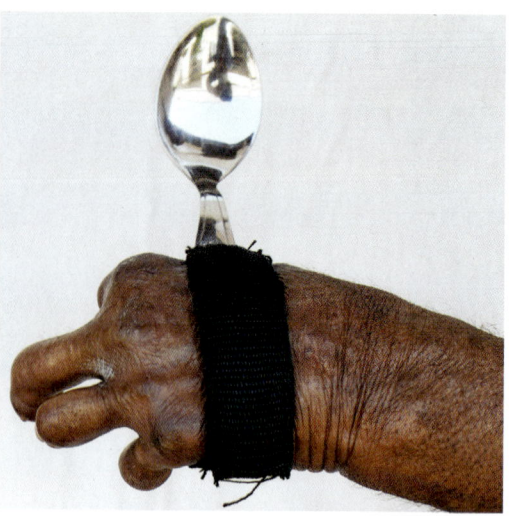

Fig. 8.80b: Universal cuff with spoon

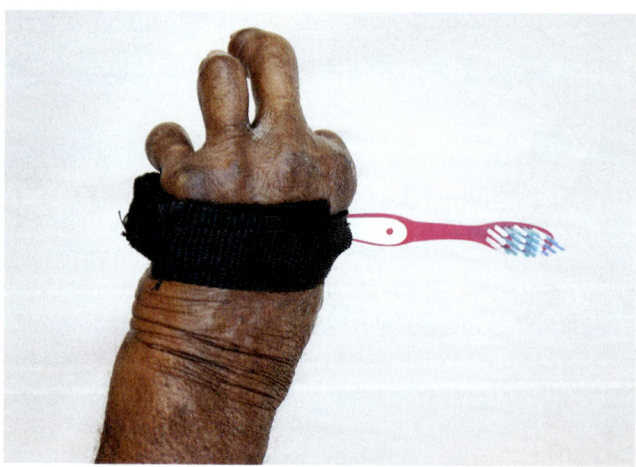

Fig. 8.80c: Universal cuff with toothbrush

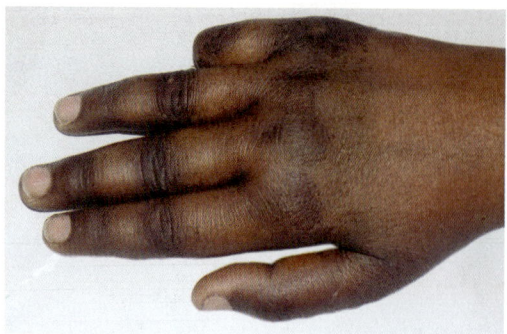

Fig. 8.81a: Cosmetic prostheses (pre)

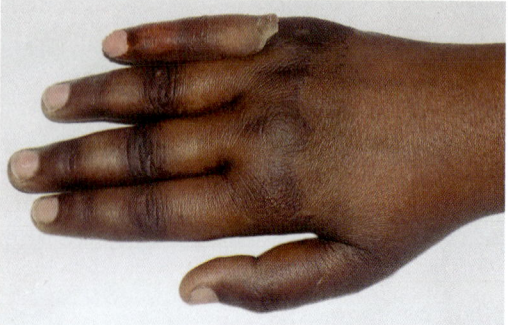

Fig. 8.81b: Cosmetic prostheses (post)

CONCLUSION

While leprosy intervention has been focused on therapeutic interventions, it is accepted that in late stages, nerve damage and consequent deformity is the most common problem faced by patients. While in certain cases surgical rehabilitation is useful, a large proportion of deformities are not amenable to functional resolution. Herein lies the use of assistive technologies, though there is an issue of an imbalance between demand and supply.

There is an emergent need to provide facilities to the needy to complete the spectrum of interventions, which is largely geared towards reducing disability at present, rather than managing ones which have already developed.

Acknowledgements

Dr Atul Shah and Dr Neela Shah for indigenous assistive devices.

REFERENCES

1. Lockwood DNJ. Chronic aspects of leprosy—neglected but important. Trans R Soc Trop Med Hyg 2018;1–5.
2. Chakraborty A, Mahato M, Rao PSSS. Self-care programme to prevent leprosy-related problems in a leprosy colony in Champa, Chattisgarh. Indian J Lepr 2006;78:3–11.
3. Lal V, Sarkar D, Das S, Mahato M, Srinivas G. A study to assess the usage of MCR footwear in West Bengal, India. Lepr Rev 2015;86:273–7.
4. Gupta P, Karthikeyan, Nathan RJ. Footwear for the person with an anesthetic foot: What options are available? Lepr Rev 2017;265–9.
5. Govindharaj P, Mani S, Darlong J, John AS. Acceptance and satisfaction of microcellular rubber ready-made footwear among patients with insensitive feet due to leprosy. Lepr Rev 2017; 88:381–90.
6. Borg J, Larsson S. Assistive devices for people affected by leprosy: Underutilised facilitators of functioning? Lepr Rev 2009;80:13–21.
7. Shah A, Shah N. Deformities of face, Hands, Feet, Trophic Ulcers and Their Management. In: Kumar B, Narang T, Dongre VV, Samanta SK, Eds. IAL Handbook of Leprosy, 1st Ed. Bhalani Publishing House, 2010;p.198.
8. Manivannan G, Karthikeyan G, Das P, Babu G. Cost effective cosmetic prosthesis for lost digits. Lepr Rev [Internet] 2015;86:117–23.
9. Atul Shah, Neela Shah, "Self-care Kit" an aid to empowerment in self-care of feet in leprosy, Published by NCLCA, Mumbai, 2004.
10. Guidelines for primary, secondary and tertiary level care by Central Leprosy Division, Nirman Bhavan, New Delhi, July 2012;pages 42 and 88.
11. NLEP Annual Report 2015–2016 Central Leprosy Division, Directorate General of Health Services, Ministry of Health and Family Welfare Government of India, Nirman Bhavan, New Delhi.

8.4 OTHER TREATMENTS

Kabir Sardana, Ananta Khurana

DRY SKIN

This is commonly experienced in long-standing cases of lepromatous leprosy (LL) and usually affects arms and legs bilaterally. Dry skin is due to lack of sweating which, in turn, is due to failure of autonomic fibers within damaged dermal nerves to stimulate sweat glands. The dry skin is less elastic and more brittle than normal skin and also if dry skin is not addressed, it breaks, forming cracks and fissures, through which infection enters and spreads, extensively damaging deeper tissues of the hand or foot and leading to disability.

Mild degrees of dry skin respond to daily soaking for about 15 minutes in warm water, followed by application of white soft paraffin (white petroleum jelly BP) to the affected regions of skin, in order to occlude water loss from the outer layer of skin.

In the tropics, where a minimum of clothes are worn, the emollient can be rubbed into the wet skin, but in temperate regions it is applied to the damp skin after light towelling. Severe degrees of dryness (ichthyosis), commonly associated with clofazimine treatment, respond better to a cream containing 10% carbamide (urea) applied to damp skin. When eczema complicates dry skin (as it often does in leprosy), a combination of 10% urea and a mild steroid is useful.

BREAST PAIN

This may occur in males who are developing gynecomastia, and is due to testosterone-estrogen imbalance, i.e. normal estrogen production by the adrenal cortex and deficient testosterone production by the damaged testes. It can be relieved by testosterone injections (*see below*).

IMPOTENCE

This is a common late complication of LL, especially if the disease was in an advanced stage when anti-leprosy treatment was instituted, or if treatment has been taken irregularly. It is due to atrophy of the *endocrine* portion of the testis. This can be suspected by finding shrunken testicles on clinical examination, and can be confirmed by finding a reduced level of testosterone in the plasma. While studies have shown that testosterone can be low to normal with elevated luteinizing hormone (LH) and/or follicle stimulating hormone (FSH) and this can be associated with signs of sexual dysfunction (decreased libido, erectile dysfunction, etc.), the measurement of testosterone is crucial for correct interpretation.[1,2] As testosterone is secreted in a pulsatile manner, two separate measurements between 7 AM and 10 AM should be taken before declaring the patient as having hypogonadism.

The treatment will depend on the testosterone levels and according to the European Male Aging Study, increased rates of lower libido and erectile dysfunction are associated with total testosterone levels <230 ng/dL (8 nmol/L) and <245 ng/dL (8.5 nmol/L), respectively.[3] Thus, administering testosterone should be dictated by its levels keeping in mind that low libido in humans is a complex interplay between excitatory and inhibitory pathways in various areas of the brain such as the amygdala, frontal cortex, hypothalamus, nucleus accumbens, and limbic systems.

Testosterone can be administered by intramuscular (IM) injections of testosterone enanthate or cypionate 75 to 100 mg weekly or 150 to 200 mg every 2 weeks respectively. Serum testosterone levels should be within the mid-normal range when measured 5 to 7 days after an injection, and the patient should be free of symptoms of androgen deficiency throughout the interval between injections. For monitoring, measure serum testosterone levels midway between injections. The optimum interval for injections varies considerably, but 10 to 17 days are usual. For oral administration, sublingual tablets containing 10 mg testosterone have been suggested two or three times a day but this is an inappropriate method of administering testosterone.[4] A monitoring protocol is given in Table 8.14. No treatment is available to correct infertility due to azoospermia.

Table 8.14: Monitoring for men on testosterone therapy

Assessment	Plan
Change in signs or symptoms	If no improvement after 3–6 months, consider discontinuing therapy
Testosterone level (for IM esters, typically check mid-cycle)	Adjust dose if needed to target the level at the mid-normal for age
Hematocrit	If hematocrit is >52–54%—withhold therapy, reduce dose or change to a different formulation; phlebotomy in extreme circumstances
Prostate-specific antigen (PSA) and digital rectal examination	If there is a suspicion for prostate cancer (PSA >4 ng/mL, increase in PSA >1.4 ng/mL within 12 months or a palpable nodule), refer to urology for evaluation
Lower urinary tract symptoms	Discontinue therapy or reduce dose if symptoms significantly worsen; refer to urology for medical or surgical management

REFERENCES

1. Guler H, Kadihasanoglu M, Aydin M, Kendirci M. Erectile dysfunction and adult onset hypogonadism in leprosy: Cross-sectional, control group study. Lepr Rev 2019;90:344–51.
2. Quyum F, Hasan M, Atiqur-Rahman M. Risk factors of testicular dysfunction in multibacillary leprosy. Lepr review 2019;90:338–43.
3. Irwig MS. How to manage men with low testosterone. Manual of endocrinology and metabolism/ [edited by] Norman Lavin Copyright © 2019 by Wolters Kluwer.https://online.vitalsource.com
4. Bhasin S, Brito JP, Cunningham GR, Hayes FJ, Hodis HN, Matsumoto AM, et al. Testosterone Therapy in Men with Hypogonadism: An Endocrine Society Clinical Practice Guideline. J Clin Endocrinol Metab 2018;103:1715–44.

CHAPTER 9

Differential Diagnosis

Pooja Arora Mrig, Kabir Sardana

While in most cases a diagnosis of leprosy is simple, if the classic lesions with hypoesthesia are present, there are situations where there can be a misdiagnosis especially in isolated lesions on the face, indeterminate cases and in pure neuritic cases. The *two signs* that may prompt the clinician to think about leprosy are:
1. Pain and/or thickening of nerves at sites of predilection as well as near chronic skin lesions.
2. Diminution or loss of either sensory (hypoesthesia) or autonomic functions (sweating and axon reflex) in suspicious skin lesions as well as in the skin areas supplied by the peripheral nerves most frequently affected by leprosy.

The disease may also often present with reactions. Leprosy does *not* affect the central nervous system; hence symptoms such as loss of reflexes, nystagmus and ataxia are absent. Also, even though the established criterion dwell on the role of slit smear, it is believed to be the weakest link in the programme. This is as finding acid-fast bacilli (AFB) in skin lesions does not by itself represent sufficient grounds for diagnosing leprosy as, in skin lesions due to environmental mycobacteria, AFB are present in variable amounts, grouped also in small masses inside macrophages (Persi et al, 1990).

To formulate a diagnosis of leprosy, a complete picture including clinical, microbiological and histopathological findings must thus be established. The pathological corroboration of clinical findings holds true *except* in type 1 reactions. Whenever a change in the immune system occurs, the clinical findings adapt to the new immunological conditions *slower* than the microbiological and histological parameters. Downgrading reactions may lead to atypical clinical pictures as well, since skin lesions usually occurring separately in different portions of the classification spectrum may be present simultaneously in the same patient.

NEUROLOGICAL CONDITIONS

Palpable Nerve Thickening *without* Anesthesia or other Signs of Nerve Damage

Excessive Muscular Development
This is generalized as in a professional wrestler, and localized as in a person accustomed to carry heavy weights on the head, with resultant thickening of great auricular nerve.[1]

Pachydermoperiostosis
A condition with generalized thickening of skin, periosteum and bone. Generalized nerve thickening was reported in the 3rd edition (1984) of this book. In addition, there

is clubbing of fingers and furrowing of the thickened skin of forehead which can easily be mistaken for the leonine facies of LL.

Palpable Nerve Thickening with/without Anesthesia or Muscle Wasting [2]

The disorders which can present with palpable nerve thickening simulating leprosy are listed in Table 9.1 and discussed below.

1. Hereditary Neuropathies

Palpable nerve thickening is seen in hereditary motor and sensory neuropathy (type 1 and type 3). These are demyelinating neuropathies which present with slowly progressive symmetric features, often with skeletal abnormalities. There is *dissociation between the paucity of symptoms and the extensive examination findings which is a typical diagnostic clue*. Diagnosis is made on the basis of mode of inheritance, phenotypic features, examination of family members and neurophysiological features.

Hereditary Motor and Sensory Neuropathy Type 1 (HMSN-1)

Inheritance: AD.

Age of presentation: First decade of life.

Symptoms: Poor motor performance, thinning of extremities, paresthesias, cramps.

Signs: Hand muscles may be affected first, while as the disease progresses lower limb is involved. Other features are distal muscle atrophy, skeletal abnormalities (hammer toes, pes cavus), graded sensory impairment and generalized areflexia with normal autonomic functions.

Nerve palpation: Generalized, smooth, uniform, non-tender nerve enlargement.

Hereditary Motor and Sensory Neuropathy Type 3 (HMSN-3)

HMSN-3 is also called Dejerine-Sottas syndrome. It is characterized by segmental demyelination of peripheral nerves, which appear *hypertrophic* as a result of concentric proliferation of Schwann cells.

Age of presentation: Infancy or childhood.

Symptoms: Delayed motor milestones, weakness and wasting of distal limbs. There is progressive symmetric weakness and deformities of lower limbs, with an equinovarus posture.

Signs: Severe sensory impairment and generalized areflexia are noted. Tendon reflexes are reduced or absent, in contrast to leprosy.

Table 9.1: Disorders with nerve thickening	
Infective	Leprosy
Hereditary	Hereditary motor and sensory neuropathy, Refsum's disease, Rud's syndrome
Immune mediated	Chronic inflammatory sensory and demyelinating polyradiculopathies
Infiltration	Neurolymphomatosis, lymphoma, leukemia, amyloidosis
Tumors of nerve or nerve sheath	Schwannoma, neurofibroma, neurofibromatosis 1 and 2

Nerve palpation: Peripheral nerves affected by the disease (ulnar, median, and common peroneal nerves) are enlarged, hard in consistency, and usually readily detectable by palpation.

Refsum's Disease

The condition is autosomal recessive and presents with ataxia, retinitis pigmentosa and hearing impairment. There is diffuse enlargement of nerves.

2. Tumors

Tumors can affect proximal as well as distal segments of nerves and are typically situated at major nerve trunks. Patient presents with gradually evolving motor and sensory dysfunction of the diseased segments. There is *pain at rest* which is a prominent feature. Electrophysiology, PET-scan and genetic testing can help in diagnosis.

3. Infiltrative Disorders

Lymphomas, leukemias and amyloidosis can be associated with palpable nerve thickening. The term 'Neurolymphomatosis' denotes diffuse infiltration of peripheral and cranial nerves, nerve plexuses or roots by neoplastic cells in patients with hematological malignancy. Diffuse infiltrative lymphocytosis syndrome is a hyper-immune reaction to HIV that infiltrates nerves to produce neurological deficits.

4. Primary Amyloidosis of Peripheral Nerves[3]

An inherited disease which begins insidiously in second or third decades and usually affects lower limbs, with impaired sensation, muscle wasting and dropped foot. Late effects are loss of tendon reflexes and trophic ulceration of feet.

Regional Anesthesia with or without Muscle Wasting but *without* Palpable Nerve Thickening

1. Syringomyelia

Anesthesia and muscle wasting develop in upper or lower limbs depending on the localization of the cord lesion. There is dissociated anesthesia (loss of pain and temperature sensation with preservation of touch) and tendon reflexes are diminished or lost. The histamine test is positive.

2. Tabes

Dysfunction of posterior nerve roots causes difficulty in walking due to loss of sensation and of position sense, and the patient has a broad-based stamping gait. Plantar ulceration is a later development. Eyes should be examined for Argyll-Robertson pupils, and CSF for syphilitic changes.

3. Peripheral Neuropathy

A mononeuropathy can result from compression of nerve or nerve plexus and may simulate pure neural leprosy, e.g. cubital tunnel compression syndrome, carpal tunnel syndrome, cervical rib and meralgia paresthetica causing sensory changes in one or both thighs.

Multiple neuropathy has a large number of causes, some of which (like diabetes) result in plantar ulceration. Depression of histamine flare in anesthetic skin is *similar* to that in leprosy, but there are *no* thickened nerves and tendon reflexes are likely to be lost.[4] The common causes of peripheral neuropathy are listed below:

HIV: Slowly progressive weakness of the distal muscles with hyporeflexia. Sometimes there may be an acute onset.

SLE: Systemic lupus erythematosus may affect peripheral nerves. The initial mononeuropathy may evolve towards polyneuropathy, where 'glove' or 'stocking' anesthesia may occur. Motor weakness is not commonly seen.

Polyarteritis nodosa (PAN): The presence of nodules with systemic features like fever, articular and abdominal pains with the presence of symmetrical polyneuropathy and slight sensory deficit, specially in the lower limbs, is suggestive of PAN though ENL is a common differential.

Sarcoidosis: While this disorder may have protean manifestations, the neuropathy is asymmetric with hypertrophic infiltration and compression of cranial nerves and, more rarely, of the radial and ulnar nerves.

Diabetic neuropathy: There is co-existent long-standing diabetes. Patients present with paresthesias and pain in the lower limbs and loss of Achilles' reflex in advanced stages. Also, 'glove' and 'stocking' anesthesia is seen with impairment of sweating and loss of vasomotor control with trophic ulcers seen on the metatarsus bones (Fig. 9.1).

Alcoholic polyneuropathy: Early symptoms are paresthesias and severe pain in the extremities. At later stages there is anesthesia displaying a 'stocking' and 'glove' distribution. The *unique* feature is the *concomitant* presence of pain and anesthesia. In *some* cases, tendon reflexes are absent, distal motor palsy may be seen, damage to autonomic fibers may occur and in late stages progressive encephalopathy is present.

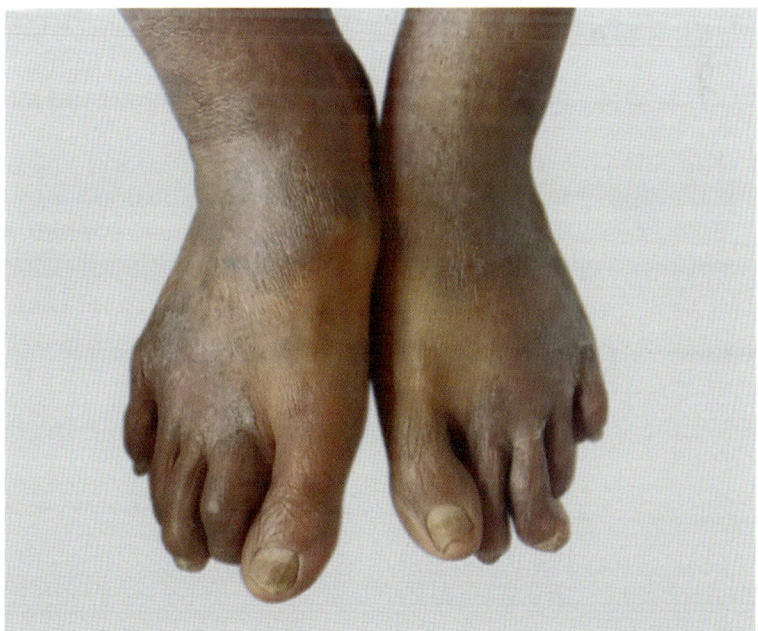

Fig. 9.1: A case of diabetes mellitus with trophic changes, dry skin and atrophic wrinkled skin

4. Hereditary Sensory Radicular Neuropathy

Loss of sensation and sweating is most severe in lower limbs, but muscular coordination is normal (vis-à-vis tabes). Chronic painless plantar ulceration is classical, together with hightone deafness. Loss of ankle jerks is usual, and X-rays of feet reveal bone changes similar to those in leprosy.

5. Congenital Indifference to Pain[5]

This is seen in children who are mentally normal. Bone changes closely simulate those of leprosy, particularly absorption of terminal phalanges of fingers and tarsal bone disintegration. Histamine test is positive.

6. Hysteria

Caution should be observed in making this diagnosis, for the original authors have treated two leprosy patients who had earlier consulted physicians in London because of regional anesthesia and had been considered hysterical. A histamine test at that time would have been negative, thus making a diagnosis of hysteria untenable.

DERMATOLOGICAL CONDITIONS

In the conditions *described* in this section the reader can assume, for it will not be stated, that there is *no* sensory loss, there are *no* thickened nerves and skin smears are *negative* for AFB. In the few instances where this rule is broken, the deviation will be recorded. Histology is not mentioned, but it goes without stating that it is essential for diagnosis in many of these dermatoses.

Lesions which are Flat and Hypopigmented

- The hypochromic macules seen in leprosy are either indeterminate leprosy or are seen in the hyperergic and paucibacillary forms of the disease. They are single or few, and usually arranged in a unilateral and asymmetric arrangement.
- Here it must be appreciated that in leprosy both erythematous and hyperchromic macules have been defined. In fact, hyperpigmented macules can also be seen and are a residual mark of cutaneous involvement in leprosy. The case history, along with the possible presence of active leprosy lesions, can clarify the diagnosis. Some cases of tuberculoid leprosy have been reported as 'primary hyperchromic' on account of the successful therapeutic response (Chattopadhyay and Gupta, 1988).[6]

1. Morphea (Localized Scleroderma)

A white plaque which may be slightly raised in parts, the edge often purple, hair growth and sweating are lost in the lesion, and when sclerosis is marked there is some sensory loss (Fig. 9.2).

2. Pityriasis Alba[7]

The circular or oval macules with fine scales (Fig. 9.3) are most readily noticed in children with dark skin. They are usually seen in atopic patients with dry skin and while they initially present as erythematous lesions, they leave a hypopigmented macule with a dried surface and occasionally fine scaling. They are usually multiple,

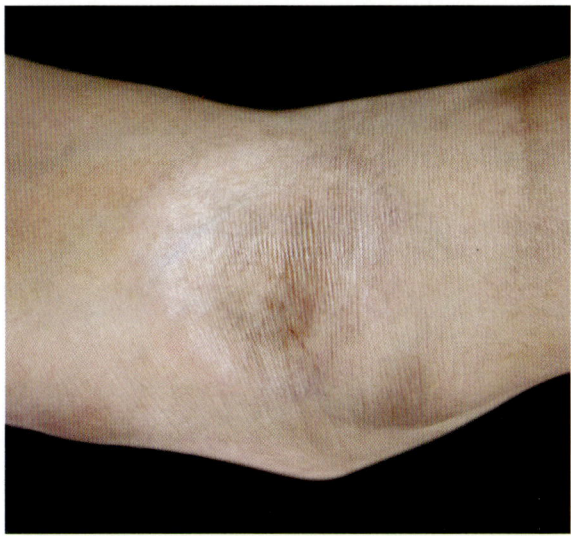

Fig. 9.2: A case of morphea with a depressed plaque and a vivid lilac border

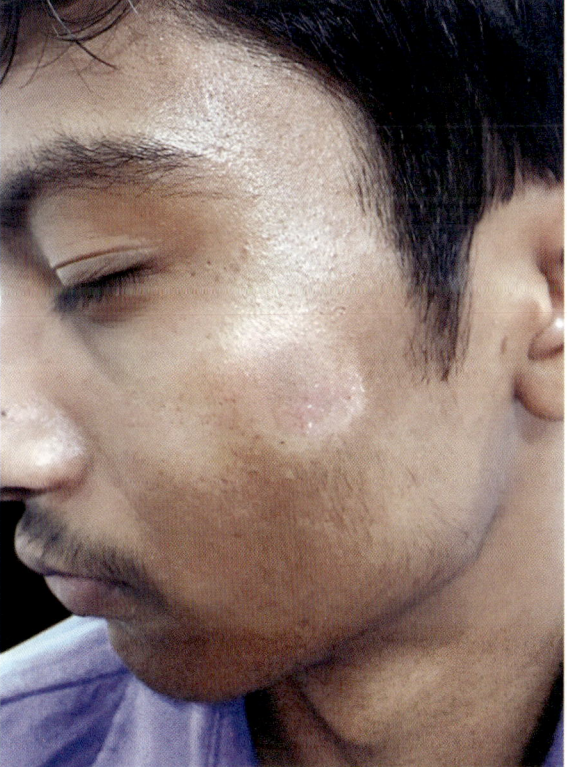

Fig. 9.3: Pityriasis alba

principally affect the face, and tend to disappear as the child grows older. Pityriasis alba may resemble indeterminate leprosy and tacrolimus is an effective option for its treatment.[8]

3. Pityriasis Versicolor[9]

Readily seen in dark skins (or in sun-tanned light skins) and favoring skin covered by clothes. Widespread involvement of the lower extremities or face should raise concern for an immunosuppressive state such as HIV. It is caused by the fungus *Pityrosporum orbiculare* that can be demonstrated in skin scrapings. The macules may appear brownish. The fine branny scaling and the finding of fungal hyphae in skin scales confirms the diagnosis (Fig. 9.4a to c). Also the lesions fluoresce under Wood's light.

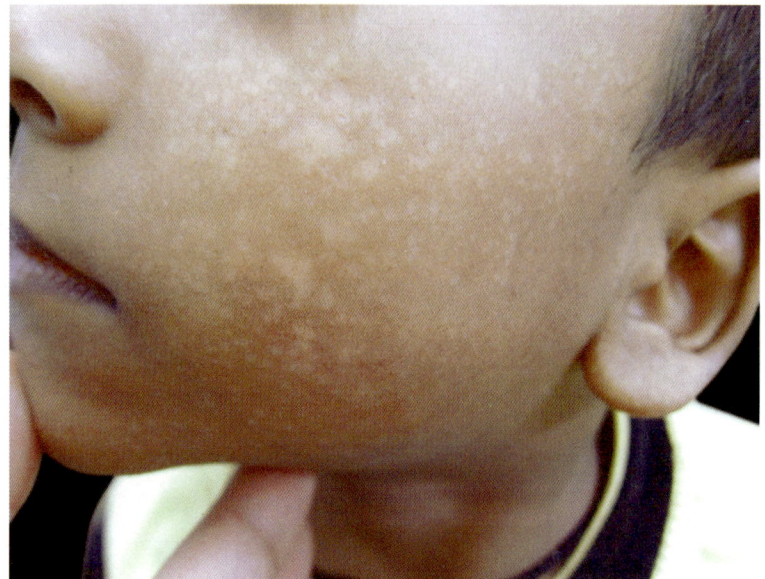

Fig. 9.4a: Scaly macules on the face in a child with pityriasis versicolor

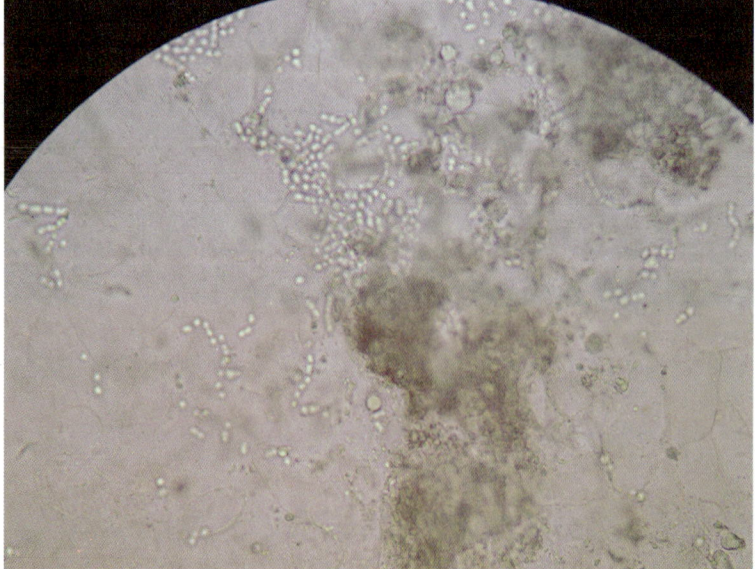

Fig. 9.4b: A KOH scraping from the patient above reveals the dimorphic morphology

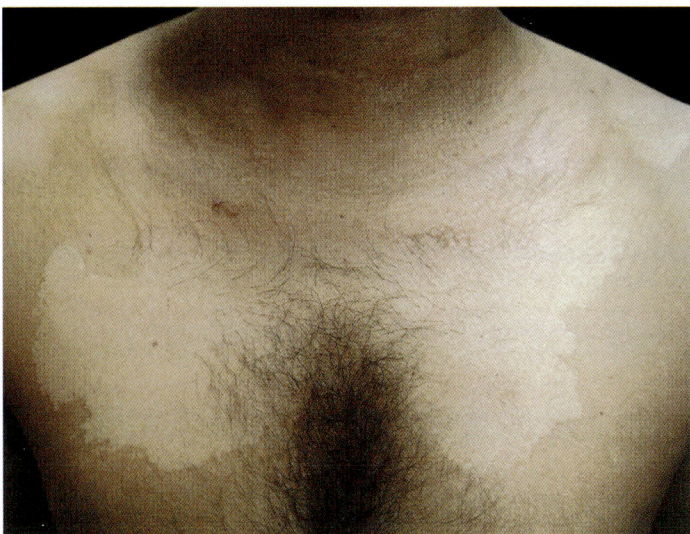

Fig. 9.4c: Pityriasis versicolor with truncal involvement which usually heals with transient pigmentary loss

4. Post-kala-azar Dermal Leishmaniasis (PKDL)[10]

Although kala-azar (visceral leishmaniasis) has a very wide distribution, this late development is largely confined to the Indian subcontinent and to East Africa.[11]

The macular phenotype can occur in either region but is more common with the Indian variant. Classically, macular PKDL presents with prominent perioral hypopigmented macules that coalesce to form well demarcated, irregular patches. The patches then spread over the malar region, followed by the forehead and scalp and then appear on trunk and limbs (Fig. 9.5). In addition, there may be erythematous

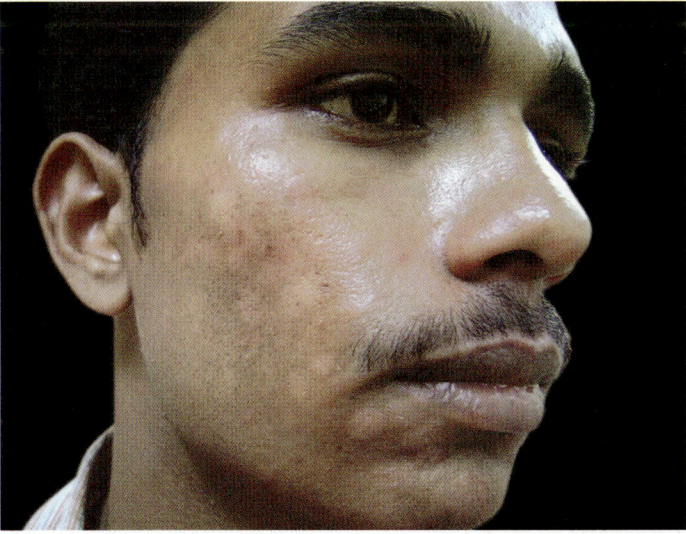

Fig. 9.5: Perioral macules with a perceptible erythema in a case of post-kala-azar dermal leishmaniasis

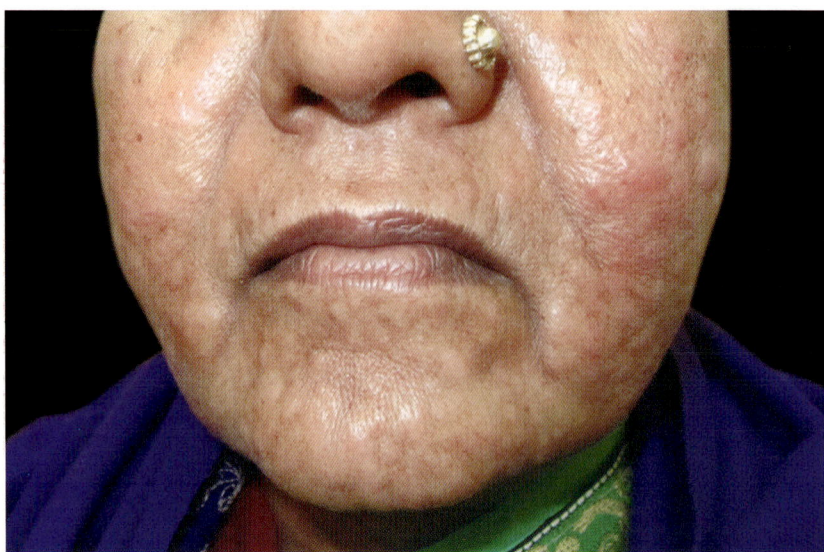

Fig. 9.6: Post-kala-azar dermal leishmaniasis: An admixture of nodules, papules and macules in the perioral area

papules and nodules on face (Fig. 9.6), less commonly elsewhere. These appear later in course of disease. There may also be facial erythema with a 'butterfly' distribution over nose and cheeks. Leishman-Donovan (L-D) bodies are present in skin biopsy.

The macular lesions of PKDL can be mistaken for macular lesions of borderline or lepromatous leprosy.[12] The arrangement in PKDL however is bilateral and often symmetric and this may by itself exclude the diagnosis of leprosy since hypochromic lesions occurring in leprosy uncommonly exhibit symmetric and bilateral distribution. Uncommonly both leprosy and PKDL can be seen in the same patient.[13]

5. Yaws

A non-venereal tropical disease caused by *Treponema pertenue*. Depigmentation is a late development and is mainly confined to hairless areas of arms and tends to be bilaterally symmetrical. It occurs chiefly in adults over 30, and other signs include hyperkeratosis of palms and soles, juxta-articular nodes, gangosa, and sabre tibiae. Serological tests are positive as for syphilis.

6. Onchocerciasis

A filarial infection confined to Africa, Central America and the Arabian peninsula. Depigmentation is usually confined to the pretibial regions of both legs, but may affect groins and buttocks. Sensory impairment is absent and microfilariae can be demonstrated in skin snips.

7. Vitiligo

There is depigmentation (achromia) rather than hypopigmentation, and hair growing in the macules may be achromic. Lesions are multiple and of varying sizes and shapes, there are no thickened nerves and the histamine test is normal (Fig. 9.7a).

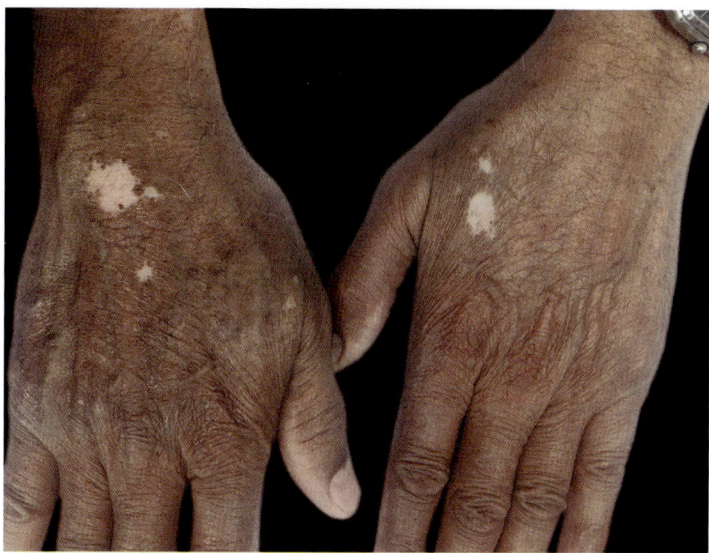

Fig. 9.7a: Vitiligo: The patient presented with milky white macules over dorsa of both hands

8. Chronic Arsenic Exposure (Arsenicosis)[14]

The pigmentary change can take the form of diffuse pigmentation, fine freckle-like spotty pigmentation (raindrop pigmentation) or macular areas of depigmentation on normal/hyperpigmented skin (leukomelanosis) (Fig. 9.7b). Mucous membrane (undersurface of the tongue or buccal mucosa) may also be involved by blotchy pigmentation. Arsenical hyperkeratosis symmetrically affects the palms and soles and can range from minute papules (<2 mm) giving gritty sensation (mild form), punctate wart-like papules of 2–5 mm (moderate form) or diffuse hyperkeratosis (severe form) (Fig. 9.7c). Malignant change is the major cause of morbidity and mortality associated

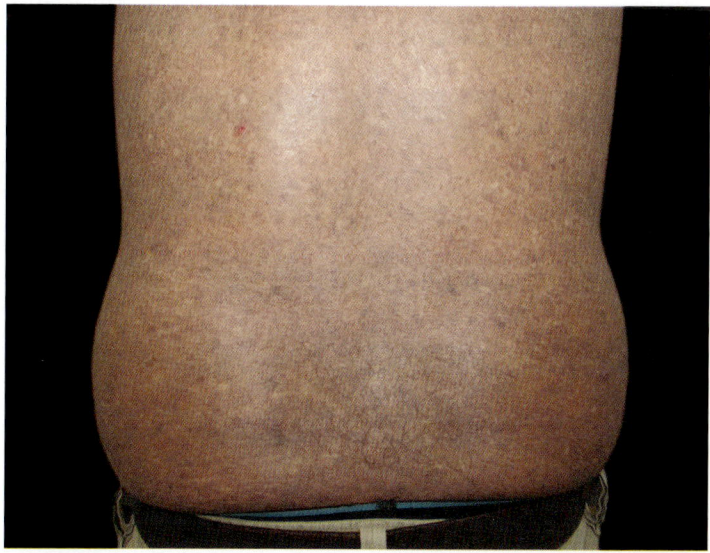

Fig. 9.7b: A patient with raindrop pigmentation consequent to intake of an Ayurvedic medicine

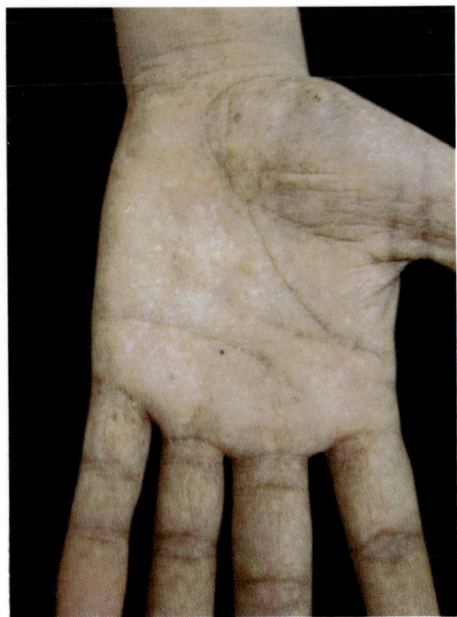

Fig. 9.7c: Chronic arsenic exposure presenting as punctate keratoses of the palms

with chronic arsenicosis and involves skin (Bowen's disease, squamous cell carcinoma, and basal cell epithelioma), lung, bladder, kidney, prostate, liver, uterus, and sometimes lymphatic tissues.

9. Chemical-induced Vitiligo

This is indistinguishable from non-chemically-induced vitiligo both clinically and histologically and results from activation of melanocyte autoimmunity by certain chemicals which include occupational as well as household use products (Fig. 9.8a and b). Hypopigmented and depigmented macules occur that simulate leprosy. However, sensation and sweat function are normal.

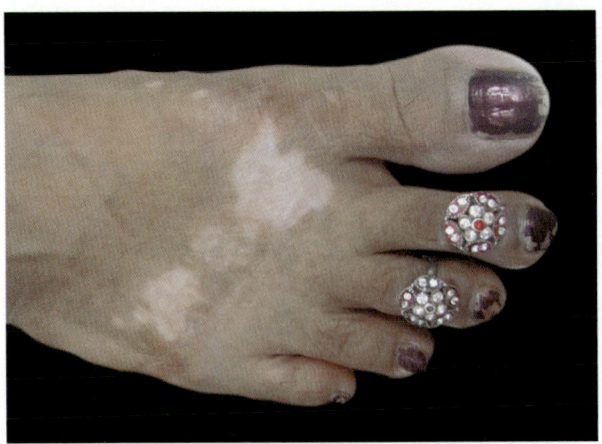

Fig. 9.8a: Chemical-induced vitiligo resulting from and following the pattern of the footwear straps

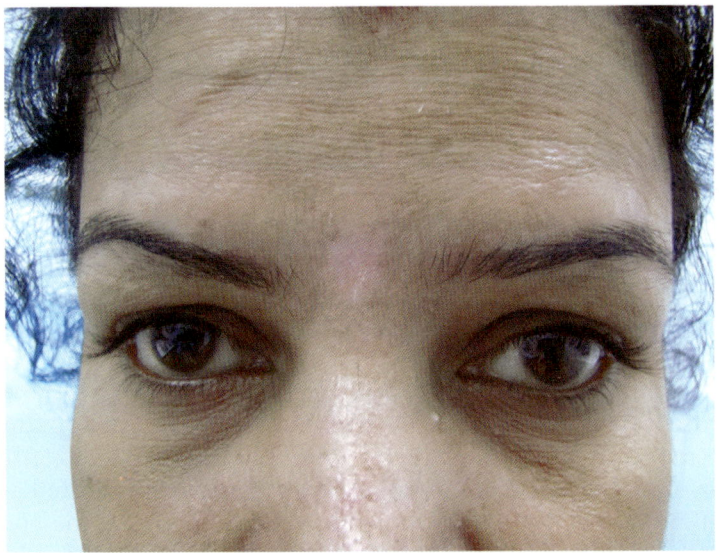

Fig. 9.8b: Chemical-induced vitiligo due to bindi sticker

10. *Nevus Depigmentosus*

It presents as a well-circumscribed hypopigmented macule that is irregularly shaped with serrated borders (Fig. 9.8c). The lesions usually appear at birth but may not be apparent then. They do not cross the midline and remain stable throughout life.

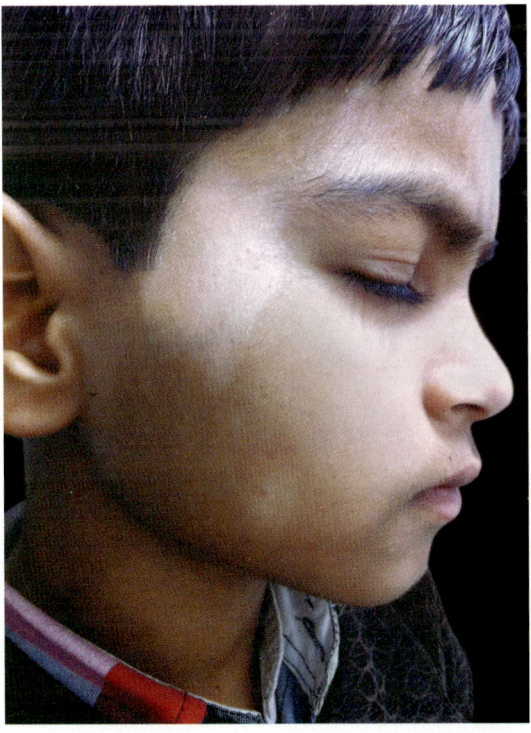

Fig. 9.8c: Nevus depigmentosus

11. Post-inflammatory Hypopigmentation (PIH)[15]

Many conditions resolve with hypomelanotic lesions, especially in skin of color patient, and may be mistaken for leprosy if adequate history is not taken (Fig. 9.9a). These include eczema, psoriasis, pityriasis lichenoides, pityriasis versicolor and sarcoidosis. Low-grade inflammation may occasionally be clinically undetectable, especially in dark skin and pityriasis alba is possibly the commonest cause of PIH closely followed by seborrheic dermatitis.[16]

Chronic sarcoidosis should be suspected in young adults of Scandinavian or African American descent with hypopigmented macules, patches or plaques, typically on the extremities, that are associated with systemic abnormalities.

12. Progressive Macular Hypomelanosis (PMH)[17]

This typically occurs in young *females*, presenting as *asymmetric*, hypopigmented, poorly demarcated, smooth macules or patches (Fig. 9.9b). However, we have seen the condition even in males (Fig. 9.9c). While *P. acnes* has been implicated as a cause, this is still not definite as therapy for *P. acnes* does not ameliorate the condition.[18] The classical site of involvement is the mid-lumbar region followed by the abdominal area. The face is notably spared.

13. Hypopigmented Mycosis Fungoides[19, 20]

Hypopigmented mycosis fungoides (HMF) is insidious in onset with a predilection for darkly pigmented skin, and in contrast to the classic MF, is seen in children or young adults. The hypopigmented or depigmented patches can have scaling and mainly

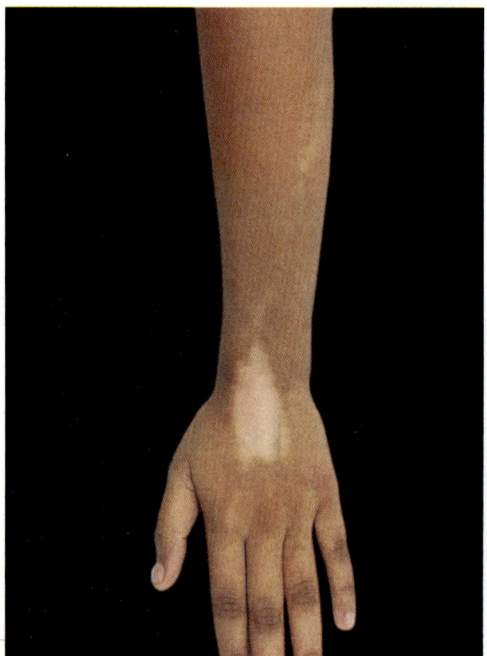
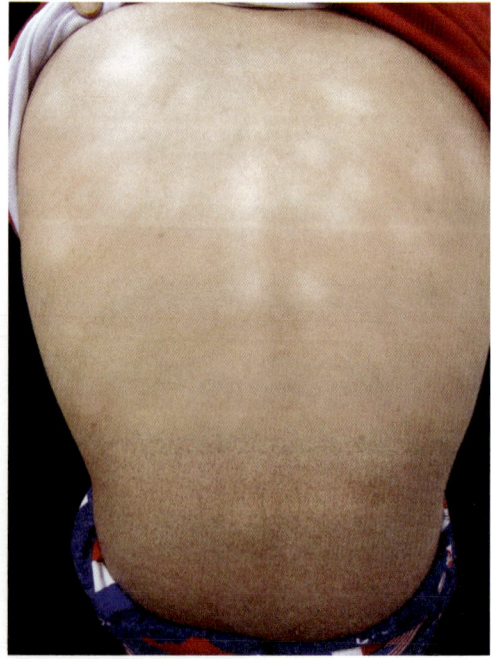

Fig. 9.9a: A young boy with post-inflammatory hypopigmentation secondary to intralesional steroid use (aka perilymphatic atrophy of skin)

Fig. 9.9b: Progressive macular hypomelanosis in a young female

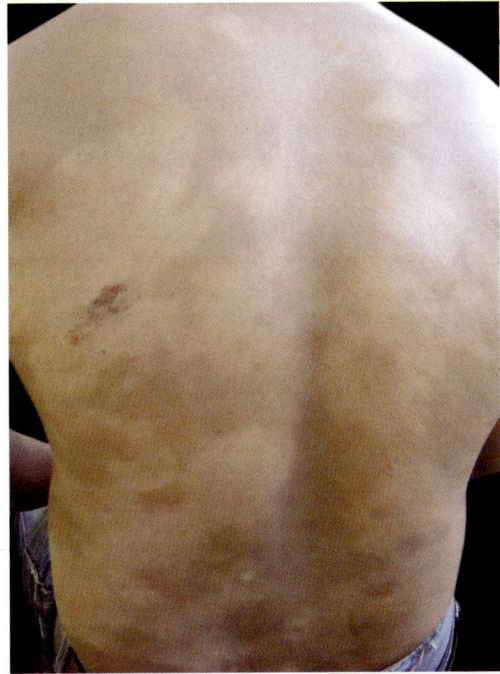

Fig. 9.9c: Progressive macular hypomelanosis with lesions in the mid-lumbar area. PMH involves the abdominal region in about 40% of cases; the face is rarely involved

involve the trunk and inner thighs, classically hip/gluteal region (Fig. 9.10). In skin of color, the lesions usually have a greyish or silver hue and both hyperpigmentation and hypopigmentation may be present, often at the same time. The diagnosis frequently requires obtaining multiple biopsy specimens, which should be obtained from steroid naïve sites.

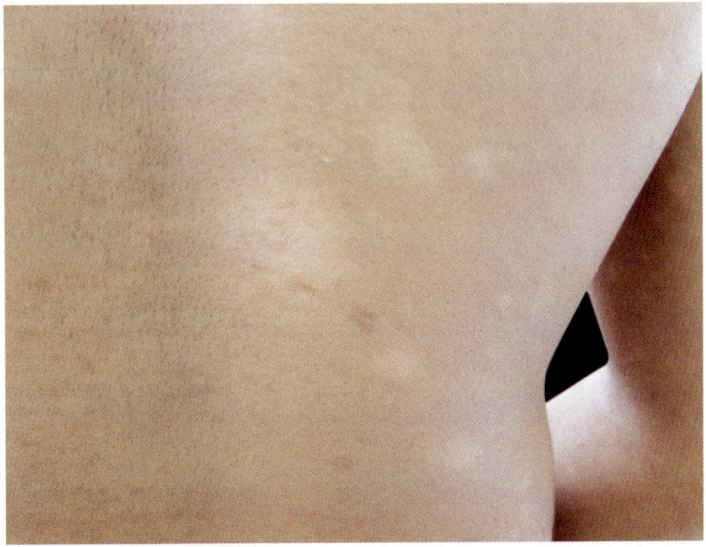

Fig. 9.10: Hypopigmented mycosis fungoides resembling lepromatous leprosy

Lesions which are Raised

Ring-shaped and circinate lesions with erythematous edges may be present in either paucibacillary leprosy (TT, BT) or in multibacillary forms belonging to the central part of the spectrum (BB). Paucibacillary lesions are anesthetic, asymmetrically arranged and may have raised edges, whereas multibacillary lesions are symmetrically arranged. In the paucibacillary portion of the spectrum, plaques may take on a well-marked and ring-shaped appearance due to central healing. In leprosy the *annular* appearance may be the result of immune areas surrounded by affected skin. In active leprosy, the *absence* of desquamation and vesiculation, together with lack of itching, allow us to exclude many skin pathologies.

Note that in the list below, numbers 4 and 18 lesions may be flat (macular), and in number 11 they may be anesthetic.

1. Follicular Mucinosis (Alopecia Mucinosa)[21, 22]

Skin-colored or erythematous plaques favor scalp, face, neck, shoulders and limbs (Fig. 9.11a). Lesions are scaly and without hair (alopecia), but hair follicles are prominent.

2. Granuloma Annulare

It chiefly affects children and young adults. The typical lesion consists of erythematous or skin-colored papules arranged in rings, and may be single or multiple (Fig. 9.11b to d). The site is commonly on extremities, and lesions run a chronic course, sometimes disappearing and later reappearing. A disseminated form is less common—consisting of papulonodules over trunk and limbs.

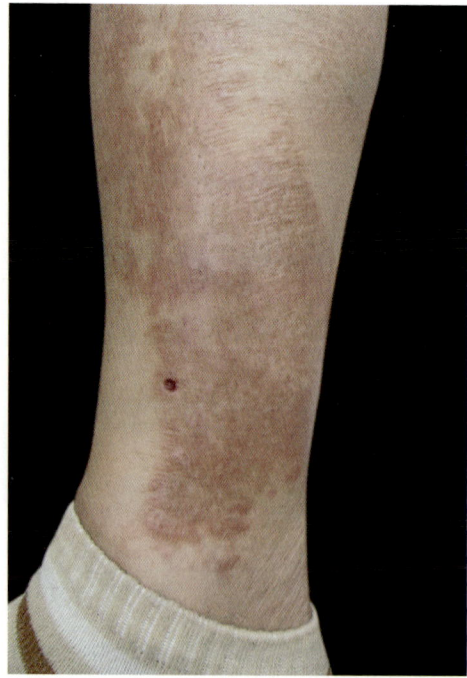

Fig. 9.11a: A plaque of mucinosis on the leg of a young girl

Differential Diagnosis

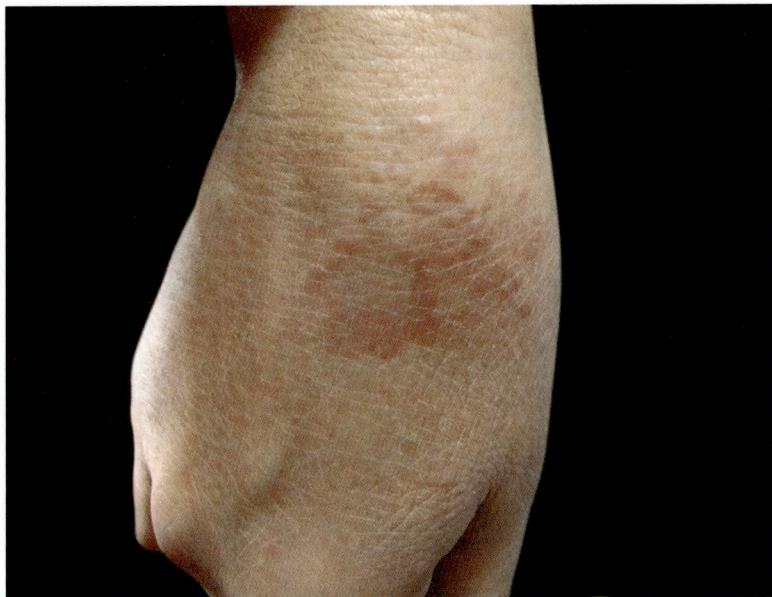

Fig. 9.11b: Granuloma annulare on the dorsum of hand

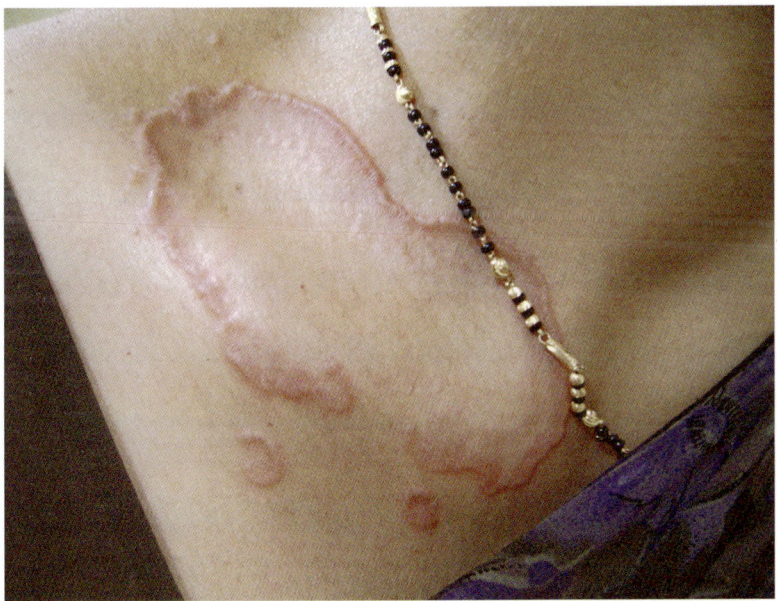

Fig. 9.11c: Arcuate annular lesions of granuloma annulare

3. Granuloma Multiforme[23]

This chronic dermatosis was first described in Nigeria, but has since been reported in other parts of tropical Africa. It has also been found in a region of Indonesia.[24] It chiefly affects adults over 40, and is never seen in children. Plaques closely simulate TT in appearance, but lesions irritate and sometimes new lesions appear while old ones subside.

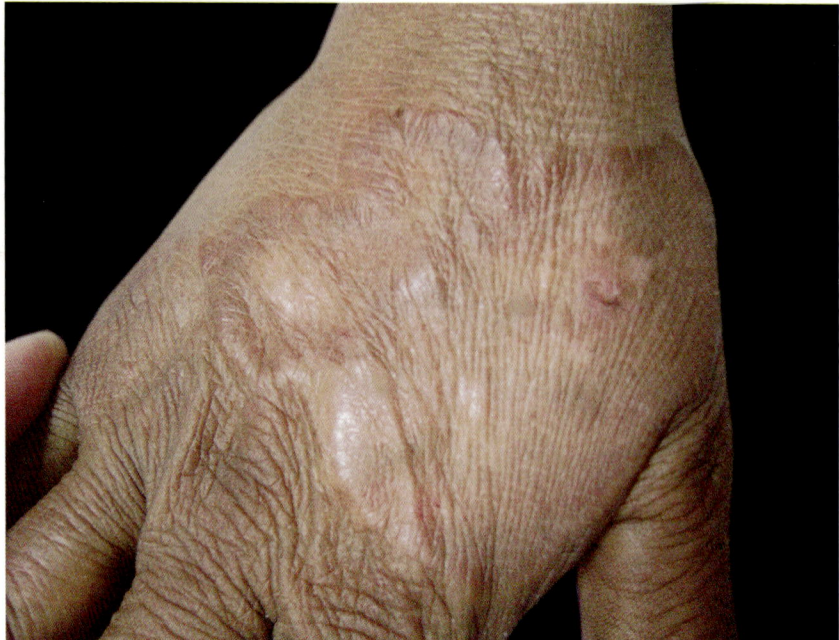

Fig. 9.11d: Granuloma annulare: Annular plaque breaking open laterally

4. *Gyrate Erythema*[25]

a. *Erythema marginatum (EM):* Macular or slightly elevated annular lesions with pink or red borders and complicating rheumatic fever, trypanosomiasis, serum sickness, or streptococcal endocarditis.

b. *Erythema chronicum migrans (ECM):* This is the first stage of Lyme disease,[26] a spirochetal infection resulting from the bite of a tick of the genus Ixodes. Within days of the tick bite, a small red plaque appears at the site and extends peripherally to become an erythematous annular lesion which may persist for months and attain a large size. Secondary lesions may appear at various sites, and the patient complains of headache and neck pains.

c. *Erythema gyratum repens (EGR):* This is always associated with an underlying malignancy and presents as multiple, macular, serpiginous bands of erythema which migrate. Pruritus is common.

d. *Erythema annulare centrifugum (EAC):* Cause is unclear, but in some cases, a hypersensitivity reaction to tinea infection is suspected. It usually affects young- and middle-aged adults who develop annular lesions with raised erythematous borders (Fig. 9.12a and b). These persist for weeks or months, and tend to recur over the years. Azithromycin has been known to be a useful therapeutic modality.[27]

5. *Kaposi's Sarcoma (Classical)*

Etiology not fully determined. In Africa, it affects all ages and males predominantly, and presents with nodules (Fig. 9.13a) and chronic edema of affected limbs. Feet and lower legs are usually involved bilaterally, and legs feel hard on palpation, as in neglected LL. Edema of legs may be the first manifestation (compare LL).

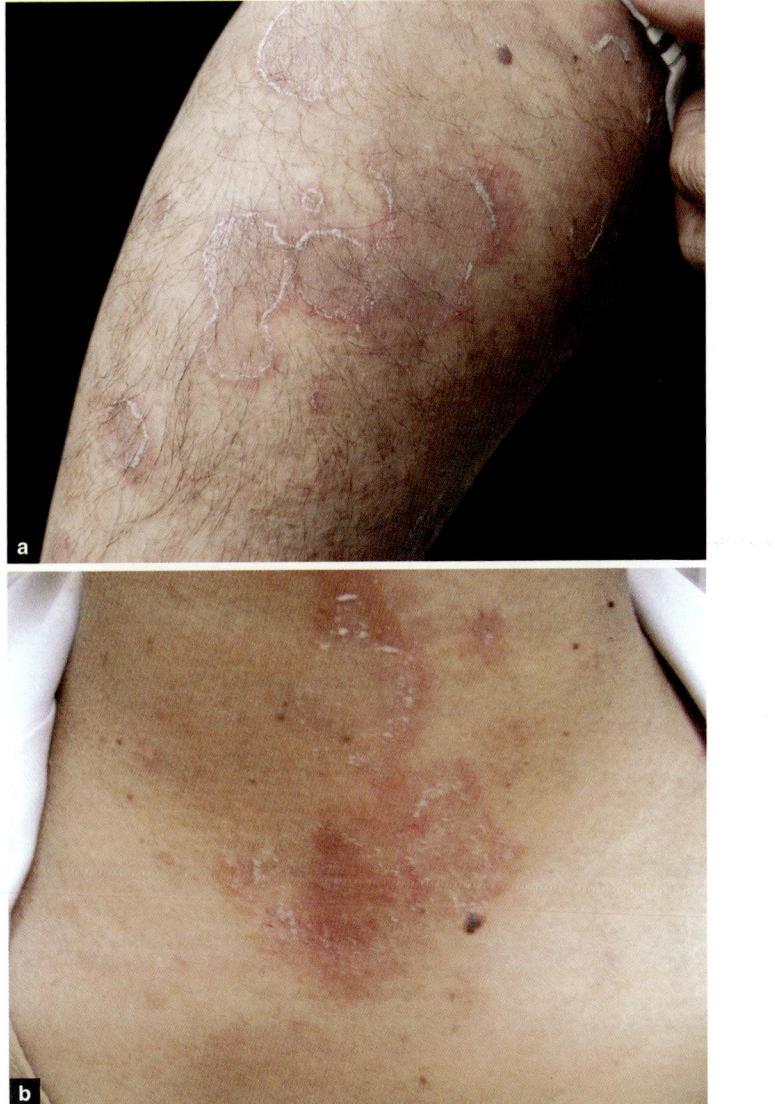

Fig. 9.12a and b: Erythema annulare centrifugum: Note the trailing scale on the inner border

6. Cutaneous Leishmaniasis

Early nodular lesions may simulate LL, but smears contain L-D bodies and not *M. leprae*. The type of cutaneous leishmaniasis most likely to be confused with LL is the disseminated anergic form, for nodules are numerous and simulate those of LL but are teeming with L-D bodies.

7. Lupus Erythematosus

The chronic localized or discoid form usually affects women of 30–50 years of age. The round or oval plaques have a scaly surface and a predilection for face, ears and scalp (Fig. 9.13b). A 'butterfly' erythema of face is common. Whitish patches with red margins may appear on the buccal mucosa, and lesions on lips look like dried collodion.

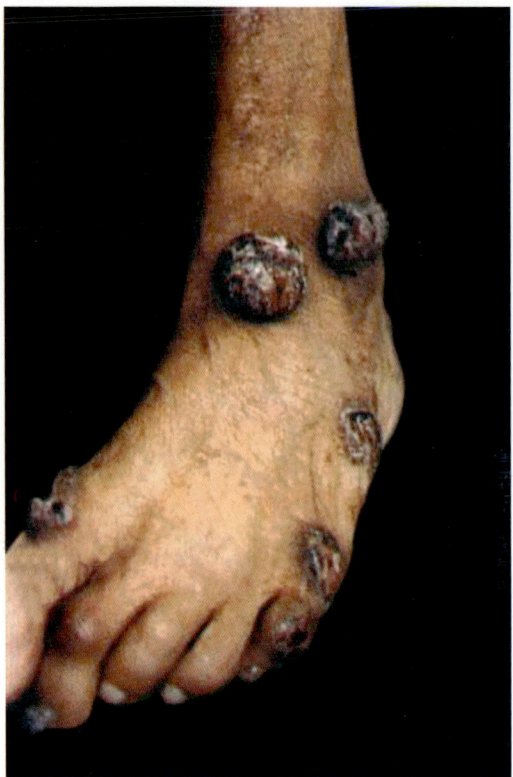

Fig. 9.13a: Kaposi sarcoma (Clin Exp Dermatol 2006;31:232-4)

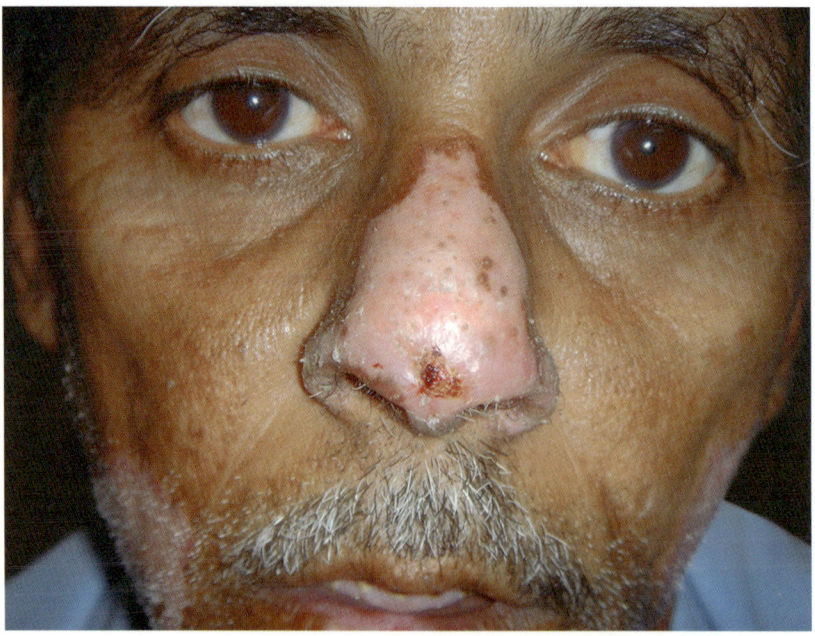

Fig. 9.13b: A plaque of discoid lupus erythematosus with follicular plugging, pigmented border and loss of pigment

8. Lupus Vulgaris

Commences as a papule which coalesces with neighboring papules to form a plaque, which is yellowish-red and irregular in shape (Fig. 9.14) (due to blanching of the vessels). The lesion becomes white when a glass slide is pressed on it, and the papules then appear as brown 'apple-jelly' spots. Occasionally, especially if the lesion is on the face, there can be a problem in diagnosis as hypoesthesia is not seen in leprosy lesions on the face and nor are the nerves consistently enlarged in this location. In this case, histological differentiation can be made from TT by the normal appearance of cutaneous nerves and caseation. If a therapeutic challenge is offered with anti-tubercular treatment a failure to respond in 6 weeks is a reliable tool in endemic areas to rule out TB.[28]

9. Mycobacterium marinum Infection ('Swimming Pool' or 'Fish Tank' Granuloma)

This is a local infection after a superficial skin injury by *M. marinum*, an acid-fast Mycobacterium which is sen in water of swimming pools or fish tanks.

Usually presents as a solitary erythematous nodule or plaque, sometimes becoming ulcerated and crusted. A skin smear from the lesion may contain AFB similar in appearance to *M. leprae*, but the organism can be cultured on a suitable medium. A skin test using purified protein derivative (PPD) from *M. marinum* is positive.

10. Mycosis Fungoides[19]

Patches of mycosis fungoides are characterized by variably large, erythematous, finely scaling lesions and can be generalized or localized and when localized, there is often a predilection for the buttocks and other *sun-protected areas* (Fig. 9.15). Scaling is variable and may also depend on previous local treatment. Loss of elastic fibers and atrophy of the epidermis may lead to a wrinkled appearance.

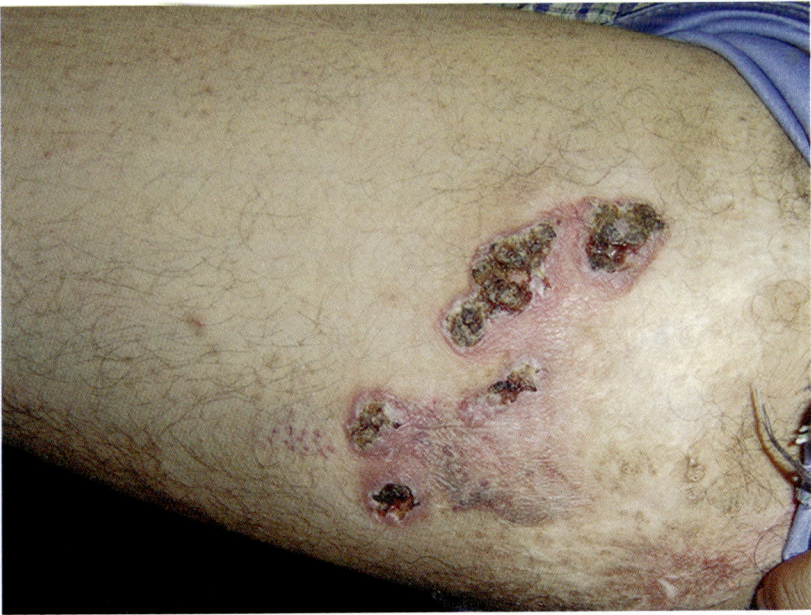

Fig. 9.14: A case of lupus vulgaris with a plaque showing activity at one edge and resolution at the other

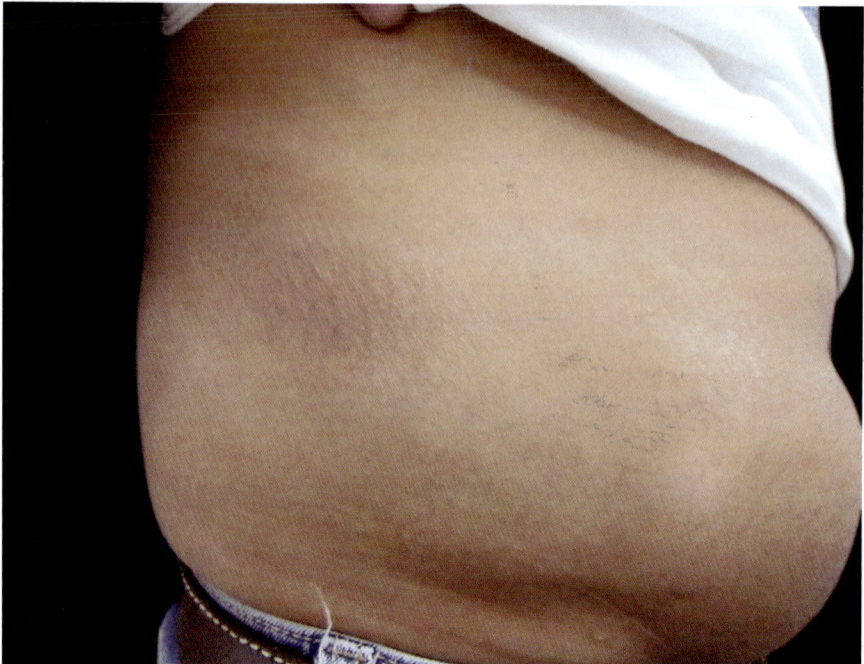

Fig. 9.15: Mycosis fungoides: Multiple plaques with atrophy marked by wrinkling of the superficial surface

Plaques of mycosis fungoides are characterized by infiltrated, variably scaling and reddish-brown lesions. Ulceration may be present but it is usually confined to a portion of the lesion; in some cases superficial crusts may lead to an impetiginized appearance.

11. Necrobiosis Lipoidica

Even though about 70% of patients have diabetes, the precise relationship of these two conditions is unclear. Dull red plaques appear, usually on anterior aspects of lower legs, slowly expanding and coalescing with other lesions to form annular or serpiginous lesions with central depigmentation and brown-red margins (Fig. 9.16). Mann and Harman have stressed the high incidence of anesthetic lesions.[29]

12. Atypical Necrobiosis of Face[30]

This occurs in adult females who are not diabetic. The annular lesions resemble borderline leprosy, but scalp is commonly involved and is diagnostic.

13. Neurofibromatosis

A congenital disorder. Nodules and oval *café au lait* (coffee colored) macules may well simulate LL. Nodules vary in size but are predominantly small (Fig. 9.17); they also vary in color and in consistency on palpation. Whereas the macules tend to appear in infancy, nodules usually appear at puberty. Bilateral and symmetrical nerve thickening has been reported[31] and there have been several reports of neurofibromatosis in association with leprosy.[32]

Differential Diagnosis

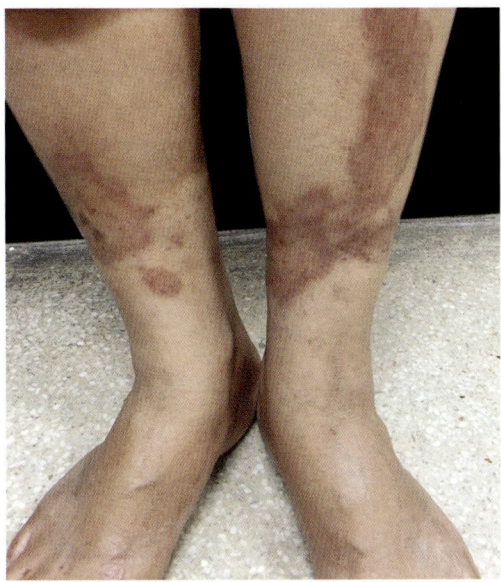

Fig. 9.16: Necrobiosis lipoidica: Depressed plaques with central hypopigmentation

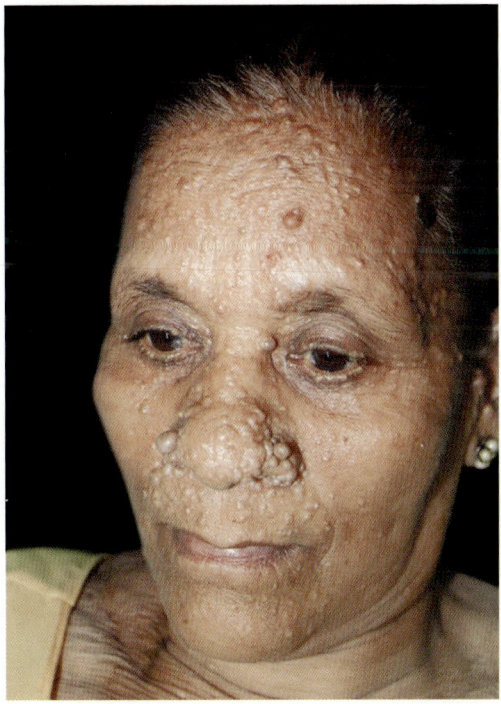

Fig. 9.17: Multiple neurofibromas on the face in a patient with neurofibromatosis

14. Pityriasis Rosea

It presents with many oval, rose-pink, slightly raised lesions with scaly surface and well defined edges, characteristically on trunk and upper half of arms and legs (Fig. 9.18). Look for the 'herald patch'. Lesions disappear spontaneously in 6–10 weeks.

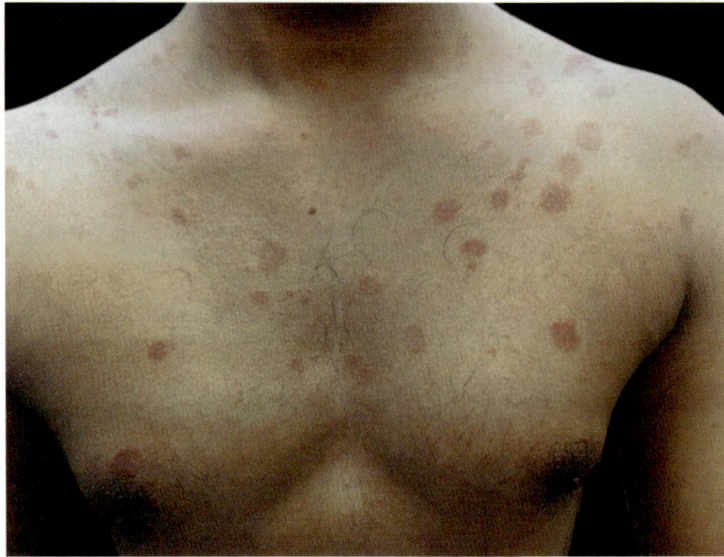

Fig. 9.18: Pityriasis rosea

15. *Psoriasis*

Well demarcated, scaly, dull red plaques simulate scaly TT, but lesions are too numerous and involve regions such as scalp and flexures which are spared in leprosy (Fig. 9.19). Fingernails may be involved.

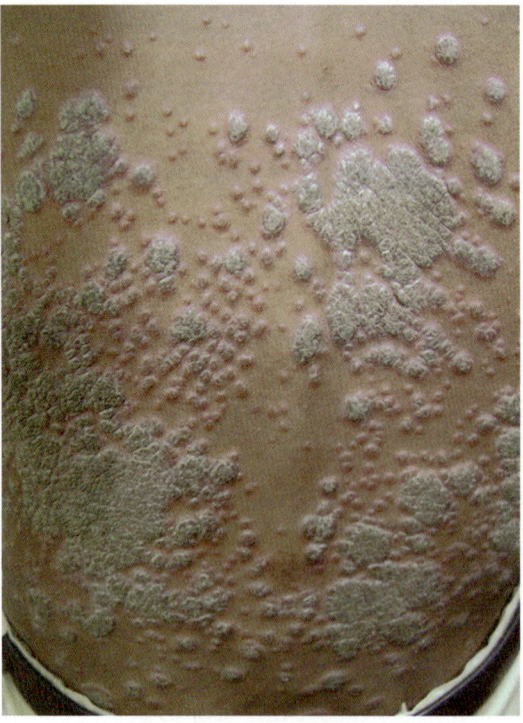

Fig. 9.19: Papulosquamous lesions of psoriasis vulgaris

16. Sarcoidosis[33]

Onset is usually in the 4th to 5th decades, and every type of leprosy lesion can be mimicked by sarcoidosis, but it is the plaque form which most commonly causes confusion (Fig. 9.20a). In fact, sarcoidosis can mimic another granulomatous disorder—lupus vulgaris (Fig. 9.20b).[34] Peripheral neuritis may add to this confusion, as may bone changes in hands and feet, the complication of uveitis (iridocyclitis), and the fact that skin lesions in both diseases may develop in scars.

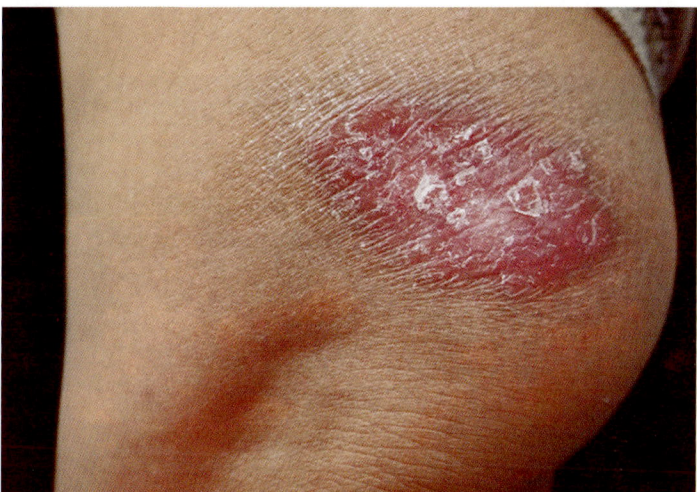

Fig. 9.20a: Psoriasiform variant of sarcoidosis

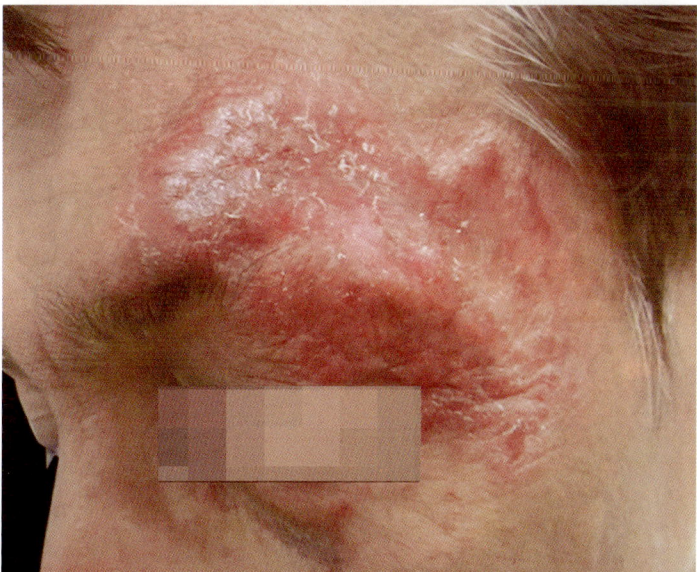

Fig. 9.20b: An erythematous plaque with central atrophy and depigmentation; showed granulomatous pathology on biopsy. The patient was treated with anti-tubercular treatment to which the lesion did not respond. Later, a diagnosis of sarcoidosis was considered and a course of systemic steroids given, which led to complete resolution. (*Courtesy*: Arora P. Dermatol Ther. 2019;32:e12968.)

17. Acquired Syphilis[35]

The brownish-red maculopapular syphilides (Fig. 9.21) of secondary syphilis, and the nodulosquamous syphilides of tertiary syphilis may be confused with leprosy, especially gummatous involvement of tongue and oral mucosa with perforation of palate, but *T. pallidum* hemagglutination assay test is positive.

18. Tinea Corporis (Tinea Circinata)

Ringworm infection of annular or plaque type may resemble leprosy, but skin scales contain the causative fungus (Fig. 9.22).

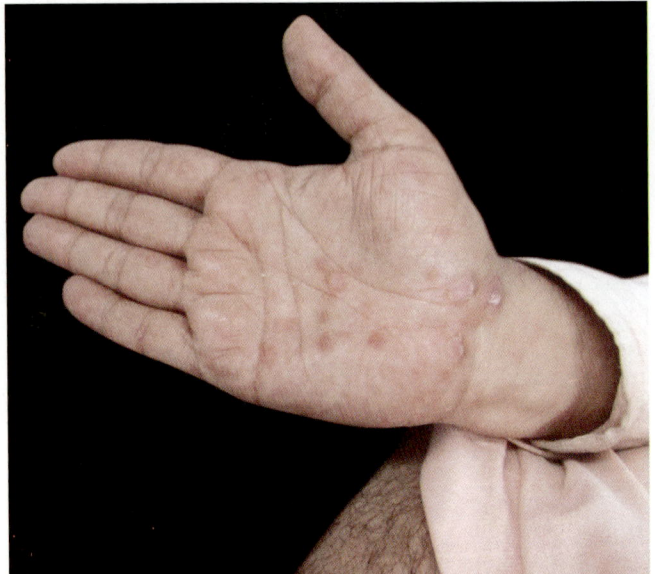

Fig. 9.21: Secondary syphilis: Erythematous to hyperpigmented plaques on the palm

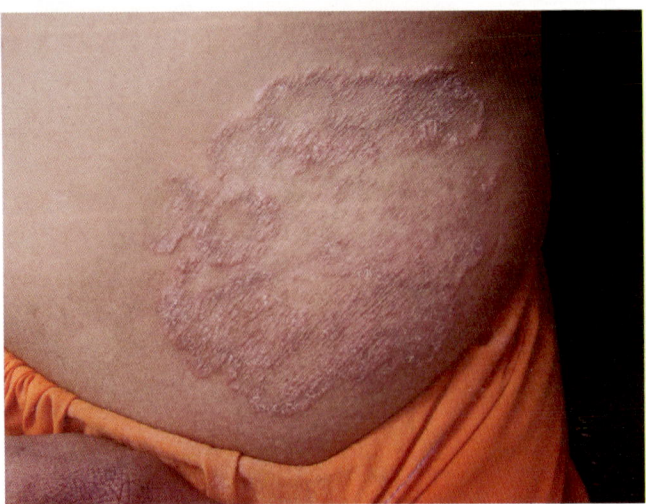

Fig. 9.22: Tinea corporis with periphery of the plaque showing prominent papules suggestive of follicular involvement due to steroid application

19. Wegener's Granulomatosis

Cause unknown, but a hypersensitivity reaction is suspected. It may be confused with LL because it usually affects young adults, begins with nasal obstruction and recurrent small epistaxes, and later develops papulonecrotic skin lesions in which vasculitis is predominant. Death frequently occurs from renal failure.

20. Subacute Lupus Erythematosus

This is a subset of lupus erythematosus (LE) with two clinical variants. The first form is characterized by squamous psoriasiform papules and the second one by annular lesions in a symmetrical distribution which enlarge and coalesce to form polycyclic configurations.

Differential Diagnosis of Nodular Lesions

1. Post-kala-azar Dermal Leishmaniasis (PKDL)

Nodular lesions of PKDL are seen on the face, neck and extremities in late stages. When present on the face, the lesions are more centrofacial as compared to leprosy where they are more on the sides and ears (Fig. 9.6). LD bodies can be easily demonstrated in the papulonodular lesions.

2. Leishmaniasis

Leishmaniasis can present with nodular or nodulo-ulcerative lesions (Fig. 9.23a and b) that can cause disfigurement. LD bodies can be demonstrated in the lesions.

3. Sarcoidosis

Papulonodular lesions may be seen in the generalized form of disease. However, other organs may be involved like lungs, lymph nodes and bone.

4. Syphilis

Nodular and noduloulcerative lesions may be seen in secondary syphilis. These nodules are few and asymmetrical compared to nodular lesions of leprosy. Biopsy shows granulomatous inflammation with abundant plasma cells and other inflammatory cells. Serological tests for syphilis are positive.

5. Leukemia Cutis

Papulonodular lesions and infiltration of skin may occur in chronic lymphatic leukemia. Face, neck, shoulders and extensor aspect of extremities are the sites of predilection. The nodules are bluish red, pruritic and rubbery in consistency. The diagnosis can be made by blood examination.

6. B Cell Lymphoma

While B cell lymphoma has variants that can be confirmed on histology, some variants have peculiar clinical features that may be mistaken for leprosy. In case of T cell lymphomas, the nodules (Fig. 9.23c)—except in mycosis fungoides—are usually localized to a specific body area. Multifocal papules and/or nodules on trunk and/or proximal extremities are seen in primary cutaneous marginal zone B cell lymphoma.[35] A middle-aged adult presenting with grouped papules, plaques, and/or tumors on

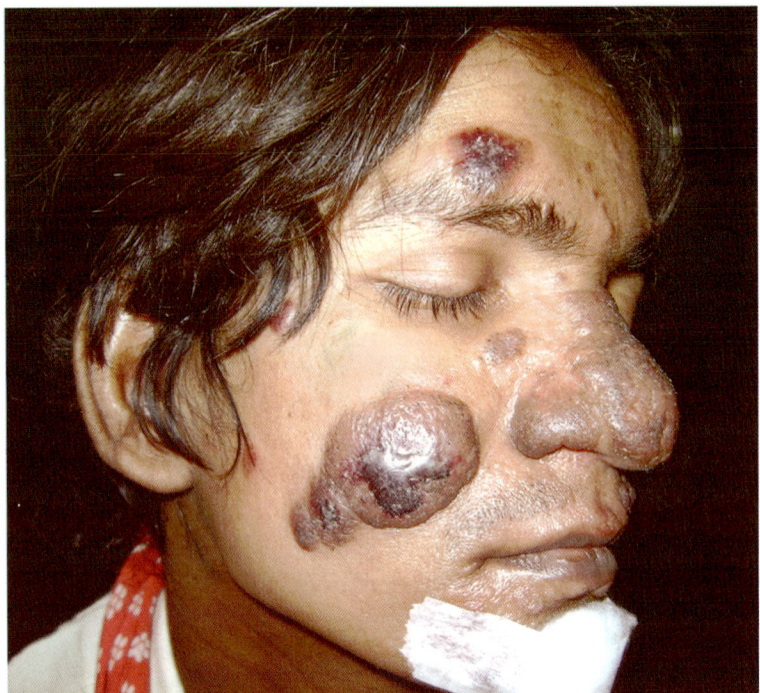

Fig. 9.23a: Nodular lesions of leishmaniasis

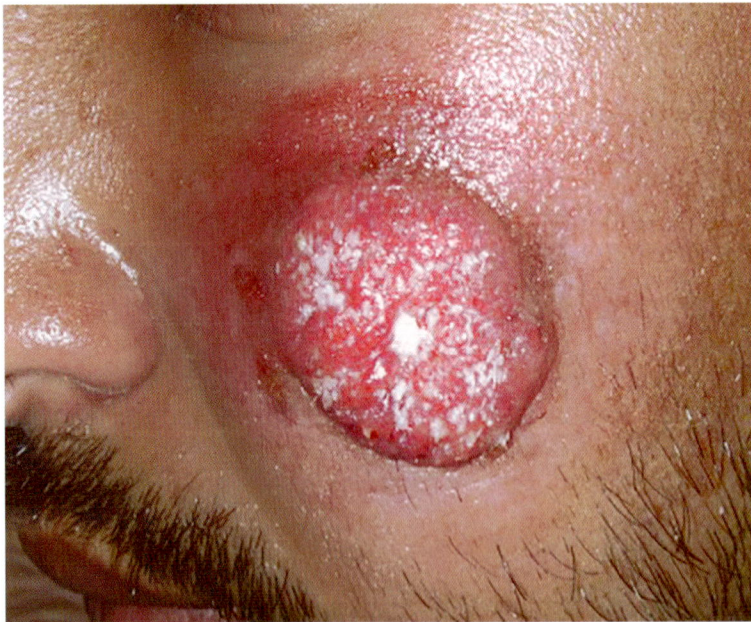

Fig. 9.23b: Leishmaniasis cutis

the scalp or back is classically seen in primary cutaneous follicle center lymphoma.[36] Thus, any markedly nodular morphology without sensory or motor deficit should raise the suspicion of lymphoma.

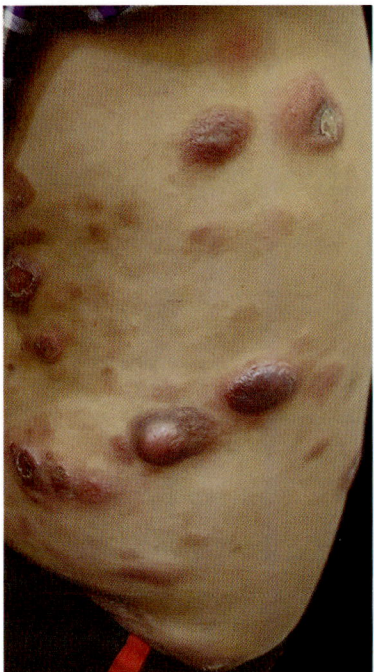

Fig. 9.23c: Anaplastic T cell lymphoma: Intact and ulcerated nodules

7. Neurofibromatosis (NF)

Neurofibromas in NF may resemble nodular lesions of leprosy. However, other features like café au lait macules and Lisch nodules will be present (Fig. 9.17).

8. Mycosis Fungoides

Plaques and shiny nodules can occur on face and trunk that resemble leprosy. The lesions are intensely pruritic.

9. Onchocerciasis

The disease may present with nodules over the lower back and extremities. Microfilariae can be demonstrated from these lesions.

Generalized Thickening of the Skin

1. Systemic Sclerosis (Scleroderma)

Cause is incompletely understood but genetic factors are suspected. The patient develops a taut and thickened skin (Fig. 9.24) which slowly becomes bound to subcutaneous tissues. Recurrent ulcerations develop at the ends of fingers, and terminal phalanges become absorbed. Polyarthritis of small joints is common, and finger contractures may develop.

2. Myxedema

A condition due to thyroid underactivity. It has many similarities to LL, like the thickening of skin, thinning of eyebrows, a hoarse voice, edematous legs, a normocytic normochromic anemia, and carpal tunnel syndrome as a complication.

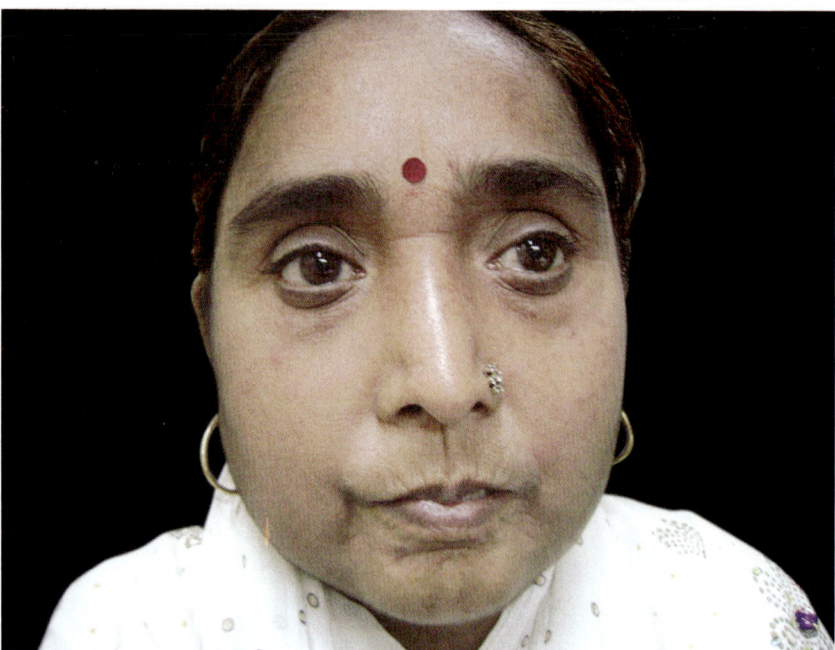

Fig. 9.24: Taut skin, expressionless face, pursed lips and telangiectasia on the face in a case of systemic sclerosis

3. *Pachydermoperiostosis*

A familial condition predominantly affecting males, in which the facial appearance, with deepening of the lines of face and forehead, closely resembles LL. Bone changes take the form of proliferative periostitis, fingers become thickened, and there is clubbing of fingers and toes.

A summary of the other differentials that may mimic the regional manifestations of leprosy is provided in Table 9.2.

Table 9.2: Differential diagnosis of regional manifestations[37]	
Deformities in upper limbs	Carpal tunnel syndrome, Scleroderma, cervical cord syndrome
Deformities in lower limbs	Trophic ulcers, cutaneous tuberculosis, atypical mycobacterial infection, diabetic ulcers (Fig. 9.25), hypertensive ulcers, sickle cell anemia, chronic venous ulcers, hereditary neuropathies, vasculitic ulcers (Fig. 9.26)
Leonine facies	Actinic reticuloid, sarcoidosis, granuloma faciale, malignancies (mycosis fungoides, leukemia cutis), mastocytosis, neurofibromatosis
Madarosis	Infiltrative pathologies like lymphomas, follicular mucinosis, hypothyroidism, secondary syphilis, alopecia areata, trichotillomania
Nasal deformities	Mucocutaneous leishmaniasis, tertiary syphilis, yaws, relapsing polychondritis, rhinoscleroma
Ear deformities	Cutaneous lymphomas, cutaneous leishmaniasis, lupus vulgaris, tumors like neurofibromatosis (Fig. 9.17)

Differential Diagnosis

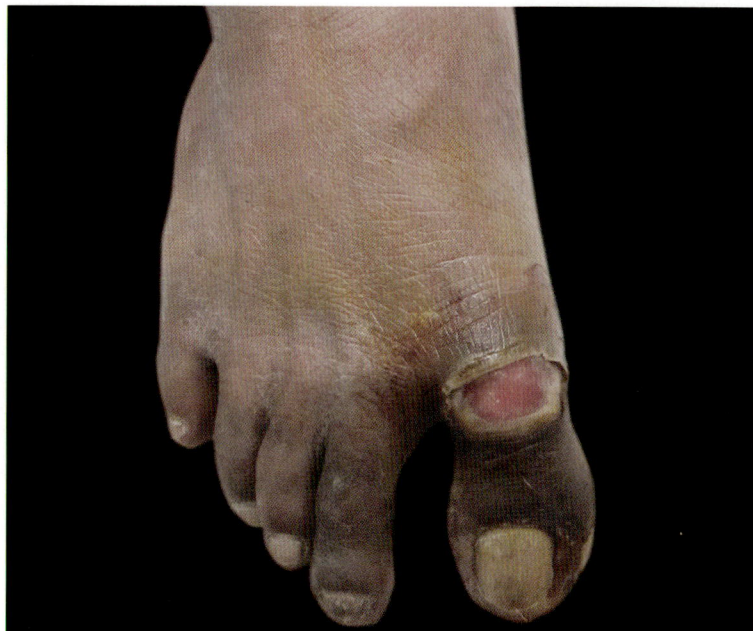

Fig. 9.25: Diabetic ulcer

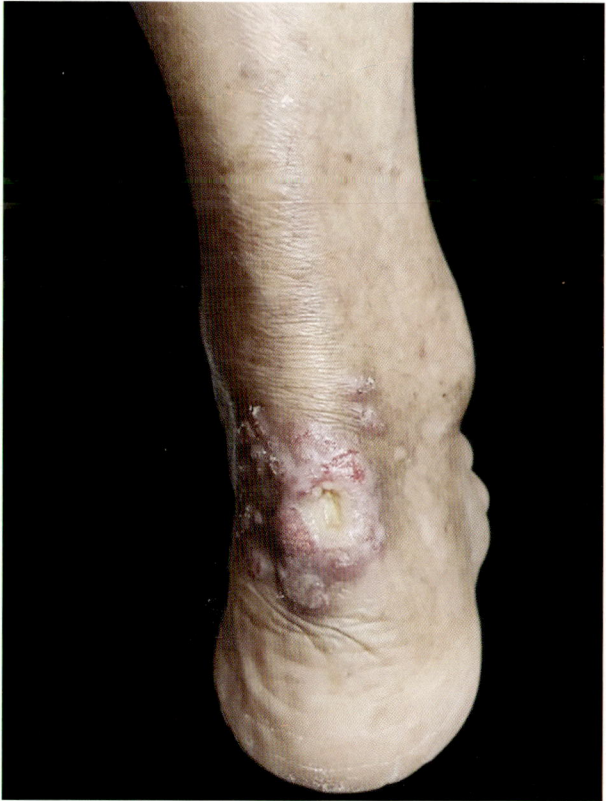

Fig. 9.26: Vasculitic ulcer in an elderly male. The ulcer was severely painful

Differential Diagnosis of Type 1 and Type 2 Reactions

These include vasculitis, panniculitis, erythema nodosum, Sweet's syndrome and bacterial, mycobacterial and fungal opportunistic infections. These conditions present with papulonodular lesions over the body and hence can resemble leprosy reactions. Type 1 reactions present with increased erythema of existing lesions along with appearance of new lesions. Constitutional symptoms and neuritis may be present. Type 2 reactions or ENL reactions present with eruption of tender nodules over extremities accompanied with fever and constitutional symptoms. However, the lesions are transient and subside in a few days leaving behind hyperpigmented macules. The transient nature of the lesions and the site can help in differentiating ENL reaction from the above mentioned conditions.

REFERENCES

1. Dharmendra. Thickened nerves in diagnosis of leprosy. Leprosy in India 1980;52:1–2.
2. Khadilkar SV. A practical approach to enlargement of nerves, plexuses and roots. Pract Neurol 2015;15:105–15.
3. Andrade C. A peculiar form of peripheral neuropathy. Familiar atypical generalized amyloidosis with special involvement of peripheral nerves. Brain 1953;75:408–27.
4. Nunzi E, Fiallo P. Differential Diagnosis. In: Hastings RC, editor. Leprosy. 2nd ed. Edinburgh: Churchill Livingstone 1994; p. 291–320.
5. Sandell LJ. Congenital indifference to pain. Journal of the Faculty of Radiologists 1958;9:50–6.
6. Chattopadhyay SP, Gupta CM. Primary hyperpigmented cutaneous lesions in tuberculoid leprosy. Indian J Lepr 1988;60:63–5.
7. Sardana K, Arora P. Disorders of hypopigmentation. In: Sardana K, Arora P, editor. Handbook of Pigmentary Disorders. Ist ed. Delhi: CBS; 2019.
8. Rigopoulos D, Gregoriou S, Charissi C, Kontochristopoulos G, Kalogeromitros D, Georgala S. Tacrolimus ointment 0.1% in pityriasis alba: An open-label, randomized, placebo-controlled study. Br J Dermatol 2006;155:152–5.
9. Sardana K, Arora P. Fungal Infections. In: Sardana K, Arora P, editor. Skin and Soft Tissue Infections. 1st ed. Delhi: CBS; 2019.
10. Munro DD, du Vivier A, Jopling WH. Post-kala azar dermal leishmaniasis. British Journal of Dermatology 1972;87:374–8.
11. World Health Organization website. Post-kala-azar dermal leishmaniasis: A manual for case management and control. Report of a WHO Consulative Meeting, Kolkata, India, 2–3 July 2012. Available at: http:// apps.who.int/iris/bitstream/handle/0665/78608/9789241505215_ eng.pdf
12. Hastings Nunzi E, Fiallo P. Differential Diagnosis. In: Hastings RC, editor. Leprosy. 2nd ed. Edinburgh: Churchill Livingstone 1994; p. 291–320.
13. Bansal S, Goel A, Sardana K, Kumar V, Khurana N. Post-kala-azar dermal leishmaniasis coexisting with borderline tuberculoid leprosy. Br J Dermatol 2007;157:811–3.
14. Skin in Systemic Disease, in. Kabir Sardana. Textbook of Dermatology STD and HIV, CBS, 2018; page 412.
15. Vachiramon V, Thadanipon K. Post-inflammatory hypopigmentation. Clin Exp Dermatol 2011;36:708–14.
16. Miazek N, Michalek I, Pawlowska-Kisiel M, Olszewska M, Rudnicka L. Pityriasis alba—common disease, enigmatic entity: up-to-date review of the literature. Pediatr Dermatol 2015;32:786–91.
17. Relyveld GN, Dingemans KP, Menke HE, Bos JD, Westerhof W. Ultrastructural findings in progressive macular hypomelanosis indicate decreased melanin production. J Eur Acad Dermatol Venereol 2008;22:568–74.

18. Relyveld GN, Westerhof W, Woudenberg J, et al. Progressive macular hypomelanosis is associated with a putative *Propionibacterium* species. J Invest Dermatol 2010;130:1182–4.
19. Mycosis fungoides. In: Skin Lymphoma: The Illustrated Guide, 4th Edition. Lorenzo Cerroni. June 2014 Wiley-Blackwell. 4th edition.
20. Furlan FC, Sanches JA. Hypopigmented mycosis fungoides: A review of its clinical features and pathophysiology. An Bras Dermatol 2013;88:954–60.
21. Pinkus H. Alopecia mucinosa. Archives of Dermatology 1957;76:419–26.
22. Fan J, Chang H, Ma B. Alopecia mucinosis mutilating leprosy. Archives of Dermatology; 1967; 95:354–6.
23. Leiker DL, Kok SH, Spaas JA J. Granuloma multiforme: A new disease resembling leprosy. International Journal of Leprosy 1964;32:J68–76.
24. Leiker DL. Distribution of granuloma multiforme. International Journal of Leprosy 1971;39:189.
25. Willis WF. The gyrate erythemas. International Journal of Dermatology 1978;17:698–702.
26. Habicht GS, Beck G, Benach JL. Lyme Disease. Scientific American 1987;257:60–5.
27. Sardana K, Chugh S, Mahajan K. An observational study of the efficacy of azithromycin in erythema annulare centrifugum. Clin Exp Dermatol 2018;43:296–99.
28. Sehgal VN, Sardana K, Sharma S. Inadequacy of clinical and/or laboratory criteria for the diagnosis of lupus vulgaris, reinfection cutaneous tuberculosis: Fallout/implication of 6 weeks of anti-tubular therapy (ATT) as a precise diagnostic supplement to complete the scheduled regimen. J Dermatolog Treat 2008;19:164–67.
29. Mann RJ, Harman RRM. Cutanous anaesthesia in necrobiosis lipoidica. British Journal of Dermatology 1984;110:323–25.
30. Dowling GB, Wilson Jones E. Atypical (annular) necrobiosis lipoidica of the face and scalp. Dermatologica 1967;135:11–26.
31. Naik RPC, Srinivas CR, Rao RV. Thickening of nerves in neurofibromatosis. Indian Journal of Leprosy 1985;57:876–78.
32. Joseph S. von Recklinghausen's disease associated with diffuse lepromatous leprosy. Indian Journal of Leprosy 1985;57:872–75.
33. James DG, Jopling WH. Sarcoidosis and leprosy. Journal of Tropical Medicine and Hygiene 1961;64:42–46.
34. Arora P, Sardana K, Gautam RK, Batrani M. Relevant diagnostic implications of the therapeutic challenge with antitubercular therapy in an unusual case of sarcoidosis mimicking lupus vulgaris. Dermatol Ther 2019 May 17:e12968.
35. Primary Cutaneous Marginal Zone B Cell Lymphoma. In: A Subtil, Diagnosis of Cutaneous Lymphoid Infiltrates, https://doi.org/10.1007/978-3-030-11654-5_41. © Springer Nature Switzerland AG 2019.
36. Primary Cutaneous Follicle Center Lymphoma. In: A Subtil, Diagnosis of Cutaneous Lymphoid Infiltrates, https://doi.org/10.1007/978-3-030-11654-5_40.. © Springer Nature Switzerland AG 2019.
37. Kundakci N. Leprosy: A great imitator. Clin Dermatol 2019;37:200–212.

CHAPTER 10

Nerve Function Assessment and Muscle Testing

Surabhi Sinha, Krishna Garg

INTRODUCTION

While WHO guidelines recommend nerve palpation for diagnosis of leprosy, it is verily impossible to predict whether the nerve thickening will improve on treatment or whether the patient will develop consequential nerve damage. Thus, the essence is "early detection" of nerve damage, for which assessment of loss of nerve function, e.g. loss of *sweating*, impairment of sensibility or *sensory loss*, and weakness or paralysis of *muscles* in the hands or feet is essential. This is because if nerve function impairment (NFI) is not treated within six months of onset, nerve damage can become irreversible and can cause permanent disability.

A patient is considered at higher risk of developing NFI if:

1. There are more than six skin lesions with or without nerve involvement (i.e. only enlarged nerve without existing NFI)
2. There is a skin patch on the face or near the eye or in the areas supplied by a palpable nerve
3. Visibly enlarged trunk nerve without existing NFI
4. There is evidence of lepra reactions (type 1 or 2) including acute neuritis, either new or treated in past six months without existing NFI
5. The slit skin smear is positive
6. The patient is classified as having multibacillary (MB) leprosy.

Established methods for nerve function assessment (NFA) are nerve palpation, sensory testing (ST) and voluntary muscle testing (VMT). The ballpoint pen (easily available) or nylon monofilament (MFT) is commonly used for ST.[3] Evidence suggests that MFT is more reliable than ballpoint pen testing. Substantial levels *(also see Section 8.1)* of underdiagnosis of sensory loss with ballpoint pen testing have been observed.[4]

For VMT, three grades (as suggested by J Watson) or the modified Medical Research Council (MRC) scale (0–5) is used *(also see Section 8.1)*.[5]

Table 10.1 mentions the time intervals for NFA. In patients with reactions, the nerve function needs to be assessed at diagnosis (baseline) and repeated every month during MDT and upon completion of treatment, thus 7 times for PB patients and 13 times for MB patients).

Table 10.1: Time interval for assessment of NFA (WHO)

All patients	• Start of MDT • Completion of MDT • Any time when there are complaints suggesting neuritis
Patients at higher risk of developing NFI	• Start of MDT • Every 3 months while on MDT • Every 3 months (until one year) after completion of MDT (Thus, 9 times during 24 months after diagnosis)
Patients with reaction	Monthly
Patients with NFI of less than six months and thus eligible for treatment with steroids	• Two weeks after starting steroids • Monthly until completion of steroid course

The principle of assessment of NFA is based on the mnemonic "LOFT":
- **Listen** to patient's complaints of pain, sensory loss, weakness or difficulties doing activities of daily living.
- **Observe** (i) eye for brightness of cornea, spontaneous blink and complete closure of the eyelid; and (ii) hands and feet for injuries, wounds and weakness in straightening fingers and toes/lifting feet.
- **Feel** for dryness, localized warmth on hands and feet and palpate nerves for pain and/or enlargement.
- **Test** (i) sensation (using graded Semmes-Weinstein monofilaments, if available), temperature, light touch (using ballpoint pen); (ii) strength of movement of eyes, hands and feet.

The suggested tools for assessment of NFI are given in Table 10.2.

NERVE EXAMINATION AND ASSESSMENT OF FUNCTION[6]

Nerve trunks are mixed nerves, i.e. they have sensory, sympathetic and motor components. Therefore, we can identify and grade the nerve trunk damage by examination for sensory loss, autonomic loss and muscle weakness.

Two components of nerve examination are:
1. **Palpation** of the nerves: For thickening, tenderness and consistency (cord-like/fibrosed).
2. Assessment of **nerve function**: Autonomic, sensory and motor functions.

Table 10.2: Tools for assessment of NFI at primary and referral centers

	Primary care center	Referral center
Nerve	Palpation	Palpation Ultrasound
Sensory function	• Temperature: Cotton swab with acetone (cold); hot/cold test tubes • Touch: 2G monofilaments • Pressure: 10G monofilaments	• Quantitative pain thresholds and temperature (QST) • Semmes-Weinstein monofilament kit • Pain scale gradation 0–10
Motor function	VMT: Strong/weak/ paralyzed (SWP)	MRC scale 0–5

Nerve Palpation (Fig. 10.1 and Table 10.3)

Tips

- Look at the patient's face while palpating the nerve gently with the pulp of the finger (not the tip of the finger) to elicit tenderness
- Always palpate *across* the *course* of the nerve
- Feel along the nerve as far as possible in both directions—a localized fluctuant and tender swelling may represent a *nerve abscess*; a hard nerve is *fibrosed*
- Nerves on the two sides must be compared to detect any abnormality
- Tingling sensation is felt when the nerve is palpated.

Autonomic Function

To find out about loss of sweating in the palms and soles: (i) Ask the patient about it; (ii) look at the palms and soles; and (iii) feel them for sweating.

Examine for presence/absence of:
- Sweating ("dry looking skin")
- Cracks/fissures

Sensory Examination

1. Look for scars of previous injuries/burns/blisters in the area of sensory loss.
2. Test for touch, pain and temperature on representative sites of palms and soles.
3. Map the area of sensory loss on palms and soles and other areas.

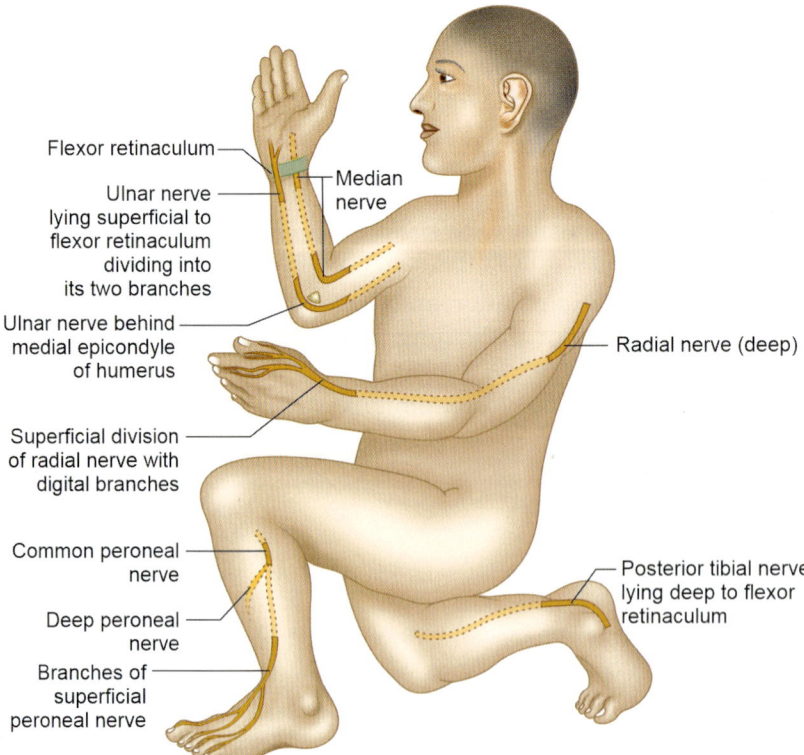

Fig. 10.1: Surface markings of all major nerves

Nerve Function Assessment and Muscle Testing

Table 10.3: Surface markings for palpation of nerve trunks

Nerve trunks palpated in leprosy	Cutaneous nerves seen/palpated in leprosy
Ulnar (ulnar groove on medial epicondyle of humerus) With elbow in flexion, the medial epicondyle is identified; the ulnar nerve is palpated *behind* and *above* it	Supra orbital (junction of medial one-third and lateral two-thirds of supraorbital ridge)
Radial (radial groove below insertion of deltoid muscle) Hold forearm with right hand in pronation and elbow in flexion. Roll the nerve in the groove in the humerus posterior to the deltoid muscle insertion	Supratrochlear (medial to supraorbital nerve)
Median (middle of wrist under flexor retinaculum) Hold the wrist in slight extension with the left hand. Roll across the center of the wrist. The enlarged nerve is palpable proximal to the wrist under the palmaris longus tendon	Infraorbital nerve (medial part of inferior orbital margin)
Posterior tibial (between medial malleolus and tendo-Achillis)	Zygomatic branch of facial (VII) nerve (zygomatic arch)
Common peroneal/lateral popliteal (below lateral aspect of knee along neck of fibula) Ask patient to flex knee and feel above and behind the head of the fibula. The first bony prominence is the head of fibula. The nerve can be traced behind the knee and can be felt even when not enlarged	Greater auricular (junction of upper one-third and lower two-thirds of sternocleidomastoid muscle)
	Supraclavicular (medial one-third and lateral two-thirds of clavicle) Radial cutaneous (anatomical snuffbox)

A diagrammatic depiction of the innervation of the palm and sole is shown in Fig. 10.2.

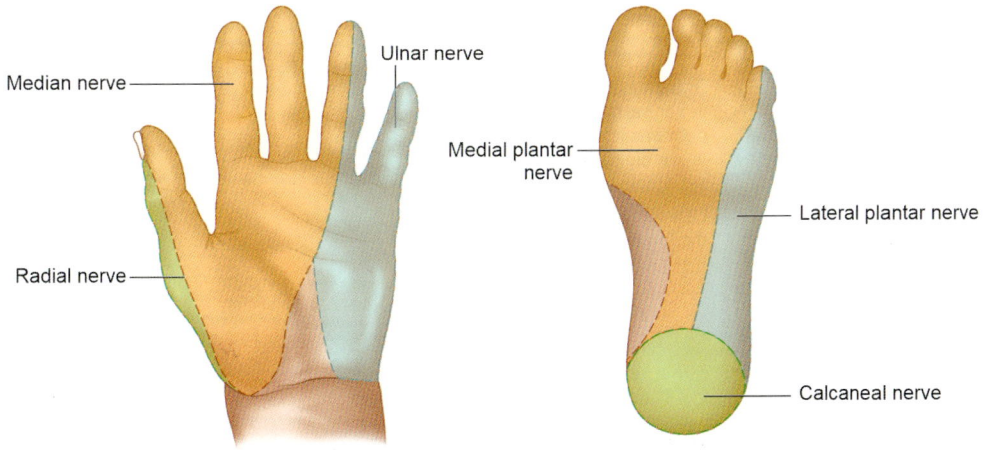

Fig. 10.2: Sensory innervation of palm and sole

As the clinician should be conversant with the course of the major nerves affected in leprosy, they are being detailed below (ulnar nerve, median nerve, radial nerve, common peroneal nerve and posterior tibial nerve) (Fig. 10.3a to e).

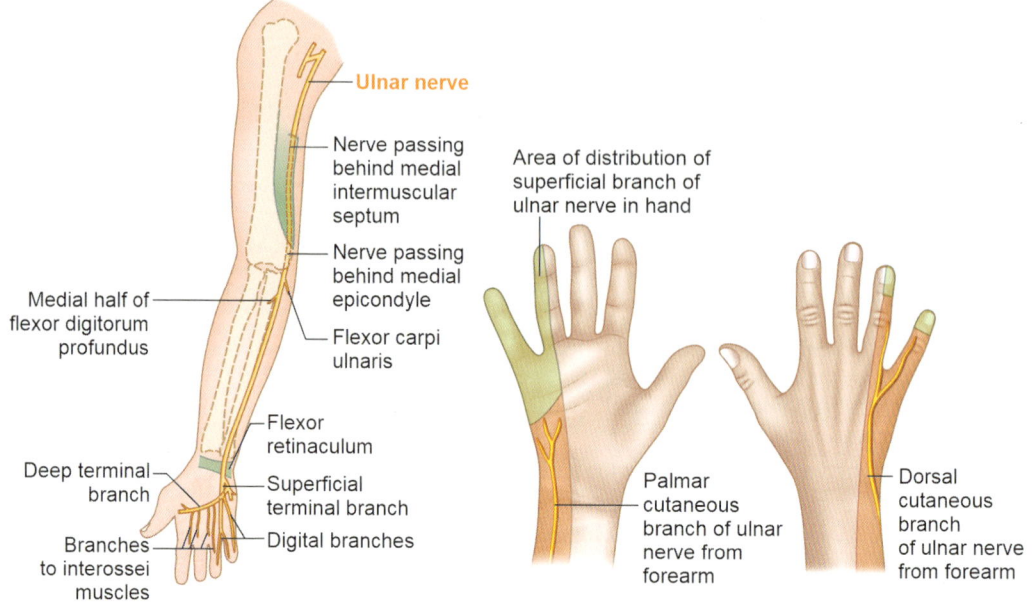

Fig. 10.3a: Ulnar nerve

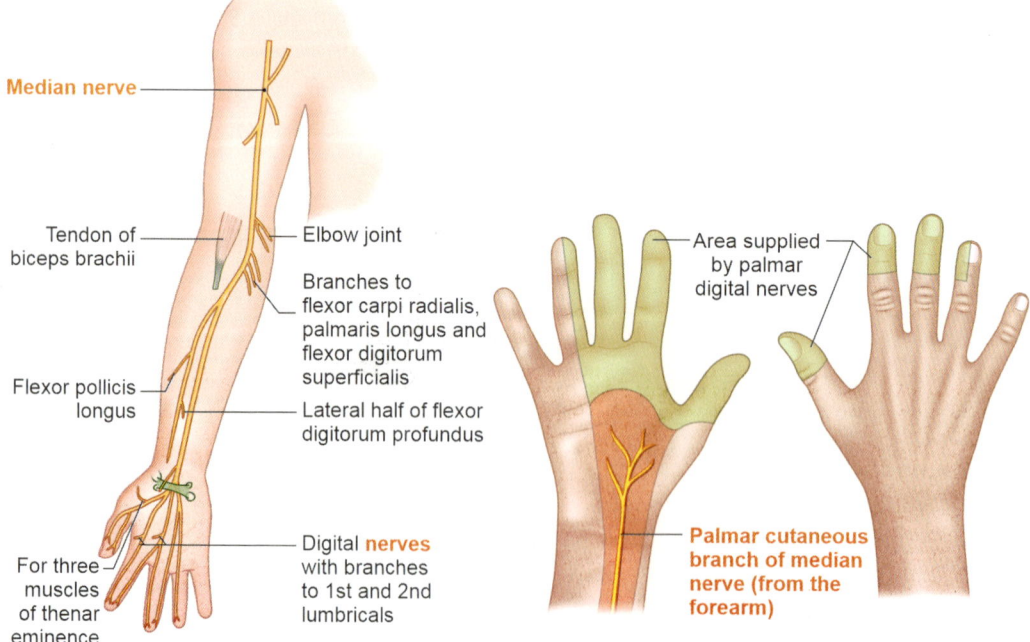

Fig. 10.3b: Median nerve

Nerve Function Assessment and Muscle Testing

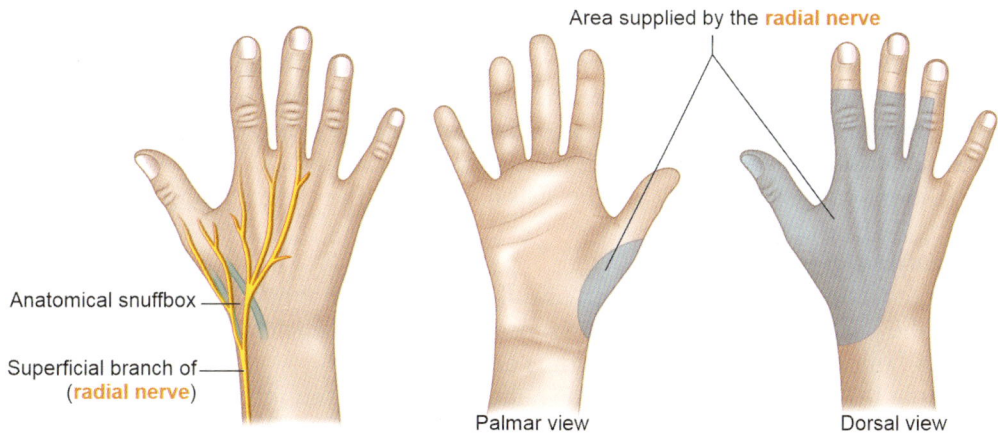

Fig. 10.3c: Radial nerve

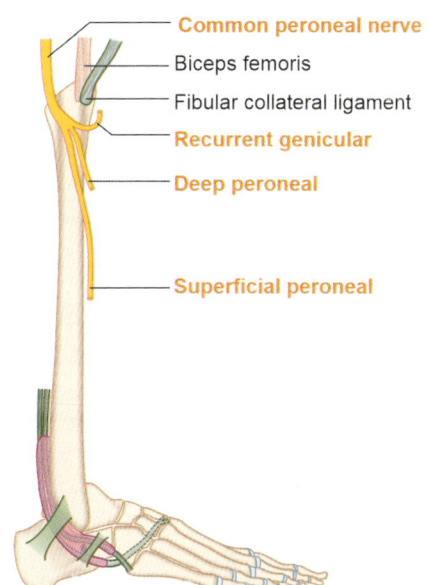

Fig. 10.3d: Common peroneal nerve

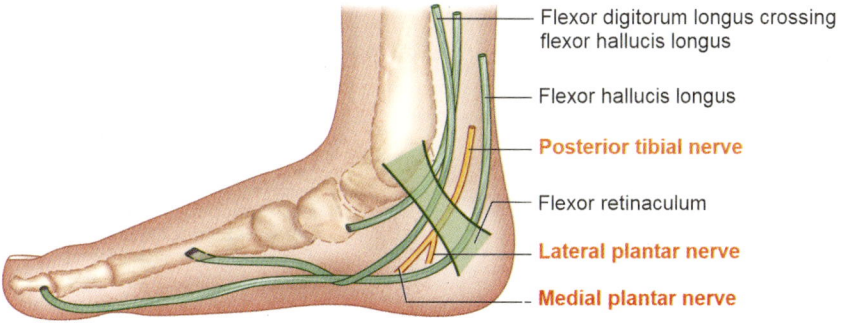

Fig. 10.3e: Tibial nerve

Tips for sensory examination

- Pain and temperature are lost *before* fine touch—test for temperature and pain for early detection. The ability to feel heavy touch, as tested using a blunt point (e.g. the tip of a ballpoint pen) is lost very late and if only heavy touch is tested in the hand, onset of nerve damage will be diagnosed late.
- To the extent possible, carry out the tests in *quiet* surroundings, to prevent the patient being distracted
- Test *normal* part first
- First test with patient's eyes open and then with his/her eyes closed
- Ask the patient to point where the sensation has been elicited. On the heel and the sole a "misreference" of about 2 cm is acceptable.
- Include 1–2 fake tests—ask what the patient feels even though you have not touched
- If using ballpoint pen, press until a slight dent appears though this may not produce the same pressure always.
- Monofilament testing is performed using five monofilaments: 200 mg, 2 g, 4 g, 10 g and 300 g. For the foot, because of known higher thresholds, the lightest, 200 mg filament, can be omitted. For monofilament, press gently until the filament bends. The same filament is not suitable for the hand and feet.

A diagrammatic depiction of the sites for testing for sensations in hands and feet is shown in Figs 10.4 to 10.6 and described below:

- For *ulnar nerve*: Test for loss of sensibility to pain, heat and light touch at two sites—(i) in the palm, 3–4 cm from the crease at the base of the little finger, along a line extending from the midline of that finger (point 4 in Fig. 10.4); and (ii) in the pulp of the little finger (point 3 in Fig. 10.4).
- For *median nerve*: (i) In the palm over the thenar eminence, about 1.0–1.5 cm from the crease at the base of the thumb and along a line extending from the midline of

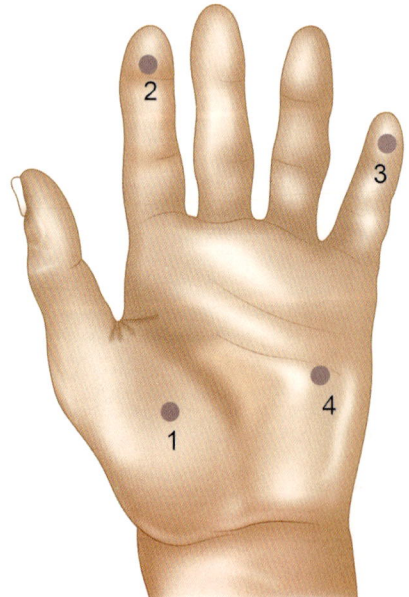

1. Thenar eminence, about 1.0–1.5 cm from the crease at the base of the thumb, along a line extending from the midline of the thumb
2. Pulp of index finger
3. Pulp of the little finger
4. Palm, about 3–4 cm from the crease at the base of the little finger, along a line extending from the midline of the finger

Fig. 10.4: Points for sensory testing in the palm

the thumb (point 1, Fig. 10.4); and (ii) in the pulp of the index finger (point 2, Fig. 10.4).
- The *radial cutaneous* and *sural nerve* can also be are tested at sites depicted in Fig. 10.5a and b.
- The *posterior tibial nerve* supplies the foot. Testing for loss of sensibility in the *sole* is not easy, because the skin is normally very thick and it becomes even more thickened in people who do not habitually wear footwear. Thus, testing for sensibility to heat or light touch in the sole is not reliable (Fig. 10.6). It is also not

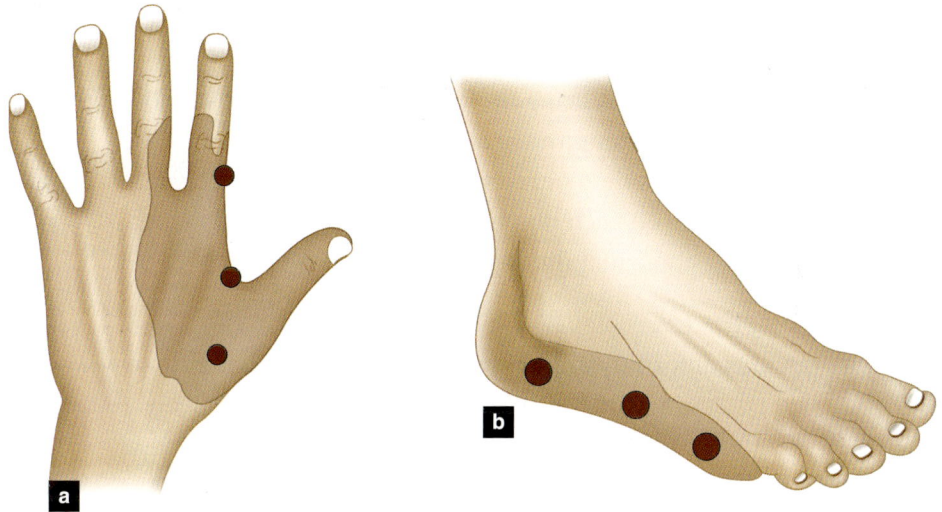

Fig. 10.5: (a) Sensory marking for radial cutaneous nerve (hand); (b) Sural nerve (foot)

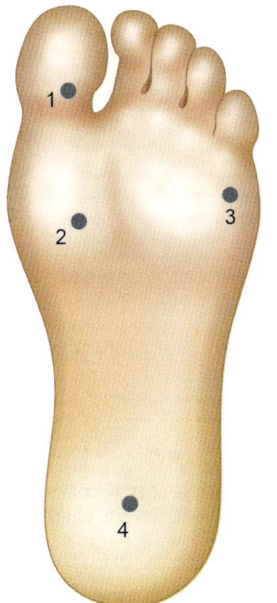

1. Pad of the big toe
2. Ball of the foot, about 3–4 cm from the crease at the base of the big toe, along a line extending from the midline of the toe
3. Ball of the foot, about 1.0–1.5 cm from the crease at the base of the little toe, along a line extending from the midline of the toe
4. Center of the heel

Fig. 10.6: Sensory testing points on the sole

possible to test for perception of pain with a sharp pin. However, perception of pressure and pain from deep pressure should be tested, using a blunt point (such as the tip of a ballpoint pen).
- *Trigeminal nerve*: Look for blink reflex. If present, check if it is as frequent as normal and does it cover the whole eye. If there is lagophthlamos, check for corneal sensation. The corneal sensation is checked by touching the limbus with a wisp of cotton/5 cm dental floss and if reflex is normal, the eye blinks.

Motor Examination

Muscle Weakness

The salient points to focus on during motor examination are listed below:
- Ask about difficulties in using the hands or in walking
- Look for deformity and other signs of muscle weakness, paralysis or wasting
- Carry out several tests on each nerve trunk
- Record normal and abnormal findings

What to look and ask for?

- Attitude/obvious deformity—little finger lies apart from ring finger/clawing/foot drop
- Bulk—thenar/hypothenar eminence flattening/wasting
- Tone—may be reduced
- Deep tendon reflexes (DTRs)—usually preserved in leprosy
- Strength/voluntary muscle testing (VMT) (using MRC—Table 10.4; or SWP system—Table 10.5).

Table 10.4: MRC muscle strength grading (in higher centers)	
Grade	Muscle state
Grade 0	No movement is observed
Grade 1	Only a trace or flicker of movement is seen or felt or fasciculations are observed
Grade 2	Muscle can move only if the resistance of gravity is removed
Grade 3	Muscle strength is reduced such that the joint can be moved only against gravity with the examiner's resistance completely removed
Grade 4	Muscle strength is reduced but muscle contraction can still move joint against resistance
Grade 5	Muscle contracts normally against full resistance

Table 10.5: SWP grading (in peripheral centers)	
(S)	**Strong** when the strength seems normal
(W)	**Weak** when the muscle can move but it is definitely weak against resistance
(P)	**Paralyzed** when there is no movement at all

1. Testing of Motor Supply of Hand

Though a detailed text is not the aim here, it is a good practice to have a working knowledge of the muscles of the palm and their nerve supply. Figure 10.7a and b depicts the muscles of the hand and their nerve supply.

A summary of the various tests of the muscles of the hand is given in Table 10.6 while the important tests are described below.

Ulnar Nerve (Fig. 10.3a)

a. *Look* for wasting (loss of bulk) of the muscles as evidenced by flattening and straightening of the little finger, side of the palm and flattening of the soft bulge of the muscle in the back of the hand between the thumb and the index finger.

b. In case of ulnar palsy, the patient is unable to keep all the fingers straight and together and the little finger tends to stay apart from the ring finger and may also be slightly bent or clawed (**Wartenberg's sign;** Fig. 10.8). The basic muscle that is tested is the *abductor digiti minimi.* Also, one must always palpate the muscle belly while testing as sometimes even when the muscle is completely paralyzed, the extensor tendon can abduct the little finger by extension.

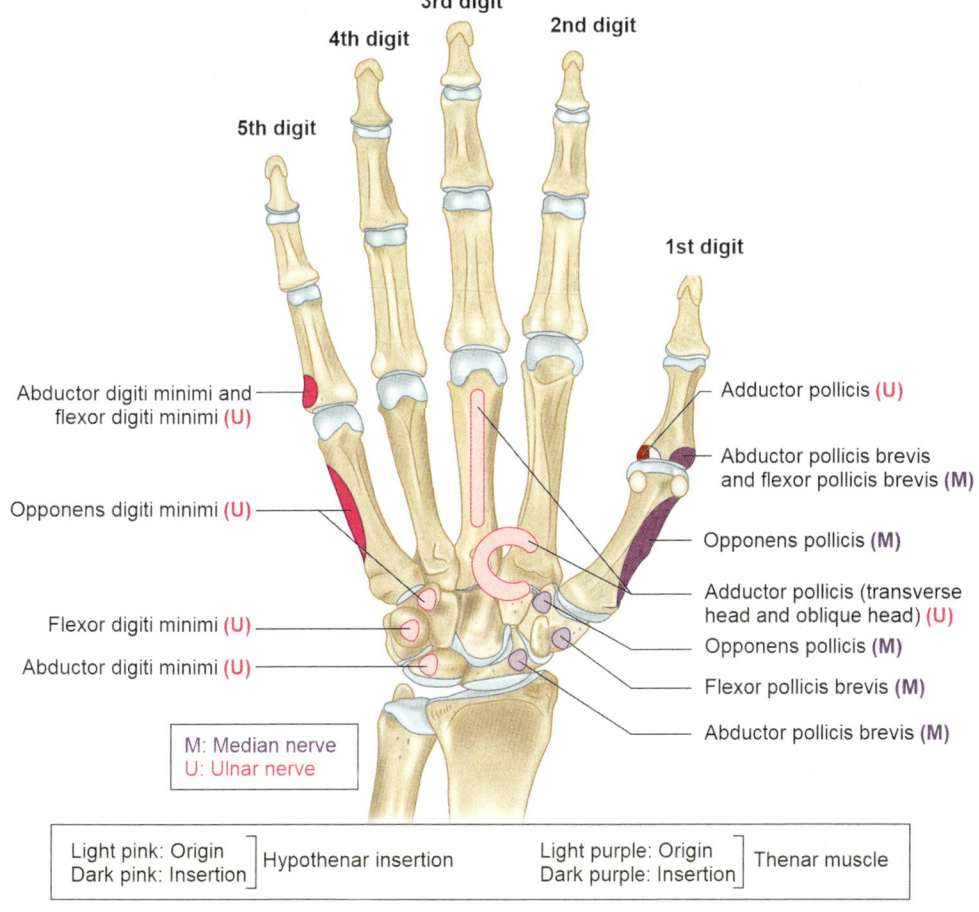

Fig. 10.7a: Muscles of hand with their nerve supply

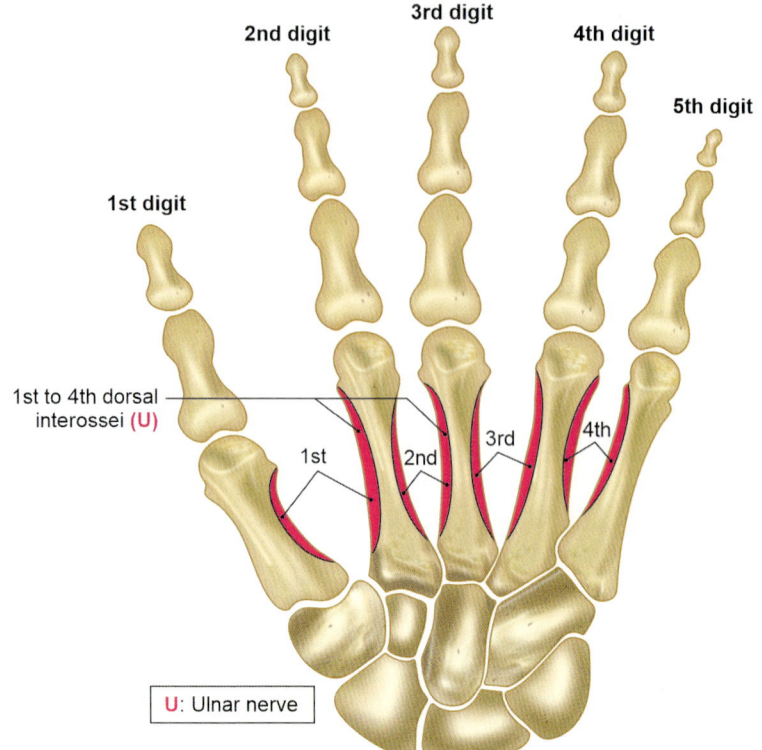

Fig. 10.7b: Nerve supply of intrinsic muscles of the hand

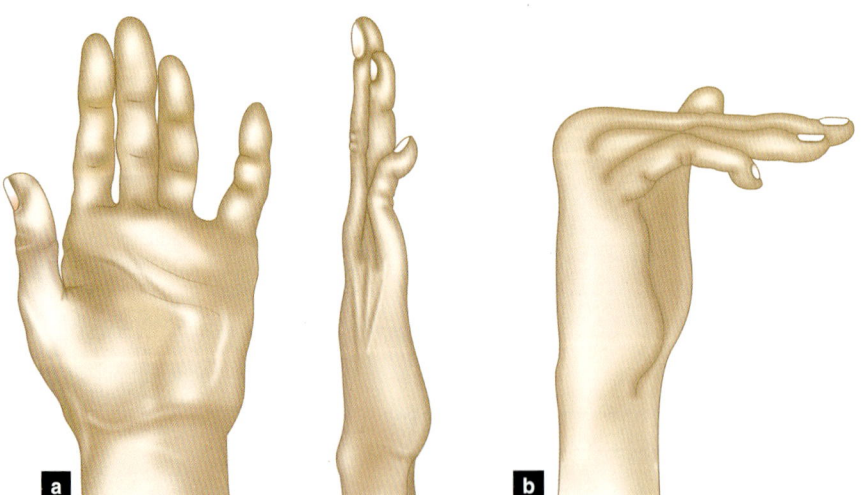

Fig. 10.8a and b: Early ulnar nerve palsy: (a) Little finger stands slightly apart from the others (Warterberg's sign); (b) It cannot be kept straight while flexing the other fingers at metacarpophalangeal joint

Ask the patient to bend all the fingers at the base, keeping the other joints straight, and to keep them like that for about 30 seconds. In early ulnar nerve paralysis, the little finger cannot be kept in this position and it will be bent.

Median Nerve (Fig. 10.3b)

a. There is weakness and paralysis of the muscles that form the bulge at the base of the thumb **(thenar eminence)**.
b. In case of median nerve palsy, a simple test is to ask the patient to stretch the hand out, with the palm horizontal and facing upwards and the fingers and thumb facing forwards. Then ask the patient to lift the thumb upwards (Fig. 10.9) and hold it in that position for at least 30 seconds. The tip of the thumb should be pointing upwards and not forwards. When the median nerve is damaged, the patient will be unable to hold the thumb in this position (due to weakness of abductor pollicis brevis).

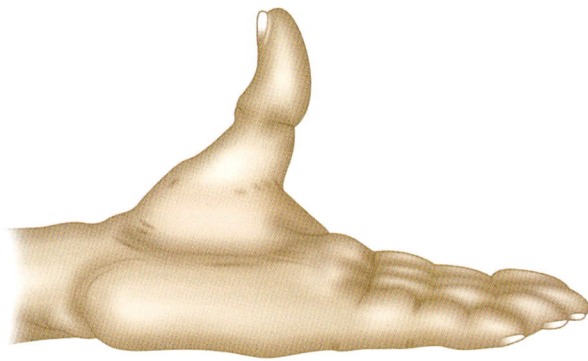

Normal, no muscle weakness

Fig. 10.9: With normal median nerve function, the thumb can be held in the depicted position, while with median nerve palsy, patient is unable to hold the thumb in this position

- Flexor digitorum superficialis muscle flexes the PIP (proximal interphalangeal) joint without flexing the terminal phalanx at distal interphalangeal joint. Hold the other fingers down, leaving the test finger free, and ask the patient to bend the test finger only at the PIP joint. If the patient has difficulty in doing this, put a pencil under the proximal phalanx of the test finger and now ask him to bend the finger (Fig. 10.10a and b). Assess the strength of the muscle by resisting the movement. If you find that the superficialis is weak or paralyzed, you should refer the patient to a specialist surgeon as the patient may be having *high* median nerve paralysis.

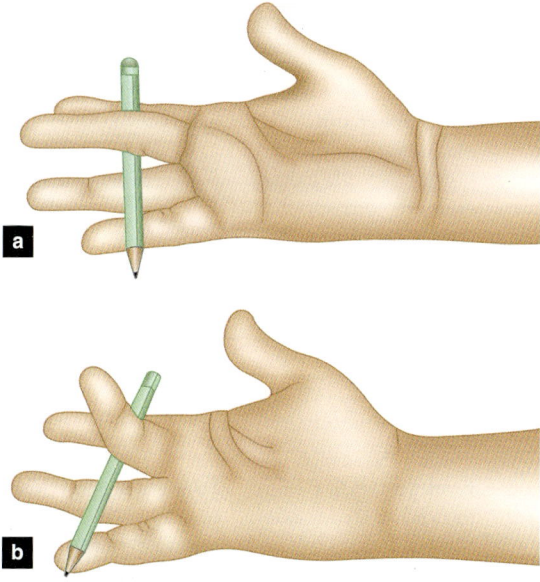

Fig. 10.10: (a) Holding PIP joint of middle finger and of that digit (high median nerve palsy); (b) Testing flexor digitorum superficialis

Radial Nerve (Fig. 10.3c)

Ask the patient to stretch both arms straight in front, holding the hands and fingers up as much as possible, and to keep holding them like that for at least 30 seconds (Fig. 10.11a). When the muscles in the back of the forearm are weak or paralyzed, the hand and fingers cannot be held up and drop down on the affected side (Fig. 10.11b).

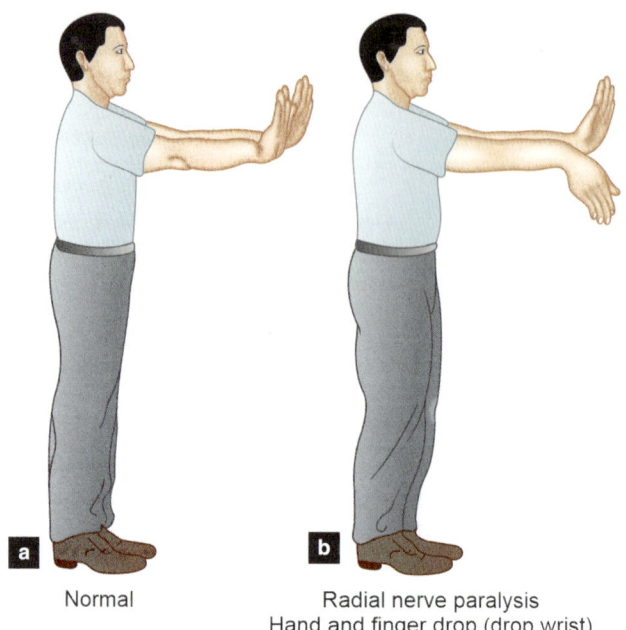

a — Normal

b — Radial nerve paralysis
Hand and finger drop (drop wrist)

Fig. 10.11a and b: Testing for radial nerve paralysis

Table 10.6: Tests for nerves supplying various hand muscles				
Nerve	Muscle	Test	Interpretation/Signs	Deformity
Ulnar	Dorsal interossei	**Little finger out test:** Ask patient to put out his hands with palms upwards and support their hand on your hand • Ask him to move the little finger out • Apply resistance at base of little finger **Egawa's test:** Test all fingers for abduction against resistance	Inability to do so	Inability to spread out fingers, guttering of interosseous spaces
	Adductor pollicis and 1st palmar interossei	**Book test:** Ask patient to hold book between fingers and thumbs of both hands against resistance	**Froment's sign:** Flexion of interphalangeal joint due to action of flexor pollicis longus (FPL) (Fig. 10.12)	Guttering of 1st interosseous space

(contd.)

Table 10.6: Tests for nerves supplying various hand muscles (contd.)

Nerve	Muscle	Test	Interpretation/Signs	Deformity
	Interossei and medial two lumbricals	Ask patient to flex MCP joints of fingers against resistance	Inability to do so	Ulnar claw hand (hyperextension of MCP and flexion of IP joints)
	Palmar interossei	**Card test:** Patient to place hand with palm up on table with fingers extended and adducted → firm paper card inserted into web space and patient to try and grasp it against resistance	Inability to hold the card (Fig. 10.13)	Guttering of interosseous spaces
			Wartenberg's sign: Little finger subtly abducted—earliest sign of ulnar nerve involvement.	
Median	Abductor pollicis brevis	**Pen test:** Patient to rest hand on table and asked to touch a pen held above the palm (Fig. 10.14)	Inability to do so	**Ape thumb deformity:** Thumb lies flat in plane of hand
	Abductor pollicis brevis	• Ask patient to keep hands with thumbs pointing towards each other (Fig. 10.15) • Ask the patient to hold his arms close to his body with elbows bent and palms facing each other • Ask him to move the thumbs away from the palm towards each other	Inability to hold them in that position for at least 30 seconds	—
	Opponens pollicis	Stabilize hand with own hand. Patient asked to touch fingertips with thumb against resistance	Inability to do so	—
	Flexor digitorum superficialis and flexor digitorum profundus (lateral half)*	**Oschsner's clasping test** • Clasp both hands	Index finger remains straight and does not flex **Pointing index/ Benediction sign**	
Radial	Extensors of wrist joint	**Wrist up test:** Close fist and dorsiflex wrist joint against resistance	Inability to do so	Wrist drop

*Affected in high median nerve palsy; not commonly seen in leprosy.

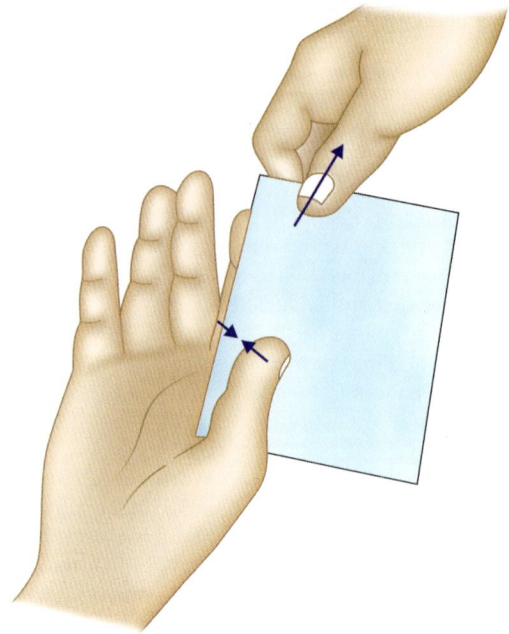

Fig. 10.12: Froment's sign while doing book test for adductor pollicis (ulnar nerve)

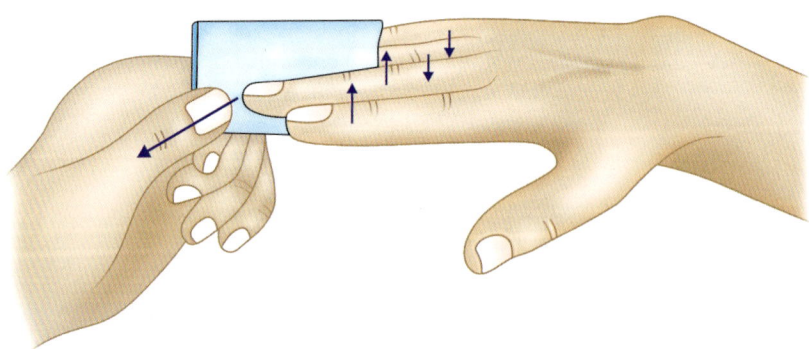

Fig. 10.13: Card test for palmar interossei (ulnar nerve)

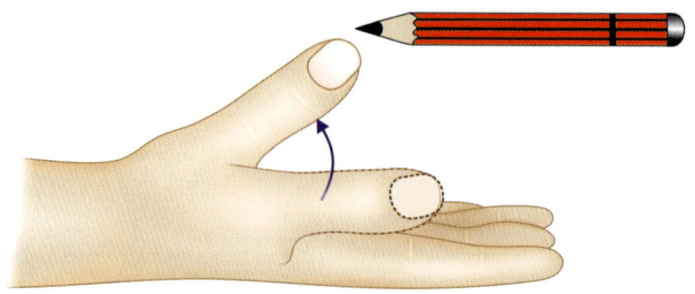

Fig. 10.14: Pen test for abductor pollicis brevis (median nerve)

Nerve Function Assessment and Muscle Testing

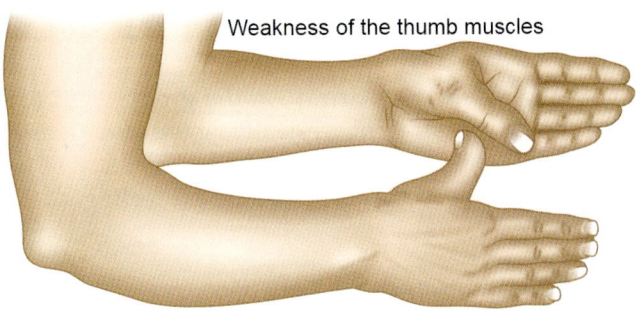

Fig. 10.15: Thumbs pointing towards each other

Test for all 3 nerves of 1 hand

Beak test
- Ask the patient to shape his fingers like a beak and move the hand to and fro at the wrist joint
- If he is able to do so—all 3 nerves of the hand are healthy.

2. Testing of Muscles of the Foot

Tibial Nerve (Table 10.7 and Fig. 10.3e)

a. Look for clawing of the toes, which occurs when the tibial nerve is damaged and the muscles in the foot are weakened or paralyzed. Instead of being straight (Fig. 10.16a, the toes become curled (clawed), so that the tips of the toes, not their pads, touch the ground Fig. 10.16b). However, this is *not* a very reliable indicator of weakness of the muscles in the foot as people who have been habitually wearing shoes often have bent toes.

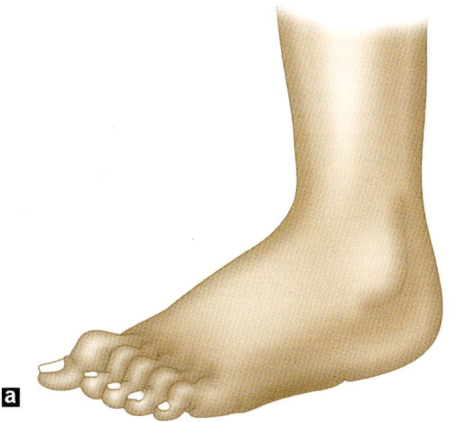

Normal toes are bent like an "S", their pads are in contact with the ground

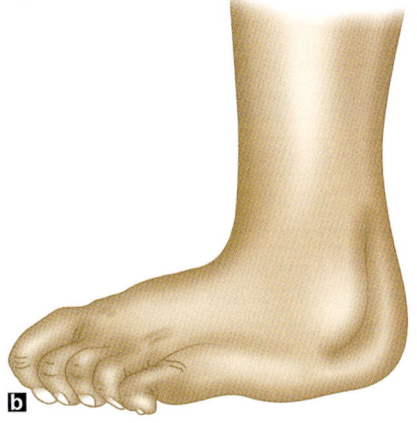

Toes are curled like "C", their tips (not pads) are in contact with the ground. This is a sign of weakness of intrinsic muscles of the foot

Fig. 10.16: (a) Normal position of toes with the pads touching the ground; (b) Clawed toes with toe tips touching down

b. Testing for weakness or paralysis of muscles in the foot is also difficult and requires some practice and its is a good practice to first try these tests on yourself:
- Ask the patient to place the foot firmly on the ground and to press the ground with the big toe, keeping it straight while lifting the other toes (Fig. 10.17a). If the muscles in the foot are weak or paralyzed, the big toe will be seen to bend as shown in Fig. 10.17b and you can confirm this by feeling it.

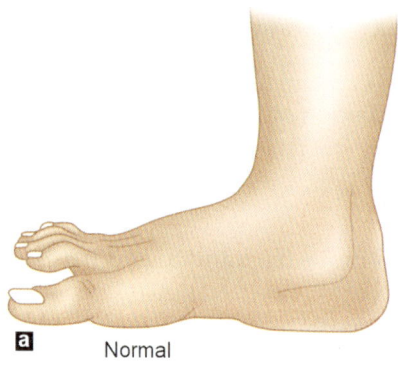
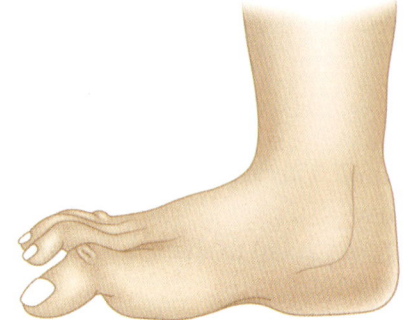

a Normal

b The big toe bends when the other toes are lifted
This is a sign of intrinsic muscle weakness due to tibial nerve involvement

Fig. 10.17: (a) The other toes can be lifted while the big toe presses down; (b) The big toe bends when the other toes are lifted

- Ask the patient to place the foot firmly on the ground, lift all the toes, and spread them out (Fig. 10.18). While the patient is doing this, watch also for the little toe moving outward. If the muscles in the foot are weak or paralyzed, the toes cannot be spread out. However, this is *not* a very reliable test as people who have been habitually wearing shoes often cannot spread their toes.

Common Peroneal Nerve (Table 10.7)

a. The common peroneal nerve supplies the bulky muscles in the front of the leg (Fig. 10.3d) that lift the foot and toes up, and the muscles on the outer side of the leg that turn the foot outward (eversion). Until these muscles are almost completely paralyzed, the patient may not have noticed any disability during walking. When this nerve is affected, the patient has a "high stepping gait"—where the patient has to lift the affected leg high up while walking. Also on examination of the front of the leg, where normally the muscles bulge out, muscles are atrophied, the bulge flattens out and the tibia is visible. For testing of the nerve is mentioned in Table 10.7.

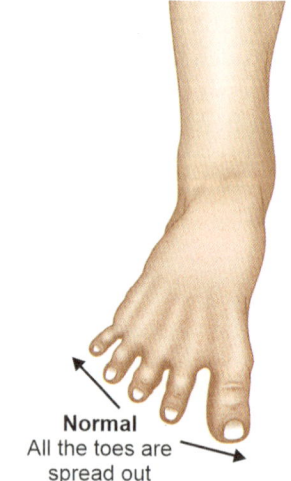

Normal
All the toes are spread out

Fig. 10.18: Normal intrinsic musculature: Patient is able to spread out the toes while placing the foot firmly on the ground

Nerve Function Assessment and Muscle Testing

Table 10.7: Tests for nerves of foot

Nerve	Muscles	Test	Interpretation	Disability
Common peroneal nerve/lateral popliteal nerve	Dorsiflexors of ankle, extensor hallucis longus, tibialis anterior	Ask patient to walk with heels up	Not possible if weak/paralyzed	Foot drop
		Foot up test: Ask patient to sit on a high stool with legs dangling and lift only foot without raising leg (support foot and apply pressure over the proximal portion of the foot)	Inability to lift up	Foot drop
Tibial nerve (medial and lateral plantar nerves)	Intrinsic muscles of feet	Ask patient to place foot firmly on ground and lift toes and spread them out	Inability to spread toes and lift them	Clawing of toes
		Ask the patient to place foot firmly on ground and retract/draw back all toes without lifting them off ground	Normally S-shaped toes on retracting but if weak/paralyzed then C-shaped—toe tips in touch with ground rather than toe pads (Fig. 10.16a and b)	Guttering, clawing of toes

b. *'Great toe up and down' test:*[5] This assesses motor function of the terminal branch of the common peroneal nerve, and the tibial nerve respectively. The "great toe up test" is performed when the patient is sitting with his/her feet flat on the ground. The patient is asked to lift the great toe only and the assessor determines muscle strength, applying pressure on the proximal phalanx.

The "great toe down test" is also called the 'paper grip test'[6] The great toe down test is the only test that can reliably test the motor function of the tibial nerve. Weakness in great toe flexion will indicate impaired tibial nerve function at ankle level involving the intrinsic foot muscles.

Tips

- All small muscles of the sole are supplied by branches of tibial nerve—medial and lateral plantar nerves.
- Sensory supply of sole is by branches of tibial nerve except a small medial area by saphenous nerve (branch of femoral nerve).

3. Testing Muscles of the Face

a. When the facial nerve is damaged, the muscles in the upper part of the face that move the eyelids and the skin on the forehead become weak. Sometimes all the muscles on one side of the face become weak or paralyzed and cause a deformity of the face.
b. Ask the patient whether he or she has any problems with the eyes. When the eyelid muscles are weak or paralyzed, there may be watering of the eye and redness and it will not be possible to close the eye.
c. Look at the patient's face. The eye on the affected side does not blink as often as that on the normal side and it may be opened wider. There may also be more tears and watering of the affected eye.
d. When the facial nerve is completely paralyzed, the affected side of the face is flattened out, without any nasolabial fold in the skin and the mouth is pulled towards the normal side by the muscles on that side.

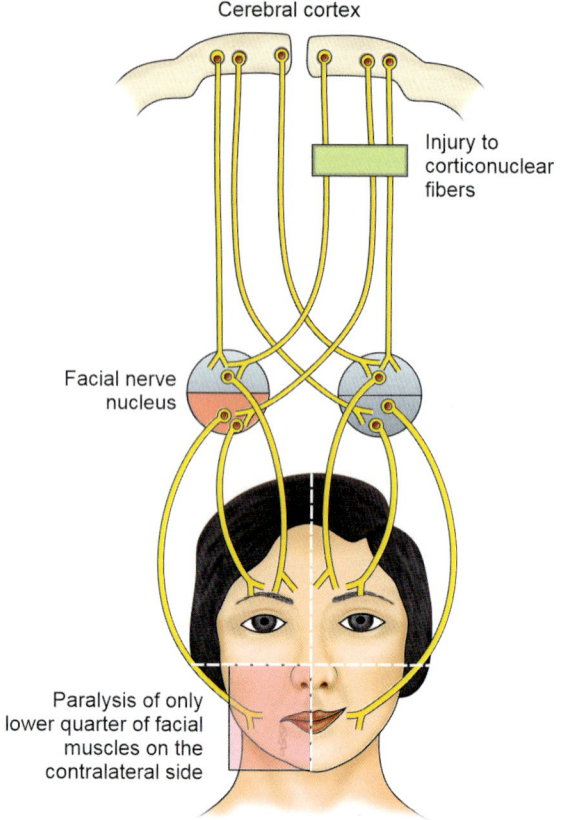

Fig. 10.19: Upper motor neuron facial palsy

Cranial Nerves

While most cranial nerves are not affected by leprosy, a few which may be affected and need to be tested are mentioned in Table 10.8.

Table 10.8: Cranial nerves examination

Cranial nerve	Function	Test of function
I	Olfaction	Test smell in each nostril with eyes closed. Coffee, vanilla, perfumed soap. Avoid ammonia—activates sensory nerves
II	Vision	Check visual acuity—finger counting at 6 m (20 ft) or Snellen chart.
III	Motor	—
IV	Motor	—
V	Sensation to face. Motor to muscles of mastication	Corneal reflex (sensory)—touch the limbus with a wisp of cotton on dental floss standing at the side of the patient → look for direct and consensual reflexes. (Touch sensation → ophthalmic branch of V nerve → motor nucleus of VII nerve → orbicularis oculi contraction → blink reflex)

(contd.)

Table 10.8: Cranial nerves examination (contd.)

Cranial nerve	Function	Test of function
VI	Motor	–
VII	Motor to muscles of facial expression. Sensation to ear canal and palate. Taste on anterior two-thirds of tongue	• Inspect face at rest for asymmetry and lid lag. • Raise eyebrows and wrinkle forehead → may be preserved on paralyzed side in leprosy • Close eyes gently → look for lagophthalmos and Bell's phenomenon Then close tightly → try to open lower lid → look for weakness of orbicularis oculi • Blow out cheeks → try to push our air → easy on weak side • Show teeth → look for deviation of angle of mouth towards normal side
VIII	Hearing and balance	–
IX	Sensation to pharynx, middle and inner ear, posterior one-third of tongue, taste on posterior one-third of tongue	Gag reflex (sensory)
X	Sensation to pharynx and larynx	Say "Ah"—uvula moves towards normal side
XI	Motor	–
XII	Motor	–

Tips

Face can be divided into right and left sides. Each side is further subdivided into upper quarter and lower quarter.

Upper face has bicortical representation. Thus, upper motor neurone (UMN) damage does not affect upper quarters of right and left sides of face (spares forehead wrinkles) (Fig. 10.19). In lower motor neurone (LMN) lesion muscles of upper and lower quarters of same side of face will be paralyzed (Fig. 10.20).

But in leprosy there occurs a *partial* LMN palsy and only temporal and zygomatic branches of facial nerve are affected.

Summary

While the above tests might sound fearsome and complicated—there is a simpler option. A list of tests given in Table 10.9 can be used to test most of the nerves and this is useful in field conditions. It does not specifically mention isolated muscles with their official anatomical names as what is tested are movements rather than individual muscles. Testing muscles in 'isolation' is, with rare exceptions, not possible and in most muscle tests there is synergistic action of multiple muscles.

A simplified version of NFA is given in Table 10.10, which encompasses the salient aspects that need to be recorded for NFA and is sufficiently adequate for most patients in clinical practice.

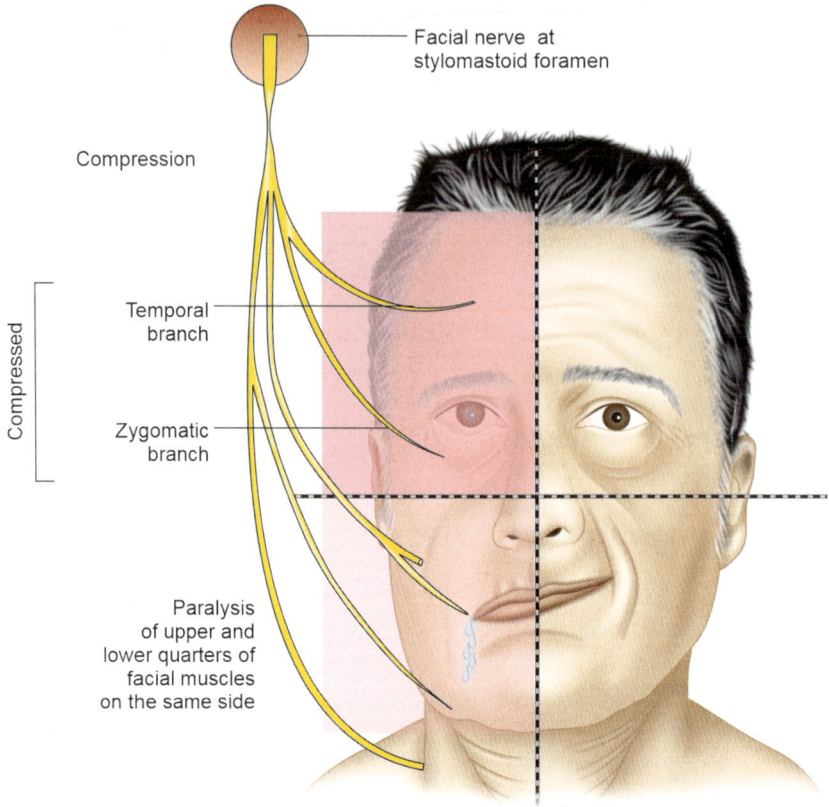

Fig. 10.20: Lower motor neuron lesion in facial nerve paralysis (in leprosy the temporal and zygomatic branch is affected)

Table 10.9: Muscle testing protocol for field set ups	
Nerve	Muscle strength testing
Facial	Eye closure
Ulnar	Little finger abduction
Median	Thumb abduction
Radial	Wrist extension
Common peroneal (CP)	Foot dorsiflexion
Common peroneal (CP)	Great toe extension
Tibial	Great toe plantar flexion

Table 10.10: Proforma for recording of NFA		
Name	Age	Occupation
	Vision and Neurological Exam	
Right	EYES	**Left**
	Visual acuity	
_____ m	Note finger count in meters 0–6 or	_____ m
_____ SC	number on Snellen chart (SC)	_____ SC

(contd.)

Nerve Function Assessment and Muscle Testing

Table 10.10: Simple recording of NFA (contd.)

Name	Age	Occupation
	Vision and Neurological Exam	
Yes No	**Corneal loss of sensation** Blink decreased or decreased sensation with 5 cm dental floss	Yes No
P W S	**Loss of muscle strength** Eye closure P: Paralyzed, W: Weak, S: Strong	P W S
_____ mm	**Lid gap: Light closure of eyes** Measure lid gap in mm	_____ mm
_____ mm	**Lid gap: Tight closure of eyes** Measure lid gap in mm	_____ mm
Yes No	Visible impairments of the eyes	Yes No
Right	HANDS	**Left**
P E N	**Nerve palpation: Ulnar** P: Painful, E: Enlarged, N: Normal	P E N
Evaluate loss of muscle strength in hands: P: Paralyzed, W: Weak, S: Strong		
P W S	Little finger out (abduction)	P W S
P W S	Thumb up (abduction)	P W S
P W S	Wrist up (extension)	P W S
	Protective sensory loss to palm of hands Light touch with ballpoint pen or 4G monofilament ✕ = Loss of sensation ✓ = Feels touch	
Yes No	Wounds on hands	Yes No
Yes No	Visible impairments of the hands	Yes No
Right	FEET	**Left**
P E N	**Nerve palpation: Peroneal** P: Painful, E: Enlarged, N: Normal	P E N
P E N	**Nerve palpation: Tibial** P: Painful, E: Enlarged, N: Normal	P E N
Evaluate loss of muscle strength of feet: P: Paralyzed, W: Weak, S: Strong		
P W S	Foot up (dorsiflexion)	P W S
P W S	Large toe up (extension)	P W S
	Sensory loss to sole of feet Light touch with ballpoint pen of 10 g monofilament ✕ = Loss of sensation ✓ = Feels touch	
Yes No	Wounds on soles of feet	Yes No
Yes No	Visible impairments of the feet	Yes No
	WHO disability grade (0, 1, 2)	
	EHF Score (0–12)	

REFERENCES

1. Brandsma JW. Basic nerve function assessment in leprosy patients. Lepr Rev 1981;52: 161–70.
2. Bell-Krotoski JA, Tomacik E. The repeatability of testing with Semmes-Weinstein monofilaments. J Hand Surg 1987;12A:155–61.
3. Brandsma JW, Schreuders TAR, Birke JA, et al. Manual muscle strength testing. Intra- and interobserver reliability of the intrinsic muscles of the hand. J Hand Ther 1995;8:185–90.
4. Srinivasan H. Prevention of disabilities in patients with leprosy: A practical guide, 1993.
5. Brandsma W, Wagenaar I, Post E, Nicholls P, Richardus J. Reliability of Clinical Nerve Function Assessment in Peripheral Neuropathies. Lepr Rev 2014;85:29–3.
6. Win de MM, Theuvenet WJ, Roche PW, et al. The paper grip test for screening intrinsic muscle paralysis in the foot in leprosy patients. Int J Lepr Mycobact Dis 2002;70:16–24.

Appendix

Gaurish R Laad

HISTORY AND EXAMINATION

Name: Age: Sex: Marital Status:
Occupation:
Address:
Residence: Kutcha/Pucca house with _____ rooms; staying _____ family members
Income: Earning ₹ _____ per month.

CHIEF COMPLAINTS[1]

i. H/o skin lesions × _____ days/months/years.
ii. H/o redness/swelling/pain/ulceration of skin lesions × _____ days/months.
iii. H/o impaired/loss of sensations over _____ (mention the part) × _____ days/months/years.
iv. H/o shooting pain in limbs × _____
v. H/o deformity of R/L hand × _____
vi. H/o difficulty in walking/chappals falling off feet × _____
vii. H/o inability to close R/L eye × _____
viii. H/o ulcer over R/L sole/hand × _____

Onset, **d**uration, **p**rogress: Patient was apparently well prior to _____ days/months/years.

1. _____ days/months/years back, he/she noticed single/ _____ (state the number) reddish/hypopigmented, skin lesions, asymptomatic/painful, showing/not showing impaired sensations to touch over _____ (part of body). These have progressively increased in size over a period of _____ .
2. If patient has diffuse infiltration of face then say patient has noticed redness, thickening and shininess of facial skin with/without thickening/skin lesion over ears × _____ (duration).
3. If patient comes with ulcer, then describe as _____ days/months/years back, patient noticed development of single/(number of) ulcers/erosions, painful/painless following trauma/spontaneously following rupture of a blister at that site over _____ (part of body). Ulcer was _____ size and showed purulent/serous,

foul smelling/nonfoul smelling discharge and was/was not associated with redness, swelling, pain in foot/hands and has progressively increased in size to present size.

4. If the patient has come with deformity of hands (claw hand/wrist drop) then describe as: _____ (duration) back, patient developed splaying of fingers of R/L hand or inability to flex the fingers/extend the wrist of sudden/gradual onset following shooting pains in that limb/spontaneously.
5. If patient complains of chappal(s) falling off feet or difficulty in walking describe as in 4 above.
6. For h/o inability to close eyes, describe as in 4 above.
   Once primary *skin* lesions as in 1 and 2 above are described, then mention that over a period of days/months/years, patient has noticed similar lesions behaving similarly, progressively involving trunk/face/upper or lower extremities.
7. If patient has presented with cutaneous type 1/2 reaction then describe as: Patient noticed development of increased redness (swelling/pain/ulceration in lesions over _____ (part) (or) h/o painful, reddish, firm, cutaneous nodules over _____ coming up in crops/few at a time, and subsiding in _____ days leaving/not leaving dark colored patches. Mention h/o fever.

After describing onset, duration and progress of skin lesions, history taking should proceed to rule out *complaints* in the following order:

a. *Precipitating factors for reactions*
   H/o cough/cold/fever/dysuria/loose motions. H/o mental stress/exertion/surgery/vaccinations/drug intake.
   In females, enquire about pregnancy/postpartum period/menstruation.
b. *Nerves*
   H/o tingling/numbness/shooting pains in upper/lower limbs × _____ (duration).
   H/o developing *numb areas in* R/L arm/forearm/leg/face, etc.
c. *Sensory system*
   H/o impairment/loss of sensation to touch (do not mention temperature, pain) of sudden gradual onset noticed by patient over medial or lateral side of R/L hand/feet/soles or any other part of body.
d. *Motor system*
   H/o difficulty in buttoning shirt/grasping pen, keys, etc.
   H/o inability to straighten fingers, inability to extend wrist.
   H/o difficulty in walking where patient has to walk by raising the foot high off the ground as compared to the opposite foot for _____ duration.
   H/o chappals/sandals falling off feet
   H/o inability to close R/L eye × _____ duration.
e. *Trophic changes*
   H/o developing blisters/ulcers/corns/cracks/resorption, i.e. shortening of fingers or toes/nail changes.
f. *Eye*
   H/o pain/redness/watering/photophobia/diminished vision of sudden/gradual onset.

g. *Nose and throat*
   H/o nasal stuffiness/blockade/crusting/bleeding/anosmia/foul smelling discharge.
   H/o hoarseness of voice.
h. *Breast and genitals*
   H/o enlargement of breast (in case of LL Hansen in males), h/o pain, swelling of testicles.
i. R_x *history*
   - H/o taking any red/brown/white capsules/tablets every month from _____ hospital for _____ duration.
   - H/o taking any R_x for reactions, h/o improvement/no improvement following R_x.
j. *Past history*: Diabetes mellitus (DM)/Hypertension (HTN)/Ischemic heart disease (IHD)/Tuberculosis (TB).
k. *Family history*
   H/o similar disease in family: DM/HTN/IHD
l. *Personal history*: Bowel/bladder habits, addictions, etc.

EXAMINATION[1]

1. General Examination
Conscious/co-operative, built, sitting/lying comfortably in bed, etc.
   Pallor/cyanosis/clubbing/icterus
   Pulse ( )   BP ( )   Jugular venous pressure (JVP) ( )
   Lymphadenopathy ( )
   Edema of hands, feet, face.

2. Dermatological Examination
a. Unilateral/bilateral/symmetrical/asymmetrical involvement of face/trunk/extremities/buttocks with/without involvement of palms/soles/genitals, etc.
b. *Lesions are in the form of*
   - Macule/plaque
   - Papules/nodules
   - Diffuse infiltration of face
   - Nodular infiltration of ears
   - Ulcers/sinuses
   - Ichthyosis
c. Diffuse infiltration—describe as shiny, thickened, erythematous skin involving _____ part of face.
d. *Macule/plaque*
   Describe with respect to the following points:
   i. *Number*: Important for classification of leprosy and progress of disease/reactions.
   ii. *Color*: Hypopigmented/erythematous/coppery red, etc.
   iii. *Shape*: Oval/round/bizarre/geographic/annular, etc.
   iv. *Size*: Ranging in size from smallest _____ cm to largest _____ cm over _____ (part of body) (you may mark lesions with skin pencil to show the examiner).

v. *Margins*: Well defined/ill-defined or well defined at places and ill-defined at places, regular/irregular, raised/flat.
vi. *Satellite lesions*: An independent lesion close to the big lesion (within <1 cm of parent lesion) (seen in borderline spectrum).
vii. *Surface*
- Dry/rough _____ Tuberculoid spectrum
- Smooth/shiny _____ BB, BL , LL
- Scaly/nonscaly
- If surface shows any ulceration then describe the same.
- Also describe the scales, if present.
viii. *Sensations*: **T**emperature/**p**ain/light **t**ouch, impaired/lost more at center or periphery of lesion or uniformly all over the lesion.
ix. *Loss of hair*: Sparsity/total loss over the lesion.
x. *Loss of sweating*: Dryness.
xi. Consistency/induration (pinch and feel)
- For small lesions—always say uniformly indurated.
- Larger lesions—whether the induration is uniform or more at the center/periphery.
- Also you may say that the lesion feels thicker and firmer in consistency as compared to the surrounding normal skin.
xii. Warmth over the lesion.
xiii. *Tenderness*: Tap the lesion and see patient's face. Tenderness over lesions is seen in reactional states.
xiv. *Local cutaneous nerves*: Run the thumb around the lesion and feel for thickened nerves. They are often enlarged in tuberculoid lesions.

e *Specific lesions*: For *annular* and *punched* out lesions: Follow the same order above but highlight:
- Central clearing
- Double margin, i.e. outer and inner, well defined/ill-defined as above.
- *Sensations*: May be lost more in the center than periphery.
- Induration will be more in periphery than center.

Mention the morphological types of annular plaques, if typical: Upright saucer—TT, inverted saucer—BL, punched out/Swiss cheese pattern—BB.

f. *Papule or nodule*: Describe as follows:
i. Number
ii. Color: Skin colored/erythematous
iii. Size
iv. Consistency: Soft/firm
v. Tendernes: ENL is tender
vi. Local warmth
vii. Level: Cutaneous/subcutaneous
viii. Surface: Smooth/shiny/scaly/ulcerated, etc.
ix. Situated over normal skin or infiltrated skin.

g. *Ulcer* is described as:
   i. Number
   ii. Size and shape
   iii. Margins—as for plaque
   iv. Edge: Sloping/undermined/punched out/everted
   v. Floor shows slough/healthy granulation tissue
      - Tender/non-tender
      - Discharge (serous/mucopurulent/purulent/blood stained/foul or nonfoul smelling)
      - Tenderness
      - Bleeding on touch
   vi. *Base*: Induration present or not
   vii. Surrounding skin shows edema/hyperpigmentation/local warmth/tenderness.
   viii. Fixed to underlying structures or not.
h. *Sinuses*: Describe as for ulcer above.
i. *Ichthyosis*: Seen in LL/on clofazimine.
j. *Clofazimine pigmentation*: Mention if seen in plaques.

3. Examination of Nerves
- Unilateral/bilateral
- Symmetrical/asymmetrical

Nerves examined in leprosy are:

A. *Cutaneous nerves*
Face and neck (supraorbital, infraorbital, zygomatic, greater auricular, supratrochlear, supraclavicular).
Forearm (medial, lateral and posterior cutaneous nerves of forearm, radial cutaneous nerve, ulnar cutaneous nerve).
Thigh (medial, intermediate, lateral and posterior cutaneous nerves of thigh).
Leg and foot (infrapatellar, sural, superficial, peroneal and anterior tibial).

B. *Peripheral nerve trunks*
Upper limb: Radial, ulnar, median.
Lower limb: Lateral popliteal and posterior tibial.
Mention whether nerves are thickened/soft/firm/tender/non-tender.
If a nerve trunk is markedly thickened, then mention:
- Segment in *cm* thickened
- Beading/spindling
- Abscesses
- Local warmth over skin
- Sinuses/ulcers/scars
- Fixity of nerve/mobility of nerve.

4. Sensory Testing (see Chapter 10)
Temperature, pain, light touch.

Hands: Palmar and dorsal aspect and corresponding forearm.

Feet: Dorsum and sole of foot and lateral aspect of leg.

Face: Full face and ears.

(Mention about any 'Glove and stocking' type of anesthesia (in LL Hansen)
Sensory loss in leprosy is always *patchy* and never *total*.
Describe as sensations impaired/lost in the distribution of _____ nerve over _____ part.)

5. Motor System (see Chapter 10)
A. *Hands* should be examined as:
a. *Attitude and deformity*
   Clawing of fingers/ape thumb/splaying of fingers/wrist drop.
b. *Muscle bulk*: Wasting of thenar, hypothenar eminences and guttering of interosseous spaces.
c. *Tone*: Hypotonia (thenar, hypothenar muscles).
d. *Power*.

B. *Feet*
a. *Gait*: Normal/high stepping gait
b. *Attitude and deformity*
   - In case of foot drop, foot will lie in a position of plantar flexion and inversion
   - Claw toes
c. *Muscle bulk*
   - Wasting of tibialis anterior/posterior.
   - Guttering of interosseous spaces.
d. *Tone*: Hypotonia
e. *Power*

C. *Face muscles* (see Chapter 10)
- Light and tight eye closure (orbicularis oculi)
- See for lid gap.
- Other tests: Frowning, showing teeth, puffing, etc.

D. *Reflexes*: DTRs (brisk/normal/lost).
   (In leprosy, DTRs are normal.)

6. Trophic Changes
Blisters/ulcers/scars/callosities/fissures/nail changes/resorption of fingers or toes.

7. Systemic Examination
Abdominal, respiratory system, cardiovascular and central nervous system.

Eyes
  i. Eyebrows/eyelashes madarosis
 ii. Eyelids—skin lesions/ectropion/entropion/lagophthalmos
iii. Conjunctiva—hyperemia/chemosis/nodules
 iv. Cornea—transparent/hazy/ulcers/sensations
  v. Anterior chamber—depth/hypopyon
 vi. Pupil—size and light reflex
vii. Iris—synechiae
viii. Lens—grey reflex cataract
 ix. Visual acuity—finger counting at 6 meters.

Nose
External nose: Skin lesions, deformity (depression of tip or bridge of nose, columellar retraction, clover leaf deformity).

Anterior rhinoscopy
- Nodules over lateral wall/septum
- Crushing/foul smellings discharge
- Epistaxis
- Deviated/perforated/nasal septum
- Atrophy of mucosa/turbinates

Mouth and Throat
Examine: Lips, gums, teeth, tongue, palate, tonsils, pharynx, larynx.

See for nodules, ulcerations, perforation (palate), loosening of incisors (upper), erythrodontia.

Breast
- Gynecomastia
- Gynecothelia
- Tenderness

Genitalia
- Skin lesions
- Testicular sensations/swelling/tenderness/hydrocele, etc.

Skeletal
Swelling/effusion/tenderness, etc.

WHO Disability Grading[2]

This is described as under.

Disability grading in leprosy	Every new case of leprosy must be assigned a "Disability grade", which records the condition of the patient at diagnosis. The grade is on a scale of 0, 1 or 2. Each eye, each hand and each foot is given its own grade, so the patient actually has six grades, but the highest grade given is used as the disability grade for that patient.
	Hands and feet
	Grade 0: No anaesthesia, no visible deformity or damage Grade 1: Anesthesia present, but no visible deformity or damage Grade 2: Visible deformity or damage present
	Eyes
	Grade 0: No eye problem due to leprosy; no evidence of visual loss Grade 1: Eye problems due to leprosy present, but vision *not* severely affected as a result of these (vision: 6/60 or better; can count fingers at 6 m) Grade 2: Impairment (vision: Worse than 6/60; inability to count fingers at 6 m) also includes (corneal anaesthesia, lagophthalmos and iridocyclitis).
EHF score	The EHF score is calculated from data already being recorded routinely. It is the sum of all the individual disability grades for the two eyes, two hands and two feet. Since the disability grade can be scored as either 0, 1 or 2, it follows that the EHF score ranges from 0 to 12. A score of 12 would indicate grade 2 disability of both eyes, both hands and both feet. The EHF score has been shown to be more *sensitive* to change over time than the disability grade itself. The simplest way to use the EHF score to measure the development of new or additional disability during MDT is to calculate the score at diagnosis (this examination is already done in the initial assessment of the disability grade) and then repeat the examination at the time treatment is completed. The two scores can then be compared.

OPINION (FINAL DIAGNOSIS)

_____ Leprosy (mention R-J classification) *with/without* type 1/type 2 reaction *with/without* disability (trophic change/claw hand/foot drop/lagophthalmos), on/not on MDT.

REFERENCES

1. Reddy NBB, Doris PG. KLEP series: Clinical Examination in leprosy. Schiettelis Leprosy Research and Training Centre Karigiri 2000.
2. Brandsma JW, Brakel WHV. WHO diability grading: Operational definitions, Lepr Rev. 2003; 74:366–73.
3. Thangaraj RH. A manual of leprosy. The leprosy mission (1989).
4. Anthony Brycesson, Roy E. Pfaltzgraff. Leprosy. Churchill Livingstone; 3rd Revised edition (1 May 1990).
5. CS Goodwin. The use of the VMT in Leprosy Neuritis. Leprosy Review. 1968; 39:209–16.
6. Richard P. Croft, Jan H Richardus, Peter G Nichollus W. Cairns S Smith. Nerve function impairment in leprosy: Design, methodology, and intake status of a prospective cohort study of 2664 new leprosy cases in Bangladesh. (The Bangladesh Acute Nerve Damage Study). Leprosy Review 1999; 70:140–59.
7. Jean M Watson. Preventing Disability in Leprosy Patients. Leprosy Mission International (1986).

Index

A

A scavenger receptor 166
A. polyphaga 159
Acanthamoeba castellani 159
Acute ENL 215
Acute exacerbation 130
Acute phase reactants 187
Acute ulcers 323
Aδ fibers 295
Adaptive immunity 167
Adductor band 360
Adrenal glands 137
Adrenals 47
Adverse drug reaction 251
Agranulocytosis 251
Alcoholic polyneuropathy 383
Alternate anti-leprosy therapy (ALT) 251
Amoebae 159
Amyloidosis 382
Anakinra 205
Anemia 251
Anesthesia 35
Annular 21
Anosmia 38
Antia's operation 337
Anti-inflammatory cytokines 164
Anti-TNF-α inhibitors 221
Ape hand 32
Ape thumb 313
Apoptosis 167
Apremilast 223
Armadillo (*Dasypus novemcinctus*) 148
Armauer Hansen 147
Assistive devices 367, 372
Autonomic function 414
Autonomic nervous 47
Autophagy 167
Azathioprine (AZA) 205, 221, 222, 273

B

Bacillus-Calmette-Guérin 286
Bacterial (bacteriological) index 99
Ballpoint testing (BPT) 297
Banana fingers 306, 308
Basic fibroblast growth factor (bFGF) 164, 170
Bell's palsy 34
Bell's phenomenon 34
Benediction sign 425
Bizarre 22
Bone 42, 134
Bone marrow 134
Book test 424
Borderline 76
Borderline borderline 122
Borderline lepromatous 122
Borderline leprosy 19
Borderline tuberculoid 121
Brand's operation 337
Breast 137
Breast pain 378
BSA 106
Buddha ears 317
Bunnel's operation 337

C

C type lectin receptors 165
Cairo classification 8
Callosities 327
Callus 328
Canakinumab 205
Capsule 148
Card test 425, 426
Cataract 39, 42, 302, 304
Cathelicidin 157
CD209/DC-SIGN 165
Cell wall 148
Charcot's foot 327
Charcot's foot or hot foot 370
Chemoprophylaxis 5, 281

Childhood leprosy 73
Chronic ENL 215
Ciclosporin 205
Ciliary body 40
Clarithromycin 253, 265
Classification 7
Claw hand 32, 306, 310, 331, 358
Claw toe deformities 323
Claw toes 32, 306, 313
Clinical aspects 10
Clofazimine 205, 219, 221, 241, 247
Clustering 158
Cock up splint 338
Coinfections 182
Colchicine 222
Cold abscess 335
Collapsed pinna 317
Common peroneal nerve 428
Complement system 166
Complicated chronic ulcers 323
Composite skin contact smear 157
Congenital indifference to pain 384
Conjunctivitis 40, 214
Contacts 158
Cornea 40
Corneal reflex 34, 430
Corneal ulcer 304
Corns 328
Corticosteroids 202, 220
Cortisol 187
Cranial nerves 430
C-reactive protein (CRP) 183
CRP 187
CXCL10 (IP-10) 186
Cyclosporine 221, 222
Cytokine milieu 194
Cytology 107

D

Dapsone 240, 244
DC-SIGN⁺ 166
DDS syndrome ("sulphone syndrome") 245
Death 46
Decompression 205
Defaulters 257
Deformities 4, 79, 306
Dehabilitation 306
Dejerine-Sottas syndrome 381
Diabetic neuropathy 383
Diagnostic tests 97
Disability 306
Disability grading 442
Dissociated anesthesia 35

Downgrading 192, 193, 198
Downgrading reaction 20, 94, 126, 192, 196, 197, 206
Drop-foot 315
Dropped foot 32
Drug susceptibility testing 230, 234
Dry skin 378
Duplex-droplet digital PCR 105
Dynamic splints 360
Dystrophin 176

E

Ectropion 40
Egawa's test 424
EHF score 442
Elbow orthosis 359
Ellis' test 214
ENL 128, 211, 212
ENLIST 215
Epidemiology 1
Epididymo-orchitis 214
Epineurotomy 334, 335
Episcleritis 40, 302
Etanercept 222
Evolution 11
Exacerbations 226
Exposure keratitis 40, 41, 304
Eyes 39, 133

F

Facial nerve 318
Facial palsy 32, 351
Facies leprosa 38, 45
Fibrosis 35, 293, 297
Finger loop splint 360
Finger orthosis 358
Fixed duration therapy (FDT) 244
Flail foot 327
FNAC 87, 107
Foot drop 306, 331, 339
Foot drop deformity 322
Footwear 367
Fowler's operation 337
Froment's sign 424, 426
Frozen hand 308

G

Gabapentin 299
Gene decay 147
Generation (doubling) time 148
Genes 147
Genetic susceptibility 148
Genome 147, 163

Geographic 27
Geographical 22
Glaucoma 39, 304
Global leprosy strategy 2
Global priority countries 1
Glomerulonephritis 214
Glove and stocking 30, 35
Glucose-6-phosphate dehydrogenase (G6PD) 245
Grade 2 disability 4
Granulocyte colony stimulating factor (G-CSF) 169
Granuloma 117
Granuloma paradox 94
Grenz zone 123
Grip-Aids 373
Growth factors 164
Gutter splint 360

H

Hair transplant 342
Hammer toes 32
Hand orthosis 358
Handicaps 306
Hansen 6
Havana classification 8
Hematology 47
Hemolysis 244
Hepatitis 251
Herceptin 179
Hereditary motor and sensory neuropathy 381
Hereditary sensory radicular neuropathy 384
High frequency 90
Histamine test 108
'Histoid' leprosy 52
Histopathology 116
HIV 93, 255, 383
Hot abscess 296
Hot foot 327
Hydroxychloroquine 221
Hypogonadism 45
Hysteria 384

I

Ichthyosis 30
IFN-γ 151, 167, 185
IL-10 169, 186
IL-17 169, 186
IL-1β 186
IL-6 186
Immune complex (IC) 185
Immune reconstitution inflammatory syndrome (IRIS) 183
Immunity 13

Immunohistochemistry in leprosy 141
Immunoprophylaxis 281, 286
Immunosuppressive 255
Immunotherapeutics 281
Impairments 306
Impotence 378
Incubation period 155
Indeterminate 11
Indeterminate leprosy 13, 76, 118
Indian classification 8
Inducible nitric oxide synthase (iNOS) 167
Infliximab 222
Instant 373
Intolerance 255
Intrinsic plus 308
Intrinsic plus toes 306
Intrinsic zero 310
Inverted saucer 21, 25
IP-10 186
Iridocyclitis 40
Iris 40
Iris pearls 40
Iritis 214, 302

J

Jagged-1 (JAG-1) 165

K

Keratinocytes 157
Keratitis 38
Kidney 46, 137
Kustha 1

L

Lactation 254
Lagophthalmos 40, 41, 304, 306, 318, 348, 367
Laminin 2, 175
Laminin α_2 chain (α_2LG) 175
Larynx 38, 134
Late reactions 206
Lateral tarsorrhaphy 349
Lazarine leprosy 53, 196
Lenalidomide 220
Leonine facies 30, 31, 36
Lepra bonita 53
Lepromata 39
Lepromatous leprosy 76, 123
Lepromatous pearls 40
Lepromin test 108
Leprosy stare 40
Leprosy vaccines 223
Leprous alopecia 31, 36

Leprous neuritis 293
Leprous stare 306, 320
LepVax 287, 288
Libido 45
Lipoarabinomannan (LAM) 166, 178
Lipofuscinosis 247
Lipopolysaccharide (LPS) 185
Liver 134
LLp 29
LLs 29
Lucio leprosy 225
Lucio phenomenon 130
Lucio-Latapí leprosy 53
Lymph nodes 46, 134
Lymphocytic infiltrate 118

M

M. indicus pranii 287
M. leprae strains 147
M. lepromatosis 6
Macrophages 163
Maculoanesthetic 20, 23, 24
Madarosis 30, 317, 342
Madrid 8
Madrid classification 8
Manila classification 8
Mce1A gene 156
MDT 252
Median nerve 418, 423, 425
Medical decompression 333
Medical Research Council (MRC) 297, 412
Mega lobules 348
Membrane attack complex (MAC) 178
Methotrexate 205, 221, 222, 274
MICA 151
Microabscess 296
Microcellular rubber (MCR) 325, 340, 369
Miliary 39
Minimal effective dose (MED) 232
Minimum inhibitory concentration (MIC) 232
Minocycline 222, 250, 266
MIP 287
Misreference 418
Mitogen activated protein kinase 178
Modulan 373
Modulan Grip-Aids 373
Molecular diagnosis 104
Monofilament testing (MFT) 297, 418
Mononeuritis multiplex 85, 293
Morphological index (MI) 101, 149
Motor examination 420
Moulded double rocker shoe 325
Mouse foot pad (MFP) 148, 230

Mouth 38, 134
Moxifloxacin 253, 264
MRC 420
MRC1 151
Multibacillary MDT (MB-MDT) 240
Multi-drug therapy (MDT) 240
Muscle 46, 137
Muscle testing 412
Mw/MIP 288
Mycobacterium habana 288
Mycobacterium leprae 6, 147
Mycobacterium lepromatosis 147
Mycobacterium vaccae 288
Mycobacterium w 287

N

Nails 36
Nasal carriage 155
Nasal epithelial cells 156
Nasal mucosa 157
Nasal secretions 155
Nasal smears and nose-blows 104
Nasal stuffiness 38
ND-O-BSA 106
Necrosis 118
Nerve abscess 23, 201, 335
Nerve biopsy 86, 104
Nerve conduction studies (NCS) 88, 297
Nerve damage 292, 294, 297
Nerve examination 413
Nerve function 412
Nerve function assessment 297, 412
Nerve function impairment 194, 292
Nerve involvement 130, 294
Nerve palpation 414
Nerve transfer 352
Neuritic Hansen 48
Neuritis 200, 297, 298
Neurolysis 334, 335
Neuropathic foot 327
Neuropathic pain 299
Neutrophils 185
New case detection 3
NLEP classification 10
NO synthase 179
NOD2 148, 151
NOD-like receptors 165
Nodular leprosy 76
Nose 38, 133

O

Ocular 302
Ofloxacin 250, 262

Onion skin 118
Opponens loop splint 360
Opponens plasty 338
Oral mucosal infection 157
Orthoses 354, 358
Oschsner's clasping test 425

P

Pachydermoperiostosis 380
Pannus 40
PAR-CRG 148
PARK2 148, 151
Pathogen recognition receptors (PRR) 169
Pathogen-associated molecular patterns (PAMP) 163
Pattern recognition receptors (PRR) 163
Paucibacillary MDT (PB-MDT) 240
PCR 88, 104, 105, 157
PCR-DNA sequencing 233
Pen test 425, 426
Pentoxifylline 219
Perineurial 118
Periosteitis 214
Persisters 240
PGL-1 166
Pharynx 38
Phenolic glycolipid 1 (PGL-1) 105, 148
Phosphoinositol 3 kinase (PI3K) 178
Physiotherapy 354
Plantar ulcers 315, 316, 323
Plastazote 370
PMM regime 253
Pointing index 425
Point-of-care (POC) tests 104
Polar LL (LLp) 9, 124
Polar tuberculoid (TTp) 9
Polyarteritis nodosa 383
Posterior tibial nerve 419
Postexposure prophylaxis (PEP) 281
Prednisolone 268, 298
Prednisone 219
Pregnancy 93, 254
Prevalence 3
Primary tuberculoid leprosy 120
Pseudogenes 147
Psoriasiform 197
Punched 22
Pure neuritic Hansen 156
Pure neuritic leprosy 85

Q

qPCR 105
Quiet nerve palsy 298

R

Radial 425
Radial cutaneous 419
Radial nerve 424
'Rat-bitten' ears 306, 317
Reaction hand 306, 308
Reactions 59, 79, 94, 182
Reactivation 59, 63
Recombinant 205
Recurrent ENL 215
Reductive evolution 147
Refsum's disease 382
Reinfection 59, 63
Relapse 59, 60, 139, 257
Reservoirs 158
Resistance 228, 254
Resistant 241, 242
Reticuloendothelial 47
Reversal 192
Ridley's logarithmic scale 99
Ridley-Jopling 8
Rifampicin 241
Rifapentine 253
Rilonacept 205
Rocker bottom foot 327
ROM 250
ROR-α 169
ROR-γt 169
Ryrie's test 214

S

Sagging face 317
Sagging skin 347
Sarcoidosis 383
Satellite lesions 21, 23, 24
Saucer 21
Saucer right way up 16, 18
Scavenger receptors 165
Schwann cell 7, 147, 165, 175, 293
Scleritis 302
Secondary tuberculoid (TTs) 9, 120
Self-care 367
Semmes-Weinstein monofilaments 297
Sensory examination 414
Serology 104–106

SFG index 101
Shepard 6
Shoulder orthosis 359
Silent 192
Single dose rifampicin (SDR) 281
Single nucleotide polymorphisms (SNP) 105, 147
Skin smears 97
Skin ulceration 52
Spleen 134
Splints 358
Split anergy 163
STAT3 169
STAT4 167
STAT6 167
Static hand orthoses 360
Static reaction 126
Stigma 3
Subpolar LL (LLs) 9, 124
Sucked candy stick 43
Sunken nose 306, 318
Sural nerve 419
Surgical decompression 333
Susceptible 241, 242
Swan-neck 306, 308
Sweating test 108
Swiss cheese 22, 27
S-W-P (strong, weak, paralyzed) scale 297, 420
Syringomyelia 382
Systemic lupus erythematosus 383

T

T regulatory cells 169
Tacrolimus 205
Temporalis transfer 350
Testes 45, 133
Testosterone 379
TGF-β 169, 170, 186
TGF-β1 297
Th1 179
Th1/Th2 167
Th17 169, 179
Th22 170
Th9 170
Thalidomide 219, 220, 270
Thumb spica 363
Tibial nerve 427
TLR1 148
TLR2 148
TLR4 148

TNF-α 151, 185, 186
Tocilizumab 205
Toll-like receptors (TLR) 148, 163
Total claw hand 331
Transmission 155
Treatment 240
Tregs 185
Triggers 182, 217
Triple palsy 309
TTp 15
TTs 15
Tuberculoid leprosy 15, 76, 163
Tuberculosis 255
Tumor necrosis factor α (TNF-α) 151, 157, 185, 186
Twisted finger 306
Type 1 leprosy reaction 94, 125, 179, 192
Type 2 reaction 94, 128, 179, 211

U

Ulnar nerve 418, 421, 424
Ultrasonography 90
Uncommon presentations 49
Uniform MDT or U-MDT 240
Uniform multi-drug therapy (U-MDT) 256
Upgrading 19, 94, 192, 198
Upgrading reaction 126, 193, 197
Uveitis 39

V

Vaccine 286
Vasa nervorum 293
Vitamin D receptor (VDR) 148, 151, 165
Voluntary muscle testing (VMT) 297, 412

W

Wartenberg's sign 310, 425
Wax bath 358
WHO 1
WHO classification 9
WHO expert committee 8
Wrist drop 338, 358
Wrist up test 425
Wrist–hand orthoses 358

Z

Z deformity 311
Ziehl-Neelsen 98
Zinc 221